T0298444

Just a GP

This autobiography from Sir Denis Pereira Gray offers a unique insight into the life and career of a hugely distinguished and influential general practitioner, from what led him to study medicine, learning his craft in the 1960s, through years of clinical practice and research to senior leadership roles within and outside the Royal College of General Practitioners.

Through detailed diaries enlivened by wonderful anecdotes, both personal and professional, Sir Denis shares candidly with the reader a lifetime of experience gained and lessons learned, highly applicable today when general practice is facing many challenges and detractors.

Both informative and inspirational, *Just a GP* is an essential read for many who have journeyed through the profession with Sir Denis and those who are in the midst of or contemplating a career in general practice today.

Just a GP
Diaries from a Career
in General Practice

Sir Denis Pereira Gray
OBE HonDSc FRCP FRCGP FMedSci

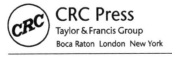

CRC Press
Taylor & Francis Group
Boca Raton London New York

CRC Press is an imprint of the
Taylor & Francis Group, an **informa** business

Cover image: Ewington Cooper Photography, London

First edition published 2024
by CRC Press
2385 NW Executive Center Drive, Suite 320, Boca Raton, FL 33431

and by CRC Press
4 Park Square, Milton Park, Abingdon, Oxon, OX14 4RN

CRC Press is an imprint of Taylor & Francis Group, LLC

ISBN: 9781032713595 (hbk)
ISBN: 9781032522722 (pbk)
ISBN: 9781032713601 (ebk)

DOI: 10.1201/9781032713601

Typeset in Times
by KnowledgeWorks Global Ltd.

To Jill

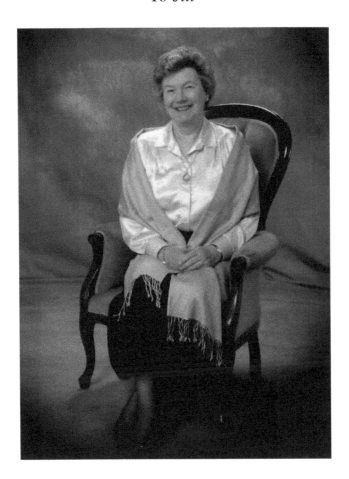

Contents

Foreword by Sir David Haslam xi
Preface... xiii
Acknowledgements... xv

Section I

1. Early Years...3

2. The Chess Story 1948–1970 9

3. Medical Student 1954–1960 14

4. Junior Doctor 1960–1962 19

Section II

5. The Practice 1962–1975..27

6. Learning the Craft – General Practice Stories 32

7. RCGP: South West England and Tamar Faculty Boards.................................40

8. Local Medical Committee and BMA 44

Section III

9. The Journal 1968–1980 51

10. The Exeter RCGP Publishing Story 1972–1997...60

11. The College Cabinet 1970–1980...67

12. The Lane Committee 1971–1974..72

Section IV

13. Department/Institute of General Practice in the University of Exeter...............79

14. Regional Adviser in General Practice/Director of GP Education.....................96

15. The South West General Practice Trust 1985–2019...................................... 107

Section V

16. The Practice 1976–1986 115

17. The Medical Annual 1979–1987 119

18. Publications Committee 1980–1981 123

19. Chair of the Communications Division 1981–1984 126

20. Educational Experiences in the Executive Committee:
    December 1980 to November 2000 129

21. Consultant Adviser to the Chief Medical Officer of the Department of
    Health and Social Security 1984–1987 135

22. The Downs and Ups of Institutional Life: 1982–1987 138

Section VI

23. Chair of Council: February 1987 to November 1990 151

24. Fellowship of the College by Assessment (FBA) 169

25. Conference of Academic Organisations of General Practice 180

26. Prison Medicine 184

27. Directorship of the Postgraduate Medical School of the
    University of Exeter 1987–1997 191

Section VII

28. Chair of Research 1993–1996 207

29. Chairmanship of the JCPTGP 1994–1997 212

30. Dentistry 225

31. The General Medical and Dental Councils 229

32. The Fetzer Institute, USA 236

33. Non-Executive Directorships in the NHS 240

34. The Practice 1987–2000 244

Section VIII

35. President of the RCGP 1997–2000 259

36. Vice-Chair, Academy of Medical Royal Colleges 1998–2000 277

37. Three National Meetings 2000 281

38. Chair of the Academy of Medical Royal Colleges, 2000–2002 286

39. Distinction/Clinical Excellence Awards for Senior Academic
    General Practitioners..303

Section IX

40. Patient Participation 317

41. The Patient Information Advisory Group/Ethics and Confidentiality
    Committee 2001–2011...320

42. RCGP Heritage Committee 2006–2012 325

43. What About The Children? (WATCh?) 329

44. The Nuffield Trust, 1993–2006...333

45. Negotiations between the Department of Health and the BMA 346

Section X

46. An Unfinished Campaign 2013–2023..355

47. Last Hurrah 362

48. General Practice as a Learning Environment 366

49. The St Leonard's Research Practice: 2002 to 2023 371

50. Reflections 385

Appendices

1. Personal Awards 399

2. Eponymous or Equivalent Lectures...400

3. Publications (in Addition to the Journal) from the RCGP Exeter
   Publications Office...401

4. Medical Annuals 409

5. Peer-Reviewed Journal Publications by DPG's Students at the
   St Leonard's Practice.. 410

6. Books/Booklets Written/Edited by the Staff of the Department/
   Institute of General Practice, University of Exeter 412

7. University Degrees/Awards Obtained from the Practice 414

8. GP Syllabus – Theory and Principles of General Practice: 20 Features 415

9. Chairmanships in the RCGP 416

10. Visitors to the St Leonard's Practice 417

11. People Met 419

12. Glossary 421

References...425

Index...447

Foreword by Sir David Haslam

"*Just a GP*". It is impossible to think of another book whose title is quite so misleading. "Just" is the word that is entirely misplaced – not merely in recounting the remarkable life and times of Professor Sir Denis Pereira Gray, but in describing the work of general practitioners as whole. That awful "just" word has been said to me on countless occasions throughout my life, typically by people who had learned that I was a doctor, and asked, "Are you a specialist or just a GP?" It is so extraordinarily illogical.

Denis Pereira Gray perfectly exemplifies the absurdity of seeing generalists as a lesser breed. His long and immensely distinguished career across the worlds of medicine, academia, and politics has been extraordinary. Throughout every step he has maintained his passion for general practice, the true value of generalism, and the immense evidence-based potential of continuity of care.

He has probably forgotten the first time that he impacted my career. Way back in the 1970s I was writing for a magazine called *World Medicine*, edited by Michael O'Donnell, and had written a satirical piece about a Royal College of Greengrocers – gently making fun of some of the more pompous aspects of the RCGP. To my surprise, I received the first of what would become a lifetime's supply of barely legible appreciative handwritten notes from DPG, then on the RCGP Council, mercifully not taking offence. Ever since, I have followed his example of sending handwritten thank-you notes. As he demonstrated, they take moments to write, and are remembered decades later.

I found this autobiography continually absorbing – both from a personal and from a professional perspective. I was intrigued to find that the behaviour of arrogant teaching hospital consultants had precisely the same inspirational effect on him as they did on me some years later – though not in the way they intended. I was fascinated by his life-long expertise in chess, and how an understanding of gameplay taught him much about the world of negotiation.

But from a professional and historical perspective, this book could not be more relevant or more important. Denis lived through, and impacted on, so many of the events and changes that have affected general practice over the past half-century. His astonishing and detailed recall reminded me of so many of the events that have moulded the development of our profession. (I can but assume that he kept a detailed diary. If not, his memory is astonishing.)

I kept on noting important phrases and sentences – such as this comment about colleagues in the 1960s who were leaving general practice, saying "This is not the medicine for which I have been trained." Denis's view – "They were only half right; they assumed their teaching hospital training had been right and the job was wrong. I took the opposite view that the job was OK, and it was the training that was wrong. This made me interested in changing GP training." Which he did.

It is easy to forget that at the start of his, and my, career, there was no expectation or need for GPs to have any additional training at all after their pre-registration house officer jobs. It was felt this was unnecessary for such a menial task as looking after most of the health needs of most of the population most of the time. For those who did undergo training, there was no expectation that their trainers knew anything about training. At the start of his career there were no professors of general practice in England. There were very few researchers. Few GPs were leading national NHS institutions. There was no place for the College on the General Medical Council. The past certainly was a different country.

The list of important, valuable, and challenging roles that Denis took on during his career is truly astonishing. He was intimately involved in the origins of so many aspects of care and medicine that we now take for granted. With General Practice currently facing existential challenges, it is truly inspirational to be reminded what determined individuals, with a clear set of intensely human values, can achieve.

And he would be the first to say he could not have done it alone. Along with the many eminent colleagues whom he writes about in this memoir, it was Jill, his wife of fifty-eight years, who made such an immense difference to his life. She too was a remarkable person – someone it was an honour to have known. This is the story of an extraordinary career during a profoundly important phase in the history of British medicine – someone who was justifiably proud to be "just a GP."

Sir David Haslam, CBE FRCGP
Past President and Chairman of Council, Royal College of General Practitioners
Past President, British Medical Association
Past Chair, National Institute for Health and Care Excellence (NICE)

Preface

I have long been hesitant about writing an autobiography but have been persuaded to do so by many friends and colleagues, both inside and outside general practice. For our four children, I hope it answers the question of what I was doing in all those meetings!

I tried and failed to write the book in chronological order as I found that, since I often had several jobs that overlapped, it did not work. The structure now consists of a series of chapters around my different roles, each describing separate stories, so that readers can dip in and out and leave those that do not interest them. It has been a rare privilege to have worked with so many colleagues in so many settings. Originally there were several chapters on our family, but these have been separated to make the length of the book more manageable and they may be produced later in a different format.

Apart from having had the privilege of holding many different roles in different institutions, I have had some special experiences such as being 'handbagged' by Mrs Thatcher, receiving a letter from Kenneth Clarke calling me "weak-kneed", being called an "academic pirate" by a university Dean, and facing an attempted ousting at the top of the medical profession.

I was fortunate to witness first hand and now describe for the first time some landmark events in the history of medicine. The three years 1986–1989 were when a fundamental change occurred in the relationship between Government and the medical profession and I was the only person in Britain who knew the academic and political leaders of the GPs, the specialists, and the Government leaders, having had meals with most of them.

This book describes the Conference of Academic Organizations of General Practice, GP distinction awards, the JCPTGP, fellowship by assessment of the RCGP, summative assessment, and the academic development of one general practice over half a century, which have not been told before.

A theme has been that general practice and GPs have been consistently undervalued, sometimes amounting to discrimination, with evidence reported both institutional and personal, hence the words "Just a GP", for the title.

Autobiographies describe the experiences of a life. Whilst references to external events are usual, multiple academic references to research are not. I have, however, included many research references for three reasons.

First, I am a GP academic, and I want to be true to both to my craft and to my discipline. For my craft, there are six chapters describing being a GP in the same general practice over a lifetime. For my discipline, I have cited many of the major research studies that were published during my life, seeking to show how many of them educated me and illuminated my experiences. During my lifetime, this research collectively came together to make general practice a new, independent, medical discipline in its own right.

Second, I am concerned that general practice, unlike specialist medicine, has largely lost touch with its own research base and relies too much on personal experience. It is the intermingling of experience and theory that makes general practice so fascinating. The core principles of general practice are surprisingly little taught in the undergraduate medical schools, in the GP postgraduate training courses, or in the training general practices. By linking much exciting medical and social science research with my lived experience, I hope to encourage medical students and trainees, who aspire to be GPs, by clarifying how interesting and how strong the underpinning theory of general practice now is.

Third, by bringing many of these references together, I hope this book may have practical use: for ideas, examples, and references, for GP trainers and academic staff, who have the privilege of teaching general practice to the most able students we have ever had. Mistakes are entirely my responsibility, and I will be pleased to hear of them.

Denis Pereira Gray
Alford House
9 Marlborough Road
Exeter EX2 4TJ, UK
Email: Denis.Pereiragray@btinternet.com

Acknowledgements

In a long professional life, I have many people to thank in the different settings in which I have worked. I have been blessed with many good colleagues over long periods of time.

I joined the St Leonard's Practice because of the example of my father with whom I was a partner for 13 years. I was joined by Russell Steele, the late Kieran Sweeney, and Philip Evans where for over 14 years we worked closely together as partners. They all understood the privilege of being independent contractors working together in a partnership, and I am grateful to them all.

Overlapping in time, I was very fortunate to be appointed to start of the Department of General Practice in the University of Exeter and to work for a quarter of a century with Keith Bolden, Michael Hall, and the late Bob Jones, soon joined by Rita Goble and Tony Lewis. Their enthusiasm, energy, and forward thinking made this a rich time in my life as we developed academic general practice and occupational therapy together. We generated much work for our administrative staff and two Mrs Smiths, Pam and Sylvia, led the teams who gave us great support.

The College of General Practitioners, which became Royal during my career, was a source of inspiration for me in the early years and enabled me to meet many remarkable general practitioners. Alastair Donald, Annis Gillie, John Horder, John Hunt, Ekke Kuenssberg, and Ian Watson, were all Presidents from whom I learned much. In my own generation, I was fortunate to work alongside the late Donald Irvine, Marshall Marinker, and Colin Waine, who did so much and who all became long-term friends. Several staff in the College, like the late Margaret Hammond, Margaret Burtt, and Catherine Messent worked with me for long periods of time and helped me greatly. The College changed the face of British medicine in the 20th century, and it was a privilege to be part of it.

In the Academy of Medical Royal Colleges, I received much appreciated loyalty from Neil Hunter in ophthalmology.

Back in the Practice in clinical retirement for a quarter of a century, with Philip Evans again, he and three successive post-doctoral colleagues, notably Kate Sidaway-Lee, made the research wing of an NHS general practice come alive as an academic unit. I much enjoyed this post clinical retirement work and am very grateful for the chance to teach, research, write, and be published 22 years after I had to retire as professor because of university rules about age.

Writing this book with so many references created much work and I have appreciated help from Beverley Berry and Melissa Wyatt, the Librarians of the Royal College of General Practitioners, the Royal Society of Medicine, and the Devon and Exeter Institution. Joy Choules played a particularly important part in checking and organising details, made innumerable helpful suggestions, and has been an important support for me for 38 years. My niece, Kate Gray, gave valuable editorial and publishing suggestions. Eleanor White, when a practice attached student, helped with editing and typing early drafts.

I thank several people who took time to read some of the chapters and advised me about their content: Diana Dean, Philip Evans, Hilla Gittins, Jonathan Gray, Kate Gray, Julia Neville, Kate Sidaway-Lee, the late John Searle, Lynn Underwood, and Patricia Wilkie.

I am grateful to James Dawson for technical advice, to Heather Heath, Archivist at the RCGP, Barbara Sweeney and Evelyn van Weel-Baumgarten for help with photographs, and to Peter Selley for help with some references. I thank the Society of Authors, which gave detailed, professional advice, and Joanne Koster, of CRC Press/Taylor & Francis, and Meeta Singh for their publishing expertise and support. I thank the many students I met over the years who encouraged me more than they ever knew.

The table below lists the people and organisations who have given permission for the use of photographs and quotations of text.

Most of all I would like to thank my wife Jill, with whom I was fortunate to share 58 years of married life, who worked with me in publishing from our home, who edited much of what I wrote, and who constantly gave me invaluable advice and support. She particularly wanted me to have a biography and helped me with it before she died.

Acknowledgements and Credits for Photographs

Figure description	Figure number	Year	Credit
To Jill			Credit to John Sculpher of Exeter
(a) With my wife Jill, my mother Kit and her father at our wedding in 1962. (b) With my father Sydney and paternal grandmother Grace Blanche at our wedding.	Figure 1.1	1962, 1982	
Jill's Exeter publications catalogue.	Figure 10.2	1995	Freddie Collins
(a) The author sitting as Examiner for PhD thesis at Nijmegen, the Netherlands. (b) Evelyn van Weel presenting her PhD thesis in public at Nijmegen.	Figure 13.3	2000	Willem van Gerwen, The Netherlands
(a) Institute of General Practice dinner (left to right) with the Vice-Chancellor's wife, Baroness Fritchie, the Vice-Chancellor and Jill). (b) Institute of General Practice Award as Centre of Excellence, with Sally Irvine (President of AMGP) Keith Bolden and Brenda Sawyer (AMGP). (c) Award to Institute of General Practice by Association of Managers in General Practice as a Centre of Excel in 1994.	Figure 13.4	1993	Justin Grainge Photography
Sir Donald Irvine the only time the President of the GMC and Chair of the Academy were both GPs, 2000.	Figure 24.1	2000	Justin Grainge Photography
Inaugural Meeting of the Conference of Academic Organizations, Initially Called the Academic Forum in 1999.	Figure 25.1	1999	RCGP Heritage Collections

(Continued)

Figure description	Figure number	Year	Credit
Visit of Chief Medical Officer to the PGMS 1993. Staff with left to right: Professor John Tooke, Professor Dame Margaret Turner-Warwick (Chair, Hospital Trust), Dr Brian Kirby, Baroness Fritchie (Chair Regional Health Authority), Professor Ernst, Sir Kenneth Calman (CMO), Dr John Tripp, Ms Pamela Mason (Regional Manager), Dr Rita Goble, DPG, Dr Michael Hall.	Figure 27.1	1993	John Sculpher of Exeter
University of Exeter, 1996. Public Orator for Sir Michael Peckham. With Chancellor Sir Rex Richards, University of Exeter. Public Orator for Sir Michael Peckham (red gown) next to Sir Rex Richards FRS (Chancellor), DPG (second left) in back row next to Sir Geoffrey Holland (Vice-Chancellor).	Figure 27.2	1996	University of Exeter
(a) JCPTGP dinner in 1997. Officers Malcolm Freeth and Justin Allen (Secretaries) with the author and Hilla Gittins. (b) Hilla Gittins and with four Chairs of the JCPTGP. Dorothy Ward Eddie Josse, DPG, Hilla Gittins, and John Lawson, 1997.	Figure 29.1	1997	Justin Grainge Photography
In 2000, (a) Kieran Sweeney Partner 1986–2000. (b) Russell Steele Partner 1976–2000. (c) Philip Evans, Partner 1987–2000.	Figure 34.1	2000	Acknowledgement to Barbara Sweeney
At the Practice the day the Knighthood was announced.	Figure 34.2	1998	*Express and Echo, Exeter.*
In 1998: (a) The Netherlands Conference on Dietary Advice. Chris van Weel on the right, wearing his Hon FRCGP tie, Bennelux Press. (b) London party with Jill where I am wearing my Cambridge half blue blazer and tie.	Figure 35.2	1998	The Netherlands Conference on diet
With Jill at Buckingham Palace after being knighted, 1999.	Figure 35.3	1999	RCGP Heritage Collections
In 1998: (a) Keith Bolden, Provost, Tamar Faculty at RCGP Spring Meeting with Professor Stuart Murray. Quay Studios. (b) Breakfast at home with Jennifer, Chris van Weel (the Netherlands) Penelope and Jill. (c) RCGP Spring Meeting. Michael Hall, organiser.	Figure 35.4	1998	Quay Studios
Welcoming King Charles, as Prince of Wales, to the RCGP, 1999.	Figure 35.10	1999	Justin Grainge Photography

(Continued)

Figure description	Figure number	Year	Credit
Gloucester. Presenting the George Abercrombie Award to Edgar Hope-Simpson (centre) in his home. The Cheltenham Newspaper Ltd. 1999.	Figure 35.11	1999	The Cheltenham Newspaper Ltd
AGM in 2000, presenting a silver bowl to the College with Dame Lesley Southgate.	Figure 35.12	2000	RCGP Heritage Collections
Presidential portrait by Carlos Luis Sancha, 2000.	Figure 35.13	2000	RCGP Heritage Collections
AGM in 2000, unveiling of the portrait with Dymoke Jowett, Provost, Tamar Faculty.	Figure 35.14	2000	RCGP Heritage Collections
First GP Chair of the Academy of Medical Royal Colleges with Jill, July 2000.	Figure 38.1	2000	John Sculphur
University of Exeter Honorary DSc, 2009.	Figure 49.3	2009	University of Exeter
Jill's obituary in the *Br. J Gen Practice*, January 2021. (With permission of the Editor.)	Figure 49.5	2021	*British Journal of General Practice*
Speech of thanks after receiving the RCGP Lifetime Achievement Award in 2022, six hours after breaking an arm and having an eyebrow stitched, aged 87.	Figure 49.6	2022	Karla Photographic Perspectives

Thanks and Acknowledgements for Permission to Quote Text

Editor, *British Journal of General Practice*	1973	Editorial, Confidentiality in General Practice *J Roy Coll Gen Pract* 1973:**23**:833–839 (Anonymous, DPG)	Confidential information is what the patient does not want the neighbour to know.
Editor, *British Journal of General Practice*	1980	Gale Memorial Lecture (1979) *Just a GP, Br J Gen Pract* 1980;**30**:231–39	Charles Peguy stated that everything begins as mystique and ends as politics.
			The Joint Committee of Postgraduate Training for General Practice – the Council of the College and the GMSC the two wings on which the plane of general practice now flies. History suggests that that it was the College which has set the direction and the GMSC which has controlled the pace.

(Continued)

Editor, *British Journal of General Practice*	2021	Evans P and Choules J (2021) Lady Pereira Gray: an appreciation *Br J Gen Pract* 2021;**72(702)**:30	Jill's obituary
Nigel Edwards, CEO the Nuffield Trust	1969	Rock Carling Lecture by Professor Sir Denis Hill	The family doctors' role is a difficult one: if it is to be sustained they must become the most comprehensively educated doctors in the NHS.
Hal Leonard	1949	*Some Enchanted Evening* 4 lines From South Pacific Lyrics by Oscar Hammerstein 11 Music by Richard Rodgers Copyright © 1949 by Williamson Music Company c/o Concord Music Publishing Copyright renewed All rights reserved. Used by Permission *Reprinted by Permission of Hal Leonard Europe Ltd*	*Some enchanted evening, you may see a stranger,* *You may see a stranger across a crowded room,* *And somehow you know, you know even then.* *That somehow you'll see her again and again.*

Section I

1

Early Years

To understand your parents' love, you must raise children yourself.

Chinese proverb

I was born at home on 2nd October 1935 as my parents' first child. This was a middle-class home where my father worked as a general practitioner (GP) and my mother taught in a junior school. Our home was a large Victorian house, bought by my paternal grandfather, also a GP. My father, like most GPs at that time, worked alone and from his home with minimal staff. Most working people seen were covered by friendly societies (an insurance system); middle-class people were private patients and my mother sent them accounts at the end of every quarter.

My parents' social life was very different from what I experienced. Before World War II, they regularly dressed for dinner in friends' homes (i.e. the men in dinner jackets and the women in long evening dresses). Many such families had servants and I had a nanny. My father was perpetually on call, doing much midwifery, often being called out from meals or social events.

For a child born in the 1930s, I was fortunate to know three of my grandparents. My mother's parents lived in Ireland, where my mother grew up. Her mother, Emma, was a Victorian mater, bringing up a family of four where there were servants rather than household machines and where the butter was served in pats. She was gentle and loving and ran a traditional home in Finisklin, Sligo, Ireland. My mother's father, John Cole, was a businessman and singlehandedly ran a wholesale sugar business. He was a Protestant in a 95% Roman Catholic community and he taught me about diplomacy. One of my mother's brothers, Jack Cole, spent his life in this business.

My father's mother Grace Blanche (née Frances, 1874–1968), lived in Exeter, England, to the age of 94. She died in 1968, after I was in practice. I got to know her well, as I used to go and see her regularly. I much regret not asking her more about my grandfather. She read a great deal and had been influential in our family by pressing hard for her two boys, Sydney and Richard, to go to Cambridge.

The one grandparent whom I never knew was my father's father, Joseph Anthony Wenceslaus Pereira (1869–1937). He was a Portuguese immigrant, born in Bombay, India, and my great-grandfather was a Portuguese civil servant. My grandfather came to Britain as a medical student, qualifying in medicine MRCS LRCP from Charing Cross in 1894. He started in general practice in Exeter in 1895, as Dr. Pereira, with very little money. He and his wife Grace had two boys, the first being my father born in June 1899. For years he did home visits to villages surrounding Exeter by pony and trap. My grandfather was politically left of centre and an active liberal in a city where most doctors were conservatives. He learned that his qualification did not mean he was a 'real' doctor and the use of the word 'doctor' by doctors without doctorates was a courtesy title. To remedy this, and most unusually, he obtained an MD by examination from Brussels in 1903. This was a remarkable example of postgraduate medical education. His photograph, in 1903 proudly wearing his MD robes, hung in my consulting room—a non-verbal signal of an Exeter GP thinking outside the box and an example to me.

DOI: 10.1201/9781032713601-2

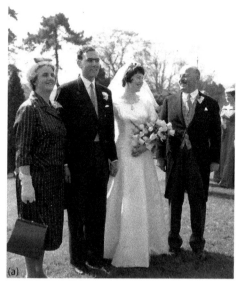 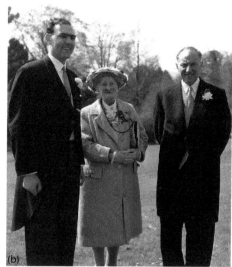

FIGURE 1.1   (a) With my wife Jill, my mother Kit and her father at our wedding in 1962. (b) With my father Sydney and paternal grandmother Grace Blanche at our wedding.

He became known as 'the poor man's doctor' as he was so good with underprivileged patients. They rewarded him in 1913 when the *Parliament Act of 1911* (known as the Lloyd George Act: The UK National Insurance Act of 1911 was a major piece of reforming legislation which provided GP care and medicines for working men, funded by the state. It was the first such health care legislation and provided a model for the NHS in 1948). was implemented by queuing for three-quarters of a mile to register with him. He acquired overnight the largest 'panel' list of patients in Exeter, and our family lived comfortably off thereafter. However, during the World War I, he suffered racial abuse, even though he was the GP with one of the largest lists of patients in Exeter. Some Exeter citizens could not differentiate a Portuguese person from a German one and nationally there were campaigns against aliens. He changed his surname by deed poll on 14 June 2018, adding Gray (chosen to sound English) to the Pereira. So, we became Pereira Grays, a formula he had used informally since 1908.

Dr. Pereira Gray died in 1937. The police lined the streets for his funeral and 12 police officers escorted him as their police surgeon. He knew me, but sadly, as I was 18 months of age, I cannot remember him. He left significant sums in his will, meaning that his two sons, my father Sydney and Richard, were comfortably off. Because he was a GP, founded the practice, took an academic approach to his practice and wrote many letters to the *Lancet* (Pereira, 1903–1915), gave the family the Pereira Gray name, and bought Holmedale for my father's home and practice, he had the greatest influence on my life of my four grandparents. I was always fascinated to hear about him and what he used to say from my patients, many who had known him (examples in Chapter 6, Learning the craft story).

My father, Sydney (1899–1975), went to Exeter School and won dozens of prizes, gained his colours for sports, and became head boy. He went straight from school into the World War I but, like many of his generation, never talked about it. He did, however, talk about learning to ride in Exeter barracks and about his horse, Tommy, to whom he was attached. He went to war as a teenager and was commissioned in the artillery to serve in France. He was in the second battle of the Somme. After the war, he went to St John's College, Cambridge and then to Bart's Hospital, London. He qualified as a doctor, MB BChir (Cantab) in 1925 and obtained the FRCSEd, a higher surgical qualification in

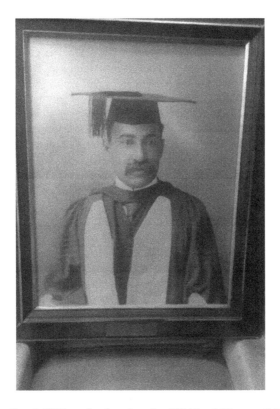

FIGURE 1.2   JAW Pereira Gray in 1903 wearing the robes of an MD (Brux). Then practising as Dr JAW Pereira.

1929, then returned in 1930 to Exeter to join his father in general practice. He went to Holmedale in 1932 as a bachelor, marrying my mother in Dublin on 1 September 1934. After my grandfather died, he worked singlehandedly from Holmedale. He was a quiet scholar and happiest at home. He loved languages, reading French, German, Greek, and Latin at home.

My father was widely read, thoughtful, and helped me greatly to avoid groupthink in later life. He thought children should learn languages and in the middle of the war with Germany quietly arranged for a German national to try to teach me the language. She did not make much progress with me, but she greatly appreciated my father's courtesy and support.

When I was about three years old, I developed pneumonia and became very ill, and my father expected me to die. Anxious consultation with colleagues led to a decision to try an experimental treatment, then called M&B 693. This was a sulphonamide and one of the first chemotherapeutic drugs used in Britain. This new treatment did me good but made me extremely sick. Soon, a later development of this product, known as M & B 760, became available. I was given this and made a complete recovery.

My mother, named Alice Evelyn but known as Kit (1907–1999, née Cole), was brought up in Ireland and became head of the primary school section of the Maynard School, opposite our home, breaking a glass ceiling by being the first married woman allowed to teach in that girl's school. She later threw herself into the practice as the first practice manager for 40 years. She ran the practice by answering the patients' phone calls and dealing with the executive council. My mother was worried about food running out, so she filled the cupboards of Holmedale with food that would keep. Current generations never have to think about food. She had great energy and wrote poetry, which was published in *Poetry Review* in 1934, and many columns for medical newspapers like *Pulse*. She gave me my love of writing and became an 'agony aunt,' or an advice columnist, for a women's magazine building this up with substantial secretarial help so that a daily package of letters was delivered by my father to the last London post at 9 pm each day. One secretary was Mrs Betty Fulford, whose daughter Joy came to work with my wife Jill and me in our home a generation later. My mother's writings paid my Cambridge fees. She remained alert throughout her later years, getting a letter published in *The Times* when she was aged 83 (Gray, 1990).

My younger brother Jonathan arrived on 6 May 1939. I can remember his birth, which, like mine, occurred at home. Although we were three and a half years apart, Jonathan bridged the gap relatively early and we spent hundreds of hours together playing games of all kinds, particularly ball games in the garden at Holmedale. He had a better eye for a ball than I did, so we were relatively evenly matched and at school he did much better in sports and in teams than I had done. Jonathan also played chess, and we played together in the school chess team and in some championships.

A Child in Wartime Britain

World War II was an experience that permanently affected those who lived through it. In terms of attitudes to sudden loss, acceptance of rationing, and conserving food and materials, the wartime generation is different from those who came after it.

One early memory is of a time when I was shopping locally in Mount Radford near our house and a bomb suddenly dropped in the neighbourhood. Looking up I could see a German bomber flying quite low, either off course or dropping his load on his way home. I was in the local post office. The motherly post office manager took me upstairs to her sitting room. This was completely illogical in terms of safety and illustrates how unsophisticated and how unprepared the Exeter population was for war.

There were several air raids on Exeter in 1942, often at night. My parents had three phases of managing their family, each progressively safer. At the beginning, we were taken to the cellar after the air raid sirens sounded; these produced a wailing noise that was easily heard. We all sat in an alcove in the cellar. Looking back, this was incredibly dangerous because if the house had been hit, we would have all been crushed inside it.

As the country experienced houses collapsing on people, the government introduced steel boxes called Morrison shelters. This was an advance on an unprotected cellar, but it is unclear if people would have been able to breathe had a big house like ours collapsed on it. In the third stage of sheltering, Anderson shelters were built outside the houses in gardens. Initially, we did not have one and when the night-time sirens sounded, we walked through a hole in the hedge to the next door garden where we shared a shelter with our neighbours. Later we had an Anderson in our own garden.

Exeter was seriously bombed on the night of 4 May 1942. This was one of the Baedeker raids, so-called from a German guidebook, retaliation on beautiful English cities, because it was claimed the Allies had bombed a German one. I was put into our Morrison shelter, then in our dining room on the ground floor. During the night I heard strange sounds like a giant walking upstairs and asked my mother what that was. "Oh," she said, "that's nothing to worry about, it's only the big wardrobes rocking!" As I was only six, this explanation satisfied me completely. Only later did I realise the force of the blasts hitting our home that night. Over 10,000 incendiary bombs were dropped on Exeter in that raid, according to Todd Gray, a local historian. My parents were up all night running around the house with saucepans, pouring water onto the wooden windowsills to try to stop them catching alight. The following morning, I remember standing in the road looking with surprise at houses nearby in Barnfield Road burning like fires. It was a mystery as to how the cathedral was not seriously damaged, as it was the biggest building in Exeter, centrally situated and lit up by the surrounding fires. One story is that a captured German pilot told nurses that he was a Christian and would not bomb a cathedral. In 2021 a 1,000 kg unexploded bomb was found after 79 years, where I had often walked. On detonation it left a crater big enough to hold a double-decker bus.

Opposite Holmedale, the Maynard School was hit by a high explosive on its tennis court and a great chunk of tarmac came across Denmark Road through our roof so hard it landed on a bed with enough force to push the bed legs through the floor. My brother and I marvelled in our sitting room below at a bed leg that was suddenly sticking through the ceiling. Fortunately, bombing in Exeter had been foreseen and stained glass from the cathedral and many beautiful historic objects had been removed to places of safety in the countryside – a rare example of preparedness.

My parents arranged for their two children to be evacuated to a village, Sticklepath, on the edge of Dartmoor. We stayed with relatives of my mother's, who looked after us perfectly well, but I was bored and just read for hours. I remember going with our host family up a hill and seeing a bright red glow in the sky, which was the city of Plymouth on fire. This was shutting the stable door after the horse had bolted, as Exeter did not experience serious heavy bombing again. I later read my mother was in tears driving back to Exeter, not sure if she would ever see her children again. Everyone expected further raids and fled their homes. My father's intense sense of duty to his patients as a GP led him to stay in our home, Holmedale, so he and my mother were alone in Denmark Road the night after the blitz (Gore, 2020).

General Practice

My father worked incredibly hard as he was responsible for both his own and his brother's general practice list of patients. This meant looking after about 5,000 patients for five years and being on call every night for all of them. GPs were allowed a petrol ration to do their home visits. His receptionist, his sole employee answered the door to patients and, before the NHS, dispensed medicines, mainly to friendly society patients. Petrol supplies held up throughout the war. He had patients over 400 square miles, including outlying farms. Sometimes on these home visits we would be given some precious eggs and a bowl of clotted cream, which was carefully carried wrapped in brown paper. This was never talked about but was much appreciated by my parents, who gave their butter ration to their children, like many families.

Family Involvement

My father's brother, Richard, had like my father qualified in 1928 from St John's College, Cambridge and Bart's and was another Exeter GP. He served as a doctor in Italy in World War II and returned to Exeter and resumed his general practice after it. My mother's brother, Nelson, was a squadron leader in the RAF, and had been appointed a wing commander, when he was killed in an accident. My mother's grief lives in my memory.

In the mid-1990s, my mother was interviewed by the Imperial War Museum as someone living in the same house 50 years after the war. I was surprised to hear her talking about children being killed by bombs locally. She protected me at the time and I never knew.

I went initially to the junior school of the Maynard, a girls' school opposite our home, later moving to Exeter School, where my father and uncle had been. Sending me to a day school was controversial, as the boys of most of my parents' friends, including a cousin, Christopher Gray, were sent away to public schools. My parents were uneasy about boarding schools. My mother was a Froebel-trained teacher and my father thought for himself. Their friends pressed them. Taking advice from an educational expert, they received a masterly statement: "The British public school system is excellent at training young men to govern India, in a way that India is not likely to be governed in the future!"

When I entered the main school I started to do very badly and was soon at or near the bottom of the class in several subjects. This was an era of corporal punishment and fagging in the boarding school and I had several beatings for breaking rules from both masters and prefects. I never won a prize of any kind and endured the middle school years. I learned valuable lessons about what it feels like to be regarded as academically inferior.

What saved me was chess and succeeding at something. I appreciated being at home the older I became. Being able to discuss matters with a liberal and tolerant father and having family discussions on controversial subjects was a great privilege. At one supper, when I was about 17, I argued vigorously in favour of capital punishment. My father kept gently raising problems, including judicial errors and the importance of the state modelling good behaviour, both of which were new ideas to me. That evening I switched positions. My father helped me to think for myself and to take positions that were often minority ones. On reaching the sixth form and becoming a prefect, I enjoyed my school time greatly. I liked biology and took zoology as a separate A-level, received good marks and was accepted by St John's College, Cambridge.

Jill

With single-sex schools, it was hard for boys and girls to meet. However, Mrs Collier started a dancing class in Marlborough Road (where I now live). She started with eight children, enabling her to teach the eightsome reel. The class was so successful that she soon expanded. Here I met Jill Hoyte, who Mrs Collier (and I) thought was the best girl dancer. We never went out together, but when she was head girl of the Maynard in 1955, she invited me to the sixth form dance where I had to dance with her headmistress! Many families also celebrated teenage birthdays with dances. At these I usually managed to have the last dance with her.

I went to Cambridge in October 1954, and she went to Bedford College, University of London, in 1956 to read English. We both went to each other's summer balls. We became engaged in 1961, as described in Chapter 4, where I recount my experience as a junior doctor.

2

The Chess Story 1948–1970

Chess, like love, like music, has the power to make men happy.

S Tartakover (1887–1956), Polish Grandmaster

No one in our family played chess, and I learnt only because my father thought boys should know how to play. He taught himself from a book and then taught me in 1944, when I was nine. Afterwards, he got me some coaching. In 1948, a chess tournament was held at Plymouth and my father discovered there was a junior section and took me. This was a new world, a proper tournament and people playing with clocks. The top section had a former world champion playing, Max Euwe from the Netherlands. It was easy to watch the master games in the same room. The masters' section was won jointly by Euwe and an Exeter star, Francis Kitto. I did badly and the junior section was won by RE Borland. I found I loved the game.

I entered the Devon boys Under-18 Championship and beat Borland in the final in 1949, thus becoming Devon Junior Champion at 13. This was a turning point in my life and opened the door to many happy hours. It gave me self-confidence when I was not doing well at school.

My parents got me another coach (Francis Kitto, 1915–1964). He was a natural chess player, with great talent, but he was very much an amateur. He had played for Cambridge on board one in 1937 and played for England in 1948 after his Plymouth success. However, he did not work at the game or even keep records. He coached me on Sunday evenings and I learnt a great deal.

Once he gave me a note for my father asking for a loan. I watched my parents analysing his relationship with me and thought the answer would be yes or no; but they decided to make the request a gift. My father said that he judged that the loan would never be repaid and then it would become a burden on our relationship. Kitto later moved to Cornwall and sadly died at the age of only 49.

Junior Championships

In the following years I defended the Devon junior title, winning it every year until the age cutoff at 18. My father took me to Newquay for the junior (Under-18) West of England Championship in 1950 where we shared a room and I won, aged 14. However, in 1951, PLT Kelly won the title after we had a 63-move draw in our individual game. I won it back in 1952, beating Kelly in the fifth round. I retained the West of England junior title in 1953, my last year as a junior. In the 1953 national British Boys Under-18 Championship, I was well out-gunned. In 1951/1952, aged 16, I won the senior Exeter Championship. At the South of England Championship, I met Harry Golombek, chess correspondent of *The Times*. A former British chess champion and a codebreaker at Bletchley Park, his OBE was the first civil honour for chess.

In the summer of 1954, I had my most serious attempt at the British boys' title, my last year Under-18. I started well, keeping among the leaders. I started the last round as joint leader knowing that if I won I would be British champion or joint champion. I played MF Collins and went all out for the win but lost, finishing fourth equal behind KD Sales.

DOI: 10.1201/9781032713601-3

Tournaments

I was selected to play for Britain in a junior tour of the Netherlands in 1954 and appointed captain, although it was my first international. We stayed in the homes of Dutch families. England won 6/6 and I scored 4/6 (BCF *Year Book 1954/55*).

Going to St John's College, Cambridge that autumn I joined the College chess club. In a first-term match against Selwyn College I was drawn on top board against MF Collins. In a small room, with no one watching, I swept him off the board. Only he and I appreciated the irony of the two results, as we alone realised I would have been the British boys' champion had our two games, only months apart, been the other way round.

I was invited by the British Chess Federation to join an invitation-only Under-21 tournament at the Hastings Congress in January 1955. They collected all the leading British juniors, including KD Sales and MF Collins. This was an all-play-all tournament. I was amongst the leaders most of the way, but had too many draws finishing second equal with 5.5/9, the only unbeaten player and half a point behind KW Lloyd. This turned out to be my best tournament result.

Cambridge

I threw myself into chess at Cambridge. The target was a half blue for chess, which meant being selected and actually playing in the match against Oxford. Happily, I was selected and in March 1955 I won on board five (out of seven). Cambridge won 4–3. I was graded nationally 194, a good county score but well below the national leaders.

At the AGM of the University chess club, I was elected honorary secretary, unopposed. This was when I first discovered that people in effect can appoint themselves to positions. This occurs not because of the election or appointment process but rather as a result of putting themselves in an unassailable position. By the spring of 1955, the fourth place in the British Under-18 Championship and second place in the British Under-21, both within the previous 12 months, meant that there was no one with a comparable record at Cambridge. Later, I saw this pattern with my professorship, with John Tooke's professorship, and later still with my presidency of the Royal College of General Practitioners.

In 1955–1956, I spent much time playing chess, often in London. In 1956, I was in the Cambridge blue team, the only Cambridge winner, on board four in a team that lost 3–4 (British Chess Federation [BCF], 1955–1956). At the AGM of the University chess club that year I was elected President for 1956–1957. This was the big job as the President alone selects all the team, the board position for all matches, and awards the half blues each year by selecting the team against Oxford. The announcement of the team was done weekly by placing names in the window of a shop opposite King's College.

In my examinations I failed to obtain grades high enough to exempt me from the second MB examination. My examiners had discovered I was reading chess rather than medicine! In the summer vacation I voluntarily went back to Cambridge — as I was a student and passed the second MB as a separate examination as an insurance. Now I was safe and could concentrate on chess even if I got a third, as the second MB ensured entry to a medical school. I was graded 4a in 1955 in the national chess system with 82 people ranked above me (1955). In 1955–1956, the Exeter Chess Club remarkably reached the semi-finals of the National Club Championship.

In March 1957, I led Cambridge in the 73rd match against Oxford, winning the toss and taking white on board one. Collins played on board two losing to David Richards. It was a close match and in a complex position where I had a rook against his two knights, I agreed a draw with HG Mutkin. The team match was also drawn (Wade, 1957). I scored 2.5/3 in my three blue games. That summer I got a 2:2 in the natural sciences and so did not need the second MB. Fifty years later, Mutkin sponsored the Oxford/Cambridge chess match.

International Chess

I was selected for the four-person British team for the fourth International Student Team Championship in Reykjavik, Iceland, on board four. With no reserve we all played every match. The USSR had Mikhail Tal on board one and a few months earlier he had won the senior USSR Championship as a 20-year-old university student. I had the pleasure of seeing both Tal and Spassky (Boris) playing for the USSR; both later became world champions.

Against the USSR, I played Gipslis. The game was unfinished at the end of the session and adjourned. I was losing but it was depressing knowing that in the gap, the grandmasters would be advising him. On resumption, I was polished off quickly. The Soviet Union won 3.5 to 0.5. I was not alone. Gipslis won the board four tournament prize, winning every game. He later became a grandmaster. The USSR won every match and 10/13 matches by three points or more out of four.

One exciting game was against Iceland. Being on board four I was placed at the end of the tables and paradoxically was the most easily watched by visitors. I had a bad game and was in difficulties. However, I then launched a sacrificial king-side attack right on the edge of the board most easily seen by the onlookers. Excitement mounted in the fast-growing audience, pressurised my poor opponent. He ran short of time and I was able to win. Britain did poorly, coming ninth out of 14 teams with five wins, one draw, and seven losses (23%). My results were four wins, three draws and six losses, also 23%.

Pal Benko, playing for Hungary, defected to the United States, later becoming a grandmaster and American champion. A report of the conference with results was published with two of my games, one win, one loss (Austurbaejar, 1957).

In 1957 there was a chess tour of Yugoslavia (then one country) by a combined Oxford and Cambridge team. I was not involved in the planning but was invited and surprised to be made captain. The tour was educational as my first visit to a communist country, then firmly under Tito's control. His picture was everywhere. After one speech of thanks to our hosts, David Richards from Oxford, translated me into German. There was warm applause. Then, since many did not speak German, he repeated the speech in Russian. There was an awkward silence. Afterwards, I asked a Yugoslav what had gone wrong? He said, "An Englishman who speaks another language well is welcome. But an Englishman speaking two languages well must be your minder from your KGB!" I went to Bart's in the autumn of 1957. I played chess and joined the University of London chess club and played for Bart's in bridge and chess.

In 1958, I attended the AGM of the British Universities' Chess Association (BUCA). The President was BH Wood, a good player who published the magazine *Chess*. An election for the post of captain was held. As past President at Cambridge and the only member there from the British team in Reykjavik, I was elected. I took this lightly not knowing what it involved. I then found myself in the middle of a national political problem. BUCA had been founded by BH Wood who saw the need and had the vision to invent a new chess organisation, becoming President. The difficulty was that this organisation was separate from the British Chess Federation (BCF), which governed British chess. Relationship problems were inevitable once student teams competed in international tournaments. Relationships between Wood and the BCF were cool.

The next World Student Chess Championship was in 1959. The first problem was being told that as captain I was expected to raise most of the funds to pay for the team! As an unsupported medical student with no secretarial help this was a tall order. Wood provided only starter funds. The BCF was not paying for a team it did not own but official international correspondence went to the BCF not the BUCA. Team selection was a big problem as both the BCF and BUCA thought they should do it. In this muddle I only survived as an inexperienced medical student because Bob Wade (1921–2008), a former British chess champion and international master, contacted me and gave great support. We met often in London cafés. Wade said he was persona non grata as he was thought to be a communist. I said I was not concerned with politics and for me only chess mattered. He suggested companies and people for me to approach, including CHO'D Alexander. I wrote the letters by hand. Most companies did not respond, but some individuals helped, so a moderate sum was raised.

Selection was complicated. I did not know who was available and the BCF thought it should select, without paying. BUCA continued to see the team as BUCA's and thought as the BUCA captain I should select it. This was solved by my welcoming information about who was available and agreeing to receive BCF advice. This led to a huge strengthening with Jonathan Penrose (1933–2021) and Peter Clarke (1933–2004). Penrose came from a brilliant family with his brother Roger (1931; later Sir and Nobel Prize winner). I selected the strongest possible team. The BCF met some costs and individual players contributed themselves. The costs of the six-person team were thus cobbled together. I'd had an unusual training in organisational politics.

This was three years after the 1956 Hungarian uprising and the country was still firmly behind the Iron Curtain. My worst moment was on the train to Budapest when a team member asked me to rearrange the suitcases so that his was at the bottom. Later, I quietly asked him why and he said he was smuggling in hundreds of razor blades! Knowing about secret police, I was shaken.

Britain was stronger than in Iceland and with more people than boards, I could rest players. The time limit was 40 moves in 2.5 hours. We came seventh out of 14, behind six East European teams with Bulgaria winning ahead of the USSR. I was disappointed, scoring only 2.5/8=31%, below the team average of 50%. I blundered twice in good positions. There were four published reports of the tournament: the official one Sajtar (1959), PH Clarke wrote one for the *British Chess Magazine* (Clarke, 1959) and mine in *Chess* (Gray, 1959) and the *British Chess Federation Year Book* (Gray, 1959/60).

University of London

Medical students at Bart's were students of the University of London so I joined the University chess club. My arrival was quite different from at Cambridge. They seemed jealous of my Cambridge half blue. They repeatedly queried my eligibility and picked me reluctantly for the first team. There was little team spirit. At examination time many people declined even for the first team; I, on the other hand, kept playing, including on the winning London team in the British Universities Team Championship. At London, colours are awarded for contributions to the team. Only later did I realise that despite playing effectively for the first team and regularly during examination times, I was never awarded a chess 'purple.'

Exeter Again

After returning to Exeter I re-joined the chess club, becoming the fourth Exeter player who had previously played for Cambridge at board one. HV Mallison (Trinity), the strongest Exeter player between the wars, ARB Thomas (St John's), and FEA Kitto (Kings) had been board one in 1937. I won a playoff for the Exeter Championship playing the risky and aggressive Goring gambit (Gray v Clapp, 1963), which was published with my notes in the *Bristol Evening Post* (1964). My note to the 18th move stated I had reached this position in pre-match preparation, indicating how seriously I was taking it. The club champion traditionally played all-members simultaneously, I won 10, drew 2 and lost 6. In another simultaneous with schoolboys at Exeter School I won 17 and lost 3.

With Thomas and Kitto on the top two boards, David Richards and me on the middle boards, and Brian Clapp, Exeter often did well in the national chess club competition, reaching the national semi-finals in 1966–1967. ARB Thomas was overall the strongest Devon player in my day. A master at Blundell's School, Tiverton, he was selected to play for England and was heartbroken when his headmaster refused him permission to be away.

The Exeter club organised a simultaneous display by Gligoric, the Yugoslavian grandmaster. Jill and I put him up in our home. When I introduced him to Jill, who was then 27 and looking great, he kissed her hand saying: "Ah! Zee English rose!" He played 24 people, polishing me off the board, losing only one game.

In the 1964 West of England Championship, with Jill watching, I finished fourth behind JM Aitken, DV Mardle and Ancell. Aitken, an international player, won. In 1965, I played the best game of my life (Hayden, 1965) and the only game I had published in the *British Chess Magazine*. I offered a bishop sacrifice which if accepted would lead to a sacrifice of 'the exchange' (surrendering up a rook for a bishop) and won in 24 moves with black. I came third equal. DV Mardle of Gloucester won with 5.5/6, drawing with me.

That year, I went to national medical meetings (the Conference of Local Medical Committees and the Annual Representative Meetings of the BMA) (Chapter 8, the LMC and BMA story), changing my life without me realising it. My last chess note was in February 1970. In the 1971 grading system, of 380 graded players in the six Southwestern counties, seven were ranked above me. However, whilst I had several draws with internationals, I never made the transition from being a leading student player to a leading adult player. Chess initially seemed part of my life, but I played it for only 23 years. After the age of 34 I never played tournament chess again.

Putin (1952) is quoted as saying that chess makes people wiser and clear thinking. Personally, I think chess is good training for life, teaching responsibility for decisions: after losing there is no one to blame. In chess the big picture counts and there is a need to weigh constantly different factors like material advantage versus space and open lines, requiring strategic judgement, as well as calculation. Serious chess is played under strict time limits—excellent training for decision-taking in the real world. Finally, chess is good training in trying to foresee the best possible move by a competitor or opponent.

ADDENDA

Jonathan Penrose (1933–2021) in 1960 played for England and beat the word champion, Tal. He was British chess champion ten times, became a grandmaster, and was appointed OBE. Devon regularly played Gloucester, usually losing, as their team included chess experts like CHO'D (Hugh) Alexander (1909–1974), a British chess champion. He led hut 8, at Bletchley Park, working closely with Alan Turing. He was recruited by Milner-Barry (1906–1995), another chess international whom I saw. I watched Alexander playing and in 1959 wrote to him seeking funds for the British student team. He gave me a donation. He was appointed CMG and CBE. The key letter from Bletchley Park to Churchill, pleading for resources, on 21 October 1941, was signed by AM Turing, WG Welchman, CHO'D Alexander and Stuart Milner-Barry (Hodges, 2014). Milner-Barry delivered the letter and was knighted in 1975, with the KCVO rather than the KCB that most senior civil servants receive. Some of Britain's best chess minds, over whose shoulders I looked, or whom I met, were at the heart of the world-leading, code-breaking team at Bletchley Park.

3

Medical Student 1954–1960

The young doctor in his early university years is still, in most medical schools, made to study man as a machine, man as a corpse, but never man as a person.

Lord Platt (1900–1978) Professor of Medicine,
University of Manchester; PRCP (1957–1960)

I was a medical student at two institutions: half the time I was at St John's College Cambridge and half the time at Bart's hospital, London. I went to Cambridge in October 1954. Gowns were worn in hall for dinner each night, which came after a Latin grace, and in the street in the evenings. University officials, proctors, patrolled the streets. The undergraduates at John's were all male. Gates were locked each evening and being found with a woman at night meant students could be rusticated; i.e. sent home.

The lectures varied greatly in quality, but the tutorials were great, being for either one or two students with a supervisor in College. Any views were tolerated, but your case had to be based on facts and argued logically. We dissected the human body for two years. This was a serious waste of effort, forming too big a proportion of a course tailored to meet the lecturers' interests and not the needs of working doctors.

I had two flatmates, Keith Mackenzie-Ross and John Doar. We wrote weekly essays. I usually wrote about six pages and was given beta+ or beta++. John Doar usually wrote four pages and was consistently marked alpha minus or alpha. From this, I learned about quality of thinking and writing.

There were 13 medical students a year at John's, about 39 in all. Jonathan (later Sir) Miller (1934–2019) was a year ahead of me, and we were often in the library together. He was exceptionally well read. He took four subjects in his finals instead of the usual three (tripos). I was told this cost him the first-class honours expected, and he was given a 2:1. [However his obituaries report that he got a first]. I went to watch Miller and colleagues at the Cambridge dramatic society. They were superb and were soon doing West End shows like *Beyond the Fringe*. He later left medicine to become an internationally distinguished dramatist.

In the year below me was John (later Sir) Grimley Evans (1936–2018) who became as passionate an advocate for geriatrics as I was to become for general practice. In 1955–1956, of 39 medical students at St John's, three were later knighted. General practice never featured as a subject at Cambridge, although the John's Medical Student Society invited John Hunt, Secretary of the new College of General Practitioners, to speak.

I became involved with university chess, which soon dominated my Cambridge life (Chapter 2: Chess). The Cambridge correspondent (1955) of Exeter School in his report on the nine old Exonians at Cambridge wrote: "Denis Gray (St John's) divides his time between chess and medicine (in a ratio of 10 to 1 one gathers)!"

In my first year examinations in 1955 I got a third class. The system was rightly telling me I was reading chess rather than medicine! In the second year I failed to get exemption from the second MB, obtaining it as a separate examination in October. This coincided with my 21st birthday when my parents came to Cambridge and gave me a dinner in London with the girl from home, Jill Hoyte.

DOI: 10.1201/9781032713601-4

I was now set up for a year's chess as the Cambridge University Chess Club President. The class of the degree no longer mattered, a third would do. I greatly enjoyed my presidential year (Chapter 2), awarding chess half blues and captaining Cambridge against Oxford. In my finals I got a 2:2.

Bart's 1957–1960

In October 1957 I found myself in a very different institution. My accommodation was in College Hall, Charterhouse Square near the hospital, which was mixed with women on the top floor. The room was pleasant and comfortable, meals were provided, and there were no restrictions about coming or going.

Opportunities for seeing patients were good as they stayed in hospital for a long time; patients with heart attacks stayed for weeks. It was possible to get to know several patients as people. Many consultants were nationally known and excellent clinicians. Bart's provided a good learning setting for physical diseases. However, mental diseases had second-class status, preventive medicine/population medicine was seriously neglected, and general practice was despised (Just GPs).

The Bart's nursing sisters influenced me greatly. They taught me what professionalism meant more than the doctors did. They were patient centred. I watched with admiration as a nursing sister would look around the ward and direct staff to see Mr X, "who does not seem quite so well today." The sisters, known by the name of their ward, knew their patients and had huge pride in their wards. One sister slept in her office when a patient was dangerously ill. The sisters managed the cleaners, who were part of the ward team, and the wards were spotless; privatisation stopped that teamwork. The disaster of the Mid-Staffordshire NHS Foundation Hospital Trust could not have occurred under those sisters. The Salmon Report (1966) introduced a management system for nurses that downgraded ward sisters and forced them, if wanting promotion, to enter management. There should have been a second system for ward sisters who wanted to remain clinicians. General practice was protected by the independent contractor status and this allowed senior GPs to continue in clinical practice while undertaking management roles, as I later did (Chapter 34, the Practice 1987–2000 story).

Many consultants taught by humiliation: at Bart's students were questioned in front of a group and then humiliated if they made mistakes. This had not happened at Cambridge and so it was a shock. This was a bigger problem for the women students, who sometimes cried, whereas the men kept stiff upper lips. I learned to keep at the back of groups and to give half answers, which whilst inadequate, made humiliation less likely. Patients were humiliated too.

On a ward round a consultant surgeon taught on an old, working-class man with a hernia. He stood the patient in the ward, without curtains, in front of a group of students and told him to take his trousers down. "But Sir," said the patient "there are young ladies present," and indeed there were, several. The consultant firmly told him again to undress, which he did. Then the consultant instructed us to examine the hernia one by one as the man stood there with his genitals exposed. I studied not the hernia but his head. The saying "he hung his head in shame," was illustrated vividly. Non-verbal communication is more powerful than spoken words and this uneducated man clearly communicated his distress and humiliation. I learned that students may learn different lessons from what their teachers think they are teaching. The lessons I learnt were: consultant power was everything; teaching was valued more than patient care; and patients' feelings, even when voiced clearly and signalled non-verbally, were deliberately ignored.

My mind turned to my father's general practice where I knew how he spoke about his patients. Previously I had taken this for granted. That day, general practice appeared more civilised than what I was witnessing in Britain's oldest teaching hospital. It was a 'light bulb' moment. I described this story in my *System of Training for General Practice* (DPG, 1977a), which was used on the Exeter GP trainers' course. Several GP trainers then told me that they had had similar experiences.

In gynaecology outpatients, women patients were brought into a large room and seated by the consultant and in front of and within earshot of about fifty medical students, mostly men. They had their gynaecological, and sometimes sexual, histories taken in public and young women were often addressed as "Topsy," a form of address that was never explained, but seemed sexist. Many patients were red-faced with embarrassment. They were then sent behind curtains and onto a couch where a nurse undressed them. The consultant examined them out of sight, but within earshot, so anything the woman said was heard by us all. A few students were given the chance to do an internal examination. After dressing, the woman came back and was given the consultant's opinion in a setting that precluded any real patient involvement or much discussion.

I sat in the back row, out of the consultant's sight, and was never once invited to participate. Years later, after learning about non-verbal communication, I realised I was distancing myself. One of the gynae consultants was very witty. These sessions fulfilled his need for an audience but met his patients' needs rather less. He was so funny that several male students told me they would never miss his outpatients as they were guaranteed "a good laugh." It is sad that such a clinic, so daunting to those patients, was for years, a model for medical students.

Consultants

One patient whom I clerked (took her history) was a 28-year-old mother of two children. I saw her every day and got to know her. She developed a nasty infection that progressed and she died. It was my first patient death and most upsetting, although I believed she got the best possible medical treatment. The only helpful comment I received was from a ward sister, otherwise students were expected to get on with it. The patient had been under a consultant, Eric Scown (later Professor Sir; 1910–2002; and professor of medicine). I had seen him try hard with drug treatment for her. Soon after the death Scown said he would teach on this 'case'. He gave an elegant exposition on bacteria, especially staphylococci, hardly mentioning that he was sorry that she had died. Neither did he think it necessary to see the young, widowed husband, who was distraught; he left that to the houseman and student. This seminar was a second 'light bulb' moment for me. Why were consultants so keen to emphasise that they were in charge of all patients in their beds, when after deaths they did not want to be involved? A disturbing thought occurred: were some consultants more interested in pathology and technology of medicine than in patients as people? Were patients sometimes just seen as the carriers of disease? General practice suddenly seemed more human and humane.

I was attached to Ronald (later Sir) Bodley Scott's firm (1906–1982), an expert on leukaemia. He was a physician to the Queen, being knighted after I left (KCVO, 1964). Virtually all his patients had leukaemia. He was a good teacher, but my experience was unbalanced. Later in general practice, dozens of my patients suffered unnecessary blood tests because I had wrongly learned that leukaemia was common. Such wards should have been used only for postgraduate teaching. Patients in teaching hospitals were becoming increasingly unrepresentative and less appropriate for medical student teaching. White *et al.* (1961) showed that only one in a thousand patients enters a teaching hospital. I later succeeded Sir Ronald as the Editor of the *Medical Annual* (Chapter 17, the *Medical Annual* story).

General practice was not recognised as a subject, with no lecturer in general practice. I was sent to a slum general practice in the East End, for a week's 'experience.' The facilities, clinical standards and teaching were abysmal. Was it arranged to put students off general practice?

A highlight was a month in Dublin at the Rotunda Hospital, a very busy maternity unit. The Irish obstetricians enjoyed having a young Englishman on their ward rounds and teased me with a smile. I never felt humiliated. "What does the young Englishman suggest?" was common. Then, whatever I said, they feigned great surprise and said they did the opposite! When I suggested admitting a woman for a D&C, they said they would do it at home. "In the slums?" I said. "Yes," they said. "And why not?" "Because these patients are mostly anaemic and will get infections," I replied. The consultant said, "Would the young gentleman from England like to see some home D&Cs and audit the infection rate?" I found myself shaving the pubic hair of poor women in Dublin slums. My audit confirmed the women were anaemic, but there were no infections among 100 patients.

In 1959, CP Snow (1905–1980; 1963) delivered the Rede lecture in the Senate House in Cambridge, a few hundred yards from St John's College, but whilst I was in London. He used the phrase "the two cultures" for the gulf of understanding between those in the arts and sciences. He made me think of other forms of two cultures. Perhaps general practice and hospital medicine are two such cultures?

The students put on a well-attended Christmas show each year, usually poking fun at the consultants. One year, I was elected to manage the beer and was astounded at how much beer I had to order. I had to get the figures checked as I had to order barrels and barrels. Even as a student I was disturbed at how much was being drunk. Only years later did I realise that drinking among medical students was a stress response. It took a psychologist to research and publish it (Firth, 1986).

There were no curfews for medics but the nurses had a curfew which precluded them going to a standard show. However, a solution was available—an open ground-floor window; so it was possible to take a nurse to a show, return after her curfew time, heave her through the window, and scramble in after her. We were then together in a dark storeroom, which was very suitable for saying goodnight! I went to the Windmill, much talked about, but I went alone as I expected it to be crude. However, it consisted of naked girls waving feathers artfully so that only an occasional bare bottom was revealed.

Attitudinal Weaknesses

Bart's suffered from four serious attitudinal weaknesses in my day: insensitivity to patients' feelings, institutional misogyny, institutional prejudice against general practice, and over-confidence.

Bart's resisted women students until forced to accept a 15% quota after the war. I heard two older consultants express regret in having them and I never saw a female consultant. Women students had a separate common room–a sign of male domination. In the United States, women officers entered their officers' mess by a side door and not, like the men, through the front door; this remained the practice until General Hay, straight after appointment as the first female general, walked through the front door of the mess.

At Bart's, general practice was second-class. Lord Moran's (1958) opinion that GPs had "fallen off the ladder," was generally accepted. It was not seen as a discipline in its own right, but a collection of other disciplines practised at a superficial level (just GPs). This attitude still existed at the top of British medicine 40 years later (Academy of Medical Royal Colleges).

The College of General Practitioners was never mentioned at Bart's, despite John Hunt, a co-founder, having worked on the medical unit at Bart's and had a consultant brother there. Hunt was so loyal to Bart's that the shield in the crest of the College is based on the Bart's crest. Bart's was inward looking. I once heard a discussion about whether a consultant was appointable if he was not a Bart's man. The gendered rigidity behind this comment was caught in the joke that "You can always tell a Bart's man; but you cannot tell him much!"

Both Cambridge and Bart's had a poor curriculum. They knew half their students would enter general practice, but little thought was given to what GPs needed to learn. I only discovered how ill prepared I was once in general practice. Lord Platt was right. Students were taught about man as a corpse and man as a machine, but not about man as a person.

Final Examinations

I crammed for finals having many suppers with Jill, who was doing a secretarial course after her English degree. I much appreciated her support but was always uneasy that she went home alone across London late at night. I was well prepared having twigged that examiners repeat questions and Jill and I analysed dozens of recent examination papers. Some questions came up again.

I went back to Cambridge for finals. The long clinical case was Friedrich's ataxia with ichthyosis– rare conditions I never saw in my life again. Were they in a qualifying examination to test students' skills or to indulge examiners' love of 'interesting cases'? I qualified MB BChir (Cantab) in July 1960 and celebrated with Jill in London. I was 24.

4

Junior Doctor 1960–1962

Some enchanted evening, you may see a stranger,

You may see a stranger across a crowded room,

And somehow you know, you know even then.

That somehow you'll see her again and again.

Rodgers E and Hammerstein O (1949) *South Pacific,* **Broadway**
Reprinted by permission of Hal Leonard Europe Ltd

I did several locum house jobs at Bart's in 1960. One lunch time in casualty a well-dressed young woman came in, very drunk, aggressive, and swearing repeatedly. She said she was not well and wanted to be examined by a nice young doctor! The casualty sister was unfazed while the woman swore at her. She steered the patient to a side room and said that if she wanted to be examined she needed to undress. The nurses managed to get her clothes off but in the melée the patient hit one of the student nurses. When I came, she swore at me and assumed I was a student, demanding a doctor. The sister patiently explained I was a doctor and the only one in the department. "F… off" was all the woman said to me.

The sister suggested I come back in an hour. When I did so, I got the same response. "Another hour!" said the sister. After two hours, the woman said she wanted her clothes back as she intended to discharge herself. Sister replied she had locked her clothes in a cupboard and she was instructed not to allow a disturbed person to leave before they had a medical examination! Then the woman said she wanted her clothes as she needed the WC. She was told to use a bedpan. After three hours the patient was less aggressive. "Give her another hour," said sister and, as I left, whispered: "she's cooking nicely!" After four hours the woman had sobered up, stopped swearing, and was anxious to leave.

"Are you now ready to be medically examined?" said the sister. The woman nodded. "Don't shake your head!" said sister: "Ask this doctor if he would be kind enough to give you a full medical examination." The patient did so. Then suddenly the sister whipped off the sheet covering her, leaving her naked and exposed. The sister said calmly "You came in asking for a medical examination by a Bart's doctor, now you will have one." Turning to me she used the phrase for consultants on the wards, "Patient ready for examination, doctor!" Halfway through, sister said, "You will remember, doctor, that Mr X [a Bart's consultant gynaecologist] teaches that a full medical examination without a vaginal examination is incomplete." As I knew he did, I asked the patient if that was all right? She said, "Whatever." I did the examination and then asked the sister to cover her up. I said I had found no active disease and thought she was fit for discharge. The patient turned to the sister, seeing who was in command, and asked if she could leave now? I expected the answer "Yes," but sister said: "No, you have two things still to do." She then summoned the nurse who had been hit. "You will now apologise to this nurse and promise you will never hit a nurse ever again." The patient did so abjectly. "Finally," said sister, "You will now apologise to this doctor. You have sworn repeatedly at him, used most unladylike language, and called him a student." The woman then emerged in a new light. I had

DOI: 10.1201/9781032713601-5

19

only heard her swearing, but now she spoke with an educated, upper-class accent. She made a fulsome apology to me that seemed so heartfelt that I said: "Thank you," and instinctively held out my hand. The woman shook it warmly. Doctor and patient were non-verbally reconciled. Finally, sister closed this unconventional consultation conventionally. She stood up, looked me in the eye and said: "Thank you very much, Doctor!" I recognised the convention of a ward sister seeing her consultant off the ward. "Thank you, sister," I said, as I was dismissed.

Such events would not happen nowadays. But, half a century on, it is interesting how one badly behaved patient had her request met precisely, although not as she anticipated. That sister generated both punishment and incentives for better behaviour and made the punishment fit the crime She extracted apologies for both a nurse and a doctor. Nurse/doctor conventions were faithfully preserved. That young woman probably learned a lesson for life.

The career advice I received was that teaching hospital posts were important for a hospital career, but clinical experience was better for junior doctors in smaller hospitals, as having no registrars, meant they could not cream off the interesting work. So, as I was planning to go into general practice, my two pre-registration house appointments were both in small hospitals without registrars. However, that advice was only half right.

Hove General Hospital

My first job was as house physician at Hove General Hospital, where I worked directly with a consultant physician, Alec Bourne. He had been a GP, was a skilled clinician, a good teacher, and I liked and respected him. He did a ward round every day, including Sundays, and was always thoughtful. I learned much in this post.

There was an 80-year-old woman whom I admitted. Her electrolytes were disturbed and I spent ages adjusting them. I proudly presented her to Bourne saying that her electrolytes were now normal. He rightly cut me down. "She's dying, Gray," he said. "For heaven's sake let her die in peace!" It was great consultant teaching. I was too inexperienced and technically minded and I learned a life-long lesson.

One of the advantages of working in a very small hospital was that house officers cross-covered for different specialties. One night, I was on call for surgery. A GP rang and told me he had a woman patient who was very ill with an acute abdomen. "I know her very well," he said, "and this is serious." When I saw her she did not seem too bad. On call all evening, I had plenty of time and used it by practising all I had read from Zachary Cope's *The Early Diagnosis of the Acute Abdomen* (now Silen and Cope, 2010). I slowly worked through every test in the book, including rarely used ones like psoas spasm and hyperanaesthesia. We chatted as I worked and she told me she had not wanted to come into hospital, but her GP had insisted. "He knows me very well," she said. "I'm sure he has my best interests in mind."

After taking the most careful history and conducting the most careful abdominal examination I had ever done, I concluded that this was not an acute abdomen. But being only a pre-registration house officer, I called the surgical registrar. He was very experienced and frequently operated at night. He examined her carefully and he too decided that urgent surgery was not necessary. He suggested putting her on the consultant's operating list for the morning. The consultant surgeon then examined her early the following morning, whilst I watched, and he too decided there was no reason to operate immediately and put her on the end of his operating list.

He opened her at about 1 pm and found that the whole of her bowel was gangrenous. All he could do was close her up and send her, dying, back to the ward. The whole surgical team was surprised, nobody more than me. How had I missed an acute abdomen when I could not have tried harder? I simply could not have done more, but I still got it wrong. I was left with an awareness of the complexity of the human body and how some conditions are simply too difficult even for caring doctors to diagnose. I acquired a life-long respect for the complexities of medical practice.

Then I re-read the GP's admitting letter, which stated that he thought she was "in mortal danger." The word 'mortal' leapt off the page. I suddenly realised that this GP had death on his agenda when none of the surgical team, even seeing her hours later, did. I understood for the first time that of the four doctors with clinical responsibility for her, who had seen her in those critical 15 hours, only the GP, without any investigations, had somehow grasped the danger she was in and the probability of her imminent death. The only clue to how this was done was his, and the patient's, repeated emphasis on how well he knew her.

I made a mental note that continuity of care seemed more important than I had understood. Years later, I had the chance of researching it as described in Chapter 49, the St Leonard's Research Practice story.

I had a woman patient with severe abdominal pain and diarrhoea and was on a ward round with a different consultant physician, who saw himself as a cardiologist. He rattled off rare cardiac conditions associated with diarrhoea. I pleaded with him to consider a bowel infection and get another opinion but he refused. The patient died. The postmortem showed massive gut ulcers. The consultant never apologised, and I learned it can be dangerous for patients to be under a consultant in the wrong specialty.

A Formal Reprimand

Late in my post, my consultant Alec Bourne, with whom I had become quite close, tipped me off that the consultants were going to give me a formal clinical reprimand for an incident in casualty. I was summoned to appear before six consultants and the hospital administrator. A pre-registration house officer alone facing six consultants was not a promising situation, but I had three advantages: I alone had been at the incident, I had two days to prepare, and the senior consultant in the chair had not prepared.

The Chair said they had decided to give me a formal, clinical reprimand for my decision to transfer to a psychiatric hospital a patient who became unconscious, i.e. an Alice in Wonderland sentence first, before the facts. I replied that any punishment was contrary to natural justice if the facts had not been established. "But they have been," the Chair said. "We have a report from a consultant psychiatrist." "But he wasn't there!" I said, "and does not know the relevant facts. You have a duty to hear my evidence." The panel conferred and I was told to describe the incident briefly. I stated that I understood this was now a committee of inquiry. They did not demur. I said the incident began about 1 am in the casualty department when a patient became violent and attacked the one nursing sister on duty. I rushed to her assistance and I thought any other doctor would have done the same. We could not subdue the man until the night porter joined us to help. I managed to give the man an injection of a tranquilliser. I rang the consultant on call, who just told me to get on with it; a kerfuffle in casualty was not worthy of consultant care. The sister and I agreed we could not keep a violent man in a medical bed as the tranquilliser would wear off and this was a very small hospital where I was the only doctor. I rang the local psychiatric hospital to ask if someone would come and see him but they refused; so I said he had to be admitted there. They did not like it and I had to push really hard. I called an ambulance, which took him with my referral note.

The panel Chair then said the man had become unconscious on the journey and had been admitted unconscious. It was a serious clinical error of mine, they said, to transfer an unconscious man and not to have escorted him. "Escorted him!" I exclaimed. "Are you really suggesting I should have left the whole hospital and its casualty department without any doctor at all?" This shook the panel visibly as suddenly they understood my dilemma. The Chair repeated that it was always wrong to transfer unconscious patients. I said the man had not been unconscious when he left Hove and three witnesses, the sister, and two ambulance men, could confirm that. I repeated that as the only doctor in the hospital I simply could not leave it without any doctor at all.

The Chair shook his head, so I switched tack. "Anyway," I said, "you have the wrong person here! I am only a pre-registration houseman, it was the consultant who was in charge; NHS regulations clearly state that consultants are responsible *at all times, whether present or not!*" The consultant who had rejected my call was on the panel and was not amused. I pointed out that after that call the consultant had delegated all decisions to me. I had to use my discretion and had done so. The panel was now on the back foot, so the Chair tried again to deliver the reprimand. I said I refused to accept it! I asked if any of the panel were prepared to come into the casualty department at night when I was next on call? If so, I would be happy to follow consultant directions. They all looked down and no one spoke. I said I doubted if the staffing in this hospital, with no medical registrar, was safe for patients. I left the room not knowing what had happened. I then received a letter stating I had made a serious error of clinical judgment. I replied in writing, rejecting the reprimand and stating that "my job description did not include engaging in prolonged physical combat with violent male patients." I confirmed I had called the consultant on call for advice. There were no further letters. Afterwards, Alec Bourne said to me quietly, "You certainly gave as good as you got!" As Hilaire Belloc (1870–1953) wrote: "Towards the age of twenty-six they shoved him into politics."

It is interesting how lightly I took it. I thought that if a complaint was received from another hospital then the consultant who was responsible should discuss it with the doctor who was the subject of the complaint. I was puzzled this never happened. Half a century later, having held senior management roles in the NHS, in a university, and in charities, I saw it differently. Here were a group of consultants clubbing together to protect one of their number facing a potential complaint when he had ducked his clinical responsibility by refusing a request for help from a pre-registration houseman for whom he had a professional duty to give "close supervision." The official NHS guidance was that pre-registration house officers, who were not fully registered as doctors, should be closely supervised. This was a classic scapegoating operation creating an audit trail in which all the blame was placed on the most junior doctor.

Royal Victoria Hospital, Folkestone

My father had rightly been insistent that I needed to do a six-month post in obstetrics. He found a six-month job at Folkestone with an obstetrician whom he knew. This post was not recognised by the RCOG for its diploma in obstetrics. My father said this did not matter; it was the experience that counted. I took the post without understanding the implications.

The Folkestone Hospital was also small. Attending two gynaecological outpatients per week and working in a labour ward gave me good clinical experience. The job had compensations. If I was called out of bed more than once at night, the staff nurse would often cook me bacon and eggs! When fractures came at weekends, I arranged the x-rays and then alternated between calling a surgeon or an anaesthetist. When I gave the anaesthetic (using halothane), a consultant fixed the fracture and when I called an anaesthetist, I dealt with the fracture.

My job included sessions in the casualty department and regularly I was the only doctor in the hospital on-call for all beds and casualty from 6 pm on Friday until 8 am on Monday morning, a total of 60 hours. This was great experience. I started well. Seeing a woman in casualty with an eye problem, I diagnosed acute glaucoma and insisted she saw a consultant ophthalmologist immediately, which she was reluctant to do. Her husband came days later saying the consultant had confirmed glaucoma, that her sight had much benefited from the prompt referral, and the consultant had never before had a referral from a casualty officer. The man tried to tip me. I diverted the money to the hospital fund.

At the beginning of the obstetrics post, I read in the hospital mess a letter in the *BMJ* (Florence, 1960) from a Scottish GP reporting neurological symptoms in patients after he had prescribed 'Distaval.' This was thalidomide, the night-time sedative of choice in Folkestone and many British obstetric wards for which there had been a reassuring controlled trial (Lassagna, 1960). House officers then chose and prescribed sedatives. Alone in the hospital, in this pre-protocol era, I decided not to use it and mercifully never prescribed it. A second letter reporting similar findings was published a month later from another British general practice (Kuenssberg *et al.*, 1961). Ekke Kuenssberg later became PRCGP and greatly influenced my career. Much more important than my reaction was the decision by Frances Kelsey (1914–2015), a medical official in the US Food and Drug Administration (FDA), the US licensing authority, who, on the strength of these two letters from British GPs, deferred approving thalidomide in the United States, protecting all American mothers.

Birth defects caused by thalidomide were a British and European tragedy due to European regulators failing to value these two GP reports. Huge numbers of mothers in the United States were completely spared the thalidomide problem thanks to just three alert doctors: two British general practitioners and Frances Kelsey in the US FDA. America understood the magnitude of the problem it so narrowly escaped. Kennedy awarded Frances Kelsey the President's Award for Distinguished Federal Civilian Service in October 1962, only the second woman so honoured. (Kelsey, photographed with President Kennedy, John F Kennedy Presidential Archive and Museum, 1962). All this stimulated me to be a regular writer of letters to medical journals.

On starting the obstetrics job the consultant said: "I do the Caesarian sections, you do the rest!" The implications escaped me. One night I was alone doing a difficult forceps delivery with neither proper training nor experience. Desperately, I asked for the consultant to be called urgently. He was in bed and came as quickly as he could, but too late, the baby died. I have rarely been so upset and was scarred emotionally. Later my grief turned to anger as I realised that a pre-registration houseman should never have been in that position. Those two consultants and the hospital management knew the risks and were exposing patients to them. Too late I realised why that department was not approved by the Royal College of Obstetricians as it had no registrar. I learned that standards of medical Royal Colleges can be very important.

A Premonition

I had stopped seeing Jill after I qualified. It was entirely my fault and was to do with the emotion of qualifying and getting my first medical jobs, which had interfered with developing personal relationships. By 1961 I had realised my mistake and was hoping to get in touch again.

Then I had a premonition, what my mother called telepathy, which she often experienced. I had a clear vision of Jill coming into a particular room in the London university student union and my seeing her looking over my left shoulder. I went to that room and with no previous contact or appointment, sat by the window and stayed looking over my left shoulder – and in she walked! I immediately asked her out for a coffee and we were together again. She wasn't exactly a "stranger," but it was "a crowded room," and "somehow I knew" that it was a turning point in my life. "Again and again" (Rodgers and Hammerstein, 1949) turned out to be 'daily' for more than half a century. We got engaged that year.

Section II

5

The Practice 1962–1975

To cure sometimes, to relieve often, to comfort always.

Hippocrates, 5th century BC

The Americans have watches: we have time.

The Taliban, Afghanistan, 21st century

I came back to Exeter and joined my father in general practice on 22 January 1962, as his assistant. However, he wanted me as a partner quickly because he was 62, so I became one on April 1st that year. My contract specified seven years to parity, as was usual. I experienced general practice as it had been throughout the first two-thirds of the 20th century. My father's style of working in 1962 was essentially the same as his father's before him. He was a single-handed GP, working from home with minimal staff (one receptionist), but with substantial help from his wife – just as his father had done a generation before.

My contract was the first used when the NHS was established. It was extraordinary by modern standards – for a fixed sum, a capitation fee, paid per patient registered, the GP was contracted to provide 24-hour care, day and night, throughout the year. If the GP was away for any reason, including sickness and holidays, the GP was responsible for paying all locum costs. This contract contained serious perverse incentives. GPs, like my father who maintained decent premises to middle-class standards, received the same capitation fee as a GP renting cheap lock-up shops, who gained a higher income. GPs were incentivised to take on as many patients as possible, regardless of their ability to look after them, and to invest as little as possible in the practice. For a practice nurse, the GP paid the salary from his/her own income. The system was competitive as patients could change GPs easily.

I had not understood this system before I entered it. I found that I was earning about £800 a year (now about £17,500), and that the practice income, even with about 3,000 patients, did not provide an income for two doctors given the practice expenses. In effect, my father was subsidising the NHS from his own income. I was not motivated by money, but I did want to bring our family up in a middle-class way. This did not seem to be possible in our practice.

By the early 1960s, political pressures grew within the BMA, which increasingly railed at this system called in shorthand the 'pool system.' That was because the government paid a pre-determined pool of money from which GPs were then paid. Faced with an unsustainable income for the future, I became politically active in defending general practice and heavily involved in the medico-political system, described in Chapter 8: Local Medical Committee and BMA.

Early Experiences

I found general practice bewildering and unsettling. Patients often did not have the diseases I had learnt about at Cambridge and Bart's but did report strange symptoms that had no obvious pathological basis that I could understand. Families seemed very important as groups but I had learned nothing

DOI: 10.1201/9781032713601-7

about either groups or family practice. In my 1969 Hunterian gold medal essay, I wrote that it had taken me about seven years to divide the body into systems which I could understand, and it had taken me another seven years to learn to put the parts together again and see patients as whole people (DPG, 1969/70). It was an uncomfortable experience, as I was constantly trying to understand what I was seeing and struggling to find a theory/explanation.

This made me committed to general practice training as there had to be a better way of introducing young doctors to general practice and protecting patients from having a succession of doctors learning their craft by experimenting on them. We had 3,014 patients when I became a partner and the practice numbers then grew steadily. The practice systems were rudimentary even to my newcomer's eyes. Letters were still handwritten, and the receptionist answered the door when patients rang the doorbell.

One of the first reforms was to ensure that letters were typed. Jill started typing my letters and my father quickly saw the advantages of this; in particular in having copies of referral letters in our records. Accordingly,he approached a patient, Marion Eyles, and she started coming to do secretarial work part-time. The first structural change was when we converted part of my mother's kitchen into an office and reorganised the paperwork. However, my mother and I still did the staff salaries, including working out the tax deductions.

Patients were seen in the consulting room, which my father had used since 1932. We started to use the dining room as a second consulting room, so that two doctors could work at once. The room reverted to family use afterwards.

One big problem facing GPs was restricted access to pathology and x-ray investigations. One of the great betrayals of GPs in London was that the teaching hospitals there lauded their new medical graduates, but their actions did not match their words. In the MRCS LRCP diploma the examiners bowed to the new diplomates. However, when new GPs settled close to teaching hospitals, they banned them from access to their pathology laboratories and x-ray departments (just GPs). As a house officer in Bart's, I saw consultants rubbishing diagnoses of local GPs, whilst simultaneously denying them the tools for the job. The College of General Practitioners (not yet Royal) campaigned against this discrimination against quality of care. The CMO, Sir George Godber (1908–2009), supported the College (Godber, 1968).

As soon as I arrived in Exeter, I asked to see the senior pathologist, George Stuart-Smith. Knowing the situation in London I anxiously enquired what access I would have to the tests done by his laboratory. He was welcoming and said that general practice was an important part of the NHS. GPs should have good access to his laboratory. He thought GPs made too little use of pathology investigations. This was a wonderful example of consultant leadership.

A more disappointing response came from an ENT consultant I asked about using an audiogram for screening for deafness. He pooh-poohed the idea. "Audiographs are not as straightforward to interpret as sight tests" (Scott, 1965). He missed the point the GP's job is to screen and detect the huge number of deaf people, some of whom play down their disability. I bought an audiogram and found the graphs from practice nurses valuable. Then 98% of my subsequent referrals led to hearing aids being provided.

When they went on holiday, my parents expected Jill and me to leave home and live in Holmedale. Jill had to cover my mother's telephone answering duty whilst I had about 4,000 patients to look after single-handed. Once our baby Peter, did not get any breakfast until 11am as the practice phone rang so regularly that Jill could not get to him. Fortunately, he was a placid baby!

My mother's generation of wives subsidised the NHS and my mother did more than most, being the practice manager for forty years. GPs usually received poor accountancy advice to make a payment to wives so low as to avoid national insurance. The accountants did not understand that the gross pay for GPs was determined by counting their professional expenses in the previous year. Understating expenses cost all GPs income. I linked up with a barrister, Pat Price, a GP's wife herself, who campaigned for proper pay for GPs' wives. She formed a company, Medical Management Services Ltd, to employ them at professionally determined rates. This was to involve Jill and me dramatically later in a big BMA meeting, described in the story of the BMA and LMC (Chapter 8).

I was the first GP in Exeter to ask the Medical Officer of Health (MoH), Edward Irvine, to attach a health visitor to our practice. One health visitor had asked to be seconded to a general practice and he paired us. Helen Chapman came as our first practice-attached professional. Irvine was a practising Roman Catholic and instructed her not to get involved in any contraceptive advice. Our practice had a long history of serving the underprivileged and my grandfather, who had started the practice in 1895, was known as "the poor man's doctor." We had many poor families where contraceptive advice was much needed. Helen referred many patients to me knowing my views well.

Her first office in the practice was in my mother's scullery, off her kitchen; it was cramped and inconvenient, but she never complained. Later, she had one of the best health visitor's rooms in the country. I saw her regularly and we had long talks about our shared patients. She taught me much about home visiting, especially homes that were 'too tidy', and I also learned her skill in organising multipronged support for some families when, as a new GP, I was sticking to physical problems. Even now, half a century later, general practice has much to learn about the social determinants of illness (Magnan, 2017), linking patients to community services and what is now called 'social prescribing'.

Working with health visitors taught me that wherever possible they should be attached to general practices. The gains are many and quick and easy confidential access with problems is immensely valuable. Attached staff help GPs, as after understanding comes care. Hence the importance of Hippocrates' maxim: "To cure sometimes, to relieve often, and to comfort always."

The GP contract changed in 1965–1966, after a political confrontation between NHS GPs and the Department of Health (Chapter 8). This removed several perverse incentives. New payments were for the rent and rates of premises. Also, GPs were reimbursed 70% of the costs of employed staff, enabling the employment of secretaries and practice nurses. A new group practice allowance encouraged three or more GPs to work together. A General Practice Finance Corporation (GPFC) was formed which provided capital at commercial rates, but which looked favourably on GPs.

Under the new GP contract, we employed our first practice nurse, which was a big success and was continued. So, in 1965, with a health visitor and a practice nurse, we were developing a multiprofessional primary care team.

Personal

Jill and I moved to Marlborough Road in July 1966 through generous help from Sheila Hoyte, Jill's mother, who was the daughter of Frederick Joseph Ricketts (1881–1945), the composer of military marches, including Colonel Bogey – she was receiving a share of the royalties. As a serving officer he wrote under the name 'Kenneth J Alford,' so we called our home Alford House.

In 1966 I came second in the RCGP Butterworth essay competition which meant I collected the prize for preventive care "Advising the Healthy" and took me onto the platform of the RCGP AGM for the first time. I was successful with the Hunterian Society gold medal for an essay on the early detection of malignant disease in general practice (DPG, 1966/67) and in the BMA's Sir Charles Hastings Prize for systematic observation and research, twice. I was fortunate to be awarded the Hunterian gold medal again for an essay on the care of handicapped children in general practice (DPG, 1969/70).

In 1968, I experienced a new emotion. I saw on television, surgeons from the National Heart Hospital reporting Britain's first heart transplant. The surgeons led by Donald Ross (1922–2014), were celebrating this considerable technical achievement, which I admired. I had until then respected unconditionally the increasing of specialist expertise, but that day I suddenly felt highly critical. Their behaviour, lack of concern for the patient, and self-congratulatory tone seemed inappropriate. This feeling grew when the patient died 46 days later from organ rejection—a problem the surgeons did not understand.

By the early 1970s, my father was over the age of 70 and the practice was growing. Retirement plans were needed. My father enjoyed the job: he was not keen to retire and there was no retiring age, but he recognised changes were needed. We therefore embarked first on a major remodelling of the house to facilitate medical practice; secondly, we sought a third partner.

I borrowed as much as possible from the GP Finance Corporation for a redesign of Holmedale. Times were difficult with 26% inflation on the RPI in 1975. The plan was to turn a Victorian family home into a purpose-planned base for group practice. I was incredibly fortunate that my brother, Jonathan, now a successful London architect, agreed to do this. I tried every permutation of rooms but could not make any design work. With dramatic architectural lateral thinking, he built a new main entrance through a cupboard in my mother's kitchen 15 feet above a path outside the house!

The new premises precisely met the brief I had given him and produced three consulting rooms, a practice nurse's treatment room, and a new waiting room. The old dining room became a dedicated office that held all the medical records; it had room for secretarial staff and a reception desk right beside the new entrance and overlooking the waiting room. My father's beautiful, large consulting room remained unaltered. In a second phase, we had a health education/health visitors' room shared with the attached district nurse, and a new trainee consulting room. A further office, called the 'quality assurance' room, was probably the first room named like this in British general practice.

This was then the biggest extension of GP premises in Devon. I was anxious when the premises were assessed by the district valuer, an independent professional, as the finances depended on the 'notional rent' he awarded. This was then paid by the NHS to the practice, to cover the interest charges on the loan. The figure was about what had been estimated: the books balanced.

We were extremely grateful to my brother, who designed this radical rebuilding while living in London. The premises gave us great pleasure. Jill made all the curtains herself in the same pattern, with contrasting colours. My brother specified top quality carpets, when most surgeries used cheap flooring, which greatly added to the ambience. The new premises lifted the morale of the whole practice team and improved our efficiency considerably. As Churchill said: "We shape our buildings, but afterwards they shape us."

My Editorship of the *Journal of the Royal College of General Practitioners* (*JRCGP*) in 1972 did not affect practice, as I edited from home where we had the journal office (Chapter 9, the Journal story). However, my appointment the following year on 1 December 1973, as part-time senior lecturer in the University of Exeter (Chapter 13, Department/Institute of General Practice) did have an impact. After 11 years full-time I started taking a day a week out of the practice.

On 1 January 1974 we started recording, using the RCGP system, the diagnoses of every consultation. We started using 'personal lists', a system of practice organisation that gives every patient a responsible GP and fosters continuity of GP care. I coined that term which is now in general use. Five years later (DPG, 1979a) I described adopting personal lists as the third most important decision of my professional career (the first two being deciding to be a GP and choosing to return to the family practice). We ran multiple internal audits of practice activity, impressing our visitors. On I July 1974 my list had 3,209 patients.

We advertised in the *JRCGP* and appointed Richard Hillier. He had recently completed vocational training, had the MRCGP and had been on a British Antarctic expedition. He joined after the conversion, with his own new consulting room. My father and I appointed with confidence, but the partnership never worked. There was never a row, but Hillier kept delaying signing the partnership agreement and it became uncomfortable. Completing his MD, he left general practice to be a director of a hospice, where he did well. Years later we met in the Royal College of Physicians. He said: "There wasn't room for both of us in the practice." We then appointed Ann Buxton in 1974.

New Understanding of Time

The challenge for GPs is to stop seeing patients as vehicles for medical problems and see them as individual people. The interplay between the physical, psychological, and social components of problems is the great intellectual challenge of general practice. Secondly, comes a deeper appreciation of time. Much medical practice is short term: GPs enjoy the longest perspectives. Coulter *et al.* (1991) researched patients with back pain after referral to an orthopaedic specialist. Five years later, 33% of those patients were still consulting GPs for back pain! Seeing girls become mothers and their mothers become grandmothers, are special experiences in family medicine, unique in the medical profession. This deeper understanding of time is a special privilege of general practice, contrasting with hospital medicine. It is illuminated by a Taliban metaphor: "The Americans [hospitals)] have watches: we [GPs] have time."

Losing My Father

In 1975, my father became ill. Cancer was diagnosed and he was operated on in the London Hospital and died on the table. It was a terrible experience, as he worked in the practice only a month before, and I was unprepared. I rushed up to London to support my poor mother. As Ann Buxton was an assistant, I suddenly became single-handed, but I admitted her to partnership the same year. The patients were wonderful, sending me many moving letters. Many cried in the consulting room and protected me by fewer consultations.

My father's death marked the end of an era. He had worked with my grandfather, been a dispensary doctor, started in general practice in Exeter in 1930, worked for 18 years before the NHS, and had responsibility for two doctors' lists single-handedly during World War II. He served for 43 years as an Exeter GP. My obituary for him was in the College *Journal* (*JRCGP*, 1975a).

6

Learning the Craft – General Practice Stories

Life so short: the craft so long to learn.

Hippocrates, 5th century BC

General practice is essentially an oral clinical discipline. The GP consultation is a human exchange in which the patient and doctor talk and listen to each other and a working relationship emerges over time. Relatively little about the patient's life is recorded in the doctor's notes, which focus on the physical elements: examinations, tests, and drugs. This oral tradition characterises general practice, so that even partnership meetings (the governing body in most practices) have relatively fewer written papers than would be the norm in the governing bodies in other organisations. General practitioners, more than other doctors, learn by listening to their patients and the stories they tell.

Narrative medicine, the formal study of verbal medical communication, was developed in the UK through academics who were mainly GPs. Narrative medicine studies, the use of language and words, shows how and why they are used, and meanings that are directly or indirectly transmitted; how similes, metaphors and phrases are used to convey meanings. Articles emerged on both sides of the Atlantic, like Greenhalgh and Hurwitz (1999) in the UK and Charon (2001) in North America, the latter stating that stories foster empathy. An important form of narrative medicine is storytelling, so doctors interested in this find themselves sharing ideas and skills with colleagues in the humanities, especially in linguistics (discourse analysis) and in processes used to study literature. Storytelling is important in all cultures and is how tribes and early humans preserved their identity from ancient times. The Bible is full of powerful stories (parables). Storytelling is a fundamental process of human communication and is an important way parents and families pass messages to their children. Stories are undervalued in scientific medicine but are how many messages are still communicated, made real, and so remembered.

The process of training medical students, particularly in teaching hospitals, requires them to cut short the patient's story and to extract key features of the 'history' that are relevant to the presence or absence of pathology and disease. Students are trained to downplay storytelling in the interests of diagnosis and 'real medicine.' GPs trained in this way have to re-learn the importance of both patients' stories and the precise words which patients use, especially metaphors and similes. It took me about ten years to do so and as I learned to understand my patients' words, so I learnt to understand them as people.

Two Frames of Reference: Pathology and Behaviour

My generation was trained to revere pathology. In Cambridge for two years I dissected the human body. At Bart's, pathology was seen as the underlying disease process which needed to be understood to explain the symptoms and diagnosis. I was told to seek "truth in the post-mortem room." None of this was untrue, but all of it is only half true. The central challenge for the GP is to understand the patient as a person, as a unique human being with individual ideas, hopes, fears, and expectations.

DOI: 10.1201/9781032713601-8

In this substantial intellectual challenge, pathology plays a lesser part, although for a few people their pathology dominates their lives. In my James Mackenzie lecture, I suggested that general practice is itself a behavioural science (DPG, 1978).

For most patients it is not their pathology but their social circumstances: their background, their childhood, their home and family, their education, and their job, which mould their lives and their health. Much pathology follows rather than leads behaviour; e.g. smoking and sexually transmitted diseases. This 'other half of medicine' has been usefully described as 'biographical medicine.' The life-course theory (Bellis *et al.*, 2017) is particularly important to GPs, as so much of what we see in the consulting room and even how many consultations adults have with us, is significantly influenced by how many adverse effects they experienced in childhood. For specialists, this information is not irrelevant, but is subsidiary. It can be dispensed with in hospital where what matters most are often investigation results.

In general practice, the situation is reversed: psychosocial factors frequently influence and may determine both diagnostic probabilities and management. The challenge is to relate them to the whole person. Since people have different ideas, this means that general practice always needs dialogue and involves listening, listening, and listening again. Only in this way can the specific individuality of each patient be understood. Since there is never enough time in any single consultation, repeated consultations over time become important. This is continuity of care and in practice is how most GPs and patients get to know each other. Patients may disclose different parts of their life story at different times for different reasons. Husbands and wives/partners often tell their stories separately and sometimes their parents and children too; family medicine dovetails with continuity of care, often reinforcing it. Sometimes one member of a family will sum up the personality of another and this may save the GP hours of analysis.

Many specialists conceptualise general practice as 'medicine outside hospital' or medicine practised in a broader range but at a more superficial level, as I describe in Chapter 38, the Academy story. Some see it as medical social work with the GP's job being to detect the relatively few people with serious disease and to refer them to specialists (Horder, 1977). Many specialists see the hospital as the centrepoint of medicine. None of these assumptions are correct. The reasons people consult doctors in the front line of the health service are different from how they present more pathological disease in the hospital service. Patients seek medical care because they have dis-ease, rather than a specific disease (Helman, 1981). It matters to GPs why patients have decided to consult. Human beings experience symptoms when they are unhappy or under pressures that may arise from their childhood, their home or their work, so the full interpretation of symptoms requires the GP to understand the patient's situation or *context*. This psychosocial mix is characteristic of general practice/primary care and gives it a distinctive intellectual edge. Sometimes, the key patient is not in the room as when, as a GP seeing a woman with depression, I too late discovered that her real problem was an alcoholic husband at home. Some children presented to family doctors are actually metaphors for their parents' anxiety.

This complicated psychosocial interaction, which is unique to each individual, can lead to symptoms being reported to GPs, which they have never heard about before and which cannot be explained by any known pathological process. So-called 'medically unexplained symptoms' comprise different entities but present a big, intellectual, clinical problem in the whole of medicine and especially in general practice. Somatisation is a syndrome when the patient reports troubling symptoms, which they attribute to physical disease but for which no physical cause can be found. Repeated investigations are negative, and referrals are usual and often repeated. Sometimes unexpected findings turn up, but a satisfactory physical diagnosis remains elusive. Many such patients resist a psychiatric approach or referral. This is quintessentially a general practice problem, which may be hugely expensive for the NHS if not managed skillfully. The scale of the problem is greatly underestimated. There are more patients in hospital clinics with 'non-cardiac chest pain' (Dumville *et al.*, 2007) than with cardiovascular pathology, and the majority of patients in gynaecological outpatients do not have a pathological basis for their concerns (Nimnuan *et al.*, 2001). GPs have to work hard with such patients, build a partnership relationship with them, win their confidence, accept their symptoms and somehow agree a *modus vivendi.*

One little understood problem is that the tests that doctors use do not behave in the same way in different settings. The effectiveness of a pathological test depends on the prevalence of the condition being tested in the population being seen. A test may be useful to a specialist in hospital, where the presence of serious pathological disease is relatively high, whereas in general practice the same test may be inefficient and generate many false positives (because the prevalence of the underlying condition is relatively rare). This explains why general practice needs to be taught by generalist doctors.

Once when I learnt that GPs were seriously underdiagnosing deafness, we bought an audiometer for the practice, which crudely measures hearing. I mentioned this to an ENT specialist (Scott, 1965) He poured scorn on this machine, speaking at length about its limitations and comparing it with the much more precise instruments he used in specialist practice. He entirely missed the point, not understanding the different and complementary roles of generalist and specialist practice. What was invaluable for GPs *as a screening test* was not appropriate for a final elucidation of deafness; but buying his instruments would have been stupidly expensive in general practice. I monitored my referrals for deafness after a positive finding on our practice audiometer – 95% led to a hearing aid being offered.

Specialist medicine, being primarily based on pathology and on specialist knowledge, is essentially hierarchical. Specialists defer to other specialists who are still more specialized, or who have greater knowledge. Generalist practice is much more egalitarian, since good general practice depends, to a much greater extent than specialist practice, on building good relationships with patients and being trusted to receive their confidences over time. Long-term relationships with patients loom larger in generalist than in specialist practice.

When I started in practice, I knew of only one book on general practice. I learnt my craft, as my predecessors had done, by experience and especially by the stories my patients and my father told me. As Hippocrates said, "The craft so long to learn." I was surprised how long it took me. Stories were particularly influential in the early years when I was in transition from being a hospital-trained and orientated doctor towards being a GP.

---

(1) Learning from My Grandfather

My father told me about how my grandfather had received a letter from a local surgeon stating he was going to operate, proposing 'heroic surgery.' My grandfather asked, "Who is the hero and does he know?" This illustrates that, 100 years ago, GPs were patient centred and cautious about specialist claims. The patient died after the operation.

I was told by one of my grandfather's patients that he used to ask questions like: "Are you tired?" and "How do you sleep?" As a recent graduate of Cambridge and Bart's, I thought I knew better and well remember expostulating with my father about how silly those questions were because most patients were tired and slept badly when they were not well. My father said mildly that such questions were useful, but I was too over-confident to take notice. It took a quarter of a century for me to receive my come-uppance. Goldberg and Bridges (1985) reported an analysis of the questions which generalist doctors could ask which correlated most precisely with the diagnosis of major depression by formal psychiatric instruments. I was fascinated that several of my grandfather's questions were there! Only because three generations of general practitioners in one family worked in succession do I know that some GPs in the 19th/early 20th centuries were skilled enough to have discovered such important questions for themselves. My grandfather was creating some modern theory, but he and his generation practised a craft, not a discipline. Little was written down or published and so carefully won knowledge died with each practitioner. General practice could not advance because succeeding generations could not build on earlier discoveries, as happens today. My grandfather was ahead of his time and had several letters in the *Lancet* between 1903 and 1915 (Pereira JAW, 1903–1915).

(2) Learning from My Father

I was called on a home visit to an old lady who had fallen and complained of hip pain. Of course, I sent her immediately to the accident and emergency department. The hospital letter reported no fracture. She called me the next day saying the pain was very troublesome. I changed the painkillers, but she called me out again in a day or two, so I changed them again. Then she phoned once more, but said she wanted Dr Sydney! My father did the home visit and when I asked what he had done he said he had her sent straight back to the accident department. "But we got a negative x-ray report," I said. "Well," he said, "her story doesn't fit with that." The next day we got another report from the hospital saying that an undisplaced fracture had been found. Then the patient rang for another home visit but said that she wanted Dr Denis! In her home she sat me down and gave me one of the most important lessons of my professional life. "I kept telling you I was in pain" (true). "You weren't really listening to me," she said. "You just concentrated on the hospital report" (true). "Your father listened when I told him exactly the same story, and he believed me" (true). "If you are going to be a good family doctor, then you have to learn to listen and to understand your patients, like your father" (true). I ate humble pie and apologised profusely. Then she said, "Come into the next room, would you like some tea?" There, she said she had made a cake for me. She said, "You made a mistake, but I'm not going to complain and I'm not going to tell your father. He has been marvellous to me for many years and I would not want him upset." I realised that I was being protected by another doctor's doctor–patient relationship. At the door, when showing me out, an elderly arm was placed on my elbow, "If you work hard," she said, "one day you can be a good family doctor too." Years later I learnt about GP consultation analysis. Then I understood the three parts of that patient-led consultation. First, was the *planned reprimand*, then the tea and cake non-verbally symbolised *forgiveness*. Thirdly, the physical touch and words of *encouragement were* the *provision of hope*. A classic triad.

Previous generations of GPs did not use the term 'non-verbal communication,' which entered general practice theory with Argyle (1975), but they certainly understood it. My father, 13 years before Argyle, advised me on home visits: "However busy you are, always take your coat off." The formal dress of previous generations of GPs signalled not just formality but trustworthiness.

Once, I was pressurised when a family desperately wanted a consultant appointment, but despite my letter and several phone calls, the consultant's secretary was unforthcoming. The family became angry with me. I asked my father what to do. He said "Cross bump!" This was his shorthand for telling me to get out of the middle-man role and so I asked the patients to ring the consultant's secretary direct. I was interested that the patient then got the appointment quickly and the family was suddenly grateful to me. My father taught me about consultants and that patients would hold me responsible for what happened with a consultant and would blame me if things went wrong. I was astonished; surely it was unfair to blame a GP? However, I later discovered this was true and it worked both ways. I had a tough consultation once when a patient was very angry because a consultant had been rude and she took her anger out on me. On other occasions, I had grateful patients when I had done no more than make a referral that led to skilled work by consultants.

Once I received a third request for a home visit in a single day. My father, seeing this in the daybook remarked: "A third request for a home visit in a single day means an admission to hospital!" This was a new idea to me. "What? Regardless of diagnosis and families?" I said. "Yes," he said, "it means you have either missed something or more usually you will have got the diagnosis right, but the family cannot cope with the care." After many years, I came to the same conclusion. Such rules of thumb are only acquired after decades of experience and form part of the craft wisdom of general practice. They have no theoretical evidence as yet but they compress years of experience. They transcend generations and show why experienced GP trainers are important.

When my father and I were sharing evening work, we were frequently called on home visits to an asthmatic child. We referred her to the hospital, but the requests continued unchanged. My father and I discussed this and noted that many calls were on Saturday evenings. Why Saturdays? What was different? Then the penny dropped—the father, who was not our patient, was then at home. The next time I saw the mother I gently explored the family dynamics. She said that the home visit requests were because of the father, "who can't bear to see her in difficulty." We saw the two parents alone and for the first time discussed what mattered – the father's anxiety that his daughter would die. Saturday evening calls greatly reduced.

General practice theory states that illness often originates in the patient's environment, whether at home or at work, or in life experiences. This story taught me how general practice is better placed to understand and manage some conditions than A&E departments. In my James Mackenzie lecture, the most important lecture of my life, I suggested that one model of the GP consultation is understanding "what the patient is feeling at home" (DPG, 1978).

The hardest teaching my father gave me occurred when I was struggling with a family who were upset with me. I told him the story, finishing with "But I got the diagnosis right." To my amazement, he then said, "In general practice, it is not enough to be right! You have to appear to be right as well." He understood that I had made the right diagnosis and made some logical decisions but I had not explained the implications and the management requirements to the family properly. I was still a pathologically orientated doctor and over-confident in diagnosis. I had still to learn that diagnoses are only preludes to management, which has to be fully explained and agreed with relatives, as well as the patient, so that everyone understands and concurs.

(3) My Own Learning from Experience

I once visited a child at home who was dying of leukaemia. He was the same age as our little boy, Peter, and looked very like him. I was in an upstairs bedroom when the young mother, in her 20s, looked anxiously at me and said, "He is going to be alright isn't he?" To my horror, it seemed that either the specialists had not told her or that she had not understood. I sat her down on a bed and as gently as possible explained. She was shattered and sobbed almost uncontrollably. I sat down on the bed beside her with tears in my own eyes, put my arm around her shoulders for several minutes and then we went downstairs and had a cup of tea together to give her time to regain control. The child died soon afterwards, and the family stayed with my practice for years. Although we did not talk much about it much, there was always a bond, as that mother knew that I knew what she had been through. This is how I learned what Iona Heath (1995) was later to call the "witness role" of GPs; being there when it mattered and really understanding the patient's feelings.

Nowadays, conventions are different. It would probably not now be possible for a young male GP to sit on an upstairs bed, alone in a house and put his arm around a young woman patient's shoulders for quite a long time.

One of the most interesting events in family practice is when girls that one has known for years grow up and have babies of their own. Suddenly the girl is a mother and often consults for her child. However, simultaneously, her mother has become a new grandmother still retaining her patient-doctor relationship with me. Then, interestingly, I noticed that sometimes these new grandmothers would send messages: "Doctor, Mary is not coping with that baby." I would then do a home visit. Invariably the new grandmother was right. Usually the new mother had postnatal depression, but twice the baby had an important physical abnormality. In 38 years of practice, none of those calls wasted my time. They improved the efficiency of the practice and my health visitor teased me about having 'x-ray eyes,' as I often got to those mothers before she did. Hoggart (1957) observed that working-class people knew the family doctor better than any other middle-class person.

Once a teenage girl said as she was leaving the consulting room: "Mum asked me to tell you that she is getting really worried about Gran, who is leaving the gas taps on." This was a three-generational consultation. These three/four-generational consultations show how families learn to use their family doctor to help other generations of their family. Family medicine across generations is both particularly interesting and, through earlier diagnoses, more efficient.

One of the special privileges of being a family doctor for more than 25 years in the same practice is that one can see not just three generations of families, but four generations. I kept a record of my families with four generations and when I retired from clinical work, 7% of all the registered NHS patients on my personal list had a four-generational relationship with me. That meant I had a baby registered, one or more parent, one or more grandparent, and one or more great-grandparent, all patients at the same time. As 7% is one in 14–15, and my average surgery session had 16–20 patients, it meant that on average in every surgery I would see a patient for whom I could picture four generations of their family. It is a rich experience being a real family doctor.

A little boy died in an accident. I knew the mother well and had looked after her through the pregnancy and had done the baby checks. She seemed relaxed, well integrated, and did not consult much for herself. However, as she stayed in the practice for the next 25 years, I watched her become a patient with chronic anxiety state, which nothing and no referral could relieve. One day, her husband, whom I also knew well, said: "She'll never stop grieving for that boy." That insight from within the family summed her up in seven words. Family doctors gain greatly from seeing several members of a family and hearing their views. This, and many other similar events, led me to try hard all my professional life to encourage different members of families to register with me. Personal lists help this and the added value is huge.

Although specialists in hospitals are best at making diagnoses of rare diseases, GPs are the main diagnosticians in the NHS. They make more diagnoses than any other kind of doctor, particularly for the 86% of patients who are not referred (Evans *et al.*, 2008). They also make diagnoses over a wider range of conditions than any other kind of doctor. GPs also make the diagnoses in more than half of the patients who are referred to specialists, as about half are for routine surgery: cataract, hip or knee surgery, or when the referral is not for diagnosis but for investigation or treatment. Sometimes GPs make diagnoses of even rare or difficult conditions, although these are not often reported. My only diagnosis of scurvy was rubbished initially by a consultant.

Narrative medicine includes the study of the use of metaphors and similes in medicine. Patients often use metaphors when they consult, as this is a standard way in which people communicate in everyday life. All doctors need to learn about patient metaphors, but especially GPs, for whom they are meat and drink. Decoding them is an important and undervalued clinical skill. One day, I saw an upper-class man with a stiff upper lip and after several minutes' discussion, I was lost and did not know why he had come. "How do you really feel?" I asked, a standard GP approach with an open-ended question. "Like a rowing boat with a hole in it!" he replied. I decoded slowly "But rowing boats with holes in them sink" I said. Then he started crying and the consultation about his depression, which he could not previously report, began.

I taught my GP registrars to "Trust your guts!" Even though I am fascinated by the theory of general practice, this a-theoretical advice was based on my experience that doctors, especially GPs, including GP trainees, absorb a vast mass of information when consulting, much of it subliminally. Intelligent and sensitive doctors continue to process such information unconsciously. Vague feelings of unease may be more important than they appear.

One Christmas Eve I did a home visit to a small baby with a chest infection. I told the parents I would call again in 48 hours, on Boxing Day. However, I awoke on Christmas morning with that baby in my mind and feeling anxious about her. I decided to do a home visit, although I was not on call on Christmas Day that year. The parents were surprised to see me but grateful as the baby had had a bad night. I re-examined her and found pneumonia. The mother burst into tears when I told her that her baby needed to be admitted to hospital on Christmas morning but she went in and did well. I believe this happened because I had picked up some cue, unconsciously, on Christmas Eve and my subconscious went on integrating the information afterwards during that night. Children when ill, particularly benefit by seeing the same GP each day, as small but important changes are then more likely to be picked up.

Research on doctor hunches or intuition from Oxford (Stolper *et al.*, 2010; van den Bruel *et al.*, 2012) followed up on GP "gut feelings." They calculated the likelihood ratio for "gut feeling" being important and found it as high as 25 times. This validates GP "gut feeling" as clinically important. As NHS policy is for more patients, including children, to be seen first by other professionals, there is a question whether they have such gut feelings too? If it is a medical phenomenon, not seeing a GP may be costly.

Some hunches are beyond explanation. I saw one patient for many consultations for vague abdominal symptoms. I had known him for over 25 years and he had been referred and fully investigated at the local hospital with a barium meal, barium enema, and colonoscopy (before scans). He was seeing an experienced consultant surgeon regularly. I had examined him thoroughly. I sat back in my chair, non-plussed. Then I had a strong feeling that he had bowel cancer, but there was no evidence. I recommended referral to St Mark's Hospital in London (which specialised in bowel disorders and this was when GPs could refer anywhere within the NHS). He declined, reasonably saying that I had no evidence and that he had confidence in the consultant. His wife, sitting beside him, asked why I was suggesting this, and I replied that I had a 'hunch.' She turned to her husband and said, "Let's back Denis's hunch!" He still declined and they started to argue, so I suggested they went home to discuss it. Next morning, they agreed to the referral. St Mark's found a Dukes Grade A carcinoma of the bowel. This is the very earliest stage with an excellent prognosis. It was removed and he was soon home. As an enthusiastic teacher, I struggled to work out how I got that hunch, but couldn't. I later discussed this referral with the patient's wife, and she said, "I just knew he wasn't right and the hospital hadn't sorted it." So, her feeling, which made the referral possible, and her own separate patient-doctor relationship with me, were two other factors, showing how family medicine can add value.

Decades later I found out that I was not alone. Smith *et al.* (2020) studied GPs with 'gut feelings' and did a systematic review of the literature. They found that GPs' intuitions of cancer had substantial diagnostic value, with a 4.4-fold increased chance of cancer being found, and that GPs who knew their patient well had more accurate gut feelings, especially older GPs.

GPs talk much about the patient-doctor relationship but those outside general practice value it less. Valuing it is difficult, but it is higher than is realised. Sometimes I was approached by families who, when moving to better, more expensive houses, would ask if the new address was in my practice area. If told that they would have to change doctors, several families decided not to move. Similarly, when doing palliative care at home, some families gave me the key to their front door, a striking non-verbal symbol of trust.

Insights from Home Visits

Before there was a medical school in Exeter, our medical students came from older medical schools, often in London. One of these came with a strong commitment to paediatrics. This student conveyed the expectation that there was nothing much to learn in general practice. One day, on a home visit to a deprived council estate, we examined a small girl with a nasty chest infection. He took a good history, did a good examination, and recommended an antibiotic, which I prescribed. I said we would call again in two days. When we did so the child was no better, indeed worse. We went out to my car where I used to teach, and we discussed possibilities. He rattled off rare complications and even tropical diseases. I kept shaking my head and when he had run out of ideas I said, "Let's go back and look behind the clock." On re-entering he found our prescription from the first visit showing behind the clock! As he realised the child had had no treatment, I saw he was about to say something that might have hurt the young mother. I quickly said, "Say nothing, sit down and listen." It's important that the patient's interest comes first. Then the mother, who knew me well, said: "I am so sorry, Dr Denis. I know I should have gone to a chemist but as you know I'm a single mother, my mother does not live in Exeter, the neighbours are awful, and there is no chemist on this estate. The rain has been heavy and I did not like to take Mary out with her chest infection." It was a moving statement about reality for the socially deprived. As we drove away, I taught that the care children receive is largely determined by their immediate environment, which GPs are best placed to understand. Later, on an NHS authority, I supported a plan to establish a pharmacy on that estate.

Most junior doctors believe, consciously or subconsciously, that the hospital is the centrepoint of medical care and that general practice means practising superficial hospital medicine outside hospital. This is wrong but it is difficult to teach the opposite. However, one home visit vividly illustrated the different perspectives of general practice and hospital medicine.

I was telephoned by a former trainee working in hospital. He sounded upset and said the hospital staff were laughing at me and the consultants were amused that the Professor of General Practice had admitted a nappy rash as an emergency! I said I would report the story at the next week's vocational release session. The trainee chair invited the paediatric registrar. The room was packed. I reported I had been on call for several practices and had received an evening call from a teenage babysitter asking for a home visit for a baby she was looking after. This was unusual. I had been in general practice for 25 years and had never had a request from a babysitter before – the first red flag. Arriving in the home around 11 pm, I found that it was in one of the poorest districts, where social problems were rife, so social deprivation was a second red flag. I was visiting a family where I did not know the baby, its parents, or the babysitter, so I had no continuity of care – red flag number three. I asked the babysitter many questions about why she was worried and why she had phoned but could not get a clear answer. She was young and inarticulate and shrugged her shoulders saying "the baby was crying." I was left not knowing why she had called – red flag number four. I asked her to undress the baby completely and did a careful examination.

There was a big nappy rash. Whilst nappy rashes are common, a big one implied that this baby might not be getting optimum care – red flag number five. There were no bruises or signs of injury, but when I flexed the hips the baby cried. I repeated this gently but every time the baby cried. Was this because of the nappy rash, or the obvious alternative that there might be a hip problem? – red flag number six. Could the ambiguous communication mean guilt, like non-accidental injury when presentations are often atypical? Could the babysitter have dropped the baby? Then the two parents came home having had much to drink. The father shouted "Who are you?" I replied I was a family doctor and had been called. "Called?" he shouted. And seeing the babysitter, shouted at his wife in front of the babysitter, saying, "Why's she here? She is not reliable!" – evidence that the babysitter was not reliable – red flag number seven. I said that the baby cried when I touched its hip so an x-ray was needed. My referral letter, presuming it would be read by the family, described "unusual social circumstances," signalling to the paediatricians. The baby was x-rayed in hospital about midnight, which was reported negative, and the baby was discharged next morning with a diagnosis of "nappy rash."

In discussion, the paediatric registrar said it was important that as hospital beds were precious they should not be used for nappy rashes! A female GP trainee asked if it had been necessary to order an x-ray at midnight? The registrar said the consultant paediatrician had requested an immediate x-ray. The trainee persisted "Could the x-ray not have waited until the morning?" The registrar snapped back "No. At that point the baby might have had a fractured hip." The room burst into laughter, upsetting the registrar because the group was laughing at him. The trainee chair summarised: "As a consultant paediatrician had decided at midnight, with the baby in a place of safety, surrounded by qualified nurses, that an x-ray was immediately indicated, then it was reasonable for a GP with the baby in very unclear social circumstances, only an hour earlier, to want one too." Later, a male trainee finishing GP training told me the incident was a turning point in his professional development. He had come, thinking I'd made a big mistake and wanting to see how I would handle it, but he had learned that GPs could assess risk in the community better than hospital-based doctors.

Stories like these helped me to learn my craft and understand general practice as a human discipline. They helped me to relate my practical experience of being a GP with the theory of general practice, which emerged during my professional career.

7

RCGP: South West England and Tamar Faculty Boards

The strength of Britain is in its institutions.

Lord Dahrendorf (1929–2009)

I joined the College of General Practitioners as an associate in 1962. There was no examination and it was an act of faith. I was soon elected a member of the Faculty Board, of the South West England Faculty, which was the executive.

The Faculty covered an enormous area, from the Scilly Isles to the Midlands. The Faculty Board met four to five times a year along a central route, from Truro to Tewkesbury. Meetings were usually held on Sundays, often involving travelling 180 miles on roads without a motorway. The business was low key. The chairs were local worthies but included Sholto Forman and RMS McConaghey (Mac), two national figures. I noticed, in my twenties, that they were more positive than those I was meeting in the medico-political world.

The Faculty Board was a support group for the few GPs in the South Western region who believed in general practice and its future and were prepared to do all they could in support. The 1960s were a grim time for GPs with much bad news. Lord Moran (1958) had given his "GPs falling off the ladder," evidence to a public body that was widely publicised. Morale was low. In 1962, the year I entered general practice, Sir Arthur Thompson (1963) delivered the annual address to the Royal Society of Health: "Is general practice outmoded?" About a third of British GPs were leaving general practice (Seale, 1964). Many colleagues, including some of my friends in Exeter, emigrated. They often used the same phrase about general practice: "This is not the medicine for which I have been trained." They were only half right; they assumed their teaching hospital training had been right and the job was wrong. I took the opposite view that the job was OK and it was the training that was wrong. This made me interested in changing GP training.

This was the worst GP crisis of the 20th century and the College was the main player in ensuring the survival of general practice. First, it and its journal were the main sources of positive thinking about general practice. The second value of the Faculty Board for me was the chance to meet older colleagues who, even in the darkest days, still strongly believed in general practice and its future and valued it as an important job. Role models matter. Third, the annual Gale Memorial Lecture brought national leaders to the South West and sometimes to Exeter. John Hunt, who co-founded the College, delivered a Gale lecture in Exeter, staying with Jill and me in our home. Pat Byrne, the first professor of general practice in England, another College President, also stayed with us. Late that night, he told me how as a senior lecturer in general practice at Manchester he had wondered how to achieve a chair and whether to push for it. He had decided to do nothing and pile up the achievements hoping a chair would come, and it did – an important lesson for me later.

Another Gale lecturer was Marshall Marinker (Marinker, 1973), whose majestic mind roamed over the boundaries of our discipline using literature and poetry. Slowly, I began to realise that general practice was producing some fundamental thinkers, not just in its own field, but in medicine as a whole.

DOI: 10.1201/9781032713601-9

The third national figure on the Faculty Board was WH (Bill) Hylton of Cleveland, Somerset. He chaired the Education Committee of the Council, which produced the historic first *Report from General Practice* (CGP, 1965), stating the case for GP training. Education was the central College activity. He and Mac reported at each meeting. The *Gillie Report* (1963) came out in my first year in practice. I was elated when I read it. It was the first positive document I had read about general practice. It was masterminded by the Chief Medical Officer, Sir George Godber, probably the greatest CMO since the war. He set up this committee, chaired by Annis Gillie, a College President and packed with College activists. This was the first time a GP had been appointed to chair a government committee. I learned that the College, young (only 11 years old), small, and politically weak, could achieve national change.

Another bonus was often travelling with David (later Professor) Mattingly, a co-opted member. He was conscientious in attending, which must often have been a bore for him, and he was the only consultant in the South Western region to do so. We got to know each other, which proved an advantage when I later applied to work in his Postgraduate Medical Institute.

Another nationally leading figure was Sholto Forman, from Barnstaple, North Devon, who had a new surgery designed around personal lists before they were so named (Forman, 1971), and who greatly encouraged me. He saw, half a century before the current fashion for bringing medical care and social work together, how logical it was. He secured funding from the Nuffield Provincial Hospitals Trust for a social worker in his practice. The attachment succeeded and the two of them wrote a book on it (Forman and Fairbairn, 1968).

RMS McConaghey (Mac) influenced me the most. He mentored me and showed me by example that the world's leading journal of general practice could be edited from a GP's private home. He became an academic father figure for me. He once said, when he realised I was active in both the BMA and the College, that I could not continue "to ride two horses." This comment later influenced my retirement from the BMA (Chapter 8, LMC and BMA story).

By 1965, the most serious medico-political crisis in general practice since the 19th century was unfolding. The original GP contract of 1948 was falling apart and I got drawn into medical politics in the BMA (Chapter 8, LMC and BMA story). I attended all the RCGP board meetings. Then in 1965, the small College Council, in the middle of this national, political storm, made two fundamental decisions which changed British general practice permanently. The College, after a big internal debate, held its first examination for membership: the MRCGP. Secondly, the College produced a small document, priced 25p, and published by Mac in Dartmouth as a *Report from General Practice*, proposing that general practice should have a formal postgraduate training programme. It was sent to every member with the *Journal* (CGP, 1965). All this in the middle of the huge medico-political storm in which the main BMA GP leader was ousted. What vision! What confidence!

The College was thinking strategically, way beyond the current organisational crisis, and to great effect. I learned the lesson that the College can make great progress even during medico-political storms, which can divert the attention of critics. I applied this lesson 32 years later when I was Chair of Council.

Tutor

In 1970, the College Council advised faculties to appoint honorary tutors and I was appointed to my first College post. I obtained a noticeboard in the postgraduate medical centre and displayed College news. I organised a study day: "New ideas in general practice," and invited the newly damed Annis Gillie (1900–1985). To my surprise, she came. At a hotel dinner afterwards there was a bomb scare and everyone was ordered outside. Sitting beside her, and feeling responsible for my VIP, I was concerned when she didn't move. "I'll just finish this," she said. "It is delicious, and they are all false alarms anyway" – and it was. As she had written a book on middle-age (Gillie, 1969) when GP-authored books were rare, she spoke to that subject with great authority. The first GP dame was a rarity and fifty years later there are still only four.

Irene Scawn, the *Journal's* business manager, after I had closed the meeting came over and smilingly said, 27 years before it happened and before anyone else said it, "I think I have seen a future College president!" By 1971 I was doing an annual lecture series in the University Department of Sociology for social workers and speaking to midwives at a conference.

The Faculty Board rejoiced, as did the whole College, when the Royal Commission on Medical Education (1968) reported. It had adopted the College's evidence (CGP, 1966) wholesale. We knew that the tide had turned. There was no anxiety at all that the Government would not accept this report. Royal Commissions have sadly gone out of fashion, but then they were authoritative and influential and the Government soon accepted the report.

Deputy Chairman of the Board 1973–1976

In 1972, as Editor of the College *Journal,* my position on the board changed – I was suddenly seen as a College leader. Mattingly was then reporting progress on the idea of an Exeter department of general practice. In 1973, the Board elected me Deputy Chairman (1973–1976) to Kenneth Southgate, from Gloucester. This guaranteed the chairmanship if I did not disgrace myself.

The Department of General Practice was established in Exeter that year. After being appointed the foundation senior lecturer in-charge (described in Chapter 13, Department/Institute of General Practice story), I became the only academic GP in the South West region. I persuaded the Faculty to hold the annual spring meeting of the College on the understanding that it would be run by College activists in the new Exeter University Department.

We made the meeting more complicated by first proposing an extra Friday afternoon so that we could showcase the new department. Secondly, we had a new idea of bussing the conference attenders into local general practices. We agreed that Michael Hall should be the lead organiser. He had outstanding organisational skills. He did it superbly with loyal secretarial support from Julie Orr. We were warned that GPs would not come on a weekday. Despite the warnings we filled the lecture theatre. We used ten-minute talks with five minutes of questions, including the four senior lecturers and some GP trainees, who stole the show. The sessions in the practice went well. The next spring meeting in Scotland adopted the Friday afternoon format. Years later, colleagues at meetings stopped me to say how interesting they had found our practice. One said he was glad to see I was a real GP! GPs don't visit each other's practices enough.

Chairman of the Faculty Board

I was elected Chairman of the Board, unopposed in 1976. My plan was to divide the Faculty into two. Younger members, whom we needed so much and who were the future of the College in the region, would not continue to travel 180 miles to board meetings. However, the Board was full of older members long used to the historic boundary. In gentle, polite discussion they could not be budged. I wrote a paper setting out the distances involved, the growing number of younger members, and their absence from the Board. I proposed a debate. This was agreed and was held in Exeter with me chairing, as Chair of the Board. No member from Devon and Cornwall would speak against dividing the Faculty, leaving the case against division to be made by members from the eastern half: Clive Richards, a former Exeter trainee then working in Somerset, and Clive Froggatt, a politically active GP in Cheltenham. The motion to divide was passed. The question went to a vote of all RCGP members in the Faculty and I wrote the paper proposing the division. The postal vote was decisive to separate in both halves of the region: in Devon and Cornwall the vote for was over 85%. The two faculties chose rivers for their names: Severn and Tamar. Severn kept the Gale lecture and Tamar established its own academic lecture, which I proposed to be called the McConaghey. I was elected the first Chair of the new Tamar Faculty Board but only to serve one year (1980), as I had already been Chairman of the old Faculty for three years.

I gave the Gale Memorial lecture for the South West England Faculty in Barnstaple, North Devon, in the closing months of that Faculty's existence (DPG, 1980a). I called it "Just a GP" and Jill gave me exceptional help with it.

Tamar Faculty (Devon and Cornwall)

The Tamar Faculty's inaugural meeting was in Plymouth on 10 May 1980. We chose Robin Pinsent, from the Foundation Council and with Devon roots, as the inaugural Provost, linking old and new. John Horder PRCGP, delivered the first McConaghey lecture and did us proud with an international approach: "From the Dart to the Tagus" (Horder, 1980). Speaking after dinner, I surprised Jill by explaining that I had previously asked to have dinner with her on her birthday, but I had not foreseen the circumstances! I presented her with flowers. Both faculties thrived and soon each had a membership bigger than the old faculty. Long after my clinical retirement, my final campaign to reform the teaching of general practice in the undergraduate medical schools, began in the Tamar Faculty in 2016 and is described in Chapter 46, the Unfinished Campaign story.

8

Local Medical Committee and BMA

About the age of 26 they shoved him into politics.

Hilaire Belloc (1870–1953)

When I came back to Exeter to work with my father in general practice, I was naïve about the practicalities of general practice and medical politics. January 1962 turned out to be an historic time to enter general practice. I joined under the first GP contract of the NHS. It was an extraordinary contract as described in Chapter 5: Practice 1962–1975. The pay was independent of the doctor's workload and the GPs' income depended on keeping patients happy. It was only when I saw the accounts that I discovered that my income was to be only about £800 a year (now equivalent to about £17,197). I was shocked to realise I had no financial future unless the system changed.

In my first year I was elected to the Local Medical Committee (LMC). I started reading the back pages of the *BMJ* each week trying to understand the complicated system that governed general practice in the NHS. The British Medical Association (BMA) is the doctor's trade union. It is a voluntary body. About three-quarters of British doctors at that time joined.

Simultaneously, there was a local medical committee system only for GPs. Every practising NHS GP is covered by an LMC, and democratic elections to the committee are held regularly. There is a national committee, which since 1948 had been called the General Medical Services Committee (GMSC) but is now called the General Practitioners Committee. There was an annual conference lasting several days where representatives of all the LMCs in the UK met. This is the policy-making body for medico-political general practice, and it sets the direction, which the GMSC then implemented. The GMSC elects its leaders from amongst its own members and because they negotiate contracts and terms and conditions of service with the DH they are called 'negotiators.'

I became more active in the Devon LMC, as I gradually became better briefed and understood the need for change. My father and I both attended the meetings, but he rarely spoke, whereas I spoke increasingly as a young militant arguing for change. By 1964–1965, I was elected as one of Devon's representatives for the National Conference of Local Medical Committees.

Medico-political Crisis

At that time there was an eruption over the evidence which the BMA had submitted on behalf of GPs about general practice remuneration which was regarded as unsatisfactory. The focal point was the absence of several important statements about general practice in the Gillie (1963) report. The GP BMA leadership had not taken College thinking into account. The conference attacked a document called SC7, demanding that more positive statements about general practice were included. The Chair of the GMSC committee, AB Davies, was forced to resign. A new Chair, James Cameron, was elected. Ivor Jones, an expert on the pool system, was swept onto the LMC leadership group by popular acclaim and later stayed in our Exeter home.

DOI: 10.1201/9781032713601-10

There were local meetings of LMCs around the country and mine in Exeter was seething with anger. GPs felt undervalued and a majority had decided that they might as well leave the NHS and practise outside it. When the crisis broke, the GP leadership called for undated letters of resignation from the NHS, so that they had a powerful bargaining counter with the Government.

The BMA was not then a trade union and had a strange system of turning itself into 'the BMA Guild,' which enabled it to carry out trade union activities legally. It organised local meetings all around the UK. I was elected Honorary Secretary of the Exeter Guild, so it fell to me to be the Exeter spokesman, the shop steward, to encourage colleagues to send these undated letters of resignation. An irony for someone with an academic career is that one of my first entries in the *BMJ* was a letter signed as a union shop steward (Edwards *et al.,* 1966).

A packed meeting was held in the Royal Devon and Exeter Hospital. I made the case for signing letters of resignation and had to answer numerous testing questions. I was at the lectern virtually all evening in my first experience of an angry political meeting. I had been "shoved into medical politics."

There are those outside general practice, and many commentators since, who believe that the 18,000 undated resignations were a bluff and that GPs would not have resigned if it had come to the crunch. My evidence is from first-hand discussions with dozens of GPs, not just at that meeting but also through numerous telephone calls. There were a substantial number of us who wrote resignation letters who meant it and, if pushed, we would have done so. GP incomes were so low at that time, and the contact rate with patients so high (even allowing for lower attendances and with fees chargeable), that even charging minimal fees and waiving all fees for the poor, would have made it perfectly possible for GPs to practise outside the NHS. I did the sums endlessly, as my income would have depended on it. I certainly would have resigned.

There were some who would never resign, but at the end of that evening I reckoned that about 80% were prepared to do so. My father and I were ready to leave. Despite having no capital, no experience of working outside the NHS and with a wife and two children to support, I was ready to risk resignation. I was fortified by the majority support for this action, which I had heard. Ultimately, general practice was more important to me than that NHS contract.

Conference of Local Medical Committees

My first meeting of the Conference of Local Medical Committees in 1965 was in BMA House and was of historic importance. The central item on the agenda was whether GPs should leave the NHS or not. The meeting was well attended and full of anger and feelings. I went into that room expecting to vote in favour of leaving the NHS.

My reading in the meeting was that there was a clear majority, backed by LMCs up and down the country, who were ready to vote to leave the NHS. The significance of this has not been understood by commentators, but the future of the NHS was in the hands of those GPs in BMA House that day. If GPs left, it would completely change the NHS, whether hospital doctors stayed in or not.

The crucial moment came with James (later Sir) Cameron's (1905–1991) speech in his new role as Chair of the GMSC. Taking on the room with courage he argued strongly against leaving the NHS and pleaded with the Conference for more time to negotiate with Government. He reported that the Fraser Working Party (of the DH) had amassed detailed evidence of much that was wrong with general practice, that the officials understood that reform was needed, and he had confidence that the (Labour) Minister of Health, Kenneth Robinson, wanted reform too. His powerful, reasoned argument for delay shook the room. There were both highly critical and supporting speeches afterwards. It was the most important medico-political speech that I have ever heard.

When the vote came, I was torn. The members of the Devon LMC had sent me to London to support their views, which were strongly in favour of resigning from the NHS. Yet I greatly admired Cameron's stand, which sounded persuasive. I felt I could not vote against my constituents, but I also could not vote to leave the NHS. So, for the first time but not the last, in a key national vote,

I abstained. Previously I had thought that abstentions represented weakness. That day I decided that an abstention was the most principled action.

I have read commentaries on those events. Most failed to appreciate the risk to the NHS. Many did not realise that most of us in BMA house that day had like me, attended seething local meetings. The significance of Cameron's brave speech has been largely missed. I believe it saved the NHS.

BMA

I had become involved in the Exeter Division of the BMA, and in 1965 I was elected Chair of the Division, at age 29. The Honorary Secretary was a fellow GP in Exeter, Jane Richards. We decided to hold a whole-day event on medical ethics and to tackle some of the most controversial topics of the time, including abortion and euthanasia. I wrote to Sir John Peel, President of the Royal College of Obstetricians and Gynaecologists and invited him to speak, and to our surprise he accepted. We had as other speakers: the Bishop of Exeter, Professor Duncan Mitchell, Professor of Sociology, and a spokesman for the Euthanasia Society.

At the committee meeting before the conference, a consultant, having seen the acceptances, suggested that he should chair the event, although he had done nothing towards it. I said that I would chair it as Chair of the Division, but it was clear that consultants expected to hold chairmanships. The attendance was greater than any other event the Division had run: well over a hundred colleagues came with many colleagues driving from Cornwall.

The next year the Exeter Division hosted a national meeting of the BMA in Exeter. This took much work, with some support from BMA staff centrally. The local committee worked hard. Jill was actively involved in an accompanying persons' programme, which lasted several days and worked well.

The Division elected me as a representative for the annual representative meeting of the BMA. This lasts a week in July and is the policy-making body of the BMA. In the mid-1960s, I was attending both the annual conferences of the LMCs and the annual representative meeting of the BMA simultaneously.

By the mid-1960s I was so active that I was asked to stand for election to the Council of the BMA. The BMA constitution then provided for one Council place for a doctor from Devon and Cornwall from any branch of medicine. That place was held by Noy Scott, a senior and well-respected GP in Plympton, Devon, a senior member of the General Medical Services Committee and Chair of the Ethics Committee of the BMA. He represented an older generation, he was not a member of the College of General Practitioners, and his experience went back before the NHS. Noy Scott and I both stood, so it was a two-horse race. It is not clear what would have happened. However, Noy Scott withdrew. He probably took soundings, discovered that I had support and could not bear the thought of losing a public election to a young upstart. So, in 1966, at 31, I became, unopposed, an elected member of the BMA Council.

In the mid-1960s, I was drawn into a curious byway in general practice politics: about how working GPs' wives should be paid? (Chapter 5: The Practice 1962–1975). By coincidence, the topic and Medical Management Services Ltd (MMS) was on the agenda for my first meeting of the Council. The BMA officers had invited a partner from its solicitors to speak which was odd as the key points were not legal.

I was invited to present the case and question the solicitor and took full advantage. Although he was a partner in a leading London firm of solicitors, I had the advantage of having had detailed briefing from Pat Price (Chapter 5) and extensive experience of what my mother did, and how our practice was operating the MMS system. I saw it as a matter of justice. It became clear that the solicitor had not given the problem serious attention. He was heavily pressurised by my questions, and his position fell apart. Several Council members were concerned to see their own legal adviser so outgunned by one of the youngest members present.

The BMA never grasped the issue of proper remuneration for doctors' wives and I never understood why not. It would have been easy for it to support the principle of formal rules and proper job evaluation and to press for rigorous external checking on exactly what work the relevant wives were doing. Meanwhile, Pat Price was riling the BMA leadership and putting backs up.

The topic came to the 1968 annual representative meeting of the BMA when Jack Henneman, representing Bournemouth and well known to Pat Price and I, proposed the motion to get it adopted as BMA policy. The BMA leadership was set on revenge and carefully planned the proceedings, with the Chair of the Representative Body, Norman Matthias, actively involved. The whole weight of the BMA leadership was deployed against Jack and me. We were publicly rubbished and the two of us were on our own. A proposal "to pass to next business," passed and our motion was killed.

Jill watched from the gallery when she was well advanced in pregnancy. Seeing her husband crushed and humiliated in public sent her into premature labour and she had to be admitted to hospital. Fortunately, things settled down and she had Elizabeth, our third child, a few weeks later. She received a charming handwritten letter from Ronald Gibson, Chairman of Council, who had engineered it all, saying how sorry he was she had to go into hospital.

This was my most bruising public experience and a lesson on how those in power can crush opposition. Jill experienced dramatically the price that wives can pay. The rights of doctors' wives and the need for GP accounts to reflect work done and practice expenses got lost in the process.

I moved a motion at the Conference of Local Medical Committees in 1969: "That the career earnings of doctors who practise the specialty of general practice should be no less than those of doctors in other specialties." It passed, becoming national BMA policy but was never implemented.

The BMA Council rejected a recommendation of the Review Body on Doctors' and Dentists' Remuneration. The Council was seething with anger and its response was to introduce sanctions and ask doctors to refuse to sign certificates. This was going through overwhelmingly with loud calls to ensure that the motion was unanimous so that the Government knew. I made a heavy speech against the proposal, strongly criticising the Review Body and supporting much that had been said about it, but as we were accusing it of breaking rules I argued it was illogical for the medical profession to break the rules in reply. Two wrongs did not make a right! I concluded that whilst I would not vote for the motion, I would not undermine colleagues who felt so passionately. I therefore abstained in the vote, alone in the room. Ronald (later sir) Gibson, in the chair, said that those who held responsibility did not have the luxury of exercising their consciences! This was the second time I abstained, alone in a national vote. A third time occurred in 1986 (Chapter 22: Downs and Ups of Institutional Life).

The Planning Unit reported (BMA Planning Unit, 1970) with Margot Jeffreys as the chair, a sociology professor, presented to the Council. Her deputy, a GP from Northumberland was Donald Irvine (1935–2018). This was the first time I saw him before we spent hundreds of hours together over the next 30 years.

Challenged by Mac that I could not ride two horses, I compared the two organisations. I was enjoying both council meetings. The BMA was much bigger and better resourced, but was geared to react, especially to the actions of governments. Its focus was what was best for doctors. The decision-making process was a majority vote. I admired the College more as it looked to the future, trying to make general practice better. Thus, 1971 was the crossover year in my life. It was my last year on the BMA Council, but as deputy editor of the *JRCGP* (Chapter 9, Journal story), I was now an observer on the Council of the College. I was attending both councils simultaneously. The College Council met at weekends and was much less formal, whereas the BMA Council met midweek and was very formal with tight standing orders and time limits for all speeches. I resigned from BMA Council.

My last responsibility was to help find a successor. I invited Jane Richards to our home and persuaded her to stand. To my pleasure she was elected to replace me. She later became the first female chair of the BMA's representative body and was appointed OBE.

Family Farewell

In 1970, I was awarded the BMA's Sir Charles Hastings Prize for systematic research and observation in general practice, for the second time. It was presented at the BMA's AGM in Leicester. Jill, with my mother and father, came to the dinner (dinner jackets and academic dress), so we were all together as a family as I left the BMA. My father wore the gown of a Fellow of the Royal College of Surgeons of Edinburgh, the only time I saw him in it. I wore the MRCGP gown.

I served for seven years on the representative body of the BMA and for four years on the BMA Council. However, it was the Royal Colleges that worked on professional standards and in general practice it was only its College that was looking ahead, planning postgraduate training, and seeking a better future.

I knew where I was going and I knew, aged 35, where I belonged.

Section III

9

The Journal 1968–1980

Reading is to the mind what exercise is to the body.

Joseph Addison (1672–1719) Co-Founder of the *Spectator*

My involvement with the *Journal of the Royal College of General Practitioners (JRCGP),* came in 1968 when the honorary Editor, RMS McConaghey (known as Mac), suddenly invited me to join the Editorial Board. I accepted at once and my name first appeared in the *Journal* as a member of the Board in the spring of 1968.

Why Mac invited me is not known, but there are several reasons which may have influenced him. We were both on the Faculty Board of the South West England Faculty. I was present when he delivered the Gale Memorial lecture in Exeter in 1964. He would have seen me as a young activist. He may well have judged my entry for the 1966 Butterworth Gold Medal Essay, where I came second. I suspect Mac had been advised to get younger members onto the Editorial Board.

Joining the Board, aged 32, was a great privilege and pleasure. I was a generation younger than all the others. I met there for the first time some of the giants who had founded the College, notably John Hunt, then Honorary Secretary of the Council. I experienced his powerful personality, his effective way of working and forceful speaking. When we were choosing a new colour for the cover of the *Journal* one option was dark brown. Hunt killed this option with a single word saying "faecal." The Board then chose blue by a big majority. The predominant colour for the *Journal* remained blue for the next 40 years. Another founding father on the Board was Robin Pinsent, who would probably have been a president of the College if he had not developed cancer of the larynx.

Mac and his small Editorial Board, backed by the College officers changed the position of general practice worldwide. They were so determined about academic standards that every GP on the original Board had an MD. The crucial policy decision was to develop a journal of record, that is one publishing original research from, on, and about general practice. He and the Editorial Board were deliberately seeking to develop an independent discipline of general practice. In hindsight that can be seen as clever: at the time it was visionary.

Of all the colleges and academies of general practice/family medicine in the world, only the Dutch College of General Practitioners did the same and it made less impact as its articles were in Dutch. All the other colleges of general practice around the world published journals with review articles, often written by specialists. Mac gave the UK a world lead. Interestingly, that was not a decision that would have been taken democratically by members of the College, which made me reflect hard about democracy and leadership.

Then in 1961, in the National Academy of Medicine in Washington, an historic decision was taken to admit the *Journal of the College of General Practitioners* to *Index Medicus,* which is the internationally recognised list of scientific journals. This was formal, public, international, recognition based on the fact that the *Journal* contained original research. A new science – general practice – had emerged. Mac created the first scientific journal of general practice in the world.

DOI: 10.1201/9781032713601-12

Change of Editors

Board meetings were always held in Dartmouth, which may not have been wise as it symbolised a degree of isolation. The *Journal* office then was a large room in the McConagheys' home. The key member of staff of the *Journal* was Miss Irene Scawn, the business manager, who worked full-time. She was later elected Mayor of Dartmouth and was appointed MBE. She ran the office very efficiently; for example, she taught me the advantage of double filing letters sent, both by topic and by date sent. The *Journal* was edited and published from that one room and printed by the Devonshire Press Ltd of Torbay. The world's leading journal of general practice was being both edited and published from one room in a GP's home.

I was sent a steadily increasing number of articles to assess, work that I found interesting and much enjoyed. By 1969, Mac had been Honorary Editor of the *Journal* for years and was coming under pressure from the College officers. He had tried having an assistant editor with another local colleague, John Burdon, a Torbay GP, who was equally committed to the College and had worked hard for it. However, apparently the relationship between Mac and Burdon did not work out and Burdon soon stood down.

The College officers were getting restless with Mac and the *Journal,* but felt hugely indebted to him as he had given years of his life to developing it. In 1970, after I had had two years on the Board, being increasingly active and winning a second Hunterian Gold Medal (DPG, 1969/70), Mac appointed me as Assistant Editor. It was a big mistake. The College officers reacted sharply. Seeing that such an appointment might prejudge the succession to the editorship, they rejected my appointment!

Mac was hurt and embarrassed, but I was not too concerned because by then I had had three years' experience on the Council of the BMA and I knew about proper procedures. Although I was at the epicentre of the problem, my sympathies were, privately, with the officers. The solution was that the post of Honorary Editor of the *Journal* was to be advertised nationally and the person appointed would work as deputy editor for a year before the handover.

Mac urged me to stand and I applied and was interviewed at Princes Gate late in 1970. It was a two-horse race, the front-runner being Ian Stokoe from Scotland. He was in his fifties, and I was only 35. He had considerable editing experience, having published a series of abstracts. I had no editing experience. In addition, he had a second Royal College membership, the MRCP. Having digested this, I wrote off my chances but decided to go to the interview to gain experience.

For the interview, the College fielded its 'A' team: the President, GI Watson; the new Chair of Council, Ekke Kuenssberg; the immediate past Chair of Council, George Swift; the Chair of the Publications Committee, John Lawson; and Mac. Of these five, four were or would become chairman or president. The interview was the toughest I had experienced, polite but probing.

I sensed intense interest when I was asked whether, if appointed, I would make, the *Journal,* a journal of the College or a scientific journal? I said the *BMJ* was an example of both at once, but the long-term trend had to be to build up the scientific base of our discipline. They were also visibly interested when I said I would write many of the editorials myself and would try to comment on topical issues. That went down well. I also said I hoped the Editor would in future be allowed to attend meetings of the Council and its Executive as editorials needed to be well informed about College thinking (Mac had not been on the Executive). After the interview I stayed in the College to wait for the result. I was astonished to hear they had appointed me. I went home to Exeter somewhat dazed, but exhilarated. I later heard that Stokoe had proposed to develop the *Journal* for abstracts.

One of the most attractive features of the appointment was that I would be an observer on both the Council and its Executive group, the General Purposes Committee (GPC), with immediate effect (Cabinet story). I was at once invited to the key meetings, in particular the GPC held the night before each Council meeting. My train was late for the first dinner and I found Kuenssberg had kept a seat on his right beside him – a powerful, non-verbal welcome.

On 1 January 1971 I became Deputy Editor and Editor-Elect. The College had taken a big risk. It had appointed as Honorary Editor someone, aged just 35, without an English degree, with only a rudimentary knowledge of grammar, and no editorial experience, to control the world's leading scientific GP journal.

During 1971, Jill and I prepared to have the *Journal* in our home. We allocated one small, ground floor room of about 100 sq ft. Jill had been advised by Mrs McConaghey never to let me use the dining room as she had done, as if she did she would never get it back! We equipped this room as an office with a separate telephone line and appointed Sheila Martin, the daughter of a College member, as the first Exeter journal secretary. As Sheila made coffees in our kitchen she got to know the family well and she later invited Elizabeth and Jennifer to be bridesmaids at her wedding.

I applied for an Upjohn Travelling Fellowship, administered by the College, to study editing and was successful. It was invaluable, as I was funded to visit the editorial offices of the *Lancet,* the *BMJ* and the *Annals of Medicine,* then the name of the journal of the Royal College of Physicians. All these Editors were welcoming and I learnt a great deal.

1972 Editorial Board

One of my first tasks was to decide the membership of the Editorial Board. Mac had terminated the appointment of all the members of his Board to give me a free hand. My BMA experience had taught me about the risks of wrong choices so I spent a long time thinking. I knew it was a once-in-a-lifetime chance and it would not be possible to chop and change afterwards. The needs were to blend academic excellence with people who would work unpaid especially on academic assessments, with political skills and to find those who would advise me honestly. There was a need to bring in young blood and freshen the appearance as well as achieve an appropriate geographical balance.

I chose: John Hunt, Donald Irvine, Ekke Kuenssberg (Chair of Council), Marshall Marinker, Geoffrey Marsh, John Miles, Robin Pinsent, John Wright and Ian Watson. I wanted the Chair of Council to ensure that he was well informed about the *Journal* because I foresaw trouble ahead as the *Journal* was consuming a very high proportion of the College's income. However, I made one big mistake, I dropped Ian McWhinney, who was a British GP who had been appointed Professor of Family Medicine at London, Ontario, Canada. It was a blunder of inexperience, a bit of little England thinking, caused by a disproportionate concern that travelling expenses for attending the Editorial Board would be an impossible cost. It was wrong to drop one of the world's leading GP academics and this decision had international repercussions. As the College *Journal* was now all British, a North American journal of general practice/primary care was soon formed with others later. Eventually, a US journal overtook the College *Journal* in the international rankings. Of course, American journals of family medicine would have formed anyway, but I accelerated that process.

Mac's achievement had been immense. He had created a scientific journal in 1958 from a roneoed *Research Newsletter* and he was Honorary Editor for 17 years – a record that will probably never be equalled. A top level College farewell was appropriate. Mac was awarded the George Abercrombie Award for outstanding contributions to the literature of general practice and received this at the 1971 AGM in his last few weeks of office.

It fell to me, as Chair of the Editorial Board, to organise his dinner in 14 Princes Gate. The first essential was to juggle dates to ensure that as many of the key College officers could attend as possible. The second question was the Editorial Board's present, and I wanted something unique. Eventually, I commissioned a sterling silver replica of Mac's final edition of the *Journal* in December 1971. I found a silversmith who constructed a silver replica of the exact size of the *Journal* with the cover on one side and the names and qualifications of Mac's editorial board on the other.

The third decision was the speeches. Dame Annis Gillie presided. This was a new phenomenon for the College because for the first quarter century after the NHS was established leading GPs who made national contributions had almost all been appointed OBE, as had Annis Gillie herself, Ian Watson, and Mac. However, four years earlier, in 1968, Annis Gillie had been appointed Dame, the first academic GP ever to achieve the Dame/Knight rank in the British civil honours system. She presented Mac with silver candelabra from the Council, saying the College had been fortunate to have an Editor with such a "cultivated mind." She warmly welcomed Mrs McConaghey who had had the *Journal* in her home throughout the 17 years. George Abercombie, the College's first Chair of Council and the first to achieve the double of chairmanship and presidency, spoke as well. I then had to make my first speech in Princes Gate, which I found daunting in the presence of several College giants. I said that the present was a thank you from all the members of Mac's Editorial Board (all had contributed generously). The silver replica was a permanent souvenir of a permanent contribution and the replica was unique as Mac's contribution had been unique, not just to the College but to world general practice. "The precious metal symbolised his precious contribution." Mac responded, thanking Irene Scawn in particular. After Mac's death, only three years later, this silver replica of the *Journal* passed to his daughter Paddy McConaghey PhD, who still lives in Dartmouth.

Editorial Work

A few days into my Editorship, a local TV station requested an interview about an article in my first issue that had been accepted by my predecessor, a scholarly analysis of trace elements in vegetables (Warren, 1972). I swotted up the figures thoroughly and went to Plymouth. The interviewer was friendly and said: "When the red light comes on you will be live for 2 million people." When the light came on he attacked. "What do you mean by publishing such an article about lead in vegetables? How dare you put local vegetable growers out of work!" This was a baptism of fire and made me cautious about the press.

I had to answer all letters, choose assessors, judge the assessors' reports, select every article, inform all those submitting of the decisions, and send each issue to the printers. I was editing the *Journal* without an editorial assistant from 1972 to 1976. The editorial process began with me, sub-editing each article, marking it up for the printer, and then proofreading every line of the *Journal* each month, first the galley proofs and then the page proofs. Proofreading inevitably clashed with family holidays, when we regularly went to Polzeath in North Cornwall. With a monthly journal, proofs could not wait, so I had to take them on holiday. Not wanting to stay alone in our rented holiday house, I took them on the beach. It became a joke at the printers when they came back sandy!

The College was not well off in those early days and only got out of debt in 1972 (*JRCGP*, 1972a). I was always conscious that at times during my Editorship, even unpaid as I was, that the College was spending as much as 20% of all its income on the *Journal*. However, the College leadership understood that to build a new medical discipline, to match specialist medicine, a published research base for general practice was the top priority. This was visionary and inspiring professional leadership. It would never have been approved democratically by the membership, which mostly then did not understand the essential need to develop a discipline. Indeed, many members did not understand the difference between a profession and a discipline (which involves establishing a new field of study by developing a body of knowledge that is peer reviewed and published, and so open to challenge). All through my Editorship I had to defend the policy of publishing original articles (as Mac had had to do before me) to colleagues who wanted review articles by specialists that told them what to do.

This was an amateur system run by an amateur. However, I was lucky as the College paid all my travel costs, including first-class train fares. The generation before me had a harder time and bore additional costs. In the early years Mac paid his own travelling expenses from Devon to London for College meetings.

Editorials

I wrote most of the editorials myself. My first, in January 1972, was a tribute to Mac: *Si memorium require, circumspice* (If you want a memorial look around you; *JRCGP*, 1972b). I never used Latin again, but this was a medium appropriate for a tribute to a traditional scholar. I judged Mac to be the greatest of the amateur medical editors and compared him to several of the great international, professional medical editors.

The editorials, as promised, became much more topical. In February 1972, "First English chair" marked the appointment of Pat Byrne as the first general practitioner professor in England (*JRCGP*, 1972c). In March 1972, my first controversial editorial was "Michael Balint." It was a tribute and finished with the words: "What Freud has become for psychiatry, Balint will become for general practice" (*JRCGP*, 1972d). This caused considerable discussion, especially at the spring general meeting in 1972. For the first time for years, people were arguing at a big College meeting about a journal editorial.

Three of my early editorials, written in my 30s, marked what proved to be three of my life-long interests. One was continuity of care (*JRCGP*, 1973a) and the other the same year on confidentiality in general practice in which I alliteratively defined confidential information as "what the patient does not want the neighbour to know" (*JRCGP*, 1973b). The next year "Patient power" (*JRCGP*, 1974a; Patient Participation story) called for "the patient to become a member of the primary health care team." Although somewhat doctor-centred by 21st-century thinking, this was ahead of its time. It marked the first of a series of actions throughout my life fostering patient participation. I also tackled topical questions such as "What is a patient?" (*JRCGP*, 1974b).

I wrote some campaigning editorials like "The maternity grant – room for reform?" (*JRCGP*, 1975b) as I had learned from some of my poorest pregnant patients that they were often excluded in the system from receiving the maternity grant. This challenged the authorities who were advertising this grant as being available to "almost all mothers," whilst excluding those who needed it most. Shaming authorities with non-aggressive rational appeals for reform is one way outsiders can sometimes achieve change. It took five years, and I expect there were other pressures, but in 1980 Lynda Chalker announced in Parliament (Chalker, 1980) that the maternity grant would be reformed and paid on the basis of residency rather than insurance contributions from 1982 onward. The Government in doing so admitted that as many as 8%, including the poorest mothers, were being excluded.

In 1975 I used the *Journal* (*JRCGP*, 1975c) to tackle long-standing discrimination in the BMA whereby GPs, however distinguished, were excluded from the presidency, the most senior office in of the Association (just GPs). Using the questioning format the editorial pointed out that every president since the War had been a specialist and one president had once said in the Council that it was "usual." (The editorial was: "Is there discrimination in the BMA?") I took some pleasure from the BMA's professional press department being unable to respond. Subsequently, several GPs were elected President of the BMA.

"Is sickness a sin?" (*JRCGP*, 1977a) was an editorial raising the new tensions in general practice where GPs were increasingly seeing illness that had been self-induced, such as smoking and sexually transmitted diseases.

Articles

It was a decision I took in the spring of 1972 which was the most controversial. I had a manuscript submitted which was severely critical of general practice. I sweated on the decision, received contrasting assessments, and finally decided to publish – and be damned! And damned I was. It was the only decision about an acceptance in nine years of editing which gave me a sleepless night, as I knew I was in for a rough ride. This article (Honigsbaum, 1972) was in July 1972 accompanied by an alliterative plea in my editorial: "Those who disagree... must like Fry justify their faith with facts" (*JRCGP*, 1972e).

The balloon went up! A national newspaper ran its front page on the story of GPs who did not have wash basins in their consulting rooms! The journal office was flooded with comment and huge criticism. Dangerously for me, heavy criticism poured into the College. Although I was a new Editor in post for only seven months, people were already calling for my resignation! In political storms, all depends on the leaders at the time. I was fortunate: the College officers were rock solid. Their line was that the *Journal* had editorial freedom, the article was not College policy in any way, and those who had a view should write letters to the *Journal* for publication. Several people told me I had made a big mistake. Others congratulated me on the decision. The great majority was highly critical. I remained convinced that general practice had to face its critics and reform where necessary. The *Journal* in the autumn carried a record number of letters to the Editor, the majority being critical of the Honigsbaum article and my decision to publish it. The furore was such that the College issued its first ever press statement about a journal article (Royal College of General Practitioners [RCGP], 1972a).

"…Mr Honigsbaum's 137 references show great industry but limited selectivity… It is therefore worthwhile to read the editorial: 'For too long papers like this have appeared in the journals of other disciplines, particularly the social sciences, where they are not read by many general practitioners. We believe it is time this type of criticism is faced openly. Either it is accurate when it deserves to be discussed or it is inaccurate, when it deserves to be answered.' …The views he expresses are his own."

One question that arose was how to handle articles that I had written myself. I sent them out for assessment to more than the usual number of reviewers and decided privately never to publish unless there were overwhelming recommendations to publish. In my nine years, this occurred three times. First, I had written a paper on "General practitioners and the independent contractor status" for the College, which then sent this paper to the Royal Commission on the NHS (DPG, 1977b). A second publication was my 1977 James Mackenzie lecture that was published in 1978 (DPG, 1978). (I never sent any of the Mackenzies for peer review, as I respected their status.) The third publication was my Pfizer lecture to the North of England Faculty, "The key to personal care" (DPG, 1979a).

In April 1979, I accepted an article by Stott and Davis (1979) describing a new model of the consultation that was so important that I placed it first in its issue. Later that year I edited a themed issue of medical audit, which drew a comment from a senior civil servant that the RCGP seemed to be the only medical royal college taking medical audit seriously.

I heard John Hunt deliver his inspirational Mackenzie lecture on the founding of the College and published it in January 1973 (Hunt, 1973), after numerous telephone calls to me when he checked almost every comma. John Hunt knew he was writing for posterity and wanted every detail correct and on the record.

Other editorial changes introduced were a revamping of the news section with much more emphasis on news. I brought in two news sections: general news and College news. I used my steadily increasing contacts in the College, in medicine, and in the university world to glean news so that readers could get an overview of what was going on across the general practice world.

In the summer of 1975, I got through the Editorial Board a paper recommending that Mac's name should be placed on the masthead of the College *Journal,* placed just under the title as: "Founding Editor, Dr RMS McConaghey." I took the proof to Dartmouth to show to him and he was delighted. However, he told me he had not been well and was being investigated. That summer he died. I was very upset by his death, as he had been very good to me. He had been an academic father figure, and I lost him only five months after the death of my own father.

The news reached me just as the *Journal* was going to press and over a weekend, with tears in my eyes, I wrote an editorial/obituary for him. This appeared in September 1975 under the title of "Mac." As so often, I expressed myself emotionally in alliteration: "He stood on the triad of the family doctor: happy at home, proud of his practice, and contented in his community" (*JRCGP,* 1975d).

1976 Occasional Papers

In 1976, I presented to the Editorial Board a paper proposing to introduce a new series of College publications called *Occasional Papers*. These were to be academic manuscripts edited to the same standard as the *Journal* but which were too long for an article. They were not to be posted to all members like supplements but were to be sold. The debate was intense, the main objection being that GPs would not buy academic publications, so they might make a loss. I am not sure it would have carried, but Ekke Kuenssberg (1976) had a manuscript he wanted published and the funds to pay for its publication. An important general principle was decided on a tactical circumstance, but that is common in politics. The policy of publishing *Occasional Papers* was approved.

Jill Appointed to the Journal Staff

By the mid-1970s, the College leadership had cottoned on to the pressures on me and my lack of staff support, with some council members quizzing Jill at meetings about this. I never asked for help. However, in 1976 the possibility of Jill working with me in the office arose. Jennifer, the youngest of our four children, was now six and at school and Jill was ready for part-time work. After getting a good degree in English, she had been an assistant editor before we married, had done editorial work on a house journal for teachers and later on worked on the letter press edition of the house journal for the Royal National Institute for the Blind, so she had professional experience.

James Wood, the College Administrator, appointed her. She was paid half-time by the College. This was a transforming development and brought much needed professional skills in editing, proof reading, and office management. Jill lifted the quality of the *Journal* and its associated publications a great deal taking a big load off my shoulders. I did a session on Tuesday mornings in the *Journal* office and we could construct an editorial from scratch. I started by dictating a draft, then Joy Choules typed it. Then Jill would give it the blue pencil treatment, then back to me for another draft, followed by retyping by Joy, and more re-editing by Jill. Several editorials were thus completed in two hours.

All the systems for receiving, recording, sending out articles for assessment, and co-ordinating the peer assessments were carried out smoothly by Jill and Joy. The percentage of articles accepted fell steadily all through the decade. The College started to give me an annual honorarium of £750.

British Journal of General Practice 1978

Leaders are always concerned as much with the future as with the present, and my approach has always been to try to look to the future and try to act so that things will be a bit better in the future. After a few years as Editor, I increasingly realised that the discipline of general practice needed a scientific journal that was unambiguously that of a discipline, not just of a college. The point was that a discipline needs strong international contributions from the leading thinkers around the world and not just from doctors. The officers of the College had asked me about this tension at my interview in 1970. A name associated with an institution has connotations of a house journal. Moreover, the *Journal of the Royal College of General Practitioners* was a bit long. Could a single stone kill two birds?

I devised the title of the *British Journal of General Practice*, which seemed to fit the bill. However, on reflection it was clear that the time was not right to try to change the title when the College was so proud of the *Journal* and paying so much for it, and when academic general practice was still relatively weak. The next question was could I protect that title and stop anyone else from pinching it? So it was that in January 1978, the *Journal* appeared with *British Journal of General Practice* as a subtitle. It attracted no comment and I did not get a single letter, but the title was there for one of my successors to adopt when the time was right.

Twelve years later, with Graham Buckley as Editor, and with more international contributions and many professors of general practice appointed, the title of the *Journal* was switched and it became the *British Journal of General Practice* in its January issue of 1991. That title has remained in use ever since.

Update Publications was doing well and had good links with College officers and particularly with John Fry. The College decided that the publishing of the *Journal* should move to Update Publications on January 1977. This meant writing papers, many meetings, and correspondence for Jill and me, but the move went smoothly and an A4 size was achieved for the first time. There was much work when the College changed the publishing system and we moved later to a big commercial firm, Longmans. I wrote the policy papers for the College, which were approved.

I tried hard to obtain subscriptions. There were only 379 when I was appointed, and I just missed my target of 1,000 before I retired. Subscriptions are a useful source of income and protect against over-dependence on advertisements. They support editorial independence. To set an example, I got to work in my own patch and I managed seven paid subscriptions from within the City of Exeter.

The early GP vocational training schemes were managed by part-time GPs with only a day to a week's time, who were middle managers, usually with no management training and minimal administrative support, and often dependent on local hospitals for advertising budgets. The advertisements were often a few lines in the *BMJ* and course prospectuses were often scruffy bits of paper. I always enjoyed integrating different parts of my life and so was able to arrange a big advertisement for the Exeter vocational training scheme in October 1974. I arranged for the inside back cover of the College *Journal* issue of January 1975 to carry a whole page advertisement for the Exeter vocational training scheme, setting a completely new level in size and prominence for such advertisements. This had a double benefit of boosting applicants for the Exeter scheme and leading other GP vocational training schemes to pay the *Journal* for their advertisements too.

Resigning as Editor

I greatly enjoyed my nine years as Honorary Editor. However, in May 1979, I gave 18 months' formal notice to the College that I would retire on 31 December 1980. Each generation is keen to avoid the mistakes of its predecessors and I was determined not to outstay my welcome, as had happened to Mac. A notice period of 18 months was bound to be considered reasonable.

I resigned from editing the *Journal* and also the editorial responsibility for all the associated College publications such as the *Reports from General Practice, Occasional Papers* and books, which we also published from Exeter (Chapter 10: The Exeter RCGP Publishing Story). I also needed to give plenty of notice to Jill and Joy Choules, the *Journal* secretary, as their jobs were both tied to my Editorship.

The College went through a full review of the arrangements for the *Journal* and its Editor. It was decided that in future the Editor should be paid with several consultant sessions per week, so the honorary tradition that Mac and I had followed for 26 years between us, came to an end on 31 December 1980.

I was put on the appointment committee after the job of Editor was advertised. There was a strong field and for me the outstanding applicant was Simon Barley. He had won the Fraser Rose Gold Medal for the highest marks in the MRCGP examination. He had emerged in 1972 writing me long critical letters. We had developed a regular correspondence and he had become a member of the Editorial Board in 1973 and worked hard there writing many good assessments of articles submitted. He knew more about the work than any other applicant and was very keen. I strongly supported him and expected him to be appointed.

Then in the discussion after the interview, Stuart Carne, there as the Honorary Treasurer, raised doubts, not about the skills, but about the man. He said he thought the Editor had to be strong and queried if this candidate was resilient enough? I was surprised as I knew Simon better than anyone else and had worked with him far more. I pressed on and he was appointed. Yet even then I had learned, mainly from my father, that older GPs over the years often acquire a deep understanding of people and their personalities. This wisdom arises from the special experience of people that GPs gain in their work. No other group of people in society sees so many people from both sexes, of all social classes, exposed and under pressure. I had noted that whenever my parents disagreed about someone's character, it was my father's judgement of someone's personality that proved right in the long term. Once we met a young couple and my mother said of the young married woman: "She's sweet!" but my father said: "Too sweet to be wholesome!" and was later proved right. Now in a College committee a similar situation arose, but I couldn't see it at the time. I was too close to the job, too concentrated on the technical skills and requirements and perhaps too young, to get under the skin of the man. Later I learnt that Carne's shrewdness had been a timely warning. Meanwhile I congratulated Simon and entered into all the arrangements about how he would succeed me.

The Annual General Meeting of the College was held as usual in November. I was presented with the Foundation Council Award, the College's highest award. My editorial for my final issue in December 1980 were "What kind of journal?" I stated that the *Journal* had become the *British Journal of General Practice* "in fact and in name" (*JRCGP,* 1980a). Having been a family doctor for families with both consultants and GPs I had learned how important and how needed that work is, so I signed off my editorship with an editorial "Family doctors for doctors' families" (*JRCGP,* 1980b). Thus I handed on the highest-ranked scientific journal of general practice in the world to Simon Barley.

The first sign of things not going according to plan came in December with the changeover planned in three weeks' time on 1 January. Simon rang me and said he could not take on the role of editing the College's other publications, i.e. the *Reports from General Practice*, the *Occasional Papers*, and some books, as well as editing the *Journal*. I had not seen this coming and Jill and I had a big rethink.

At three weeks' notice, I offered to keep the Honorary Editorship of the College publications if Jill could keep her part-time editing/publishing job and if the College officers agreed I could continue as an observer on the Council (which I did not need at the time having just been elected to the Council). The officers agreed, especially as Stuart Carne was one of them. Thus the editorships of the *Journal* and College publications separated.

Simon Barley gave Jill and me a generous tribute in his first issue as Editor of the *Journal* in January 1981 (Barley, 1981). The College dined us both in 1981 and we were presented with an elegant carriage clock. Six months after my retirement as Editor, I was appointed OBE in the Birthday Honours list. We did not know why, as there are no citations for OBEs. Jill and I presumed it was recognition for editing the *Journal* without a salary for nine years for a registered charity. We took Peter and Penelope with us to the investiture at Buckingham Palace.

ADDENDA

EDITORIAL BOARD

After leaving the Editorship I remained on the Editorial Board under Simon Barley, Graham Buckley, and Alastair Wright and left in 2001 whilst David Jewell was Editor; in all, I experienced six editors and had 33 years on the Board.

MEMBERS' ATTITUDE TO THE *JOURNAL* 1997

Seventeen years after leaving as Editor I became involved in one last *Journal* incident. The Midland Faculty ran a survey of the views of the *Journal* by their members (Wilkinson *et al.,* 1997; Does the *BJGP* need more fizz and pop?) stating "that the *BJGP* is not relevant to the non-academic GP." This opened the fact that a scientific journal of record exists as much for the discipline as for the readers. The Editor at the time was Alastair Wright, a lovely, gentle man but not a political animal. As Honorary Editor of RCGP publications and a member of the Editorial Board of the *Journal*, I mobilised the whole Editorial Board to sign an article in response to counter what might develop into a threat to the *Journal*. As I had drafted the text I was the first author (DPG *et al.,* 1997d).

McCONAGHEY MEMORIAL LECTURE 2022

The Tamar Faculty invited me to deliver the 2022 McConaghey Lecture in Exeter on the occasion of the 70th anniversary of the College's foundation. Happily, Mac's daughter, Dr Paddy McConaghey PhD, and his grandson, also known as Mac, were able to come and hear my final tribute to Mac.

10

The Exeter RCGP Publishing Story 1972–1997

The chief glory of every people arises from its authors.

Samuel Johnson (1709–1784), 1755

RMS McConaghey (Mac), a GP in Dartmouth Devon, started publishing for the College when in addition to the *Journal* he published some manuscripts which were too long for a journal article but for which he was able to obtain sponsorship to cover printing and posting. These were *Supplements* with the same editorial standards as the *Journal*. They were also individual expressions of opinion by the authors and did not represent College policy. They were published in orange covers and were posted with an issue of the *Journal* to all members of the College. Later they went on public sale.

Secondly, he introduced *Reports from General Practice,* which were publications representing College policy. Some of these reports, in blue covers, were extremely influential, such as the call by the College for formal vocational training for general practice (*Report from General Practice No 1,* College of General Practitioners, 1965) and *Report No 5*, the College's evidence to the Royal Commission on Medical Education (College of General Practitioners, 1966). They changed the face of medical education in the UK. Like the *Supplements*, the reports were posted to all members with the *Journal* and they too were sold. Thirdly, he had the imaginative idea of publishing a facsimile copy of William Pickles' (1939) *Epidemiology in Country Practice*, one of the classic books by the first President of the College (Pickles, 1984).

These were the publications I inherited on 1 January 1972 when the *Journal* office moved to our home in Exeter. Initially I continued exactly as Mac had done, as my main aim was to learn the job and get it done.

The first new publication, apart from the *Journal,* came in my first year with *Teaching Practices,* a report on GP training in the Northern region where the regional adviser in general practice and author was Donald Irvine (1972). This became *Report from General Practice No 15.* I was both Editor and publisher as Mac had been before me. The 1970s were to be a decade of dramatic advances in the thinking and development of vocational training for general practice and both the *Journal* and its associated publications reflected this.

I was able to secure sponsorship for several *Supplements,* including two by Ann Cartwright, a leading sociologist. *General Practitioners and Abortion* was her evidence (Cartwright and Waite, 1972a) to the Lane Committee (1974), which was reviewing the 1968 Abortion Act (Lane Committee story). *General Practitioners and Contraception* showed that GPs were providing much contraceptive advice in 1973 before it became available through the NHS (Cartwright and Waite, 1972b).

When John Horder became President of the College in 1979, preventive medicine was his strategic priority. This was a visionary move, which changed the role of British general practice. He obtained substantial sponsorship, which enabled the publication and distribution of a group of *Reports from General Practice,* produced by a series of working parties, which he had set up on different aspects of preventive medicine. These became *Reports from General Practice Nos 18–22* and were sent free to all College members.

I had been co-convenor and draftsman of the working party on children (Experiences in the executive), which became *Report for General Practice No 22, Healthier Children—Thinking Prevention*

DOI: 10.1201/9781032713601-13

(RCGP, 1982), and I was even more heavily involved with *Report from General Practice No 25, The Front Line of the Health Service* (RCGP, 1987a), drafting it just before I became Chair of Council (Ups and downs of institutional life; Chair of Council story). It was approved by the Council in January 1987 and Jill and I published it.

Occasional Papers

The RCGP *Occasional Papers* (OPs) began in 1976 when the Editorial Board approved my proposal (*Journal* story) and we got the first three published the same year. Kuenssberg's report became *An Opportunity to Learn, Occasional Paper 2* (Kuenssberg, 1976). This was the year that Jill started working in the *Journal* office half time and it was a baptism of fire for her, after 15 years out of publishing and having had four children, she started to deal with three *Occasional Papers* while she was still learning how the *Journal* itself worked (*Journal* story). One new job for her was getting estimates from two or three printers for the separate publications and then to recommend one. She did not always recommend the cheapest if there were other factors such as speed of turn-around.

The series continued with progressively increasing interest and sales. I became involved as an author when my entry for the Hunterian gold medal, which I was trying to win for the third time, was rejected (curiously the Hunterian Society made no award that year). I submitted it to the Editorial Board, which unanimously recommended publication. It came out as *Occasional Paper 4, A System of Training for General Practice* (DPG, 1977a, 1979a). The words 'a system' came from a chess book, Nimzowitch's (1950) *My System,* which had much influenced me. This was when vocational training schemes for general practice were developing across the UK and the English-speaking world. It sold well and was the first *Occasional Paper* to go into a second edition two years later. Eventually it became the bestselling of all the *Occasional Papers.* Being rejected for the Hunterian medal was the best thing that could have happened to me as *Occasional Paper 4* made my reputation as a GP educationalist. I had another rejection, which also proved beneficial many years later (described in Chapter 46, Unfinished Campaign story).

Several *Occasional Papers* charted new developments in general practice, such as patient participation (*OP 17*; Pritchard 1981), teamwork (*OP 33*; Jones, 1986), and enablement when John Howie *et.al.* (1997, *OP 75*) showed how GPs can "enable" i.e. empower (give more confidence in self-management) large numbers of their patients.

We published 75 *Occasional Papers* from the Exeter office with two going into second editions in the 21 years between 1976 and 1997. Taken overall the sales of *OPs* covered their costs. as I managed to get many sponsored. Jill retired in 1997 and I edited three more, the last being No 78, before I retired from their Editorship when President. I got much pleasure from selecting authors and working with them to produce the *Occasional Papers,* which I hope contributed to the development of the discipline of general practice.

Later, the College abandoned the *Occasional Papers.* Professor Rodger Charlton was then Editor and was told that financial success was required for each one separately (Charlton, personal communication, 2017), whereas I had been allowed to treat them as a series. They are a big academic loss and general practice, as the broadest branch of medical practice, particularly needs outlets for interesting new ideas and developments. I believe that the assumption that putting papers on the Internet has the same outcome is not true. Losing the *Occasional Papers* was one of several steps the College made in the 21st century away from having a primary academic focus.

Books

Once the *Occasional Papers* were established the next idea was to identify and reprint the great classic books on general practice that had gone out of print, and so make them available to the new generation of GPs. The aim was to create a distinctive series of classic books all in the same format.

I chose white covers with the College crest in colour on the front, the earlier format of the College *Journal*, which had inspired me in the 1960s. I hoped they would eventually appear as a set in medical and general practice libraries.

We published by photo reproduction, which was cost-effective. It was easy to choose the books as I had read them all; trickier was getting permission to reprint from the original publishers. I was pleased that the status of the College as a registered charity made this possible. Prices were based on estimated sales and with the aim of recovering costs. Most sold for about £15. We published 14 books in the white cover series (Appendix 5). Their success led us to publish some books conventionally.

There were four groups of our books. The first were those which advanced the discipline of general practice, like Kenneth Lane's (1992; first published, 1969) *The Longest Art* and Frans Huygen's (1990; first published, 1978) *Family Medicine: The Medical Life History of Families.* Both have enduring power and 30 years later are still influencing medical students and young doctors. Another classic was *Doctors Talking to Patients* (Byrne and Long, 1984; first published 1976). HMSO, the publishers, were helpful in granting permission to republish. Although this was about audio-recordings of GP consultations it showed how GP consultations, later studied by video-recordings, could be analysed objectively, transforming the quality of GP teaching.

The success of Huygen's book led Richard Grol (later Professor), an academic psychologist also from the University of Nijmegen in the Netherlands, to offer us republication rights of a book he had written. This book provides an insight into one of the special roles of GPs. Alone in the medical profession seeing the very first presentation of illness, GPs have the privilege of being able to steer patients towards a healthy response and may be able to prevent them becoming locked into, or 'fixated,' on their symptoms (somatic fixation). Although translated into English, the text was so stilted that I thought I would have to reject it. However, the subject was of great importance and Jill did a great deal of work on it, virtually rewriting the text. The title was also unsatisfactory, and she produced in 1988 a brilliant new title, *To Heal or To Harm?* In five words and with alliteration this caught the essence of the book (Grol, 1988; first published, 1981). Grol was ahead of his time and even 40 years later the importance of his work has not been fully appreciated.

When the *BMJ* stopped republishing the *Future General Practitioner—Learning and Teaching,* I obtained the rights for the 25th anniversary of its publication in 1987, and so bring it where it belonged—in-house (RCGP, 1987b).

The second group comprised three books, which were the outcome of research undertaken in single general practices. The first was William Pickles' (1984) *Epidemiology in Country Practice,* a classic which made Pickles' name in 1939 and contributed to him being elected the first President of the College. The second book was *Psychiatry in General Practice* by Arthur and Beatrice Watts, who wrote the first book on mental illness in general practice (Watts and Watts, 1994; first published, 1952). The third book was a tribute to Ian Watson, a College President whom I much admired. He was an expert in viral diseases and described to me ways of detecting different infections clinically. I had never met anyone else who could do this. He had great dignity and was a superb after-dinner speaker, the first I ever heard delivering a witty and politically astute after-dinner speech to a Secretary of State without notes. (I asked him afterwards how he did it, and he said: "Three weeks' hard work!") He lifted my expectations and understanding of such speeches more than anyone. He died prematurely and we were sent his papers. Jill created a book from them, and we published it posthumously: *Epidemiology and Research in a General Practice* (Watson, 1982).

Writings from single general practices, like John Fry (1961), Julian Tudor Hart (1971), and Geoffrey Marsh (Marsh & Kaim-Caudle, 1976) influenced me greatly. Whilst most of the professors of general practice in the 21st century studied big databases, I remained convinced there was a continuing role for single practice research (as described Chapter 49, the St Leonard's Research Practice story).

Another group of our books were biographies of three GP leaders, two of whom were presidents: William Pickles (Pemberton, 1984), James Mackenzie (Mair, 1986) and Patrick Byrne (Findlater, 1996). Pickles' book contains a photo of him receiving an honorary doctoral degree from Leeds in 1950, breaking a glass ceiling by being the first GP to receive an honorary degree after 1948. John Findlater, a partner of Byrne's, wrote the last book in the white cover series, which Jill and I published in her last year in the Exeter office. We have a copy of it signed by Pat Byrne's widow, Kathleen, an FRCGP herself.

The final group of books we published were 'one offs.' *Trends in General Practice Computing* (Sheldon and Stoddart, 1985) illustrated how a college could lead an important development in clinical practice. This was years before British hospitals seriously considered computerising their records. *The Pursuit of Quality* was a tribute to Professor Avedis Donabedian (1919–2000), a US expert on quality of care in medicine (Pendleton *et al.*, 1986).

We published *Milestones*, a commercial success in its original format by Pan Books. It is a unique, witty description by a GP trainee of his feelings going through the 'developmental milestones' of his GP trainee year (Stott, 1991). It contains some profound insights into adult learning in medicine. Whilst it sold well, sadly the GP deaneries in postgraduate GP education did not ensure it remained available for trainees after our edition sold out.

John Horder and Stephen Pasmore (1987) co-wrote a book *14 Princes Gate: Home of the Royal College of General Practitioners*. This was a pleasure to publish with over 40 photographs, including one of a world-famous banker, Pierpont Morgan, who had lived there. HM King George V1 and the Queen are shown visiting. Two American presidents are shown, Hoover and Kennedy, and the latter is shown in the garden when the house was the home of the US ambassador, JF Kennedy's father. The building was stormed by the SAS in 1980 after the Iranian embassy next door was captured by terrorists (Chapter 11, College Cabinet story). We were given photos of the SAS camping in the building from where they launched their successful rescue operation. Jill was under orders to black out their faces as some were serving soldiers. Horder's inscription to Jill was: "We made a success of this together."

The most substantial book we published was *The Writings of John Hunt*, who had co-founded the College (Horder, 1992). John Horder was a great President who cared passionately about the College and its history, for which he worked all his life. He had known Hunt personally and worked with him. This was a labour of love and Horder pulled all the text together as editor. Jill put it in hard covers – the only time we did. We produced a small, limited edition, which was inevitably expensive at £55. We had a deadline as it was to be presented to HRH the Prince of Wales when he visited the College for its 40th anniversary in 1992. We made the deadline and John Horder presented the book in person to HRH. We were introduced to Prince Charles, now King Charles (Figure 10.1) and Jill curtseyed beautifully!

We also published *Balancing Dreams and Discipline* by Sally Irvine (1992), the College's general manager. This was published in a smaller A5 format along with the successful *MRCGP Examination* (Moore, 1994). Finally, we published some booklets including *Prevention and the Primary Care Team* written by a joint working party of the College with nursing colleagues (RCGP, 1986) and Jill published catalogues of all our publications (Figure 10.2). How the Exeter office took on the publishing of the College's annual reports is described in Chapter 18, Publications Committee story. For 15 years, from 1982 we published the annual *RCGP Members' Reference Book* (RCGP, 1982–1996).

As Editor, I could invite at my sole discretion, leading activists to write chapters on new ideas and growing points in general practice. I commissioned about 20 articles a year and chose keen, emerging, younger GPs to write these. They brought energy into the book, but I always selected them with an eye on the likelihood of them delivering on time. Between 1982 and 1996 I was rarely let down. Sterling paid top writing rates for these articles and Jill edited them all. A price of the new arrangements was that Sterling Publications negotiated 'advertorials,' i.e. text designed to advertise some products which

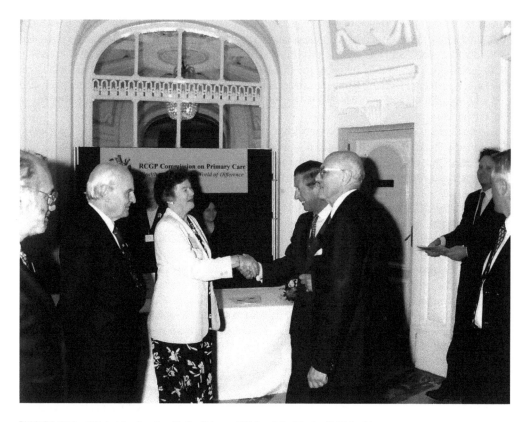

FIGURE 10.1   Jill shaking hands with the Prince of Wales. John Horder (left), looking on.

were an unattractive feature of the book, but all the production costs, i.e. the substantial printing and postage costs, were paid for by these advertisements.

Workload

The *RCGP Members' Reference Books* were large, typically 450 pages, and the extra work for the staff in the Exeter office was considerable. Not only was there a large amount of copy to be prepared, i.e. all the sections of the College's annual report, 33 faculty reports, and all the articles (usually about 20), but the many deadlines needed to be monitored, chased where necessary, and then everything had to be edited. Inevitably there were laggards but over the years Jill built good relationships with the authors involved so that we always met Sterling's schedules. Their manager, Molly Fox, was there the whole time we published; she and Jill got on well with Jill enjoying an annual visit to London to see her.

Our final edition was in 1996. That *RCGP Members' Reference Book* carried the 18-page annual report for 1995 from the Joint Committee on Postgraduate Training for General Practice (1996a) which I had drafted as its Chair and which had been approved by the JCPTGP. It explains why and how the JCPTGP had introduced summative assessment of general practice (Chapter 29, JCPTGP story) and the JCPTGP's (1996b) second position paper.

After a few years, the work of editing the *Journal*, the separate publications, and now the *RCGP Members' Reference Book* put pressure on the small (120 sq ft) office. So, we built an extension to the house. We moved into the new office in 1985 and this coincided with a change of secretary, and

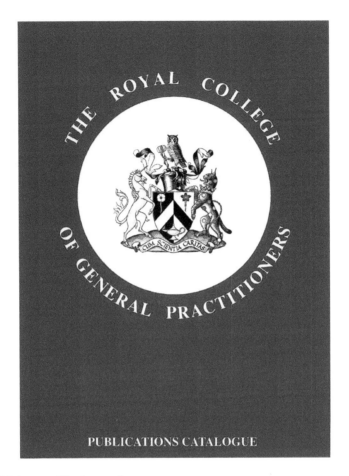

FIGURE 10.2 Jill's Exeter publications catalogue.

the arrival of Joy Choules who worked for us for over ten years. She developed editorial interests and proofreading skills. Jill got her promoted to editorial assistant, which helped as the number of publications kept increasing. The College officers said the College should pay rent for a room being exclusively used for the College. A chartered surveyor valued it and the College paid his recommendation.

Accountability to Members

I was Honorary Editor of the *Members' Reference Book* for 15 years (1982–1996) and estimate that this saved the College at least £750,000 through savings on printing and distribution costs. While the financial savings to the College were valuable, they were not the main reason for my editing the book for so long. I hugely admired John Hunt (later Lord Hunt of Fawley) for his model of the *Annual Reports*. He carefully ensured that each year the work of the College was fully documented, and the reports went to every member. This was real accountability by the leadership and a visible mark of respect to each individual member. Every fellow, member and associate could see exactly what was being done, what was achieved, who was doing what, and how their subscriptions were being spent. It provided comprehensive information for most of the members who never came to London, which was why we called it *The RCGP Members' Reference Book*. John Burdon from Torbay edited the annual report after Hunt and in his style. The RCGP is unusual amongst medical royal colleges in having a complete series of detailed *Annual Reports* covering 43 consecutive years (1953–1996), which hopefully will provide source material for research and when future histories of the College are written.

Documented annual reports did not last. After I retired the College stopped them, producing short 'impact reports' which were long on smiling faces in colour but shorter on facts. Then it stopped sending them to all the members and just made copies available to those attending AGMs. The College is much richer than in my day, but College members are relatively less well informed and less aware of exactly what the College is doing or who is doing what.

Jill's 60th birthday was in May 1997. She enjoyed the job very much but was ready to stop. I could not continue without her, so we gave advanced notice to the staff and the College. The Exeter publications office closed in November 1997. The College gave Jill a farewell lunch and retirement presents.

Conclusions

We had a college office in our home from 1972–1980 for the *Journal* office, and 1981–1997 for the College publications, 25 years in all. I edited 108 issues of the *Journal* and six supplements to the *Journal,* 12 *Reports from General Practice* (Nos 15–27) and three *Policy Papers,* sending them all to the whole RCGP membership. After 1976 we then edited and published 75 *Occasional Papers*, about one every 15 weeks. I edited three more after the Exeter office closed, 12 white cover books, four other books and an assortment of booklets. We had been turning over more than £100,000 pa. We edited 15 editions of the *RCGP Members' Reference Book* (1982–1996) vetting each advertisement and with responsibility for about 7,000 pages. In addition, Atalink published a book for the College, *Forty Years On: The Story of the First Forty 40 Years of the Royal College of General Practitioners* (DPG, 1992a), a history of the College written by me, and a series of articles which I commissioned (Appendix 5).

The challenge for the College in the 20th century was how to achieve influence when it was a younger, smaller body than the BMA. How this changed the balance between generalist and specialist medicine and revolutionised postgraduate education is a story for another day, but visionary national GP leadership in the 1960s–1970s was one important reason. College publications were another factor as the views of successive councils and leading GP thinkers came personally to every College member. These publications decisively influenced the Royal Commission of Medical Education (1968) and repeatedly the DH. They were one way that the College punched above its weight.

The end of my Editorship coincided with the arrival of the internet, and nowadays policy documents, instead of being published and posted, are put on the web at very much lower cost. However, it is not clear if ordinary College members are as well informed as they were in the past or whether they feel as involved with the College as they did when personal copies of the annual reports and College publications arrived through their letter boxes.

As inventing, editing, and publishing the *Occasional Paper* series was one of my contributions to the College, and introducing Fellowship by Assessment was another, for my Presidential portrait in 2000, I arranged for *Occasional Paper 50* (RCGP, 1990), which describes the story of FBA, to be in my hands to depict symbolically my giving the *Occasional Papers* series and FBA to the College.

ADDENDUM

Jill died in September 2020. The Editor of the *BJGP*, Euan Lawson, generously gave her an obituary, written by Philip Evans and Joy Choules, with a photo of her in our office in our home (Evans and Choules, 2021).

11

The College Cabinet 1970–1980

There are no bad seats at the cabinet table.

Chrystia Freeland (1968–) Deputy Prime Minister of Canada

All organisations need a way of taking day-to-day decisions between meetings of the governing body. The subgroup usually emerges as a leader group and undertakes strategic thinking and policy development. In the RCGP, the governing body is the Council and the executive group was called the General Purposes Committee (GPC) and later the Council Executive. I had requested observership in my interview for the Editorship. This was granted, and the observership on the Council and GPC were invaluable. Observers receive papers, attend meetings and can speak, but not vote.

As Editor-elect at the end of 1970, I became an observer in the College cabinet. Here I was amongst national leaders with 20 years more experience than me. This College cabinet has a chapter for two reasons. First, I had the privilege of serving there for longer than any other British GP, 27 years. Secondly, being a member of that group was one of my most powerful forms of continuing education. The College brought together many of the most enthusiastic GPs in the country. Being in that 'cabinet' in any role was a great privilege. As Chrystia Freeland was later to say: "There are no bad seats at the cabinet table." On arrival on GPC, I was 35, young and junior, but not alone as the College appointed Donald Irvine as Secretary of the Council. He was four months older than me, so I was 'the baby.' The College was deliberately bringing on the next generation.

Leader groups set standards: for knowledge of what the facts are, standards of analysis of those facts, standards in speaking and communication, and crucially standards in writing papers. Writing is the essential method of communication and standard setting in universities and in big institutions. Having one's writing rejected is usually painful. How people react is a test of character too severe for some who withdraw. Learning painful lessons and improving drafting needs emotional strength as well as technical skill. Leader groups require papers and their members are regularly asked to write them. This is how people are tested. It is a good rule that if you want to know somebody's ability, get them to write a policy paper and all will become clear. My own limitations in writing had been exposed in the Lane Committee (Chapter 12, Lane Committee story).

Leader groups hear confidential information. Leaders become better informed than the average member. The British honours system is usually thought of as recognition for jobs well done, particularly service to the public and to charities. However, in addition, the record of civil awards over time gives a public indication of the status of the organisation with which the individual is involved in the eyes of the British establishment. The multiple grades and hierarchical structure give Britain more scope for subtlety than with honours systems in many other countries. The rise in status of general practice over the years was faithfully recorded, step by step by the British honours system.

When John Hunt finished his Presidency in 1972 there were private hopes in GPC that he would be knighted. This was thought to be appropriate recognition for him, but it also would help the status of the College and general practice. Annis Gillie had been appointed a Dame in 1968 after her Presidency, the first such award to an academic general practitioner. John Hunt had done more, having co-founded the College and being an outstanding Honorary Secretary for 18 years, a record.

DOI: 10.1201/9781032713601-14

Twenty years on from its foundation it was clear that the College had substantially influenced the Royal Commission on Medical Education (1968) and was a success. In 1967 it had been awarded its Royal Charter as an institution, a signal from the establishment. New medical Colleges were forming. However, Hunt was offered a CBE. This is a high civil honour at national level, and was awarded to William Pickles, the first President. CBEs are still often awarded to Royal College presidents. The College leadership was disappointed and some advised him to reject the honour. However, he wisely accepted it. There was a widespread feeling that he would have been knighted in any other branch of medicine as every president of the RCPLondon and the RCSEng was being knighted. It was thought that even John Hunt was seen as "just a GP." The disappointment registered outside the College and, uniquely, Hunt was appointed to the House of Lords, taking the title of Lord Hunt of Fawley. He was the first, and remains the only academic GP, ever appointed to the House of Lords. He then played a major role in debates on the 1978 *Medical Act*.

I had a ringside seat in a tight Council election for the presidency. There were two strong candidates and the Council was evenly divided. One was George Swift, a successful Chair of Council who had pioneered the most important development in postgraduate medical education for general practice, as the first regional adviser in general practice. Secondly there was Patrick Byrne, the first professor of general practice in England and so was pioneering undergraduate teaching of general practice. I heard many discussions over meals as Council members analysed these two. I had no vote as an observer, but I expected Swift to win. However, shortly before the election I was at a conference with Swift in the chair. Suddenly I realised, as did many others, that he had had too much to drink over lunch. Byrne was elected President. I learnt that in elections for top offices, people judge candidates on all their behaviour, and not just on their professional successes.

Royal President

At the beginning of the 1970s, the College officers exploited a special feature of the RCGP constitution, i.e. allowing a non-medical president. This is possible because in the RCGP it is the Chair of Council who is the policy lead, equivalent to the prime minister. The President is head of state and equivalent to the monarch. In the specialist Royal Colleges, the president is both head of state and prime minister, in the model of the American constitution.

Thus the RCGP could have a Royal President and as a result of some very skilful footwork between the officers and the Palace, HRH the Duke of Edinburgh took this role for the year 1972–1973. I attended a big dinner in London, packed by members of the College from all over the UK welcoming him.

The Royal College of Obstetricians and Gynaecologists was founded in 1929, the third medical royal college in England. Its establishment was bitterly opposed, in a battle with the Board of Trade, by the RCP and RCSEng. The older Colleges lost and the obstetricians got their College. The three Medical Royal Colleges in England, the Physicians, the Surgeons, and the Obstetricians and Gynaecologists soon started to work together, forming a triumvirate which ran much of British medicine between 1930 and 1952. The Presidents of these three Royal Colleges met regularly. The PRCP often emerged as the leader and they had been crucial in 1945–46 when the PRCP, Lord Moran, with the support of the other two Colleges, outmanoeuvred the BMA, by dealing directly with Aneurin Bevan, and securing multiple privileges for specialist doctors (Pater, 1981).

When it became clear that plans to form a College of General Practitioners were serious, Sir Russell Brain (1951) wrote a classic "just GPs" letter on behalf of the three Colleges (letter in the RCGP archives) informing John Hunt that they had decided that there would not be a College of General Practitioners, but suggesting they might have a subordinate role as a Faculty! For arrogance and misjudgement this is hard to beat and is evidence that the three Royal Colleges were more interested in their own status than in the public interest or developing education and standards for GP colleagues, who needed these the most.

With great skill, the GP leadership formed the College in secret and once it existed, opened it up as I described in my history of the College (DPG, 1992a). The new College of General Practitioners acquired 2000 members in its first six months. I learnt that top-class leaders have to be able to think laterally and sometimes devise innovative solutions.

It is understandable that those three Presidents in 1952 might have felt miffed when the GP College formed and might have found it hard to invite the RCGP to join them. However, after they had all been replaced, the reason for excluding GPs disappeared. In 1967, after 15 years, much longer than several other medical colleges, the College of General Practitioners was granted its Royal Charter, implying that the establishment was having some difficulty in accepting that a GP College was in the same league as specialist Colleges. However, with Royal status awarded in 1967, the logic for the GP College joining the meetings with the three Colleges was overwhelming. However, it was still excluded (just GPs).

The challenge for the College leaders of the now Royal College of General Practitioners was considerable. How do you persuade three independent Presidents of three independent Medical Royal Colleges to issue an invitation that they do not want to make? The solution was elegant and effective. Using the year when the Duke of Edinburgh was President, an invitation from him, *as PRCGP,* to dinner at the RCGP home in 14 Princes Gate was sent to the other three College Presidents. The three specialist Presidents could hardly refuse a Royal invitation and of course it was an RCGP dinner. A steer from the Duke over that meal that regular meetings and good relationships between the Presidents of the Medical Royal Colleges seemed desirable, did the trick. The President of the RCGP was then invited to the regular meetings with the other Presidents.

I was in the cabinet when the *National Health Service (NHS) Act* of 1977 became law, which introduced mandatory vocational training for general practice. This was the College's biggest ever political achievement, as this *Act* occurred only 12 years after the College had published a little booklet, price five shillings (25p), advocating this policy in 1965 (CGP, 1965). [Strictly speaking it took only 11 years as there had been a lowkey *NHS Vocational Training Act* in 1976, which is little known.] The Conference of Local Medical Committees voted to oppose vocational training for years, finally agreeing it in 1974, and then by only two votes. I learned that big changes in medicine, including Acts of Parliament, could be achieved with skilful preparation.

James Mackenzie Lecture 1977

The Awards Committee of the Council took a risk in 1976 in giving me 18 months' notice to deliver the 1977 James Mackenzie lecture. This, the most prestigious College lecture, is delivered annually at the AGM, and 1977 was the 25th anniversary of the foundation of the College. I do not know why I was invited as I was only 42 at the time and the youngest ever Mackenzie lecturer.

I understood the challenge and read several books and dozens of articles in preparation. I then poured it all out and virtually wrote a small book, which was ridiculous for a one-hour lecture. In those days there were no word processors, so it was all dictated and then endlessly retyped. Jill spent hours editing and cutting and forcing me to choose between different ideas, and she gradually imposed order bringing it to length. She then rehearsed me for several hours, coaching me about length, emphasis, and cadences.

Just before I started, Kuenssberg became worried about its length, which the College had not specified. "Cut it down!" he said. "Just keep the purple passages!" It was far too late to change a word, so I smiled and said nothing. Although I was a university senior lecturer, my legs shook behind the lectern. The lecture was a plea for personal preventive medicine and home visiting. Three original ideas were that instruments would become 'miniaturised,' that general practice would be seen as a behavioural science in its own right, and that understanding what the patient is feeling at home was a new model of the consultation.

My conclusion was rhetorical and emotional: "25 years ago this year...25 years ago this month...25 years ago this very day..." underlining the significance of the 25th anniversary. I finished by playing on the words of my title that a new model of the consultation was GPs learning to understand what the patient was "feeling at home." I heard a strange gulping sound as I was winding up and was startled to realise that several women in the audience were crying with emotion. When I finished, I was given a warm standing ovation, which was so forceful that I could feel waves of air coming down from the tiered lecture theatre. Jill and I had not foreseen this and we had not prepared for it, so I did not know what to do. I stood up and bowed to the audience. Afterwards Kuenssberg said, "It was all purple passages." The College allowed me to invite several family members, so Jill, Peter, and Penny came to hear the lecture and also came to the lunch afterwards.

The James Mackenzie lecture was published (DPG, 1978), four months after my *System of Training for General Practice* had been published (DPG, 1977a) and I had also had an article defending the independent contractor status (DPG, 1977b). The College gave me the George Abercrombie Award for "exceptional contributions to the literature of general practice" in 1978. The next year, my lecture to the North of England Faculty "The Key to Personal Care" was published in the *Journal* (DPG, 1979a), followed by my 1979 Gale lecture, for the South West England Faculty "Just a GP" (DPG, 1980a). I became known in general practice through these five publications in four years.

Childcare in General Practice

The Court Committee (DHSS, DES, Welsh Office, 1976) report, *Fit for the Future,* created big problems for general practice by proposing the creation of a "general practitioner paediatrician (GPP)" who would spend "70% of their time" with children. Professor Court (1912–1994) was a distinguished paediatrician from the North East. I gave evidence to the Court Committee submitting my Hunterian gold medal essay on the care of handicapped children (DPG, 1969/70). When he came to Exeter, I met him face-to-face saying that children should be cared for in general practice in a family-centred, continuity-based service by generalist doctors. He was unimpressed.

Colin Waine and I wrote a paper (unpublished) against the GPP. In March 1977, a big debate ensued in Council. Although the report received some support from officers, the views of Colin and I prevailed, so the RCGP rejected the GPP. This led the GMSC to reject it too. The GPP was dead. The College realised it should be positive on childcare in general practice. Alastair Donald was elected to chair a working party with Stuart Carne, Colin Waine and me. The working party's unanimous report was adopted by Council as College policy (RCGP, 1978). This valued childcare in general practice and sought to develop it. A longer and even more positive report, *Healthier Children – Thinking Prevention,* was produced later (RCGP, 1982) with Colin and I both involved (Chapter 20, Experiences in the Executive Committee).

Later, I received a letter from Sir George Godber (1993, personal communication), retired as CMO, saying that he had set up the Court Committee, but he supported the RCGP position. He wrote that the paediatricians had been "blinkered." Parts of the Court Report were implemented, like a National Children's Committee, and Professor Brimblecombe from Exeter was appointed to chair it.

Professor Court was disappointed. I met him several times and he was elected an Honorary Fellow of the RCGP. Despite being previously appointed CBE, he was never knighted. He was a nice man but naïve, seriously underestimating the RCGP. He, like many specialists, did not understand the generalist role and he undervalued the fact that children were seeing a GP 35 times on average by the age of five, whilst most British children never saw a paediatrician after being born.

The College paid for Jill and me to go to the WONCA conference in Switzerland if I agreed to select and edit conference papers for an *Occasional Paper* and if Jill chaired a session on doctors' families. She later wrote an article and chapter on this subject (Jill Pereira Gray, 1982, 1984) and gave many lectures on it. Her session was expected to be small, but it coincided with a dull plenary. People poured into her meeting giving her 600 doctors whom she handled beautifully. I spoke from the audience microphone, announcing myself as the chair's husband: "May I congratulate you, Madam chair, on managing 600 doctors as well as you manage six of us at home!" to applause. Jill's response was:

"I'll deal with you later," which drew more applause. The selected papers formed *Occasional Paper 10* (RCGP, 1980a).

The Iranian Embassy Siege 1980

In April 1980, I was in a meeting in Princes Gate for the budget of the Exeter journal office. Alastair Donald was in the chair and heard a noise that disturbed him. The committee thought it was a car backfiring. Donald proposed adjourning the meeting, but I delayed that by pushing for approval of a typewriter! It was nodded through and we went downstairs. To our amazement the building was full of men with guns. We were rounded up and ushered out of the building immediately. As I did so, I was shouted at: "Keep your head down – you are in range!" We had no idea what was happening. Outside the police were cordoning off the road and we were directed away from the building. I was soon told that terrorists had seized the Iranian Embassy, which was the next-door building. They had taken hostages, including a policeman. I rushed to a phone box to ring Jill "I'm OK," I said. "Why shouldn't you be?" said Jill, as the country did not yet know.

The SAS occupied the College, drilling listening probes in the walls. The incident was on the international news. During the ensuing days the world watched it live on television. A hostage was murdered and the SAS, commanded by Lieutenant-Colonel (later General Sir) Michael Rose (1940–), were authorised by the Home Secretary to assault. They used the College building, jumping from our balconies and dropping from the roof on ropes. Tom MacDonald (Mac) jumped off our front balcony into the room I had so often used, killing two terrorists within 30 seconds (*The Times*, 2020). The hostages were rescued. At a College dinner later, an SAS officer presented a shirt to the College emblazoned: "Do not mess with the SAS!"

The College AGM 1980

The AGM in November was a challenge. My resignation as Editor had lost me my two observerships on the Council and the GPC. After 10 years, I appreciated GPC greatly but membership on it meant being a member of the Council.

Council elections for the national places were voted on at the AGM. I sat with Jill at the back of the room, anxious, with more candidates than places and national GP leaders like Donald Crombie and David Morrell, standing. There were only four places. The vote was counted during the meeting and I came top of the poll. My position in the College changed dramatically and I felt hugely empowered. I at once became a member of the Council and at the first meeting of the Council I was elected to the GPC.

12

The Lane Committee 1971–1974

I'm against abortion. On the other hand I believe in a woman's choice.

Nancy Reagan (1921–2016) First Lady of the United States

In 1971, the Secretary of State for Department of Health and Social Security (DHSS), Sir Keith Joseph (conservative), decided to review the working of the *Abortion Act*. I was rung in the Practice by Sir George Godber, Chief Medical Officer. He asked me if I was a Roman Catholic and when I said no, he invited me to serve on this new committee. I was very surprised.

Background

The Abortion Act 1967 had followed years of discussion. The previous legislation was the *Offences against the Persons Act* 1861, which made abortion illegal. In a test case in 1938, Joan Malleson, a family planning doctor, referred a 14-year-old girl who had been gang raped to a gynaecologist, Mr Aleck Bourne, who aborted her. In court, Malleson gave evidence for the defence and Bourne was acquitted by the jury. This case illustrates how case law can lead statute law.

The immediate background had been many press reports, described as "feverish" and often critical of the *Abortion Act*. It was claimed that large numbers of foreign women were coming to Britain to have abortions. There were reports of adverse medical consequences of abortion. Norman St John-Stevas, had proposed a review of the *Act* with support from as many as 250 MPs. The *Act* came into effect in April 1968, so this reaction had occurred relatively quickly. The Lane Committee was established because of concerns about the *Act* and there were expectations that restrictions were needed.

The problem was that the two positions on abortion: that it should be a woman's choice and that it was murder were both strongly held by influential groups and were incompatible.

Membership

The key figure in the Chair was the Hon. Mrs Justice Lane (1905–1988) known as Dame Elizabeth, who had become the first female High Court judge. She was the oldest member of the committee and old enough to be my mother. This committee was unusual in being the first government committee to have a female chair and a large majority of women members, 10 out of 15. Doreen Rothman, a medically qualified secretary to the committee, and on the staff of the DHSS, said that this was decided in the DHSS.

The Secretary of State was actively involved in the choice of members with the Chief Medical Officer, Sir George, ringing both GP members personally. Of the 15 members, six were doctors: two consultant gynaecologists, Miss (later Dame) Josephine Barnes (1912–1999) and Professor (later Sir) Alexander (Alec) Turnbull (1925–1990), then of the Welsh National School of Medicine, but soon to move to the chair at Oxford; Professor (later Sir) Ivor Batchelor (1916–2005), professor of psychiatry; Rosemary (later Dame) Rue, a regional medical officer (management role); and two GPs, Derek (Tim)

DOI: 10.1201/9781032713601-15

Wilson and me. It was also unusual to have more than one (token) GP. I was the youngest doctor. There were two nurses: Rachel Worsley, a chief nursing officer and ME Munro, a ward sister at St Thomas's. Mrs Kate Barratt was a headmistress. Eight members were health professionals. There were two lawyers: Dame Elizabeth and a Scottish QC, Mr Johnston, as well as two from social work: Eva Learner, a social worker and Juliet Cheetham a lecturer (later professor) in social administration at Oxford. Rupert Hughes was the senior civil servant.

Working of the Committee

The secretariat usually write the drafts for such committees, but Dame Elizabeth said she would write the drafts herself. As a judge she was used to this. She thought women should be treated equally. She said that if she was a man the committee would use the phrase "Mr Chairman," so she instructed us to address her as "Madam Chairman," which we all did.

The committee had 33 meetings, starting in June 1971, spread over two and a half years, and included visits to 15 institutions, mainly hospitals, around the country. The committee received a wide range of evidence, often conflicting. Many were invited to give evidence in person, including Sir Stanley Clayton, President of the RCOG. Women who had had an abortion or been refused one were also invited to give evidence, and some gave moving testimony.

Dame Elizabeth was always firm, impeccably courteous to all witnesses, and fair in allowing dissenting opinions. Of the 15 members, about two-thirds were active and influenced thinking and the wording of the report, and about one-third were relatively quiet. At the beginning, I was out of my depth in terms of analysis and drafting skills. Once, after writing a draft section, the Committee tore it to shreds. Summing up, Dame Elizabeth said: "Oh, Dr Pereira Gray, what can I say? Perhaps 4 out of 10 for trying!"

Evidence from the RCGP

Kuenssberg, Chair of Council, asked (told) me to write the RCGP evidence. My heart sank. With fiercely held opposite positions, I would be bound to annoy colleagues. I demurred saying I was not an expert on abortion. Kuenssberg insisted: "Even if you are not an expert now," he said: "soon you and Tim will have read more about abortion than any other British GPs!" I wrote the draft evidence with medical professionalism as the theme using my Hunterian essay's "three-dimensional" approach GPs, take a physical, psychological and social approach (DPG, 1969/70). This was over a decade before the publication of the same idea in the United States by Engel (1977), who called it a "triaxial" approach. The RCGP emphasised the unique role of the GP as the only doctor with continuity and understanding of the family. The draft called for gynaecologists to have better training in general practice and community care – the first time the RCGP had called for better training of specialists. The College approved my draft as the evidence and sent it in. The evidence was published (RCGP, 1972b). Mercifully, it attracted little comment. The RCGP's evidence was well received by the Lane Committee. Kuenssberg's skill in making a member of the committee write it paid off as I often referred to it. Whilst the committee was meeting, the most important decision on abortion ever taken in the United States was a ruling by the US Supreme Court (*Roe versus Wade*; Supreme Court of the US, 1973), which liberalised abortion across the United States.

Safety

One big question was the safety of abortion, as there were reports of significant adverse effects (Stallworthy *et al.*, 1971) and Stallworthy was the professor of obstetrics at Oxford and Vice-President of the RCOG. Turnbull led a rigorous analysis of the published evidence, which concluded that abortion was safer than was being claimed. Later, this was confirmed when it emerged that it was safer for a woman to have an early termination than to have full-term pregnancy, which was particularly important in the light of the wording of the *Abortion Act*: "risk – greater than if the pregnancy continued." During the committee's meetings abortion was the biggest cause of maternal deaths in Britain and about two-thirds of abortions were in the private sector.

Differences between Two Medical Royal Colleges

In the early 1970s, two kinds of doctor were central to abortion: GPs because every woman had one, and gynaecologists who did the terminations. A difference was revealed between the evidence from the two medical royal colleges most involved: the RCOG and the RCGP. Gynaecologists saw themselves as the experts because abortion was a surgical procedure, so surgeons should decide. The RCOG opposed the "social clause" whereby the woman's mental health was to be considered. It urged restriction of the "approved places" where abortion could be done and any questioning of consultants' views on abortion at appointment. This College gave forceful evidence in person by its President, Sir Stanley Clayton, stating the cut-off date should be reduced to 20 weeks. In contrast, the RCGP evidence supported the social clause in Section 2 of the *Act* on the grounds that it fitted GP theory of whole person medicine. The RCGP did not send a deputation, or a chief officer, simply replying that its evidence had been formally approved and published.

Whilst the Lane Committee was sitting, the RCGP *Journal,* which I edited, published two booklets: *General Practitioners and Contraception* (Cartwright and Waite, 1972a) and *General Practitioners and Abortion* (Cartwright and Waite, 1972b) – independent research by Ann Cartwright, a leading social scientist. They showed that GPs were then ready to give contraceptive advice and half were raising the topic of contraception routinely with their patients postnatally. Both these journal supplements were circulated to every College member.

The RCOG lost its recommendations. The Lane Committee helped change the balance of power in the medical profession. When the Committee started in June 1971, the RCOG was one of the three senior English medical royal colleges, working closely with the RCP and the RCS(Eng). These three were the power in the medical land and together had tried to stop the RCGP forming 20 years earlier (Brain, 1951; Chapter 11, College Cabinet story). Every President of the RCOG was then appointed a knight or dame. However, after the Lane Committee reported, the standing of the RCOG was diminished as it looked out of touch with patients, GPs, and society. The RCOG Council gave Josephine Barnes a chilly reception when she reported on Lane (Wivel, 1998). The RCGP started to overtake the RCOG in terms of influence. By the 1990s, the RCOG president was no longer being knighted routinely although those of the RCP and RCSEng were. The honours system reflected the establishment view. Later, an RCOG gynaecologist thought the RCOG had been taken by surprise by the strong views of patients and general practitioners and had been inward looking.

My Role

My role in the committee changed as I mastered the evidence. Ivor Batchelor (1916–2005) took me under his wing, teaching me much. Dame Elizabeth said, in what I presumed was a compliment, that I could have been a barrister! I was elected to handle the press. At the press conference, Jill represented the *JRCGP*. She was amused to hear someone ask who I was and being told, "I don't know, but he's an articulate kind of guy!" The press was surprised when we described the *Abortion Act* as a "humane piece of legislation." I was on *News at Ten,* speaking on the report. A civil servant crouched beside me out of sight. I slipped up in one sentence. He stopped the camera and the interview was re-run! Television interviews are not as spontaneous as they seem.

Conclusions

The Committee's report was published in three volumes: two volumes were facts and evidence adding to its authority (Lane Committee, 1974 Volumes 1,2 and 3). The non-verbal message was: "Here are the facts, conclude differently if you can." Mrs Justice Lane (1905–1988) was the key figure. She started with conservative views stating restrictions on abortion were needed. However, she gradually changed her mind as evidence appeared. She called her autobiography: *Hear the Other Side* (Lane, 1985) and certainly did so in the Committee. My respect for her rose as her powerful intellect, impeccable courtesy and open mind emerged. Later, she came to Exeter on the judges' circuit inviting Jill and me to dinner with several lawyers. Later still, when she was next in Exeter, Jill and I returned the dinner in our home.

An Abortion Amendment Bill was later presented to a Select Committee of Parliament proposing limitations. I was asked to advise and drafted a defence of the Lane proposals. The College (RCGP, 1975) published this.

ADDENDUM

In 2017, on the 50th anniversary of the 1967 *Abortion Act* a conference was held at the RCOG. I was invited, being the only surviving medical member. I suggested that the authority of the Lane Report was partly because it was unanimous despite the great controversy of abortion. I suggested that the key person preventing a dissenting minority report was Dame Josephine Barnes, since despite having a leading role in the RCOG, she had in effect sided more with the RCGP evidence than that of her own College.

Civil honours, especially knighthoods/damehoods, are rare. However, members of the Lane committee were subsequently honoured in an unusually high proportion. Cheetham, Wilson, and I were appointed OBEs; and Barnes, Batchelor, Turnbull, Rue, and I were all later appointed dames or knights.

With hindsight the Committee was too optimistic and confident that education and free contraception would reduce abortions. We did not foresee that 50 years later abortions would number about 250,000 pa.

Section IV

13

Department/Institute of General Practice in the University of Exeter

Everything begins as mysticism and ends as politics.

Charles Peguy (1873–1914) French essayist

I was appointed in 1970 as a college tutor by the South West England Faculty of the College and was on the Devon Local Medical Committee, which elected me one of its representatives for the national conferences. I was elected a member of the BMA Council and so was beginning to think on a wider canvas. In 1966 I wrote a paper proposing that a department of general practice be established within the Exeter Postgraduate Medical Institute (PGMI). David Mattingly, Director of the Institute, warmly encouraged this (Chapter 27, Postgraduate Medical School story).

The LMC and the Faculty of the College endorsed the idea and it went to wider consultation. The Cornish GPs were enthusiastic, writing to Bristol that they wanted a centre in Exeter as Bristol was too far away (170 miles from Truro). This reflected the geographical reality of the Southwestern region.

An influential consultant paediatrician in Exeter, Freddie Brimblecombe, took a great interest in the PGMI and actively supported my paper. I now faced the same situation that Fuller had done in Exeter a decade earlier – general support for a good idea but who would pay? Brimblecombe took me to see Gordon McLachlan Secretary at the Nuffield Provincial Hospitals Trust, which had funded the PGMI. Would the Nuffield fund this extension? For reasons that were never explained the proposal was turned down.

My appointment as honorary Editor of the RCGP *Journal* started on 1 January 1972 with the journal office in our home in Exeter (Chapter 9, *Journal* story). This brought many of the world's original general practice articles to my home and greatly strengthened my position in Exeter, giving me new academic status.

First Postgraduate University Department of General Practice

Lobbying for the proposed Exeter department was effective. The Royal College of General Practitioners (RCGP) supported it strongly with a letter to the Department of Health and Social Security (DHSS). The University briefed the Exeter MP, Sir John Hannam (conservative), who lobbied his colleague Sir Keith Joseph, Secretary of State for the DHSS (conservative). A formal bid went to the DHSS from the University of Exeter.

The DHSS invited the University to a meeting in London. The university team was: Professor David Mattingly, Professor Lesley Reed, representing the university senate, Barrie Behenna (administrator), and me. The meeting went well.

Subsequently the university's plan for an academic department of general practice was turned down but the DHSS offered to fund some GP lecturer sessions. Discussions took place about the grade and scale, and subconsultant scales were suggested. I objected strongly (letter 2 May 1973), pointing out

DOI: 10.1201/9781032713601-17

that the GP regional adviser scale was the top point of the NHS consultant scale and giving multiple examples of academic GPs on the consultant scale. Eventually, the NHS clinical scale was agreed. I was quite happy about the separate sessions rather than a practice as it gave flexibility and fewer administrative complications.

In 1973 the DHSS agreed to fund a department of general practice in the University of Exeter with 1.5 full-time equivalent senior lecturers in general practice and secretarial support for five years. The University advertised the lead post at half-time.

I applied, with eight others, including Keith Bolden. The interview committee was chaired by the new Vice-Chancellor, Dr Harry Kay, and George Swift, a recent Chair of the RCGP Council, was the external adviser. Both the Faculty of the College and the Devon Local Medical Committee were represented. I was appointed and started on 1 December 1973. On arrival, David Mattingly welcomed me but said he had no office for me so would I please work in the library! I learned quickly that resources were tight.

My appointment that day is a good example of an event appearing different at the time from the perspective of hindsight. At the time I was enthusiastic, excited and full of hope and ideas. In hindsight I was, with my one half-time post, alone for 11 months, the only academic GP in the whole of the Southwestern region with 3 million people.

Vocational Training for General Practice

The new Department was funded to develop vocational training for general practice. The background was a unique set of events and timing. In April 1968, the Royal Commission on Medical Education had recommended that general practice postgraduate education should be on the same basis as the medical specialties. This greatly enhanced the position of general practice. The Government soon accepted the Commission's report. In doing so it created a problem: postgraduate specialist medicine was entwined with the NHS – how was this to be matched for the largest branch of medicine which had no history of postgraduate teaching? The DHSS was on a hook and felt vulnerable. It would have to facilitate a national training scheme on a bigger scale than ever before without an understanding of what was involved. The DHSS was not in the business of funding university departments. It had never done so before and it did not do so again. My good luck was that our proposal arrived in the narrow window of time after the Government accepted the Royal Commission's report and the DHSS was involved and needed ideas. A department of general practice, in a new university, strongly backed by the newly Royal (1967) GP College was a way of developing GP training at low cost.

My first big decision was to request that the whole-time vacant lecturer's post be divided into three-thirds, instead of, as expected, two halves. There were high level doubts that there were enough local GPs of the necessary quality available, reflecting a lack of confidence in general practice. However, David Mattingly started as he was to continue, saying it was my call. So it happened. I was confirmed as Senior Lecturer in-charge.

My first task was to set up the Exeter vocational training scheme. The easy bit was planning the half-day release course in term time as I could control that. The problem was negotiating with consultants that their senior house officer posts be used for GP trainees. In those days consultants appointed their own house officers. In most areas GP course organisers were disadvantaged by the status system. High status specialties like internal medicine had no incentive to use their posts for GPs as they could easily fill the posts, so they usually refused. However, consultants in geriatrics and psychiatry had great difficulty getting good junior staff, so they mostly agreed. The geriatricians became my most co-operative consultant colleagues.

I was privileged with consultant support from David Mattingly, now in 1973 the first medical professor in Devon and Cornwall, and from Freddie Brimblecombe as they gave me their SHO posts in medicine and in paediatrics. I had the VTS set up in four months and accelerated the process by agreeing one-off ad hoc combinations of jobs. The first Exeter GP trainee, Adrian Jacobs, started on 1 April 1974. I was grateful to the relevant consultants to be able to link four, three-month posts in A&E, ENT, gynaecology, and ophthalmology, giving trainees wide experience in a single year. Advertisements drew strong applications. We offered every consultant whose post was involved, and every GP trainer involved, a place on the interview committee. "Which consultant is to chair this?" asked one of the consultants and was surprised to be told that, as we were selecting future GPs, the GP Department would do so.

I started the three-year programmes on 1 August so that trainees entered general practice for two months to see it first-hand and learn what they needed to learn most from their hospital posts which began on 1 October. I taught the half-day release each week on my own from April to November.

The University got strong applications for the three part-time senior lecturer posts. We allowed applications from general practices up to an hour's travel away. We shortlisted eight and appointed Keith Bolden, Michael Hall, and Bob Jones. Keith had had articles published in the *Journal of the Royal College of General Practitioners (JRCGP)*. They came from very different practices and all three started on 1 November 1974. I found experienced senior secretaries Mavis Huckle and Pam Smith and by then we had offices in the Exeter postgraduate medical centre.

Michael Hall, who had many great ideas, acquired a seedling from the tree on the Island of Kos, where it was reputed Hippocrates had taught. We were able to arrange for the President of the RCGP, Professor Pat Byrne, to plant it. In 2003, Professor Ruth Hawker, Chair of the Royal Devon and Exeter NHS Trust and I, later had a plaque erected to mark the occasion.

The prospectus for a typical vocational training course usually consisted of a cheaply produced sheet of paper. We produced a properly printed booklet with formal aims (i.e., to develop multi-disciplinary training – perhaps the first such aim in a British GP scheme) and included a recommended reading list for trainees (University of Exeter, Department of General Practice, 1979). This was accompanied by a whole-page advertisement in the RCGP *Journal*.

In 1974 I attended the first year of the RCGP Nuffield course for course organisers run by Paul Freeling, a leading GP and Suzie Barry, a social scientist. The six one-week modules formed the most important course I ever attended, and I learned much, especially how to tune in to the hidden feelings in an interactive small group and what it feels like to be an adult learner.

One element was providing an educational event locally in front of Paul and Suzie, so I volunteered to give a lecture on medical education in the Exeter postgraduate medical centre to a big audience. I rehearsed the theory of the Nuffield course and the educational paradigm. It was badly received. All the comments at the end were negative and hostile. Even friends said they did not see what relevance this had, and it ended by a leading local GP saying he had come to hear their new senior lecturer in general practice speak and had expected he would actually speak about general practice! The event was an unmitigated disaster and the biggest educational failure of my life. I retreated to my office with Paul and Suzie and was surprised to see tears in Suzie's motherly eyes: "You tried so hard," she said, "and they destroyed you." I had let the Department down and spent ages reviewing it all. I realised I had broken a golden rule of not starting and understanding where the audience was. I knew I would have to teach that same material for years ahead.

Afterwards when faced with 25 prospective GP trainers with the same subject in the same lecture theatre I did it differently. "Educational theory," I said, "has followed general practice! We would always give blood pressure treatment only after taking the BP, educationalists call this pre-course assessment. We always have a target BP in mind. Educationalists call this an educational aim. Then later we would always measure the BP to see if the treatment had worked. Educationalists call this post course assessment. The three together make a 'training triangle' (DPG, 1977a) which, by the way, educationalists call the "educational paradigm." This time the GPs lapped it up.

The senior lecturers shared the teaching on the course and experimented freely. In particular, we developed interactive small group work, ie using the behaviour of the group to illuminate feelings and attitudes. It needed skilled group leadership which Keith, Michael, and I learned on the Nuffield course (*JRCGP*, 1975e). We developed a trainee group, encouraged them to make suggestions and take responsibility. I had lunch with the trainee chair regularly.

We hosted the 1978 Spring general meeting of the RCGP which moved around the country. Michael Hall took lead responsibility and did a great job. We introduced two innovations. First, we started the meeting at 2 pm on the Friday by showcasing the Department in the Exeter postgraduate centre through a series of ten-minute talks, followed by five minutes of questions. Two trainees spoke and stole the show. Secondly, we bussed the whole conference to our practices. This proved popular and colleagues spoke to me about it for years afterwards – although one did say he was interested to learn I was a real GP!

We soon ran out of space and were grateful to the architects in the Regional Hospital Board for designing an extension. However, the NHS would not fund it. The RCGP rescued us and Ekke Kuenssberg, Chair of Council, used his contacts. The Dorothy Mackenzie Trust (Sir James Mackenzie's daughter) kindly donated the remaining capital from Sir James Mackenzie's initiatives. This did the trick and we got an invaluable extension.

When our scheme was inspected by a College team, led by John Horder, he asked why we were not offering trainers' courses. We had not thought about it. He said quietly he could not see any group better placed. We were impressed by this peer review, which identified our collective blind spot. We started offering one-week residential trainers' courses, which were soon over-subscribed and are described in the regional adviser story.

Multi-Professional Staff Team

Rita Goble was a dynamic leader. She was an occupational therapist and she skilfully built links with two other allied professions, physiotherapy and speech therapy. She joined the Department as a Research Fellow, whilst holding the important post of Principal of the St Loye's School of Occupational Therapy in Exeter, the biggest such school in England.

She obtained a grant of £100,000 from the King's Fund, London and led a programme of educational developments for these three professions. This programme ran a series of educational sessions for them. Once she had her PhD, she was appointed Senior Lecturer in the Department in 1986. We appointed a tutor in each of the three professions as much was being done as a three-profession group. She was the first of us to initiate a research programme enabling nine therapists to obtain research degrees, MPhils and PhDs and she did all the supervisions. She led the country and her profession.

Rita wrote several articles in the allied professions' field. However, as head of department, I did not do enough to encourage her to write for medical peer-reviewed journals. I was too hands-off and a marker article on developing the allied health professions was never published in an influential medical journal. Once I realised this gap I wrote an article myself with Rita and colleagues in four professions (DPG *et al.*, 1993), but it was too late.

One of Rita's PhDs was appointed to a professorship in Canada and another, Jill Ashton, a social worker, was appointed Chief Executive of the Exeter Primary Care Trust. Anne Walker (1990) a senior physiotherapist, did an excellent study of GP-based physiotherapy, finding positive results for patients, the physiotherapist, and GP satisfaction compared with patients receiving physiotherapy in hospitals. This did not get the national recognition it deserved.

We were trying to empower our trainees and were offering them leadership training. The most dramatic example of trainee empowerment was when we got Angela Douglas, an unknown trainee in her twenties, elected democratically to the GMC (described in Chapter 16, Practice story, 1976–1986).

I was appointed OBE in the birthday honours list of 1981, the third GP OBE in Devon since the war, after McConaghey in Dartmouth and Sholto Forman. This was a boost for the Department of General Practice. At the 1981 department dinner I said: "Some people think OBE stands for Officer of the Order of the British Empire but you know it means: "Other B.......s' efforts!"

In 1981 the words "British empire" went unremarked. Today one in 50 people decline the honour mainly because of them. It is disappointing that the name of the order has not been adjusted to be the "Order of British Excellence" as suggested by a Select Committee of Parliament on Public Administration (2004).

Publications

The *Lancet* published two different anonymous editorials about us. The first in 1978 was "General Practice Training – Exeter Style" and was a tribute to our system for postgraduate training for general practice (*Lancet,* 1978). The second, two years later, on my article "The key to personal care," was headed "Personal doctoring" and was very supportive (*Lancet,* 1980). No other university department of general practice got such treatment, which gave us a big boost.

In 1977, my booklet *A System of Training for General Practice* was published as RCGP *Occasional Paper 4*. This described the principles of the Exeter vocational training scheme. It included the first report of interactive group work with GP trainees, interpreting some non-verbal behaviour in the group. It also described a trainee rebellion against the system and how the GP lecturers responded by doing a "home visit," i.e. going to the juniors' mess.

This publication became a calling card for the Department as it was one of the first accounts of how to organise vocational training in general practice. It went onto most reading lists in GP training schemes in the UK and many abroad, bringing several international visitors to the department, including a President of the Royal Australian College of General Practitioners. *Occasional Paper 4* made a second edition in 1979, with several appendices giving more details.

The publishers Croom Helm Ltd approached us and agreed to publish a book on general practice management. The book was written by the four of us and was called *Running a Practice*. The staff meeting assumed that I would be the lead author, but I proposed that it be Bob Jones (Jones *et al.,* 1978). It went into three editions with Bob leading each one (Appendix 6).

I was approached by Macdonald and Evans, a local publisher in Plymouth, and agreed to write a book, as sole author, on vocational training for general practice. I was too inexperienced and should have gone to a bigger national publisher but they produced the book, in 1982, *Training for General Practice,* satisfactorily (DPG, 1982), but with much too little marketing.

Michael Hall edited a book on ideas and techniques for GP training *A GP Training Handbook*. All four of us wrote chapters with other colleagues. He rightly went to Blackwells, who promoted it well and it went into three editions (Hall *et al.,* 1983), selling 5,500 copies.

My article in the *BMJ* on GP trainers set out core principles and how general practice training differed from training in specialist medicine. It noted how GP trainers had to undertake training in teaching methods, and how being formally selected for a senior position did not confer the right to teach. GP teaching was an additional professional responsibility needing time and so should be paid. Several characteristics of trainers were described (DPG, 1984a).

Keith Bolden, with Barbara Tackle one of the practice nurses in the Exeter Mount Pleasant practice, wrote the first *Handbook for Practice Nurses* (Bolden and Takle, 1984). This was also published by Blackwell and went well. By 1988 all the four senior staff were first authors of books.

Keith Bolden and two course organisers wrote another book describing the running of a vocational training course (Bolden *et al.,* 1988). All three of the early books on training for general practice had come from the Exeter Department. We had fulfilled the hopes of the funder and produced the first two books on general practice nursing as well (Damant *et al.,* 1994).

Declan Dwyer from Plymouth was one of these Exeter course organisers and he founded a new journal for GP course organisers, which he edited for some years. It is now called *Education for Primary Care*, the second general practice journal developed in Devon. Useful educational publications continued, such as how learning styles influence learning (Lewis and Bolden, 1989) and the report of an innovative course mixing GP trainers with practice nurse trainers (Bolden and Lewis, 1990), both in the *BJGP*. Bob Jones edited RCGP *Occasional Paper 33 Working Together – Learning Together* (Jones, 1986) and was the first of us to do qualitative research. Jones *et al.* (1993) studied carers' experience in breast cancer (163 citations). Then Jones and Greenwood (1994) studied how breast cancer patients' views of their symptoms compared with their GPs' understanding. By revealing a "mismatch" between patients and doctors he showed the need for and then fostered patient-centred medicine.

Keith Bolden led on advanced analyses of consultations and did further training on the Myers Briggs personality type, running courses for trainers on it which were soon in demand outside the trainer system. He also taught transactional analysis. Russell Steele joined him in many of these courses.

The Exeter Department's GP training course was unique in having four GP senior lecturers running and continually analysing it. A difference was we subscribed to university values, including research and writing. Our aim was that the trainees should, be future leaders, learning thinking and writing. They had many good ideas. We encouraged all who were interested to research and write. One way was to include a half-day a week in their practice timetable making it clear a project was expected. Some trainees made substantial research contributions.

Richard Westcott (1977) first showed in the *JRCGP* that patients with emotional problems had longer consultations (50 citations) Roger Peppiatt *et al.* (1978) was one of the first as a GP trainee to observe how many patients at weekends had consumed large quantities of alcohol. He measured this and published the findings years before this became a national issue (45 citations). Three trainees, Clare Ronalds, Angela Douglas, and Peter Selley *et al.* (1981) were co-authors of the report of the *Fourth National Trainees' Conference,* which the Exeter trainees organised and published as RCGP *Occasional Paper* 18. It included two new research findings identified by our statistician, Ian Russell, that trainee satisfaction was associated with the trainer holding the MRCGP and providing three hours a week or more of teaching. Over a dozen trainees achieved publications in the peer-reviewed literature. No other GP vocational training course in the UK had as many.

The initial grant from the DHSS expired in 1978 and the DHSS reviewed the Department. Diana Walford, later Medical Director of the NHS Executive, inspected us. She was brisk and efficient, with probing but always fair, questions. At the end of the day, meeting with David Mattingly, university officials and me, she said she was completely satisfied with the quality of the work and satisfied we were providing value for public money. The grant was renewed for a further five years. Alone with me in a car, she opened up. She was sure NHS general practice was the highest priority for academic leadership and said we were doing well. When I thanked her she said that the decision was easy: "You are doing all this on only one and a half consultant posts!"

Later, she co-opted me on to a DH working party reviewing the huge NHS sums SIFT paid to medical schools for medical education. General practice was excluded (just GPs). Walford, used me whenever resistance to reform appeared. John Howie in Edinburgh tackled this problem with the Scottish ACT. The Walford Group fed into the Winyard report (1995) *Sift into the Future* opened the door to SIFT funding for general practice education in England.

In 1981 I had a lecture tour in New Zealand and thanks to Jill's mother child sitting, Jill came. The programme was full and once I had three sessions in two different towns on the same day. Our cases went missing once and Jill was stuck in travel clothes for dinner in a smooth hotel. We were seated behind a pillar. When leaving on a local flight in a tiny Cessna plane we were carefully separated from US colleagues. Later we were told they thought the Americans would have complained!

Eponymous Lectures

I was privileged to give several eponymous lectures including the leading general practice one, the James Mackenzie lecture of the RCGP (DPG, 1978). I eventually gave 22 in three countries (Appendix 2). Keith Bolden delivered the Australian equivalent of the Mackenzie, the Connolly lecture, of the Royal Australian College of General Practitioners.

Academic General Practice at Keele

The Department was recognised as an important model when I was invited to visit the Vice-Chancellor of the University of Keele in 1979 meeting also with local leaders. Keele then established an academic GP department with a senior lecturer and two lectureships, all like my post, part-time, but unlike Exeter they secured regional health authority funding. The Wolstanton practice in Newcastle-under Lyme provided farsighted leadership including the first Senior Lecturer, an RCGP Honorary Treasurer, Douglas Garvie and Peter Croft who like me was later appointed a professor. The Keele story is important as it replicated developments in Exeter and so provides evidence of the latent talent in general practice, which can blossom if given a fair chance (Fisher and Croft, 2022).

It also has implications about how best to develop general practice nationally. It vindicated the RCGP cascade strategy of the central Nuffield course, delivered by GP leadership, and inspiring and up-skilling regional GP leaders. I met Alistair Ross, the first Senior Lecturer and Mike Fisher an activist, there. Both Exeter and Keele maintained strong links with local general practices.

World Health Organisation 1983

The Department's high profile led to invitations for me to several WHO seminars as a "temporary adviser" or "consultant." One was in Yugoslavia and another in Czechoslovakia. I spent a week in the WHO head office in Geneva.

Then the Department received an invitation to host a week-long WHO seminar in 1983 and I was invited to chair it. Detailed briefing included a requirement that the WHO flag should fly on the highest local public building, in our case the Royal Devon and Exeter hospital. I forwarded this to the hospital chief executive who replied that the consultant staff were not happy about flying this flag for a general practice meeting. I informed WHO; the latter then reminded the Foreign Office of international agreements; the Foreign Office informed the DH, who informed the hospital. The WHO flag flew all week.

WHO brought a dozen deans of European medical schools plus Sir John Reid, CMO Scotland, and other medical internationalists. The topic was the future of medical schools in Europe, which was a delicious irony as WHO had chosen a university as host that did not have an undergraduate medical school. We took the seminar to the St Leonard's Practice and demonstrated our computer records. The deans had been talking about the importance of preventive medicine and taking a population approach and we were pleased to demonstrate both in an NHS practice. They were ignorant about general practice and none of them had departments of general practice like ours.

WHO required two evenings' entertainment for the seminar but provided no budget. I was rescued by the Chair of the Exeter Health Authority, Murray French, who funded a meal, the price being my having to make a speech standing halfway up some stairs. Jill rescued me for the other evening laying on a full dinner party for all the members of the seminar in our home. I was in the chair for the week and worked hard to keep everyone together and get conclusions supporting the development of general practice/primary health care.

Sir John Reid (1925–1994) was KCMG (an unusual honour as civil servants usually receive the KCB; it recognises international diplomatic achievements). He was a great internationalist and a former Vice-Chair of the International Board of WHO. He helped throughout the week with skilled comments. He said he had never seen a WHO seminar dine in a private home before and later invited me to accompany him as the one of the UK representatives for a few days to the WHO Health Assembly held in Geneva. This was a fascinating experience and gave me several meals and discussions alone with him when he taught me a great deal. I think he saw this as a way of returning Jill's and my hospitality. His premature death, aged only 69, was a great loss.

I was the first GP to chair a WHO seminar and was in the chair all week taking detailed notes. I was pleased the way the discussions went and I sent a paper to the WHO regional office summarising the meeting. To my horror, a document was sent back which reported the meeting with a very different emphasis. Crucially, it stated that undergraduate medical training produced GPs – an irony to send this to a postgraduate university department of general practice. This had been written by the WHO staff officer who had attended the seminar. I wrote a careful rejection and referred him to my note and paper. He refused to change it, stating it was his report.

I sought advice from Sir John Reid who confirmed my paper was accurate. However, nothing would make the official budge. Sir John and I had always worked in a British culture in which the Chair is in

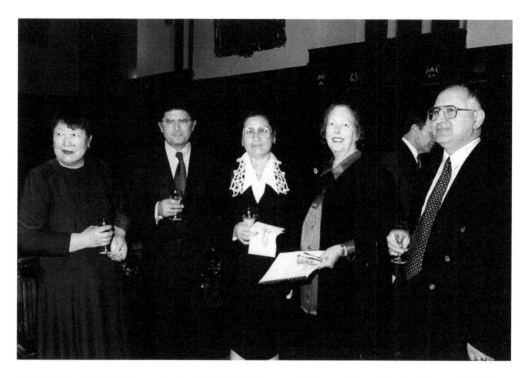

FIGURE 13.1 Rita Goble (second right) with WHO visitors at the Institute of General Practice, Exeter Guildhall.

charge of the meeting and is responsible for the minutes/record. However, the official saw the secretariat being responsible for the record and the chair as a figurehead. I had to decide whether to escalate the problem in the WHO hierarchy and wage a war with an international institution a thousand miles away or to let it go. We could not reach agreement, which was a spectacular defeat for me. WHO duly printed and published a report, with minimal changes, which was a travesty and gave harmful messages about GP training. I was profoundly disappointed. The pleasure and achievement of holding and chairing the first ever WHO meeting in a university department of general practice turned to dust. I never put the publication (WHO, 1984) on my cv or ever referred to it. WHO sent another team to the Institute in 1997, which was a happy social visit.

Staff Team

I chaired the staff meeting of the four of us, which we had every week after the vocational training course finished at 5 pm, or at other times in the vacations. This raised questions about leadership style. Commentators often draw analogies with the cabinet but there are important relationship differences. Prime ministers are in a stronger position vis-a-vis their cabinet colleagues than any professional leader in a university or royal college as they appoint people to the cabinet and can sack them at any time. In the professional world, leaders have to work with colleagues who have either been appointed, like my three fellow senior lecturers, or elected like officers in medical royal colleges. Political life is short term. Governments are elected for only five years and the average shelf life of a government minister is only two to three years. Government policies are often rushed with a focus on quick results. However, I was appointed senior lecturer aged 38 and Keith Bolden was younger, we planned to work until we were 65. Taking the long-term view was therefore easier.

My leadership style was therefore deliberately long term and sought to build up the leadership team and keep it together. We were nicknamed the "gang of four." This style was comfortable as it matched clinical general practice where GPs seek to empower their patients and partners and work to build and maintain good long-term relationships with them. I went out of my way to ensure credit went to others and showered colleagues with thank you cards.

However, this meant I sometimes went along with policies with which I disagreed but were important to the others. Twice a clash came when I proposed introducing another colleague on the staff. First, I proposed John Preece, a GP in Exeter who had an outstanding reputation as a conscientious and caring GP. Academically he was the first author of an article describing the first time a GP anywhere in the world had gone on-line with computerised medical records. He had laboriously entered all the computer records himself (Preece *et al.*, 1970). This had been published before the Department was established. However, my suggestion was not welcomed. In balancing a strong team feeling amongst the four and their feelings that I was not a dictator, John Preece's appointment was lost. I regretted that for ages and believe not offering a post to the only GP in Exeter who had published an article that was a world first was a serious failure of my leadership. In 2020, fifty years after Preece's article, the second author in that author team, Dennis Gillings CBE, was knighted. He had led Quintiles in the United States and became a British billionaire. He and his wife became the biggest single donor to the University of Exeter. Similarly, I proposed Wilf Selley, a local dentist with the FDS, with a postgraduate qualification and writing skills, as a dental senior lecturer in general practice. This too was opposed and never happened (Chapter 30, Dentistry story).

However, the gains were huge and the four of us and our wives became good friends and colleagues and a real team. In 27 years I only exercised formal authority in the face of strong written opposition within the lecturer team twice: first to establish the Exeter MSc, and secondly when deciding to stop my personal teaching on the GP vocational course and concentrate on research. Both were high level strategic policies, both were strongly disputed within the leader team. Ultimately, leaders sometimes have to decide, alone.

We steadily expanded the academic staff team over the years, like Rita Goble as a senior lecturer in 1986. It was a big step to have a non-medical colleague in the leadership team. She was very energetic and proved to be a good colleague. Tony Lewis, a GP in West Cornwall, did fellowship by assessment

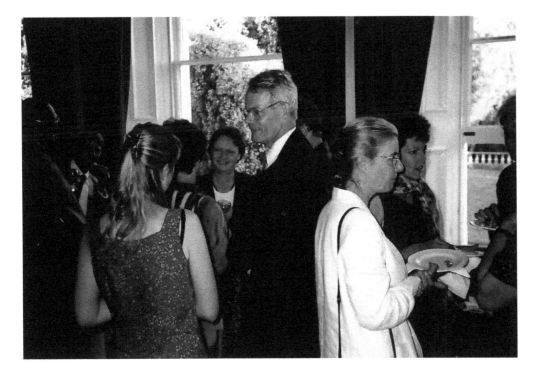

FIGURE 13.2 Tony Lewis, Senior lecturer in general practice in 1999.

of the RCGP in the first wave in 1989 and moved to be nearer the Department. He completed an Open University degree and was a skilled teacher. He became another senior lecturer in general practice.

We also later recruited Alan Hooper as another non-medical senior lecturer in leadership. He had senior experience in the armed forces and in the leadership centre in the University. Martin Marshall was the first of our master's students to progress to an MD, which I co-supervised and he too was later appointed a lecturer.

MSc in Healthcare 1986

During the mid-1980s we had much discussion about launching an MSc. First, general practitioners and occupational therapists were (and still are) seriously short of opportunities to undertake higher university degrees. Secondly, the degree courses that were available were generally in specialist medicine or epidemiology. Thirdly, many were whole-time, and in effect impossible for working GPs. We constructed a six-module, part-time course with a compulsory dissertation. I wrote leadership module It took 18 months to get through the university committees. We were approved in the spring of 1986 with me as course director. It was the first master's course in health care in the UK that was multiprofessional, part-time, and located in a university department of general practice. British universities were then remarkably controlled by Whitehall with each university being told each year exactly how many students it was allowed to enrol and punished financially if it either under- or over-recruited. But part-time master's degrees were outside this system. We were free to recruit as we wished. Some professors were jealous.

We started in October 1986. The response was moving. People remortgaged their homes to pay the fees and one of our early MSc students, Brenda Sawyer, a practice manager, was driven from Southampton by her husband. We had two GPs, including my partner, Ann Buxton, several nurses and a hospital chief executive. When I was unexpectedly elected to chair the RCGP, the next year, I stood down as course director and Keith Bolden, now converted to the course, took over as director and developed it well. It became one of the biggest master's courses in England bringing valuable income to the Department.

Computers in General Practice

In 1983 the DHSS with Department of Trade and Industry launched the "Micros for GPs" with 149 volunteer general practices, a scheme to encourage the use of computers. Several of us were accepted. Practices paid half the cost and ours transformed my clinical practice. Michael Hall led this locally and Bob Jones was active on the national GP Computer Group. The Department did the user survey. Bob got the national appraisal evaluation, *Micros in Practice* to be co-authored by our Department [DHSS, Joint Computer Group and Exeter University, 1986]. A *Prescription for Change: A report on the longer term use and development of computers in general practice* (Fitter MJ *et al.,* Sheffield and Jones RVH, Exeter, 1986) was the DHSS position paper. Quietly the Department emerged in a leading academic position on GP computing.

In discussions in London I benefited from this lead and the Department was appointed in 1989 as the national centre to develop the care card. This project meant putting the GP medical record onto a card like a credit card, which patients could carry. All depended on Robin Hopkins, an Exmouth GP with rare IT skills. He obtained an MPhil, which I supervised, and became Senior Lecturer in General Practice to lead this project with Michael Hall. He did well and made it happen so the cards could be read through card readers in surgeries and pharmacies. The NHS Management Executive (1990) DH gave an evaluation of the project, which was favourable, and recommended a further trial. Two booklets and an editorial in *J Med Systems* (Hopkins, 1990) were published. This could have modernised the NHS if the DH had followed up this research the UK would have had a world lead. Sadly, the Blair government was later persuaded otherwise by management consultants who advised a huge £20 billion top-down system which never worked, losing a great opportunity.

Bob Jones noting how much support was available for cancer patients and how little for patients with similar problems through serious physical diseases established a new charity to support them. This was called Continuing Care at Home CONCHA (1986) and did much useful work.

Professorship

In 1985, the Vice-Chancellor of the University of Leeds invited me to apply for his chair of general practice. This was pretty strong encouragement and that Department was much better resourced than Exeter, where we were living on our wits. Indeed, we were appealing for funds through a new charitable trust (Chapter 15; South West General Practice Trust story). Jill and I had a hard think about priorities as it would have meant the family moving. We both had mothers in Exeter and it meant leaving the Practice as well as the Department; I had many 23-year relationships with patients and a personal list. I took the letter to Dr (later Sir) David Harrison (1930–2022) Vice-Chancellor.

The question was would I ever get a chair in Exeter as my head of department, David Mattingly, had not proposed me? Harrison asked for my cv and said it merited the right to apply myself, but the Exeter process required eight external assessors, one from overseas, and took an academic year. I declined the Leeds Vice-Chancellor's invitation and applied to be a professor at Exeter. One of my friends, trying to be helpful said he hoped it would be noted that I was a GP and doing a full share of out-of-hours and night calls. He was told: "No. He will be judged like everyone else on academic criteria, particularly publications, grants won, and leadership." My friend realised that clinicians competed with full-time academic colleagues whilst working only half-time. However, my name went to the July 1986 Senate for approval of a personal chair, from 1 October; so I became a professor virtually on my 51st birthday.

I became the first professor of general practice in the University and in the Southwestern region. The senior lecturers generously gave me an engraved sherry decanter. All the lecturers received invitations to teach abroad and I was appointed to the Government Committee on breast cancer screening, chaired by Sir Patrick Forrest (1923–2021; Forrest Committee, 1986).

A Big Surprise

In the summer of 1986, I was visited by Robert Hart, a consultant microbiologist and Chair of the Joint Medical Staff Committee (JMSC) of the Royal Devon and Exeter Hospital. His message was one of the most surprising of my life. The hospital consultants wanted me to be the next Director of the Postgraduate Medical School. I had not considered this as there was a deputy director in post. I consulted the senior lecturers, who were unanimous that I should apply (Chapter 27; Postgraduate Medical School story). I was appointed and took up the Directorship on 1 April 1987. We all thought this was for only five years, so I kept the leadership of the Department of General Practice.

Focus on Research

With the departmental teaching going well, I increasingly reflected on our research role. The problem was that we were mainly a teaching unit and there was a huge need for research in the Department and in general practices. When I suggested I stop teaching on the GP training course I was pressed hard to stay with a group that were pioneering teaching methods and enjoying it. Eventually, I did withdraw from vocational training and started offering supervisions for general practitioners who wished to undertake a research degree, the MPhil Exeter. Its regulations allowed it to be taken part-time and the fees were reasonable, so GPs could do the degree while working full-time in their practices.

I started with Jonathan Stead, a former trainee, so we knew each other. He studied practice nursing. Another early recruit was Robin Hopkins who, remarkably, from a small general practice in Exmouth had gained admission to the committee, which was drafting standards for computers across Europe.

Moving from teaching to research supervision was a big change. GP teaching was people orientated, full of groups, with constant analysis of everything that was happening. There was a buzz which I much enjoyed. The research supervisions were different. I was alone in a room with a colleague for about three-quarters of an hour. There was no peer group and I had to work on a subject chosen by the student, when I often initially knew little about it.

I soon learned that GPs were often very intelligent and frequently had exciting ideas for research. Generalists by nature think broadly. However, they had great weaknesses in not understanding research methods and most of them had little or no training in critical writing. The supervisions were therefore an exercise in personal encouragement and empowerment, helping them to read and understand the principles of research articles and theses while in the process giving personal examples about their own data and writing. After each supervision, I wrote a long letter summarising the position and giving advice.

GPs often follow even radical innovations once they see a working model by a local colleague. I was encouraged when two of my partners, Kieran Sweeney and Philip Evans, both registered for an MPhil and asked to have me as their supervisor. This showed confidence in our partnership relationships in the practice (Chapter 34, Practice story, 1987–2000). Phil Evans was interested in high blood cholesterol. I encouraged GPs, to undertake projects using clinical data from their own computer systems. This had the advantage that it enabled them to refine the data, check it in their clinical time, saving time gathering data outside the practice. Philip discovered that the recommended practice of heavily investigating everyone with hypercholesterolaemia produced few findings. His article was published in the *BMJ* (Evans and DPG, 1994). This encouraged him and he joined the RCGP working party on high cholesterol in general practice. Philip and I served with leading lipidologists and first learned that atheroma was reversible (Waine report, 1992)-. This was later confirmed (Nissen *et al.,* 2005) and was and is big encouragement for GPs learning they had the power reverse atheroma with statins. Kieran Sweeney was interested in miscarriages. He had many ideas and developed an original patient-centred perspective on a problem then being relatively ignored. He became very patient-centred in his later writings. I supervised two doctorates and 12 GPs for MPhils.

I was an external examiner for doctoral degrees in the universities of Edinburgh, and London and two in Nijmegen in the Netherlands. In Holland I learned the importance of celebrating academic success through big parties after a thesis is awarded (DPG, 1992b; Celebrating a thesis – the Nijmegen way). We started celebratory dinners for new graduates, their spouses, and sometimes their mothers. Both Philip and Kieran got their MPhils (Evans, 1995; Sweeney, 1996). Both became lecturers in general practice and had successful academic careers. Both became professors.

I recruited one MPhil student, David Kessler in Bristol. He had started a career in psychiatry and held the MRCPsych. He was well read and had a thoughtful mind. He wanted to research how symptoms are attributed (understood) by patients. The Institute then held a research grant to study depression in general practice, so the study was to analyse prospectively how GPs diagnosed or missed depression, assessing this by standard questionnaires. A new feature was asking the same patients to complete a symptom attribution questionnaire. This classifies people as "normalisers" who attribute (rationalise) symptoms to external events, "psychologisers" who worry about symptoms, or "somatisers" who attribute symptoms to disease. Our findings were fascinating. GPs rarely missed depression in psychologisers or somatisers but did so more often in normalisers. The attributions of those depressed patients "it's only the weather, doctor" steered the GP away from a diagnosis. GPs were sensitively tuning in to their patients' thinking but were then colluding with them. This is important to GP theory as it explained for the first time why the GPs, who are most sensitive to patients, may miss depression. I described this collusion as a new adverse effect of continuity of care. Kessler *et al.* (1999), with 597 citations. David Kessler too later became a professor.

International contacts were a great pleasure. I visited Professor Huygen, in the Netherlands as the father of European academic general practice. He was charming and told me about how in 1944 his starving patients were fed by food drops by the RAF. He gave me one of his pictures. I was an examiner for two doctoral theses in the University of Nijmegen, held in public with big attendances.

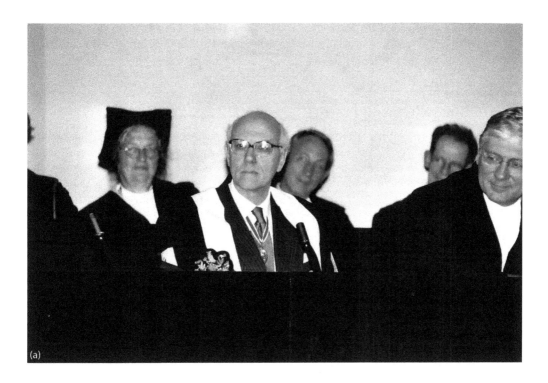

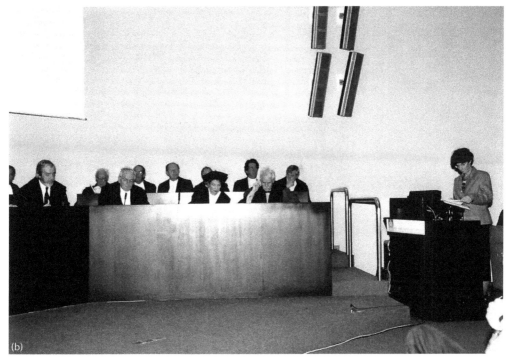

FIGURE 13.3 (a) The author sitting as Examiner for PhD thesis at Nijmegen, the Netherlands. (b) Evelyn van Weel presenting her PhD thesis in public at Nijmegen.

Roger Bulger, the Head of the Institute of US Teaching Hospitals came to visit the practice and said our computing system was ahead of anything in the United States. Over dinner with some Exeter trainees he told them they were "the future."

First Institute of General Practice

The Department was now firing on all cylinders. I was re-elected Director of the Postgraduate Medical School in 1992 (Chapter 27, Postgraduate Medical School story) and had high level discussions in the University. John Tooke, now a professor, proposed a new institute of clinical sciences, which I actively backed. I was then campaigning for the Department to be made an institute. With reluctance in high places about two institutes, I pointed out the University was contributing minimal funding for academic medicine and nothing to the Department of General Practice. We should be allowed titles that would best support us. Two institutes were created in 1993 within the PGMS. The Department became the first Institute of General Practice in Europe and an Institute of Clinical Sciences was

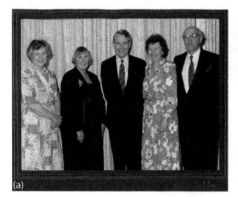
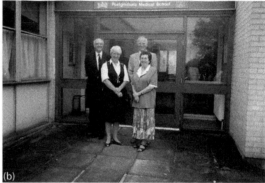

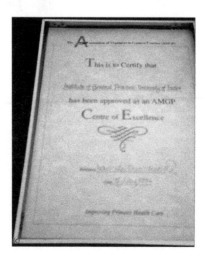

FIGURE 13.4 (a) Institute of General Practice dinner (left to right) with the Vice-Chancellor's wife, Baroness Fritchie, the Vice-Chancellor and Jill. (b) Institute of General Practice Award as Centre of Excellence, with Sally Irvine (President of AMGP) Keith Bolden (He is at the back on the right) and Brenda Sawyer (AMGP). (c) Award to Institute of General Practice by Association of Managers in General Practice as a Centre of Excellence in 1994.

also formed (University of Exeter, 1995/6). The Institute's influence on NHS administration helped to develop a local hospice. Our annual department dinner, although a subdepartment of the medical school attracted the Vice-Chancellor and his wife and two chairs of the Regional Health Authority. The Institute was recognised as a Centre of Excellence by the Association of Managers in General Practice.

Harkness Fellowships are elite travelling fellowships, designed to balance the Rhodes scholarships, run by the Commonwealth Fund of New York, enabling British citizens to spend a year in a leading US centre. No GP had won one until Kieran Sweeney broke this glass ceiling. He had an exciting year in the US with his wife Barbara and their children. He came back to the Practice fired up with energy and ideas. This was a personal triumph for him but good for the Department. Soon Martin Marshall, another Exeter trainee, was also awarded a Harkness. He too had a stimulating year. Few GPs later received a Harkness.

The Department/Institute consciously gave leadership training, not knowing if we were succeeding. However, three of us, now all over 80, have witnessed some interesting careers. Angela Douglas was twice elected in national ballots of all English doctors to the GMC. Kieran Sweeney sadly died at the height of his intellectual development, but achieved a personal professorship. Michael Dixon LVO OBE became the head of NHS Alliance, Chair of the College of Medicine, and the first GP ever to be Head of the King's Royal Medical Household. Domhnall MacAuley became a professor E E and Editor of the *British Journal of General Practice.* Martin Marshall CBE became a professor and Chair of the RCGP Council. Nick Cooper was elected President of the Academy of Medical Educators. Sarah Purdy became the first GP Dean of the Bristol Medical School.

As Michael and Keith approached retirement, I tried hard to get them promoted to reader. The University's policies were too rigid. Michael had brought a whole succession of assets to the university

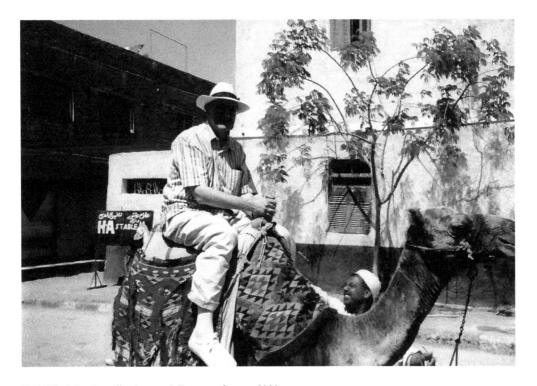

FIGURE 13.5 Travelling by camel, Egypt conference, 2000.

and been an invaluable colleague and senior teacher. He was the first GP to chair the trustees of a major national charity, the British Diabetic Association, bigger than the RCGP. Keith had written three books and several academic articles. He negotiated funding from the 'Knowhow' fund which brought Hungarians to the Exeter MSc. He had successfully negotiated with the Egyptian government and the Institute was appointed to train Egyptian family doctors who came to Exeter, and we provided GP teaching in Egypt including a first conference on family medicine, where I first travelled by camel! That million pound grant was then the biggest in the history of the University. I was deeply disappointed that neither got readerships and believe they both should have done. Today 'readers' are, 'associate professors' and much more readily appointed.

Bob Jones was, sadly, the first of the 'gang of four' to die in 2005 (Hall and DPG, 2005).

Retirement

I was to retire on 30 September 2001. I sought permission to continue researching, funding myself completely from grants. This was declined by the Head of the School for Sport and Health Sciences, advised by the Personnel Department. An appeal to the VC was unsuccessful. The University's rules were rigid and it could not envisage successful research after age 65. So I retired on that date. The Institute organised a farewell seminar with many colleagues and former trainees speaking, several movingly. It was like a festschrift, uncommon in the GP world.

They gave me a dinner and presented me with a beautiful, silver bowl and a generous cheque.

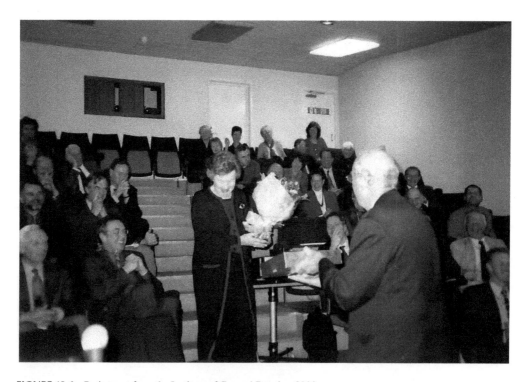

FIGURE 13.6   Retirement from the Institute of General Practice, 2000.

ADDENDA

In forced academic retirement from the University I switched to doing research in the St Leonard's Practice (Chapter 49, St Leonard's Research Practice story).

A merger of the Exeter and Plymouth postgraduate medical schools formed a new undergraduate 'Peninsula Medical School.' The new Director of the Exeter PGMS introduced a reorganisation dividing research from teaching and closed all the departments. The Institute lost control of its big grant. The substantial financial cushion for general practice that the 'gang of four' had accumulated for their successors was lost to general practice. The Institute did not last after I left and closed on 31 July 2002. It existed as first the Department of General Practice and after 1993 as the Institute of General Practice for 28 years.

The huge enthusiasm and identity of general practice, expressed as the first British Institute of General Practice in a European university, can, in Peguy's words, be seen as a kind of mysticism and, as he perceptively wrote, sadly ended in politics. The Institute of General Practice died. It has been one of the big disappointments of my life that this Institute in the University of Exeter was not allowed to continue.

14

Regional Adviser in General Practice/Director of GP Education

Human history becomes more and more a race between education and catastrophe.

HG Wells (1866–1946)

In 1948, the medical schools did not teach general practice as a subject and thought they were producing 'safe doctors' after only an undergraduate education. General practice had no postgraduate educational system. There was no professor of general practice in the world and no sense that general practice would become a discipline in its own right.

The BMA established two working parties on general practice, both chaired by Sir Henry Cohen (1900–1977), the second recommended postgraduate training for GPs for the first time (Cohen Committee, 1950). The College of General Practitioners formed in 1952 being the single most important step in reform.

The Nuffield Provincial Hospitals Trust's conference in Oxford in 1961 (Chapter 44, Nuffield Trust story) set the scene for decentralising medical education away from London. (Pickering, 1962) It proposed local postgraduate medical centres, many built close to hospitals. The Exeter one opened in 1970.

The new College of GPs developed three influential policies: first was the principle of "special vocational training" being needed for general practice (CGP, 1965); secondly, it gave evidence, to the Royal Commission on Medical Education (CGP, 1966); thirdly, the College established in 1965 an examination for membership (MRCGP), the first general practice examination in Europe.

In 1967, the General Medical Council (GMC) with Henry Cohen (later Lord Cohen) as President, decreed that undergraduate medical education was only preparation for postgraduate training (GMC, 1967). It thus steered the Royal Commission on Medical Education (1968) to recommend postgraduate training for general practice, which it did. The Government accepted the report of the Royal Commission. However, its problem was how to establish postgraduate training for half the medical profession from scratch. It was impossible to copy specialist medicine, where the relevant royal colleges had led, because the College of GPs was still young (14 years old) and small (with about a third of GPs as members).

A unique educational experiment started in 1965 in Wessex in the UK, which did not occur in any other specialty or in any other country (Swift, 1968). The politically powerful BMA GP Committee firmly opposed compulsory postgraduate GP training. The solution was innovative. The DHSS (1972) directed each regional hospital board to fund one part-time GP, one per region, to lead GP education, initiating postgraduate training. It was imaginative as these were *hospital* boards. The posts were in the postgraduate medical departments of medical schools, accountable to postgraduate deans. The BMA GP committee was offside and had no way of stopping this.

In the Southwestern region, the first GP regional adviser appointed was Michael Lennard, a Bristol GP. He was the obvious choice as he had the best credentials. He formed a new GP committee in 1973 bringing together all interested in GP training across the South West. These committees were soon

DOI: 10.1201/9781032713601-18

empowered to appoint general practice trainers, instead of local medical committees. As a College activist, I was offered a courtesy place, but after I had been appointed to lead the Exeter GP department in December 1973 with a remit to develop vocational training, I had an ex officio place. So I was present at the very beginning of the South West region's GP educational developments.

Regional Adviser in General Practice

By 1975, the Department of General Practice at Exeter was running one of the most innovative vocational training schemes in the UK. Joe Cates, Medical Postgraduate Dean at Bristol, invited me to become an associate regional adviser to Michael Lennard. I declined, saying I thought that the post ought to be a full regional adviser. I said that David Mattingly, my boss in the Exeter Postgraduate Medical Institute, was a professor in an independent university and was not accountable to the Postgraduate Dean. (Later I learned that Cates had previously manoeuvred against Exeter having a university medical department.)

I gave him examples, like the northern region, which had more than one GP adviser. Michael Lennard still preferred to have an associate adviser. Impasse! It was not the easiest time, as my father, who was my partner, died in harness in March 1975 and so I had suddenly become singlehanded in the practice. Cates was a strategic thinker and often cited Napoleon to me. Privately, I think he thought I might one day split Devon and Cornwall away from Bristol's control. This happened in the 21st century, but not through me. Then Michael Lennard invited me to a private dinner, steered by the Dean. We thrashed out a *modus operandi*, agreeing that I would confine my activities to Devon and Cornwall and this would be reinforced in my title. I would not interfere in Gloucester, Avon and Somerset and would support Michael as the 'senior' regional adviser. In return he agreed to me being a second full regional adviser in general practice. In July 1975, Joe Cates appointed me Regional Adviser in General Practice (Devon and Cornwall), part-time in Cates' postgraduate department of the University of Bristol, which was reimbursed by the regional authority. I got a part-time secretary in the Exeter Department of General Practice. I became a regional adviser two years after the role was formalised.

I devolved much of the teaching of the Exeter vocational training course to Keith Bolden and Michael Hall, while trying to visit every GP who applied for approval as a trainer in their practices. This was unusual as trainer appointments in many regions were by interview in medical schools. My philosophy was that the practice was the key setting and needed to be visited as well as assessing the trainer as a clinician. Visits took time. Exeter to Penzance and back is 200 miles, so a visit there was a serious commitment.

My first finding was that whether the trainer held the MRCGP or not was important. It often indicated an attitude to taking general practice training seriously. After these visits I sent detailed written reports back to the trainer and practice, setting out their strengths and making suggestions. This is a powerful educational process. The key elements are a visit in person to the practice and the ability to make direct personal observations and then a follow up letter/report in writing. This enabled face-to-face discussions with the partners and staff in the practice on their home ground and was capitalised on by confirming the key messages 'in writing.' Fifteen years later, this process came to be known as 'academic detailing' (Soumerai and Avorn, 1990).

That autumn I set up a particularly important dinner in Plymouth. I invited all the course organisers in Devon and Cornwall to dinner. All but one came, and I chaired a pleasant meal. At it I offered a plan to create a group that would meet regularly, share information, form common policies, give each other mutual support. They readily agreed and what was to be a major educational group emerged. From then on, we met quarterly, and all paperwork and preparation were done in the Exeter regional adviser's office. This leader group proved a source of many ideas and was important in disseminating information, leading GP trainers and supporting its members.

Once the course organisers' group was established, I initiated an annual Devon and Cornwall trainers' conference to build-up the trainers into a coherent body. It had two aims: to spread high-level teaching skills and to develop trainers so they developed an increasing pride in their role. These conferences were financed by Section 63, an educational fund paid for by the DHSS and administered by GP regional advisers. They were held in four-star hotels in Devon and Cornwall, such as Saunton Sands at Braunton, North Devon.

We had outside speakers and did group work, splitting up the trainers from the five vocational training schemes, so they met each other and shared ideas. The residential nature (Thursday lunchtime to noon on the Saturday) gave good opportunities to socialise and relax. Much peer learning took place in the bar! Soon, each of the five trainer groups took turns to run it. In later years international speakers like Nigel Stott, the GP professor in Wales, and Professor Chris van Weel from the Netherlands, spoke.

The regional adviser service was developing quickly and there was more and more work. We started appointing associate advisers, part-time (one or two sessions per week) at each end of the region. They assisted the two regional advisers, but in Devon and Cornwall we developed 'functional' associate advisers who led on some important educational issues, such as assessment. Keith Bolden and Michael Hall applied, were the best qualified, and were appointed. The three of us worked even more closely together.

Over time, the educational and management responsibilities steadily grew, I resisted creating whole-time jobs and instead kept trying to involve more GPs in different roles. This broadened the team and shared expertise. Multiple course organisers became necessary for the bigger vocational training schemes. We invented the role of a 'peripatetic' course organiser, Alun Edwards, from Barnstaple, became highly skilled in leading practice visits and writing constructive reports fostering developments in the training practices.

Single trainers in practices were usual, but one GP trainer died in a car crash. This was very sad and I was forced to find another practice for the GP trainee at short notice. This was tricky as our standards were strict and we had few reserves. The advantages of having two approved trainers in a single practice became obvious to insure against such disasters and also countering the isolation some trainers felt, when seeking educational expenditure within practices on practice libraries and equipment. Multiple trainers, with permission for only one trainee at a time, helped to build up training practices.

In 1976, the Joint Committee for Postgraduate Training (Chapter 29, JCPTGP story) was formed as the controlling national body for GP training with UK-wide responsibilities and its guidance was important to regional committees. Once appointed to it in 1981 I kept the RGPEC fully informed of national thinking.

The RCGP review of the Exeter scheme led to it providing trainers' courses for the region (Chapter 13, Department/Institute of General Practice story). Our first course was run by Keith Bolden, Michael Hall, and me, with 25 prospective trainers. We started on Sunday evening and finished at noon on the Saturday. This first course was very hard work. Sunday evening started with a battery of assessments, including personality tests, like the Myers Briggs Type Inventory (MBTI) (Myers Briggs, 1993). On Monday I did a session on educational theory from my *System of Training for General Practice* (DPG, 1977), followed by Keith leading them to assess each other's teaching using video recordings. In the evening we went to a local pub. There the course members engaged vigorously with the tutors and we would regularly be surrounded by a group challenging us sharply on everything we were doing. Fears that we were trying to change them (yes, we were), that we weren't following teaching hospital methods (yes, true), etc. The three of us had to have reasons for everything. It was a big advantage editing the College *Journal* and knowing many articles on vocational training.

One technique was to give the next day, to those who had been arguing with me, photocopies of the references of the evidence on the subjects they had raised. These intellectual battles were for the heart and mind of the discipline of general practice. These were working doctors who had never thought there was any theory about either general practice or teaching. They only had their hospital consultants as role models and most of them had been taught only on ward rounds/in lecture rooms, often, they told me, being humiliated. Most had never before been taught before by GPs. They had no concept of general practice as an independent discipline and most did not read the College *Journal* seriously. We were seeking a revolution in attitudes with colleagues, often older than us. An aim of the course was to learn how it feels to be an adult learner. We gave them the chance to practise teaching with volunteer trainees. We drew parallels between the teaching process and the clinical process in general practice and taught that the doctor–patient and trainer-trainee relationships were similar and illuminated each other as described in my book *Training for General Practice* (DPG, 1982). At the end of the week, we gave them a big handout with notes and references.

Good working relationships and friendships were formed. Once, when teaching about Michael Balint to a very sceptical group, a course member suddenly gave me strong support and said he had regularly attended Balint groups himself in London, driving up and down from Cornwall! This was Geoffrey Smerdon – one way of finding a new course organiser. If human history is a race between the catastrophe of the GPs' situation and education, we were providing the education.

Deep emotions were sometimes released. Once, a trainer alone with me said, with tears in his eyes, how our course had transformed his attitude to general practice and given him new respect for and enjoyment of the job. After one trainers' course I got a phone call from the wife of one of the course members. "I want to thank you" she said, "for sending my husband back a different man!......We were drifting apart and I was thinking of divorce and now he is sensitive again – like the man I married!" Then she started crying and rang off.

It was possible, but difficult, to lead standards from London. The alternative was to develop standards in the regions. Donald Irvine in the Northern region was the first in Britain to secure the policy that all trainers should hold the MRCGP.

New Regional Adviser Organisation 1983

Michael Lennard retired in March 1983. The Postgraduate Dean, now Michael Roberts, said that as I was a full regional adviser, I was the obvious successor. However, I was anxious as I knew the Southwestern region and its GP training better than anyone. It is the longest region in England, spread over 250 miles. I thought I could not do the job as it needed to be done. Lennard had had great difficulty in coming westwards, hence my own appointment.

Moreover, the two regional adviser model had worked very well, so why change it? I devised a completely new structure which would have three full regional advisers in the South West region: one four-session per week adviser for Gloucester, Avon and Somerset, one with four sessions for Devon and Cornwall, and a third regional adviser with just two sessions per week, who would be senior to the other two. This one would have responsibility for relating to the Dean, speaking for the region on all relationships outside the region and chairing the Regional General Practice Education Committee. The total was only ten sessions, i.e. less than one 11 session whole-time equivalent. Michael Roberts quizzed me hard on this as there was no UK precedent. He was brave enough to approve it and then appointed me to the all-regional role.

Two adviserships were advertised and competitive appointments made of Roddy Hughes for Gloucester, Avon and Somerset and Keith Bolden for Devon and Cornwall. Both appointments were extremely successful and I was fortunate to have two such colleagues. Roddy led his half of the region by example with quiet and effective standard setting and a good eye for developing GPs. Keith Bolden was also a good manager and developed high-level teaching skills with expertise in transactional analysis and the MBTI. (Chapter 13, Department/Institute of General Practice story). I chaired the three-adviser group, which met quarterly before the RGPEC meeting to ensure close co-ordination.

I was co-opted to the South West NHS/Universities Liaison Committee, the first time a GP had been present since 1948. It had powerful people on it like the Chair of the Regional Health Authority and the Vice-Chancellor and Dean of the University of Bristol with the Regional Medical Officer. I was intrigued that meetings took place as if general practice did not exist. RHAs had no responsibility for general practice and ignored it. The NHS was equated with hospital practice. My chance to speak came only in response to asides; for example: "All these patients GPs keep sending in!" I could then report the national statistics, i.e. that GPs were only referring 5% of the patients they saw. These facts made an impact, as they were quite new to that group.

I listened to the language, as GPs practise what was later called narrative medicine (Greenhalgh and Hurwitz, 1999). A recurring phrase was: "If there are 100 GPs there will be 100 different opinions." Why did they think this? Gradually it became clear they had no evidence, but all of them believed this firmly! Did it matter? I worked out that such a belief was a good excuse for not engaging with general practice and taking no notice of it (Just GPs). After a few years I became accepted in this committee. I was in effect "Mr General Practice," as they realised I was head of the only university department of general practice in the region, the all-Regional Adviser in General Practice in the University of Bristol and was the recent Chair of two RCGP faculties.

Unusually I was invited to join the regional NHS officers on a visit to Professor Donabedian's university department in Ann Arbor, Michigan, USA, to study quality assurance. My stock rose as none of them had heard of Donabedian but I told them I had read his classic article on structure, process and outcomes (Donabedian, 1966) and had incorporated this thinking into our GP trainer assessment system. Also, I had edited and published a book, *In Pursuit of Quality* written around him by the RCGP (Pendleton *et al.*, 1986). This US visit illustrated the aphorism that much of the value of meetings occurs outside the meetings themselves. I learnt nothing about quality assurance, but the long flights and numerous meals over three days were invaluable in cementing working relationships at the top of the regional NHS.

Martin Reynolds, Regional Medical Officer, soon asked me to lay on a tour of general practices. He stayed in our home for two nights and I drove him around Devon visiting practices providing quality of care and enthusiasm, including rural and inner-city practices. I discussed many of the principles and facts about general practice. We developed a warm working relationship. However, he soon left for a job in another region. You can't win 'em all!

Regional Plan for General Practice 1984

In 1984, I realised that a regional plan was needed for general practice. I therefore wrote one, building it around the academic need for two secure university departments of general practice. I took it to the RGPEC. It was approved with little discussion. One leading member asked me why I had written it. He said he thought it was a waste of my precious time and it would not lead to anything useful. I realised how poorly trained many GPs were in leadership and management. I was isolated in my own committee.

Michael Roberts took the plan to the regional Postgraduate Medical Education Committee, which he chaired. The predominantly specialist members were not interested and were familiar with regional plans in their specialties. The small number of GP members had all approved it previously in the RGPEC. "That was a non-event," one of them said to me. "Not at all," I said. "It was a key step. Now Michael can send it to the Regional Authority." That was the point. He did and the Southwestern Regional Health Authority endorsed it. It became formal policy of the NHS in the South West. This ensured support from successive regional medical officers, a commission to write a planning document. Crucially, it led to a new charity forming with profound consequences, as later, the South West regional authority produced £800,000 to implement it (Chapter 15, South West General Practice Trust story).

I paid great attention to the RGPEC. This was a strong, regional committee with representatives from both the two RCGP faculties, all the local medical committees, and every vocational training scheme in the region. The Medical Postgraduate Dean always attended. It met quarterly, and travel expenses were refunded by the regional health authority. I sought to build it up as much as possible. All decisions on standards and criteria for the appointment of trainers were taken in the RGPEC as were all decisions on which GPs were to be appointed or not appointed as trainers. In later years, the Committee delegated approvals to the regional advisers, but decisions not to appoint or not to reappoint were always taken by the full Committee.

Declining to (re)appoint a GP as a trainer caused a stir. We had inherited trainers appointed under a previous system by local medical committees with no educational criteria. Those early trainers often saw trainees as free assistants and did not hold with the new educational approach. They often refused to comply with the new criteria and when it received reports of this the RGPEC declined to re-appoint them. As some were influential GP leaders this was talked about. Word got round that we were serious. All trainers had a right of appeal to a central body but our documentation was so tight that in 25 years we had only one appeal. This widened the gap between general practice and hospital practice, where it was assumed that all consultants could and should teach and removing teaching privileges from a consultant was unheard of. I summarised some of these developments in the *BMJ* (DPG, 1984a).

After practice visits we updated tables in the regional office in Exeter where the percentage of trainers with each feature was recorded. It was gratifying to see steady progress. I initiated a succession of innovations such as having two trainee representatives with full voting rights, one from each end of the region. Having such experience and real responsibility can be formative. One of those trainees was Andrew Blythe, now a senior medical educator in the Bristol Medical School. We were also early in having a patient representative.

We developed a system for grading GP records on how well they were put in order. Thus, we steadily raised the standards for new trainers until eventually every new trainer had to have all their medical records in chronological order. A positive finding was that the non-training practices, over which we had no jurisdiction, soon followed suit. A major advance was to categorise this standard. The committee agreed that all the regional standards were minimal, so that every trainer had to have all of them. However, once 51% of trainers had some feature, we categorised it as a 'usual standard.'

By continually disseminating how many trainers had these standards the trainers were steadily informed about how their colleagues were developing and were quietly educated on standards. This ensured quality improvement. When some special arrangement or facility was found we identified this as a 'good idea' and disseminated these as well. South West trainers were thus continually learning from their peers. It was a pleasure watching good ideas move to being 'usual' standards and then to be mandatory standards over several years. This was a standards escalator producing slow but steady improvements in standards, at a pace the profession could handle and support.

Sir William Osler remarked that postgraduate doctors move to where there is intellectual energy and interest, so I closely watched GP recruitment as trainees in the 1980s could choose where to train. In 1985, the Southwestern region was the eighth largest among 14 NHS regions for the number of "unrestricted general practitioners" but had 166 of 1,758 GP trainees, the largest number GP trainees of any English region (*OHE*, 1987).

A *BMJ* article listed a league table of all UK regions of GP vocational training classified by their pass rate in the MRCGP (Wakeford *et al.*, 1993). As the MRCGP was the accepted national endpoint for vocational training this was one measure of the quality of teaching. Severn was placed in the top six regions in the UK, and Devon and Cornwall was top in the UK. This was powerful national recognition. Some big city regions and their advisers were not happy, as some complacency was punctured. The table was included in the *RCGP Members' Reference Book* 1994. This was a triumph for the Devon and Cornwall GP trainers who were often teaching in isolated rural practices.

The regional plan for GP education underlined the need for two properly resourced university departments of general practice. With the plan formally approved the three regional advisers initiated discussions on founding a charity. Since 1983, I had responsibility for the whole region. I came round to the idea of forming one registered charity with two aims: to establish a GP department at Bristol and secure the finances of the Exeter department. The charity was launched (Chapter 15, South West General Practice Trust story).

The new Regional Medical Officer was Alastair Mason. He understood the importance of general practice. He wanted to follow up the regional plan and took the idea to the regional primary care committee, chaired by Michael Hall, of a more detailed plan for the development of general practice/ primary care in the Southwestern region. It was agreed that a planning document be written, with an all-regional perspective. The Exeter Department of General Practice was commissioned to write it, without a fee, but with agreement that the South West Regional Health Authority would pay publication and circulation costs. This made it possible for the plan to be negotiated across the region.

I wrote the plan filling it with national and regional references, which I had in my files. The Regional Primary Care Committee was happy and initiated a consultation process sending it to the RGPEC, both the RCGP faculties, and all the local medical committees in the region. I submitted it privately to the assessors of the *Occasional Papers*. We received many comments, but they were virtually all on minor points; Michael Hall and I accepted them all as none of them affected the main policies of the paper. The RCGP assessors recommended the paper as an *Occasional Paper*. The RMO honoured his agreement, paying for all the printing costs for *Occasional Paper 52, Planning Primary Care* (DPG, 1992c) and reimbursing the costs of distributing it to all GP organisations in the South West region. As *Planning Primary Care* was agreed after widespread consultation and was formally approved, I never heard anyone say again: "For every 100 GPs there are 100 opinions."

Just One GP Registrar?

Michael Roberts always treated me fairly making me an Associate Medical Postgraduate Dean and often involving me in specialist medicine. Once I was on a group allocating a new block of anaesthetic registrars. I was irritated as the DH had arbitrarily given anaesthetics a year's extra training, whilst the needs of general practice were much greater. The 1992 NHS executive letter on quotas for registrars (Walford, 1992) was the worst example I had seen of how the NHS discriminated against GPs. It outlined how the NHS and specialist academic specialist medicine were intertwined in providing as many as 4,617 paid registrar training posts in specialist medicine in the NHS with not one for general practice (Just GPs). I sat silently all afternoon whilst the allocations were decided. At the end, Michael asked if I had anything to say? I said: "As the representative of the largest branch of the medical profession it would be nice if we had just one GP specialist registrar!" There was an uncomfortable silence, which Michael broke by saying, "OK, we'll give one place to general practice." All agreed and I thanked them. Two days later, London officials telephoned me. Whitehall rules prevented even one registrar going to general practice.

Although this protest failed, I was learning how systems worked which helped with the Distinction awards (Chapter 39). The big picture was that a few GPs, mainly professors and regional advisers by the late 1980s/early 1990s, were, for the first time since 1948, penetrating the NHS power structure and were seeing key information that general practice had never seen before.

In May 1994 I was elected Chairman of the JCPTGP. This empowered the Southwestern region as I reported fully all the big developments, decisions and new ideas to the RGPEC, the trainers and course organisers. This made it easier for local colleagues to prepare for changes (Chapter 29, JCPTGP story).

Directors of GP Education 1996

In the mid-1990s a senior DH official told the regional advisers that the DH was planning to take over the postgraduate deaneries. The setting was CRAGPIE, the Conference of Regional Advisers in General Practice in England and not the UK Conference of Regional Advisers, as the latter included advisers from Northern Ireland, Scotland, and Wales. This proposal was for England only.

When postgraduate medical deans were first established after World War II, they were placed in medical schools. They were usually part-time, all consultants, and usually accountable to the dean of the medical school. Their salaries were reimbursed by the NHS through the regional health boards (later regional health authorities). Mostly, they had great autonomy. In 1972–1973, when regional advisers in general practice were established, they were appointed in deaneries with the postgraduate dean as head of department. All but one, including me in 1975, had contracts with a medical school; for me, the University of Bristol. The exception was the East Anglian Regional Health Authority, which employed its deanery staff directly.

There was an obvious reason for placing these deaneries and posts in medical schools since they involved organising postgraduate medical education, and education is a core function of universities. Medical schools provided undergraduate education up to qualifying medical degrees, most commonly MB BS or equivalent. Universities and medical schools also provided higher postgraduate qualifications like masters' degrees and doctorates. Importantly, the universities are also the main source of research in the UK, so placing postgraduate deaneries in institutions where research was being done ought to foster the spread of new knowledge. In addition, many believed in a continuum of education with undergraduate and postgraduate education fitting together. Finally, universities have a tradition of independence and inculcating rigorous thought based on facts and evidence.

The postgraduate deaneries in England, Northern Ireland, Scotland and Wales grew and flourished. In particular, they successfully developed postgraduate training for general practice and built it into a comprehensive national system for the largest branch of medicine in only ten years, between 1972 and 1982. This system certainly was not broken, so why fix it? And why only England and not in the other three nations? Several pressures were operating.

First was the constant wish of both politicians and the civil service for control. The desire for control is in the DNA of senior civil servants. The deaneries ran on public, taxpayers' money, so the piper could call the tune. Such control was emerging in other walks of life sometimes to a remarkable degree. At this time civil servants decided how many places to fund in each British university and then devised financial penalties for any university that over or under recruited. The cult of management was further developed in England than in Scotland where education was more valued. Government is functionally closer to institutions in Scotland and personal contacts are stronger. Many Scots in top jobs have attended one of only five leading Scottish universities. A consensus can be built across Scotland in the same way that we built a consensus across the Southwestern region. The population of Scotland is similar to a big English region. However, in England, London politicians and civil servants are more remote from professional leaders around the country.

Secondly, in my view, the universities unwisely provoked the DH by charging on-costs. Of course, if university medical schools are paying staff, supplying accommodation and dealing with employment problems, then there is a real cost. The principle of an on-cost charge was reasonable; the issue was its size. From the early days the regional health boards/authorities paid an on-cost charge. By the mid-1980s, when as the Adviser for the South West and building good links with the regional health authority, I became concerned at the size of on-cost charges. Michael Roberts and I discussed this and he sought moderation. Then British universities, led by Universities UK, decided that universities should charge full on-costs, at 40%. This was implemented so the NHS bill for deaneries rose sharply. The decision about what percentage to charge was far above my pay grade or the Dean's. I doubt if those universities analysed what they had, what it was worth, and what they stood to lose.

What the medical schools had was valuable: huge contacts with the medical profession at all levels, and much goodwill (quantified in the South West General Practice Trust story, Chapter 15). After the DH moved nurse training schools into universities, new possibilities for collaboration between the health professions within universities emerged. Such possibilities had value to universities and should have been reflected in on-costs lower than 40%. As a staff member of the NHS, I heard regional officials bemoaning on-costs and wondering what could be done. Doubtless such wonderings went up the line.

The third factor in the take-over was the dissolution of the regional health authorities and their replacement by regional outposts of the NHS executive. These were smaller bodies which were less independent, more managerial, and much more political outposts of Whitehall. The change-over followed the NHS Act of 1990 and I regretted it. In my view the UK was already too centralised, and more decisions should be taken locally in the regions. The old regional health authorities used to sort out many NHS decisions within their region using local knowledge. Diverting more decisions to London inevitably means decisions taken by less well-informed and more remote individuals.

Although on-cost payments might be the same whether paid regionally or nationally there were close working contacts and much sharing and collaboration within the region between the universities and the RHAs: witness the Southwestern RHA taking me to the US as a university-employed doctor. People knew each other. All this induced a give-and-take attitude and more sharing. Once RHAs were abolished, everything went to London. Suddenly the 40% overheads from all the regions appeared a big sum creating a new incentive to review. This was DH money. Could it be better spent? East Anglia did not pay overheads and paid the deanery staff directly, a precedent existed.

Postgraduate deans and regional advisers were to become civil servants for the first time and would become entitled to a civil service pension, which seemed a bit better than the NHS or University Superannuation Scheme (USS), which the advisers had. Pay would go up a bit and a new title was proposed – Directors of GP Education. Whole-time posts were offered, reversing the long-established tradition that regional advisers did clinical practice. Some advisers were keen to go whole-time as some did too little clinical practice to enjoy it.

I tested the water diplomatically as I was the adviser most critical of the proposals; but it became clear that there no real resistance from either the postgraduate deans or the regional advisers and indeed several advisers were positive about the proposal: better pay, a better pension, and a better sounding title. These were difficult meetings for me as I was 60 in 1995, the age when many civil servants retired, but was full of beans and looking ahead.

My reservations grew for three reasons. I believed the step to full-time working was fundamentally wrong. A regional adviser working in general practice, even part-time, is a professional medical leader. A full-time director of GP education doing no clinical practice is a medical manager with experience of general practice. Secondly, a civil servant owes a contractual duty to obey ministers (Hart, 1995) For me this is incompatible with fully independent professionalism. Finally, a national take-over of the whole of postgraduate medical education seemed to damage medicine as an independent profession. I had argued with colleagues for various standards in general practice, sometimes winning and sometimes losing, but always as clinician to clinician and because I believed the evidence. Directing colleagues because of a minister's policy did not appeal. The devolved nations did not pursue this civil service takeover so differences between England and the other nations grew.

However, with CRAGPIE agreeing, it was clear it was going to happen, and my thoughts turned to my personal position. Could I fend it off? By coincidence, the official managing the transition was called Ms Exeter. I took this to be a good omen! She came to see me and I explained that I thought it was inappropriate for me to become a civil servant. I produced two special factors. First, I was the elected Chair of the JCPTGP (Chapter 29, JCPTGP story) and it was essential that a professional leader of an independent, professional, regulatory body should not be accountable to a minister. I should be able to give independent advice and even disagree with ministers if necessary. I was the only doctor in the UK in that chairmanship. Naturally, she said she would have to take advice. I said I hoped I would not be made to resign, as it would be rather public. I fired a second barrel. I gave her a photocopy of a letter in the *Lancet* from a former permanent secretary of the DH, Graham Hart, which stated that professional leaders should not be civil servants, as they needed to have independence (Hart, 1995). I have often been teased in my family about keeping press cuttings. Twice in the 1990s, as here, they proved of great value.

These moves worked. My case was escalated to the Medical Director of the NHS Executive, Graham Winyard. He was well placed to decide as he had been the medical postgraduate dean for Wessex and we knew each other. He could judge if my resignation if forced, would make waves. He knew my age and that I would have to retire at 65. The compromise was that I would become Director of GP Education for the South West, retire at 65, and have one session per week of my pay moved from the University to the Regional office, i.e. the NHS, and would be treated in the regional office like other GP directors, seeing confidential documents, but would not become a civil servant. I would not have to sign the official secrets act or a civil service contract or have a civil service pension. Unlike all the other postgraduate deans and regional advisers in England, I had a few more precious years of full professional independence.

Being Externally Reviewed

In my new role, I sat on a management group in the South Western NHS Management Executive. The agenda did not interest me as the items were mainly about London-based political initiatives. Moreover, the meetings were held early in the morning in Bristol. I asked for permission to send a deputy and was refused, as I was the only GP in the region cleared to receive confidential civil service information. As this was not about developing general practice, I stopped going. An NHS official in the region set up a regional review of my work. I presumed that this was a management ploy to find some serious weakness or error that would force my resignation. The region appointed Jacky Hayden, the first British GP to become a medical postgraduate dean, and David Percy, my opposite number in Wessex, to be assessors. Both were national leaders and good choices. Of course, all three of us knew each other well in the small world of GP postgraduate education. The risks were high, and my reputation was on the line as both assessors were very able.

I wrote a long, heavily referenced paper setting out chapter and verse of what GP education in the South West region had achieved. Dynamic organisations need to benchmark their performance against the leading units nationally. I was always doing this. This paper was approved by the RGPEC. We had the greatest number of GP trainers in England, our management costs were the lowest of any English region, and our trainees had the highest pass rate in the MRCGP in the UK (Wakeford *et al.*, 1993). Jacky was on the Council of the RCGP, so we showed how the South West had more RCGP fellows by assessment than any other region. David Percy was interested in higher education, so I reported how the South West had established in Exeter one of the largest master's courses in primary care in Britain. Several GPs had MScs plus, unusually also several GPs had research master's degrees. Most trainer applications were arriving with a video of the doctor teaching mostly showing skilled teachers. General practice had quietly overtaken hospital-based teaching in both skills and attitudes.

The assessors were courteous and correct. I kept smiling. Their problem was that the South West was outperforming both their regions. Their report was factually correct and made administrative proposals. They thought I was over-concerned with benchmarking (!) and advised that after retirement I be succeeded by a full-time replacement. The official, who had set up the review, congratulated me on my knighthood saying (Chapter 35: President of the RCGP): "You keep surprising us, Denis!"

All leaders are exposed and putting one's head above the parapet always means being shot at sometimes. Once on the platform with 100 trainers, a critic, sitting at the back, asked if I recommended Berger and Mohr's (1968) *A Fortunate Man?* I sensed a trap but said yes. Then he said, in a carefully prepared ploy, that the GP in the book had committed suicide so he was no role model! Seeing me caught on the hop the whole room went quiet. I said that, as fellow GPs, we should have compassion for a colleague with severe depression. van Gogh's paintings were masterpieces, despite his suicide.

In 1996 the Exeter trainers' group, running the trainers' conference invited me to give the keynote lecture. My problem was that I had a key commitment in London that evening with the conference being held in North Devon. I urged the organiser to run very tightly to time so that there could be a long question session. I prepared as for a national eponymous lecture, analysing the blurring of boundaries in the new post-modern age (DPG, 1996). To my horror, the conference ran late so I started at the end of the morning. There was time for only one question and I had to race to Taunton for the London train. The trainers were not just disappointed, many were angry with me. The feedback was highly critical, not for my content, but for walking out on them. Whilst national lecturers often leave conferences after their lecture, those trainers saw me as one of their own. I had spent 21 years, 1975–1996, building them up; leaving without staying for lunch was discourteous. My commitment in London, chairing a seminar went well so both my tasks for that day were completed; but process trumps task and for once my multiple roles clashed seriously. It was 21 years before another Exeter group ran that conference, and with no memory of 1996, invited me to deliver the keynote lecture in 2017.

The Conference of General Practice Educational Directors (COGPED) in 1998 saw figures for the 23 regions in the UK. The South West had the fewest Director/Associate director/tutor sessions of any English region in relation to the GP population and the lowest cost to the NHS per doctor in England. The South West was the lead deanery in recruiting GP registrars in most of the previous ten years. It was the leading region in terms of NHS GPs holding the MRCGP (*RCGP Members' Reference Book*, 1996). For the RCGP fellowship by assessment (Chapter 24, Fellowship by Assessment story), the South West had 18% of all FBAs in the UK and was the lead region. Three GPs obtained MDs.

At my last meeting with the advisers and course organisers I warned them that postgraduate education was about to change. My successor, Michael Ruscoe was well prepared with both fellowship by assessment and an MSc. However, he was to have a full-time post and so would be a medical manager in Bristol and do no clinical practice. It would not be possible for him to lead on clinical standards. I encouraged them to support local GPs to obtain fellowship of the RCGP by assessment, to encourage GPs to obtain higher degrees, and to ensure that clinical standards were fostered locally. Clinical development needed running medical audits. As I finished some were in tears.

Regional Advisers as a Group

There is no academic analysis of the regional advisers in general practice, which is overdue. The role was unique to the UK as in other European countries, like the Netherlands, vocational training is run by the university departments. The regional advisers produced several national leaders. There were only 18 at any one time. Two were elected to the two highest posts in the medical profession: the Presidency of the GMC (Irvine) and the Chairmanship of the Academy of Medical Royal Colleges (DPG), and a third became Chief Inspector for General Practice of the Care Quality Commission (Field). Several became postgraduate deans. In the RCGP, eight were elected to the Chair of the Council, including remarkably five between 1976 and 1990 (Lawson, Donald, Irvine, Hasler, and DPG). The advisers were the dominant group in the JCPTGP in its 30-year existence. Three were secretaries (Irvine, Hasler and Styles) and six were chairmen (Lawson, Josse, Donald, Irvine, DPG and Toby). They were effectively the executive arm of the RCGP. Interestingly, they had relatively little executive authority and did not control hospital posts directly or control many resources. Their skills were negotiation and leadership The regional advisers developed a whole new postgraduate training system for the largest branch of the medical profession in only ten years, 1972–1982, whilst all working part-time. By 2018, it was the most effective postgraduate training system in the medical profession (Paice and Smith, 2009; Goldacre *et al.*, 2008; GMC, 2018).

I retired on 30 September 2000, virtually on my 65th birthday. The Regional General Practice Committee gave me a generous send off and a present of a still life, now in our hall. I knew how lucky I had been. I had been the first regional adviser in Devon and Cornwall for eight years and then had all-regional responsibility for general practice education for another 17 years. I was the longest serving GP adviser/director in the UK and the last regional adviser/director/postgraduate dean in England who was not a civil servant.

I had learned an enormous amount from enthusiastic colleagues, who had become some of the best medical teachers in Britain. It was a huge privilege.

15

The South West General Practice Trust 1985–2019

Fortis fortuna adiuvat (Fortune favours the brave)

Terence (190–159 BC)

The 1983 reorganisation of the regional adviser system in the South West region made me the senior Regional Adviser in General Practice with all-regional responsibility for policy (Chapter 14, Regional Adviser story).

I was also in-charge of the only general practice university unit in the Southwestern region at Exeter. I therefore had a seat on the South Western Regional Health Authority's (SWRHA) Liaison Committee with the two universities in the region. I was the first GP to sit on this since 1948 and the only one there. Here I got to know personally all the key movers and shakers in the SWRHA, notably the Chairman, Sir Bernard Seccombe, the Regional Manager, Pamela Mason, and the medical officers, Martin Reynolds and later Alastair Mason.

The outstanding academic problem for general practice in the region was the absence of an undergraduate department of general practice in its only undergraduate medical school, at Bristol. There were longstanding anti-GP attitudes, which I had experienced as an RCGP leader when a professor of medicine had said that a department of general practice in Bristol would be: "over his dead body!" ("Just GPs.") A later professor of medicine, Alan Read, showed no enthusiasm either. The Vice-Chancellor at Bristol was a distinguished mathematician, Sir John Kingman FRS, who was theoretically orientated and did not value general practice – the ultimate practical medical discipline.

It was therefore a daunting challenge for GPs outside the University, who were suffering from its policies. How do you make an independent Vice-Chancellor and an independent medical school change their minds?

A Regional Plan for General Practice

I realised that what was needed was a formal policy and so the first step was to write a regional plan for general practice. I did this and included in it the need to develop academic general practice in both the medical schools in the region and to develop the discipline with improved standards of care by general practice across the Southwestern region (Chapter 14, Regional Adviser story). I took the plan to the Regional General Practice Education Committee (RGPEC), which I chaired, where it was approved with little discussion. I did explain to all who were interested that the idea was to pass the plan upwards into influential places, but most GPs either did not think that it would work, or that if it did progress, nobody would do anything much about it. I was on my own.

However, the Medical Postgraduate Dean, Michael Roberts, took it to the Regional Medical Education Committee, which he chaired. I was on this committee. It was also approved there after desultory discussion from its predominantly specialist membership. However, I noted that many consultants on that committee understood what regional plans were about as some had been involved with plans for their specialties. I got all I wanted but was left anxious about how much better educated

DOI: 10.1201/9781032713601-19

the consultants were than my GP colleagues. I realised I needed to put in place additional education, specifically for GPs. These ideas later matured into fellowship by assessment (Chapter 23, Chairman of Council story) and a programme of research degrees for GPs (Chapter 13, Department/Institute of General Practice story).

Michael Roberts took the plan to the South West Regional Health Authority (SWRHA), now endorsed by the whole of educational medicine in the South West. This had three beneficial effects. First, it offered the RHA a coherent rational plan. Second, it showed that general practice had got its act together and had agreed a single, all-regional plan. Third, it provided policy authorisation for regional officers if any opportunities were to arrive.

University General Practice in Bristol and Exeter

By 1984 the Department of General Practice in Exeter was an obvious success; it had acquired a national reputation and had even been appointed by the World Health Organisation (WHO) to host a week-long seminar on the future of Europe's medical schools (Chapter 13. Department/Institute of General Practice story). However, its major weakness was that it had no secure funding and after 1983 it was a self-funding unit within the University of Exeter.

Clearly this was unsatisfactory and there was an urgent need to give it some financial security. With an energetic leadership team at Exeter, which included Keith Bolden and Michael Hall, the idea kept coming up of launching an appeal, which I supported, and it was becoming clear it would have to happen. At the same time, it was clear that nothing was happening to develop a university department of general practice at Bristol. There were some tentative suggestions about launching an appeal for that as well. These suggestions, however, were less well-developed, and the GP leadership in Bristol did not have an established organisation from which to launch it. I spent ages mulling over this problem. I judged an appeal for Exeter would be a relative success, but I had some anxieties about the Bristol appeal and whether it would do as well. The Exeter Department had built up strong working relationships with the GP trainers and training practices right across Devon and Cornwall. A failed appeal at Bristol might do harm in allowing the enemies of general practice to claim that there was no strong groundswell of support. Furthermore, to have two appeals running for academic general practice in one region at once would be needlessly competitive and would tend to drive Exeter and Bristol GP colleagues apart. Eventually, I decided the logic was to have one South West England all-regional appeal to support both academic departments of general practice in Bristol and Exeter simultaneously.

We had some careful discussions in the Exeter Department, where we all realised that there was no precedent for such an appeal and that it would seem odd to appeal simultaneously for two GP departments in two separate universities. We also realised that such an appeal might weaken the success of a straight appeal for the Exeter Department. Keith Bolden and Michael Hall were fortunately by now both associate advisers in general practice for the Southwestern region. Both were leading members of RGPEC and both had a deep understanding of, and contacts with, the Bristol general practice community. They were both generous and positive and both agreed to the wider view. We agreed to offer our Bristol colleagues a joint appeal. The key GPs in Bristol were Michael Whitfield, who had long campaigned for a university department there, and in key positions in the Deanery Roddy Hughes, the Regional Adviser in General Practice for Gloucester, Avon, and Somerset and Dick Bruce, Associate Adviser in the northern half of the region. They welcomed a joint appeal.

I consulted privately with some senior colleagues in academic general practice, mainly professors of general practice. They were universally opposed to the idea. One professor of general practice told me that it was simply silly to appeal to GPs, who were independent contractors, to raise funds for universities when they had no responsibility to do so. This was disappointing advice, which made me rethink my position but in the end it was a matter of belief. I believed in academic general practice and I had personal experience of the strong working relationships that the Exeter Department had made, particularly with GP trainers. One wife rang me after a GP trainers' course for making her husband so much more sensitive and in tears she thanked us for saving her marriage. I judged GPs would support us in our hour of need. This advice, however, explains why the SWGPT is unique.

A Registered Charity

We carefully mulled over the structure of the appeal, as it could have taken several different forms. A registered charity looked by far the most satisfactory, as it would be legally separate from both universities and we could ensure GP control. If it was part of either university, there was danger that the university hierarchy might take control or take the funds (as happened later to GP funds in Exeter). It would also be easier to have a single registered charity if it were to relate to two different universities. I took advice and was told about a local solicitor (Adrian Miller) who was interested in charities and charity law. Adrian was good to work with and soon offered us a draft trust deed to discuss. The legal process of setting up a registered charity was not difficult. However, the politics of who the Chair and the Trustees should be was exquisitely sensitive and would determine the success or failure of the appeal. I used my national contacts to approach Lord Richardson, who had just retired as President of the General Medical Council. He knew me a bit as he had seen me speaking at national meetings but he had no record of being involved with GP organisations, and I doubted if he would accept the chairmanship. However, to our great pleasure he did, and he proved an outstanding first Chairman.

We carefully constructed a team which would balance the Bristol and Exeter halves of the region. We had Trustees from Cheltenham in the east and Padstow in the west as we knew how areas distant from main centres feel cut off and excluded. We were pleased to have the two leading consultants in medical education in the region: Michael Roberts FRCS, Medical Postgraduate Dean, and David Mattingly FRCP, Director of the Exeter Postgraduate Medical School. The initial Trustees were Lord Richardson (Chairman); Keith Bolden, Exeter; Dick Bruce, Cheltenham, Gloucester (Honorary Treasurer); Frederick Difford, Bristol; Kenneth Gay, Padstow, Cornwall; Michael Hall, Shebbear, North Devon; Roddy Hughes, Bristol; David Mattingly, Exeter; Denis Pereira Gray, Exeter (Honorary Secretary); Michael Roberts, Bristol; and Michael Whitfield, Bristol. We signed the deed on 22 May 1985.

I drafted a letter, approved and signed by all the Trustees, and sent to all general practices in the Southwestern region launching the charity and requesting donations. We requested covenanted donations as additional tax relief would greatly increase their value and would also give the trustees stability in planning. We sent the agreed regional plan, a covenant form, a pre-addressed, stamped reply envelope, with a covering letter signed by all the Trustees.

We knew there were many GPs mainly orientated either to a department of general practice at Bristol or to the existing one at Exeter. We wanted to capitalise on strong local feelings but also to give the Trustees as much discretion as possible. We gave donors three options: donate so that all their funds would be used to support a new department at Bristol; donate so that their funds would be used in support of the existing department at Exeter; or donate to a general fund where the Trustees would have discretion to use the funds as seemed best in their judgement.

I always slept well, and difficult decisions have not kept me awake. However, accepting the Honigsbaum article for the College *Journal* in 1972 (Chapter 9, Journal story) had given me a bad night as I foresaw the coming storm. Now, 13 years later in October 1985, I slept badly again after the letters were posted. If the appeal fell flat and drew only derisory sums, I knew all the Trustees would be damaged professionally, but I was "Mr General Practice" in the region at the time and my reputation would be damaged most of all.

Response to the Appeal

The response from GPs was quite magnificent and beyond our expectations. Letters and cheques poured in and many were for £500 a year, covenanted for five years. This sum in 1985 was equivalent to £1,535 today. Many practices were giving the Trust the current equivalent of £7,500 over five years and we would get tax relief in addition. We sought £250,000 and approximately succeeded. I suddenly had a major job on my hands as Honorary Secretary writing heartfelt letters of thanks! Fortune favours the brave. Donations came from all parts of the Southwestern region. The biggest sum was to support a new Bristol department, but a significant proportion was donated to the fund for the Trustees' general discretion. This was empowering for the Trustees, because it indicated both great generosity from GPs, who were much less well paid in 1985 than nowadays, but also trust in our leadership.

After the launch, my lobbying in the NHS Universities Liaison Committee was vigorous. I kept saying that as GPs themselves had raised so much for a department for which they had no responsibility, that it was shameful the authorities were leaving a gap in Bristol. I repeatedly stated that Bristol was "falling behind" other medical schools in the UK. Members of the RHA were impressed by what the GPs had achieved and that a single co-ordinated plan had been agreed and now had significant resources to support it. All this convinced the Regional Chairman, Sir Vernon Seccombe (1928–2014) and the Regional Authority. DH policy increasingly supported academic general practice. It then was ahead of many university medical schools in appreciating the role of general practice and its significance in the NHS.

One day, Sir Vernon told me that he had negotiated over £800,000 to initiate a university department of general practice at Bristol. However, he was near the end of the financial year and the financial rules of the NHS did not allow funds to be carried over financial years. "No problem," I said with a smile. "Registered charities are not bound by such rules." The RHA transferred over £800,000 to the SWGPT on the understanding that we would use it for the Bristol University Department. So good were the working relationships and so great the mutual trust that the Regional Authority staff never even asked the SWGPT to guarantee that the money would go to Bristol.

The Trustees held a unique event at a midpoint in the region and invited both Vice-Chancellors of the two universities to attend: Sir John Kingman (1939–) FRS for Bristol, and Dr (later Sir) David Harrison (1930–) for Exeter. Both virtually had to come. Lord Richardson courteously handed over two cheques, a very big one for Bristol. Sir John Kingman then had to say in public, when accepting, that he would establish a department of general practice in Bristol, which he did. We treasured that moment. Initially, Michael Whitfield led this department, but a chair was advertised and Debbie Sharp appointed. Thus, complete victory was achieved. The GPs across the Southwestern region can take great pride as it was their donations that conquered the Bristol citadel.

Continuing Role of the SWGPT

Although forcing Bristol to accept a department of general practice was always a major objective, the more general objectives of the SWGPT were to enhance and develop academic general practice throughout the region, particularly through the Bristol and Exeter medical schools. The SWGPT continues 39 years later giving both university departments flexibility. They can apply to use it to maintain staff between grants or to fund staff for particular roles. Trust funds contributed to two general practice buildings, one in Bristol and one in Exeter and supported innovative educational events in the UK and abroad. The Trust has enabled some junior doctors to attend conferences. Several publications have acknowledged Trust funding. Although currently, interest rates are low, in the past they produced useful sums. Professional investment advice increased the funds. Endowment funds have advantages including receiving interest and being a vehicle for donations, although registered charities must comply with charity law. The SWGPT has managed on only two trustee meetings a year and clear delegated policies. More endowed charities for general practice are needed.

There has been no fundraising since, but other funds became available enabling 'reserve funds' to be established for specified functions. A profit was made on a trainee conference in Exeter, which was generously transferred to the SWGPT as a reserve fund to support GP trainees. Numerous educational GP meetings have been funded and also equipment. The SWGPT has provided flexibility for both GP researchers and teachers in a time of tight budgets. A reserve fund was established to honour Michael Lennard, the Bristol GP who was the first Regional Adviser in General Practice in the South West.

The SWGPT operated with minimal expenses. It never had a full-time member of staff. The Trust's administrator for many years was Joy Choules, who worked with Jill and me for years in the RCGP *Journal* office in our home. She became a member of staff in Professor John Campbell's Department of Primary Care in Exeter, whose support for the Trust was much appreciated.

After Lord Richardson (1910–2004) died, the Trust had three further Chairmen: John Clubb, a GP from Oxford, Professor David Mant OBE, Oxford, and currently, Professor Roger Jones OBE. There have been three honorary treasurers: Dick Bruce, Fred Difford and the current one, Philip Evans of Exeter. The trustee membership changed over the years but the balance between Bristol and Exeter, east and west was maintained. The funds as I left were about £750,000.

I was the last Founding Trustee and helped to sustain the memory of the great generosity of working GPs in the region who made it all happen. I retired as a Trustee and the Honorary Secretary on 30 September 2019 after 34 years. Joy Choules stood down too. The Trustees gave us both generous presents and hosted a lunch for Joy and me in 2021 asking me to report how the Trust had been formed and to make some suggestions for the future. I offered the thoughts in Chapter 46, Unfinished Campaign story.

Section V

16

The Practice 1976–1986

Medicine is not only a science, but the art of letting our own personality interact with the individuality of the patient.

Albert Schweitzer (1875–1965)

After a difficult time in the practice with the big building conversion, a partner leaving, and my father dying, the next 10 years were about regrouping and developing.

After my father died, we interviewed Russell Steele, who came with his wife Kath to lunch with Jill and me in our home. There was a problem as their dog and our rabbit did not get on very well! I appointed him as an assistant with a view and as a partner in January 1976. He became a stabilising anchor in the practice for almost 25 years. He was a committed member of the College, became a GP trainer, and worked hard as an examiner for the MRCGP.

I published in the *JRCGP* Julian Tudor Hart's (1975) prize-winning essay on hypertension. He obtained the blood pressure of every patient, raising our practice's expectations and fusing clinical and population medicine.

Vocational Training 1975–1981

This was the decade when the Practice became heavily involved in GP training. Trainees then chose their training practice. Our first trainee was Adrian Kratky at the end of 1975. I was the only trainer to start with and set up a system in which trainees had a one-hour tutorial every week with telephone-protected time. Each trainee was given a half-day each week for a project, which was a powerful motivator, normalising a trainee project, and underlining its importance. The computerised practice records provided a wonderful laboratory of information for trainee projects.

My most radical innovation was accompanying GP trainees on every night call. The trainee entered the house first, did the consultation with me watching silently, and we then went to the bathroom to discuss it; the trainee then completed the consultation. Although time-consuming for the GP trainer, night calls provided an ideal setting for education and sometimes empowerment. A night call often indicates fear in the family. The whole family is often present and the doctor has unusual control of time. It is an ideal setting to disentangle the physical, psychological, and social factors that make general practice so interesting. The trainee and I went together in one car and we often ended up in our kitchen over a hot drink for more discussion.

On one night call Angela Douglas commented that the GMC consisted mainly of older men. I thought highly of her and valued her intelligence, Could I help her to develop nationally? I suggested that she might stand for election as a member of the GMC. She said she would never be elected. Eventually she agreed to stand and I supported her candidacy as Chair of the RCGP Faculty, getting her jointly nominated with Michael Hall. RCGP members were asked to use the single transferable vote system and vote for these two in any order. When Michael was squeezed out, a big block of votes transferred from him to secure her election. West country GPs got their representative and Angela

DOI: 10.1201/9781032713601-21

became the youngest elected member in the history of the GMC (Chapter 31, GMC and GDC story). The trainees told me this night call teaching was unusually valuable and I believed it was particularly effective. I always intended to write it up, and certainly should have done so, as I did it for six years, but sadly it was one of the ideas that I did not complete.

The trainee project idea worked well. The first trainee audited my diabetic care in the *JRCGP*, which showed up significant deficiencies in my care of diabetes at that time (Kratky, 1977). A good number of subsequent trainees were also successful in both doing projects and getting them published: (Richard Westcott, 1977; Roger Peppiatt *et al.,* 1978; Clive Stubbings and Gowers, 1979; Roger Peppiatt, 1980; Angela Douglas, 1981; Ronalds *et al.,* 1981; Nicholas Bradley, 1981, 1983a; Mollie Donohoe and Philip Courtney, 1982; Lindy Colmer and DPG, 1983). I know of no other general practice in the UK that had nine GP trainees who authored 11 publications in the peer-reviewed literature over nine years.

Some of their research was influential. Richard Westcott first showed that patients with emotional problems had longer consultations (51 citations). Nicholas Bradley (1983a) showed how easy it was for children to obtain cigarettes, which led to a Home Office national crackdown and new notices in shops across England. Ronalds *et al.* (1981) found that trainees' satisfaction was significantly related to how many hours of teaching the trainers provided. I had 13 personal trainees – eight men and five women. Eight achieved publications (Appendix 3) and three obtained a distinction in the MRCGP. Many became friends.

One trainee was caught in the middle of a clash of opinions. We were relaxed and sitting together in our common room with a young consultant psychiatrist visiting at our weekly Friday lunch. A call came in from a woman in a 'phone box saying she was thinking of committing suicide. The trainee was first on call. The consultant said: "Let her sweat." For the only time in 38 years, as the trainer and second on call, I reacted sharply and raised my voice at the poor trainee: "Ignore him! Go straight away as an emergency!" The trainee looked at the consultant and back to me and then left without a word. After she had gone, I asked the psychiatrist how many of his patients had committed suicide. "None," he said. "Well," I said: "Don't give advice like that until you have had two suicides, like me, and beware of judging patients you have not seen!'"

Once Russell Steele had completed his trainer's course and shown that he was keen on teaching, I stood down as trainer. My last trainee, Mollie Donohoe in 1981, organised a delightful surprise party for me. I went with Jill to what I thought was going to be a supper with Mollie and her husband, Phil Courtney, but I found that Mollie had brought together most of my former trainees. It was a really special evening.

A Partnership Difficulty

A difficulty arose in the partnership about claiming of night call fees. GPs who did night calls were entitled to an item-of-service fee of about £40. However, the GP had to get the patient to sign a form, which was distasteful. One partner particularly disliked claiming these fees, finding it an unpleasant chore at the end of a night call and often did not do so. The other partners resented the loss of income as they complied and were entitled to a third share. After repeated discussions, no change occurred and I found myself in a partnership meeting with tensions rising and wondering how to sustain the partnership. I proposed that we changed the system so that the GP who actually did the night call was paid the whole fee rather than it going into the partnership pot. This was agreed and implemented the next morning. Problem solved.

Visitors

After our new premises had been completed, we were able to start inviting visitors and, in effect, showcase general practice. Two special features were the gracious consulting room with a view looking across to the Cathedral, which made a magnificent setting for discussions, and the quality assurance room where we could demonstrate a series of internal professional audits.

I used the growing number of contacts I was making in the region and in London, to invite colleagues to come and see the practice for themselves (Appendix 9). Visitors included the Medical Postgraduate Dean, Sir Brian Bailey, a chair of a Health Education Authority, and many senior colleagues. These visitors included David Ower (GP lead in the DHSS) and Sir Donald Acheson (Chief Medical Officer, DHSS) who stayed with Jill and me in our home, which helped build relationships and allow frank discussions in private. I was always grateful to Jill for willingly having a succession of strange doctors to stay.

Personal Lists

I became converted to personal lists in the early 1970s when I found that even with partners as close as I was with my father, with good personal and professional relationships, difficulties can arise when a single patient gets different advice from two GPs and it was unclear which GP was clinically responsible. Personal lists link every patient with a responsible GP, increase continuity and clarify clinical responsibility. We introduced personal lists on 1 January 1974 and all succeeding partners inherited the system. A major insight by Albert Schweitser is that in general practice we need to learn to integrate our personality with the individuality of the patient. That needs continuity.

However, the system was little understood, so I used the practice data to present the case for personal lists in my lecture to the North of England Faculty in Newcastle. This was when I coined the term "personal lists," a term now in general use in British general practice (DPG, 1979a). The Faculty also invited me to give the after-dinner speech when I teased Donald Irvine, the then young guru in that faculty, about turning the headquarters of the Royal College of General Practitioners into "the biggest branch surgery in the British Isles!"

On 16 February 1980, the regulations for vocational training were implemented, stopping untrained doctors entering general practice. Our assistant, Margaret Mitchell had worked for years with my father. The three partners asked her if she would like to be a partner. She accepted and became a partner just before the open entry gate to general practice closed.

As a partner her consultation rates were audited, like the other partners, and a graph displayed in our common room. Her patients consulted at about twice the rate of the three other partners, whose rates were similar. She asked about this at our weekly partners' lunch, which led to discussions about how often to bring patients back and techniques for empowering patients to look after themselves more. We discussed how some patients could become dependent on GPs. Even though she was in her late-50s, some of these were new ideas for her. Interestingly, the rate her patients consulted her fell steadily and after 18 months were indistinguishable from that of her three partners. I learnt that internal audit and peer discussion, in private, can be a powerful form of continuing medical education and that doctors in their late-50s are well capable of learning new consulting techniques and applying them. Private discussions of personal performance with trusted colleagues are the key.

In 1983, the WHO invited the Exeter Department of General Practice to host a week-long seminar on the future of European medical schools. (Chapter 13, Department/Institute of General Practice story). The deans all came to the practice. We put them in the big consulting room and gave a prepared seminar on the facts and figures about general practice. We emphasised the Alma Ata Declaration (WHO and UNICEF, 1978) and showed them detailed practice audit information from our practice computer. Those deans had never seen anything like it. However, there is no evidence that it influenced their medical school curricula.

Kieran Sweeney

After Margaret Mitchell retired, I was approached by Kieran Sweeney, an Exeter trainee who had recently completed the scheme where he had been exceptional. Once as a trainee he had asked for a year out to work in France. Knowing how strict the French authorities were, I blithely told him I would fix it if he got the necessary French consents. To my surprise he did, so I kept my promise and he worked for a year speaking French in hospitals and earning his keep playing the piano in cafés. This was a man with many talents. He arrived in 1986, the first partner vocationally trained in Exeter and the first to ask about research opportunities. I offered him the idea of studying broken continuity of care in general practice, which he subsequently did (Sweeney and DPG, 1995; 107 citations). This was the first ever study of discontinuity of GP care. Professor Barbara Starfield (1998) described it as "interesting" and it stimulated several studies in the USA on discontinuity (Kahana *et al.*, 1997).

Soon after Kieran arrived, an RCGP crisis pitchforked me into the Chair of Council (Chapter 22, Downs and Ups of Institutional Life). I had fully informed my partners about the impending change in the Directorship of the Medical School, but was only able to give them the two weeks' notice that I had myself of the College Chair. Fortunately, Russell, an active College examiner, understood how angry the examiners were and how serious the crisis was for the College. All three partners and the manager were very supportive, which I always appreciated.

17

The Medical Annual 1979–1987

Of all the needs a book has, the chief need is that it is readable.

Trollope (1815–1882)

The *Medical Annual* was a well-known textbook published annually by John Wright & Sons, Bristol when, in 1978, the publishers approached me and asked if I would write a chapter on general practice. This was not a new idea as the book had previously had a chapter on general practice written by Professor JDE Knox. However, I would be the first non-professorial GP and from a younger generation The Editors were establishment figures: Sir Ronald Bodley Scott FRCP (1906–1982) and Sir James Fraser Bt FRCS (1924–1997). Bodley Scott was a distinguished consultant physician on whose firm I had been a medical student at Bart's about 20 years before (Chapter 3, Medical Student story).

I wrote the chapter and, looking back, see my first words were "The discipline of general practice" (DPG, 1979b). This was in the 1979/80 volume of the *Annual*, which was then described as in its "ninety seventh year." I was asked to write the chapter again in the following four years.

Then, unexpectedly, I was approached for a meeting with the publishers, who told me that Sir Ronald had died suddenly in a car accident in 1982, just after he had edited the 100th anniversary volume. They asked if I would like to take on the whole book as Editor. Jill and I discussed the idea, which had been a surprise. The work was attractive as I enjoy writing and editing, and I would have the sole discretion in choosing who would write the different chapters. I thought it would be a substantial gain for general practice if this well-established book changed its orientation completely towards general practice. The other great advantage was that Jill and I could do it together and she could be named on the title page as Assistant Editor. We hoped we could identify interesting growing points in general practice and help our readers to be more informed, and hopefully better doctors.

The payment offered was moderate but was welcome, as all my College work was unpaid and we had four children at home with university costs still to come. I negotiated a satisfactory contract with John Wright, which gave me sole discretion on everything that mattered.

I re-orientated the book towards general practice and used the framework of the RCGP's classic book *The Future General Practitioner – Learning and Teaching,* published in 1972 (RCGP, 1972c). This divided general practice into five areas: (1) health and diseases, (2) human development, (3) human behaviour, (4) medicine and society, and (5) practice organisation. I hoped to reinforce the thinking in *The Future General Practitioner* and it would be a convenient framework.

By 1982, I was well placed to know who was who in British general practice, both the intellectual leaders and those who were up and coming, and who would be able to write good chapters. The second judgement to be made was always whether or not selected authors could be relied upon to deliver their manuscript on time. The aim was to produce a book that was interesting and readable, as Trollope noted, which would be relevant for thoughtful GPs, especially candidates for the MRCGP examination, and GP trainers. Hence, it had to contain either good summaries of important topics, or descriptions of new ones, and important new developments. Such developments could be clinical, organisational, political, or cultural. To ensure the books reflected the enthusiasm and dynamism of youth, I invited a good proportion of younger GPs to write.

DOI: 10.1201/9781032713601-22

First Edition 1983

The first volume to come out under our editorship was in 1983 and so was the 101st in the series. It was well produced as John Wright & Sons had agreed to increase the size of its pages and to give it a smart hard cover. Jill and I liked the new, more distinctive, presentation. The title was re-orientated to calendar years, whereas the first 100 editions had been across two years; i.e. my last chapter in the old style had been in the 1982–1983 volume.

There were 28 separate chapters running to 284 pages and included a professional index provided by the publishers. I wrote the preface explaining the new editorial plan and I also wrote two chapters myself, one of which was on training for general practice, drawn from my book of the same name (DPG, 1982). Similarly, the chapter on healthier children drew on the work I had done as co-convener of the College working party of that name (RCGP, 1982; Chapter 11, College Cabinet story). The main achievement was getting Sir George Godber (1983) to write a chapter on general practice. He was then recently retired as Chief Medical Officer for the Department of Health and Social Security and many consider him one of the greatest chief medical officers since the war. He had always been supportive of general practice and the College when in post. He was just as supportive in this chapter. He and I corresponded for years, usually with him sending me a list of books he thought I ought to read.

The authors were a mixed group and included several consultants, two of whom I had served with on the Healthier Children Working Party. Other consultant authors included two outstanding national leaders: Professor Michael Shepherd (1983) from the Institute of Psychiatry, who was the country's leading expert on the treatment of mental problems by GPs in the community. He concluded that: "the primary medical care team is the keystone of community psychiatry."

Chatting with him in the RCGP one day, I was intrigued to hear that this leading psychiatrist was jealous of the influence that Michael Balint had had in general practice. Although a leading epidemiologist, Shepherd was weaker on the human side of medicine and especially the doctor–patient relationship, on which Balint (1957) was so strong. I was so surprised that I said nothing. Epidemiologists prioritise numbers over people and groups over individuals. They therefore tend to undervalue the human side of medicine and the importance of individual patients and their relationships with their doctors. GPs are the lead standard bearers within medicine for a professional relationship with an individual patient as a person. As Professor of Epidemiological Psychiatry, Shepherd could never match Balint's (1957) fundamental insights into the GP–patient relationship, which have permanently empowered GPs.

We had a chapter by Professor Norman Tanner (1983), the national expert on human development. Jim McEwan (1983) on my Communications Division wrote on preventive medicine. The College was well represented by its President, John Lawson (1983) and by Colin Waine and Margaret Hammond (1983), College librarian, who wrote jointly on the literature of general practice. The College's leader on the examination, Professor John Walker (1983), wrote a chapter. A notable chapter was on patient participation by Peter Pritchard (1983), when the topic was still new, soon after I had initiated a patient group in the RCGP (Chapter 19, Communications Division story). Three younger authors had trained on the Exeter training scheme. One, Nick Bradley (1983b), wrote a thoughtful analysis on time in general practitioner consultations, linking the annual consultation rate and the average length of consultations, which has not been clarified even 40 years later.

1984 Edition

The 1984 edition had 25 chapters, of which I wrote three myself. I introduced the idea of writing a chapter surveying the events in general practice during the previous 12 months which were of academic, political, and social interest, including major GP appointments. With this "The Year in General Practice" (DPG, 1984b), I was introducing into the new format the chapter I had previously written each year for the old-style *Medical Annual*. My other chapters included one on auditing the amount of the personal preventive care provided in our practice (DPG, 1984c) and one on the World Health Organisation and general practice, enabling me to write about the Alma Ata Declaration (WHO and UNICEF, 1978). I had missed the significance of this declaration when editing the College *Journal* (DPG, 1984d).

Authors in this edition included the future RCGP President, Stuart Carne (1984). Marshall Marinker (1984) Director of the MSD Foundation, where I was on the Advisory Committee (Chapter 20, Experiences in the Executive), wrote on the development of video-recording and analysing consultations in general practice. A chapter on child development was written by Margaret Pollak (1984), who had been a GP before becoming a consultant paediatrician at King's College, London. Jill wrote a chapter, on the health of doctors' families, having chaired a session attended by 600 doctors at the World Conference of Family Doctors (WONCA) in 1980 and written an article in the *Journal of the Royal College of General Practitioners* in 1984 (Jill Pereira Gray, 1982, 1984). This attracted attention and led to her receiving several invitations to lecture on the subject around the country.

1985 Edition

The 1985 edition, which had 31 chapters, was the biggest of the five years.

The overview of the year in general practice continued. A highlight was a chapter by Lord Young of Dartington (1985; 1915–2002) one of the great innovators in post-war Britain. He had drafted the Labour Government's successful manifesto for the 1945 general election in Dartington, Devon and led the creation of the Open University. Another highlight was a chapter by Professor Desmond Pond (1985; 1919–1986), then the Chief Scientist to the Government and a former PRCPsych. On retiring he became one of my patients. This was the first edition of *The Medical Annual* with international authors, with chapters from Professor Chris van Weel (1985) from the Netherlands and Professor Yair Yodfat (1985) from Israel, both internationally distinguished academic family physicians.

Two British GP professors charting innovations were Hamish Barber (1985) from Glasgow, on higher university degrees for general practice, and Brian Jarman (1985) who had developed a computer programme enabling GP patients to determine what benefits they were entitled to. This increased uptake and he and I hoped that this innovation would roll out in general practices, especially in deprived areas. But sadly, it was not then followed up. Similar ideas were developed 30 years later. A College dinner led to a chapter by Mary Talbot (1985), Chair of the Practice Managers' Association. I gave encouragement to a group that needed all the support that it could get. One of my chapters suggested that general practices produce an annual report (DPG, 1985), which our practice did for years. This fosters forward planning still sadly lacking in general practice. I wrote two and a half chapters myself, sharing one on small groups (DPG and Bolden, 1985).

1986 Edition

One chapter by a GP, Edwin Martin (1986), on prison medicine, prepared me for a later role (Chapter 26, Prison Medicine story). Sally Fountain (1986), soon to marry Donald Irvine, wrote a chapter on management, as the General Manager for the RCGP. My two chapters were on AIDS, as I had been the only GP on the DH Expert Advisory Group on AIDS, and on "Nakedness in Medicine," which attracted considerable attention (DPG, 1986 a,b). I wrote a chapter jointly with Brian Jarman on the importance of GPs as examiners in the final examinations in medical schools (Jarman and DPG, 1986).

1987 Edition

In the 1987 edition I wrote the usual chapter on the year in general practice and two others. Other authors included two colleagues who were later elected both Chairman and also President of the RCGP: David Haslam (1987) wrote about behavioural problems in children. Michael Pringle's (1987) chapter was on assessing consultations in general practice. Sally (later Baroness) Greengross (1987) wrote on the care of the elderly. An unusual system of paying GP partners by personal lists was described by Robert Walton, a GP, and Brenda Sawyer (practice manager; Walton and Sawyer, 1987), whom I visited. We later used a modified version (Practice 1987–2000). My chapter on breast screening (DPG, 1987c) followed from being a GP on the Forrest Committee (1986c), which had recommended this.

In 1986/87 John Wright decided to stop the *Medical Annual*. The book had a loyal following, but they were not making as much as they wanted. They pressed us to make new arrangements. However, in the RCGP in 1987 I had suddenly become Chair of Council (Chapter 23, The Downs and Ups of Institutional Life). We would have had to resign anyway. I was elected Chair of the College on 10 February 1987, so the 1987 edition came out during my Chairmanship.

Summary (Appendix 4)

I wrote the review of general practice chapter for four years, 1979–1980 to 1982–1983 and in the four years 1983–1987 that Jill and I edited. The five books averaged 27 chapters. Of the 137 chapters, I wrote 13 alone, two were written jointly, and Jill wrote one. We wrote 11% of the content over the years. Eight authors became College/Faculty presidents, including Sir Desmond Pond PRCPsych, and six became PRCGPs: Carne, Drury, Haslam, Lawson, Pringle, and me. Jim McEwan (1940–) later became President of the Faculty of Public Health Medicine and 18 years later, in the most important election of my life, voted for me (Chapter 38, Chairman Academy story).

Professorial authors included Paul Freeling, David Haslam, Conrad Harris, Peter Higgins, Brian Jarman, Mike Pringle, Chris Van Weel, John Walker, and Yair Yodfat. The first five separate chapters in the original format of the *Medical Annual* entitled "The year in general practice" (1979–1980 to 1982–1983), with the four chapters of the same title in the 1984–1987 editions, form a contemporary record of general practice in the UK over almost a decade. It proved possible to identify growing points in general practice. However, several have not been followed up as hoped. GPs are still the branch of the medical profession with the smallest proportion of higher university degrees, and practices still do not have computer programmes informing poorer patients of their social security entitlements. Most general practices still do not produce annual reports, and general practice is still not taught and examined in medical finals as a distinct, research-based discipline.

Although the fee Wrights paid authors was not exciting, virtually everyone accepted and delivered their manuscripts on time. It was a privilege to be able to take a helicopter view of general practice and to invite colleagues, senior and junior, generalists and specialists alike, to explore the growing points in general practice: clinical, organisational and societal. Jill and I enjoyed our five years working together on the *Medical Annual*.

18

Publications Committee 1980–1981

Annual reports help planning, transparency and accountability

Denis Pereira Gray (1985) *Medical Annual*

On 1 January 1981, I had left the Editorship, which had dominated my professional life for a decade. Having been elected a member of the Council for the first time, rather than being an observer, a few weeks earlier at the 1980 AGM, I was now eligible for the first time to hold a committee chairmanship and Council elected me Chair of the Publications Committee. The new Editor of the *Journal*, Simon Barley, was also on the committee ex-officio. To ensure proper governance we agreed that as Honorary Editor of RCGP publications I would be accountable to the Chair of Council.

Annual Reports of the College

The College had always published an annual report. John Hunt edited all the early ones himself and set a standard of meticulous recording of facts and referencing. He was succeeded as Honorary Editor of the annual reports by John Burdon, a colleague I knew well because he worked in Torbay, Devon.

When Burdon indicated that he wished to stand down, I started to think seriously about the College's annual report in my capacity as Chair of the Publications Committee.

I have always been an obsessive reader and I noticed advertisements of a new development in the publishing world, whereby commercial publishing companies undertook quite expensive publishing in exchange for the right to sell and place advertisements in these publications. I pursued the possibility with a firm called Sterling publications. At the time Penny was looking at medical schools and I fitted this in with taking her to Bart's where my father and I had been students. Both she and I expected that she would wait in a waiting room, but the Managing Director of the firm invited her to come into the room whilst we talked. This was the only occasion in my life when I did serious negotiating on behalf of the College with one of our children watching.

I was able to establish that Sterling Publications was prepared to publish the whole of the RCGP's annual report, including the reports of all the faculties, and bear all the postal costs to every fellow, member, and associate of the College. The price was them obtaining and including both advertisements and advertorials, which are commissioned text plugging some commercial products. I spent much time clarifying the degree of control that the College would have on both.

Sterling was prepared to offer me an absolute veto on all advertisements and advertorials. As the College's annual report was costing the College about £30,000 a year to publish and distribute to every member there were big financial gains to be had. I knew that prominent advertisements would be a high price to pay, but the degree of College control looked attractive. Then it emerged that Sterling would want articles on various clinical topics, as pegs on which they could hang their advertisements. We negotiated that the College Editor would be able to choose the authors of such articles and, moreover, that Sterling would pay them the then the current commercial rate. Sterling understood that they

DOI: 10.1201/9781032713601-23

would have to pay the Editor, and I had to manoeuvre carefully so that they did not pay me and I did not become their employee.

I suggested that they paid the College directly and was confident that this editorial fee could go towards paying for Jill's job in our home. Finally, there was a need for an Editorial Board, and it was easy to agree that this would be chaired by an RCGP figure. Colin Waine was the obvious choice as he was active in the publications committee and soon succeeded me as its chair. It was agreed and that Michael Summers and I would both be ex-officio members of the Editorial Board of the reference books and this Board would meet annually in the College.

A final development was the possibility of printing the entire college membership in the book. This was attractive because it would let College members see their name in print, be a quick way of letting College members check who was and who was not in the College and was an open and transparent process.

I got this offer confirmed in writing and then took it to the College officers. One or two were slightly incredulous, but the key figure was Douglas Garvie, the Honorary Treasurer, who was shrewd and with whom I got on well. He did a serious job in talking through the issue of editorial control and it was of course his budget that was going to benefit to the tune of £30,000 a year. He supported it strongly and the officers approved it unanimously.

So the annual *RCGP Members' Reference Book* was born, and the first edition was sent to all College members in 1982. I was its Honorary Editor until 1997 and estimate that this system saved the College at least £750, 000.

The Work of the Reference Books

The *RCGP Members' Reference books* were big, typically 450 pages. There was much work for Jill and our secretary in the Exeter office in monitoring and chasing all the items to be reported. Each section of the College reported as part of the Council and all the 33 faculties did so too. All this meant Jill was building good relationships with the administrative staff at the College HQ, and in the faculties. Inevitably there were laggards, so she had to jog them with great patience. The College officers stopped including the list of members in later editions on privacy grounds.

Another bonus of this system was that I could invite at my sole discretion leading activists to write chapters each year for the book and have them paid at professional rates. I was able to select about 20 each year preferring the able younger GPs coming up in general practice.

Transparency and Accountability to Members

The financial savings to the College were valuable, but, in addition, my aims in editing this publication for so long were empowering ordinary members. I hugely admired John Hunt (1905–1987, later Lord Hunt) for his model of the *Annual Report.* He ensured that each year the work of the College was fully documented and was posted as a separate publication to every College member. This was real transparency and accountability by the leadership and a visible mark of respect to ordinary members. Every fellow, member and associate could see exactly what was being done, who was on what committee, and how the College's money was being spent.

The College was running on members' subscriptions, and, like Hunt, I wanted every member who was interested to be able to see exactly what was going on and why. These full annual reports were read by a reasonable number of members as some talked to me about the contents at meetings. Most members never go to college meetings in London. As I became more involved with other Royal Colleges, I checked discreetly what kind of annual report they sent to their members. No other College came anywhere near providing ordinary members with the level of detail that the RCGP was doing.

Since Burdon edited exactly in Hunt's style, the RCGP is unusual in having a complete, published series of annual reports, detailed and referenced available from 1953 to 1996 — 43 consecutive years. These should prove useful sources when future articles and histories of the College are written.

Full annual published and distributed reports sent to each for member did not last. After I retired the College abandoned the fully documented annual report and moved to much shorter 'Impact reports,' which were long on smiling faces in colour and much shorter on facts. Then the College stopped sending these to all the members and just made copies available to those members who came in person to annual general meetings. Ordinary members were no longer so informed.

As the Internet developed the RCGP, like many other organisations, increasingly relied on "publishing" information on-line, so saving substantial printing and distribution costs. However, less information is made available than the reference books contained and, in my discussions with members, College members are now less well informed and less aware of what the College is doing, who is representing them, and in what way.

Perhaps just as there is unexpected power in continuity and personal care in general practice (DPG, *et al.*, 2018) there was power and effectiveness in supplying in writing College information and ideas to each member individually in their own home or practice?

End of the Chairmanship

My chairmanship of the Publications Committee ended unexpectedly after only one year when Alastair Donald, Chair of Council implemented a big reorganization. This created four new divisions and one of them, the Communications Division, was organised to include other committees like the publications committee within it (Chapter 19, Communications Division story). The Council elected me to chair this division, precluding me chairing the publications committee, so I resigned, and the publications committee elected Colin Waine to succeed me.

ADDENDUM

Jill and I edited the *RCGP Members' Reference Book* from 1982 to 1996.

19

Chair of the Communications Division 1981–1984

Skate to where the puck is going, not to where it has been.

Wayne Gretsky (1961–) Canadian Ice Hockey Player and Coach

In November 1979, Alastair Donald (1926–2005) was elected Chair of Council. He, like me, was a third generation GP following father and grandfather, and like me he was born at home over the shop. We both went to Cambridge where Alastair won an athletics blue and I got a chess half blue, then we both went back to our respective family practices. Both of us developed a deep commitment to general practice and expressed this through GP education. We both thought that making after-dinner speeches that made important points whilst making people laugh was a leadership skill that had to be learned. He was the first regional adviser in general practice in South East Scotland and I was the first in Devon and Cornwall. We both gave Mackenzie lectures and later both of us were Chair of Council and President. We got to know each other well on the College's Nuffield course in 1974.

Donald created four "divisions" or super committees for two reasons; first, to group existing committees which had common elements together, and second, to widen the College's leadership team. The latter aim was unusual in the College and unusual in national institutions, including government, where the norm is to concentrate power centrally. There are personal and organisational reasons for this. Many leaders (and managers) have controlling personalities, which they express in their leadership roles. Secondly, when things go wrong in institutions the usual reaction is to introduce a new protocol to stop the incident recurring and to control people more.

The adverse effects of increasing control over people are not well known, but include lower morale and less innovation. Jarman (2000), in his Harvean oration of the Royal College of Physicians, noted that increasing the numbers of hospital managers was associated with increased mortality in patients, whereas increased numbers of hospital clerks and administrative staff were associated with reduced patient mortality. Donald believed the RCGP was over-centralised and that that there were many more good ideas about in the College than just those in the mind of one Chair of Council.

His four divisions were: communications, education, membership, and research. In November 1981, the Council elected me Chair of the communications division, with a three-year term.

Donald said to me: "Think of yourself as a quarter Chairman of Council!" which was remarkably empowering. I wanted to look to the future and as Wayne Gretsky, a professional ice hockey player and coach said, "move to where the puck is going." At my first meeting of the division in December I proposed several new College activities that I hoped would strengthen the College in the future.

A Patient Group

I had been interested in the patient's perspective since I found out in my practice how important and valuable it was. I wrote about this twice. First in January 1974 as College Editor, when I wrote an editorial published anonymously, called "Patient power" (JRCGP, 1974a). By today's standards this was not very good and rather doctor centred. It concluded by seeking to "include the patient in the

DOI: 10.1201/9781032713601-24

primary health care team." However, it introduced the subject. Then I had an article in one of the medical newspapers (DPG, 1980b). This argued, for the first time, that patients should have their own committee within institutions like the RCGP. I could now make it happen.

Recently there have been some alternative versions reported about how the patient group in the RCGP started and when. This is because the event has historic significance being the first patient group formed in any British medical institution. Hence the background is fully described here – the date was December 1981 when the new communications division approved my proposal to establish a patient group in the College.

The main problem was that this idea did not have a mass of enthusiasts to develop it. Hence, identifying who should lead a new group within the communications division was tricky. I chose John Hasler for several reasons. First, we were both regional advisers and we got on well. Second, he was an excellent administrator and had been a good Secretary of Council. Third, he was broad in his leadership of the GP deanery in the Oxford region and had notably incorporated a clinical psychologist, David Pendleton, in his leadership team. Finally, and crucially, I discovered that he supported the idea of developing a patient group within the College. Once he agreed, I proposed him in the division to lead a new patient group, making it clear to him and to the division that, whilst a skilled GP leader was needed to initiate this project, the firm aim was to ensure a lay appointment; i.e. a patient chair for the group, as soon as possible.

I replicated the hands-off relationship that the Chair of Council had established with me and said I would not interfere as long as he and the group reported progress to every meeting of the division. John Hasler did well. He in turn invited Nancy Dennis, a patient advocate and they worked in partnership. The group was called the Patient Liaison Group and it developed well.

An International Group

RCGP had no organisational focus overseas. The word 'organisational' was key as there had been several individual RCGP members who had had a strong international awareness and had been actively involved, Stuart Carne, Ekke Kuenssberg, John Lawson, and Lotte Newman were all examples. However, there was no group or focus within the College promoting or integrating international activities.

By 1981, I had also become aware after eight years as a senior lecturer in general practice, that in the British academic community there was a strand of little Englander thinking. Overseas research in family practice was not well enough known or respected; I sometimes heard important overseas research being undervalued because the work had "not been done in the NHS."

I had been fortunate that the College had sent me to two world conferences of WONCA (World Organisation for Family Doctors): Canada in 1976 and Switzerland in 1980, and I had been with Jill both times. That very year Jill and I had been on a three-week lecture tour in New Zealand. I was a committed internationalist so I therefore proposed that a new international group be established within the communications division. This too was approved.

I had difficulty in selecting a chair and eventually chose John Lawson, as this new group would need authority and an internationally experienced chair. He was surprised, as a former Chair of Council and it was not then customary for past council chairs to chair committees afterwards However, he accepted and then did well in getting this group off the ground. I did not foresee that the precedent of a past council chair taking on a committee chairmanship would be a precedent for me (Chair of Research).

New Members' and Trainees' Groups

I also established a new members' and a trainee group in the College. This idea came from my experience in the College's Nuffield course, which was the most important course I ever attended (JRCGP, 1975e). It had sensitised me for life to the perspective of the adult learner. Our experience in Exeter of GP trainee representation had been encouraging and we had also arranged for trainee representatives to serve on the Southwest Regional General Practice Committee, which selected GP trainers. I hoped these experiences would be replicated in the division.

I asked Clare Ronalds, the Exeter trainee who had chaired the fourth national trainee conference recently held in the Exeter Department of General Practice and the first author of the report of that conference (*Occasional Paper 18*; Ronalds *et al.*, 1981). Clare was by then at Manchester and she accepted. I was also able to get David McKinlay, an emerging leader who was later to become a regional adviser, to lead a group for new GP principals.

Progress

All three of the new groups prospered and developed well. Indeed, so much so that momentum for the patients group led to the division proposing it be established as a group reporting to the Council. This was approved in 1983 and remained the position for the next 40 years. This meant that the patient leader obtained speaking rights in the Council, the College's governing body. The energy in the young principals and trainees group led to a paper from its chair, McKinlay, proposing in September 1984 in my last meeting that two separate groups be formed, recognising that both young trainees and trainees could develop separately. The outcome was that four groups were effectively promoted to a being active units in the Council in their own right rather than remaining in the communications division.

The patient group formalised its organisation and introduced advertisements for its new members. It provided patient assessors for many years whilst fellowship by assessment was operating (Chapter 24: FBA). It later changed its name to the Patient Partnership. It is still consulted on all RCGP policy papers.

The International Committee went from strength to strength and developed many contacts and mutual support systems around the world. Notably, the RCGP developed MRCGP international, a culturally sensitive examination, which led the medical profession and has been widely used in the Middle East.

The new members' group developed so well that there are now big meetings to welcome new MRCGPs, like university graduations, where they come with their parents. The College developed the trainees' group so much that trainees have become "associate members in training." All three of the groups owe much to their three initial chairs who led them well. My three-year Chairmanship of the Communications Division ended in November 1984 and the Council elected Colin Waine to succeed me.

20

Educational Experiences in the Executive Committee: December 1980 to November 2000

In medical education, as in other kinds of education what matters most is not the knowledge imparted to a man but what the man himself becomes in the course of acquiring the knowledge.

Plato

My membership of the RCGP Council Executive fell into three parts. The first decade, 1970–1980 (Chapter 11, College Cabinet story) has been described. That was followed by a decade (1980–1990) when I held various offices and then, after a gap of three years (1990–1993), a final seven years (1993–2000). This was an important part of my continuing education.

The Joint Committee on Postgraduate Training for General Practice (JCPTGP) was the national regulator for general practice training (Chapter 29, JCPTGP story). In 1981, I was first elected to it by the Council mainly on the strength of my regional advisership and the *System of Training for General Practice (Occasional Paper)* 4 then in its second edition (DPG, 1977a, 1979).

Healthier Children – Thinking Prevention

John Horder was the President who changed British general practice by developing the GP's role in preventive medicine. In 1980, he set up several working parties and chaired the co-ordinating group himself (RCGP, 1980b).

One group was on child care, and he made Chris Donovan its convener. However, when its report came to Council, I savaged it in debate so severely that the Council rejected the report outright. Then I had my arm twisted by Horder as I had never had it twisted before. He was irritated. He pointed out that I had written a gold medal essay on child care in general practice (DPG, 1969/70), had been a member of the Council's working party on child care (RCGP, 1978) and had said in debate that I thought child care in general practice was important, so I ought to put my time where my mouth was. He pressed me to join his child care working party. I was then resigning from the Editorship of the College *Journal* and declined. Horder increased the pressure and I faced a President, whom I greatly admired, fighting for his top priority on preventive medicine in general practice and a subject that I had emphasised in my Mackenzie lecture.

I surrendered, provided I became co-convener and Colin Waine and Freddie Brimblecombe joined the group. I wanted Colin since he was a hospital practitioner taking paediatric emergencies in his local hospital and I thought he was more experienced with children's emergencies than I was. I wanted Brimblecombe, from Exeter, whom I knew, as a general consultant paediatrician, as it seemed unwise to have all the consultant input through child psychiatry. Horder agreed all this.

The report took two years and much work. I took three months' sabbatical leave in 1982 to write the report. The two consultants, Freddie Brimblecombe (1919–1992) and Philip Graham (1932–), a child

DOI: 10.1201/9781032713601-25

psychiatrist and soon to be Dean of the Institute of Child Health in London were both supportive. The report was approved by the group and came to the Council in September 1982.

I started the debate with every advantage: Horder, as President, and Alastair Donald, as Chair of Council, were both supporters. A spectacular debate ensued. I had the advantage in proposing the motion and having the right of reply. In the debate all the RCGP heavy hitters came out on my side including six members of Council who had been or who would chair the Council. However, the rank and file of council members dissented in numbers. I was one of the strongest debaters in the Council and I gave my winding-up speech everything I had, but lost the vote. *Healthier Children* was not approved. This was the biggest defeat in a College debate I ever experienced. I was shattered. This bruising experience made me reflect for years about leadership and democracy.

Alastair Donald commiserated with me. "Don't worry," he said: "It's a good report and will be seen as such in time. It is like *The Future General Practitioner — Learning and Teaching* (RCGP, 1972c) which was also never formally approved by the Council and was also well ahead of its time." "What about publication?" I asked, since *Reports from General Practice* represent College policy. "Publish it as a report!" he said: "Chairman's action!" Leadership indeed! So Jill and I published *Healthier Children — Thinking Prevention* as *Report from General Practice* 22 (RCGP, 1982). Horder had obtained funds to post this and his preventive care reports as *Reports from General Practice* to every member.

College publications, whilst going free to the College membership, were made available for sale. *Healthier Children* sold so well that that it became the best selling of all the five reports on prevention and ran into a second edition. Research showed later that it was one of the few College publications that altered GP attitudes significantly. Paediatricians wrote favourable reviews of it. Later the Government altered the GP contract to increase child care prevention work in line with proposals in *Healthier Children*. It did prove to be ahead of its time and, on the day, Alastair Donald judged it right.

It was appropriate that, as Colin Waine and I were the two GPs in the UK who did most to kill the Court report's proposed general practitioner paediatrician, we were then the two who did most to construct a positive GP policy on the care of children in general practice. GPs care as much about children as paediatricians, whilst knowing the children and their families much better. At the time, the average child in Britain saw a GP on average 35 times between birth and the age of 5 (Loudon *et al.,* 1998; table), whilst most children never saw a paediatrican after birth. GPs care for children using continuity and family perspectives, as parents are usually patients too.

Serving under Irvine as Chairman

In November 1982, Donald Irvine took office as Chair of Council. He led the College into a high-profile confrontation with the GP BMA committee, then called the GMSC, over GP out-of-hours, with the College taking a strong line in favour of GPs retaining responsibility and discouraging the use of deputising services by GP trainers. The GMSC was chaired by John Ball, one of the most able of the BMA GP committee chairs. This was the first clash of policy between the College and the BMA GPs since the College had been founded. It dented relationships between the two leaders and the two houses.

The trend towards more use of deputising services continued, but the College intervention ensured that doctors participating had to have a certificate of satisfactory completion of training for general practice. This achievement was designed to protect patients and attracted little notice at the time, but exploded into public consciousness years later when a patient died after negligent care out- of-hours from an overseas doctor who had never been examined in the UK.

Irvine launched a "quality initiative," a programme encouraging GPs to report the work in their practices and what they had achieved in quality of care (Irvine, 1983). This was strong, professional leadership, reinterpreting the College's traditional focus on "standards of care in general practice" into something practical and applicable in every general practice. Irvine got good support from members of Council and support in some faculties. Bill Styles, as secretary, and Sally Fountain, (later Irvine), as head of the administration, published a quality newsletter disseminating good practice in the College.

A spring meeting of the College was held in Cambridge in 1985, and I was invited to a debate proposing the motion "That British general practice is the best in the world!" It was opposed by Professor Vuori, a Finnish international expert with the World Health Organisation. Before the event I was teased about an impossible task. Several hundred people came. The room was packed. Jill was there, but Penny, our medical student daughter, sadly could not come. I opened traditionally with a summary. Professor Vuori did a good job pointing out British problems and his seconder, an Irish GP, backed him up wittily. Vuori closed for the opposition, and I sensed he was winning. For my five minutes right of reply as proposer, I quoted text from Vuori's book about private general practice (abhorrent among College GPs) and complained loudly about why he had not mentioned this? For the Irish seconder, I asked the room why he had kept quiet about his GP training? The reason I said was that he had come from Ireland to a British training practice since he knew that British general practice was the best in the world! The audience laughed and voted agreeing the motion.

Poor Professor Vuori was culturally non-plussed, and I felt sorry for him. The customs of British debate and knockabout humour were outside his experience. They were however appreciated by Nicholas Pisicano (1924–1990), the Executive Director of the American Board of Family Medicine, who said he had enjoyed the debate and promptly invited me to become a member of the Editorial Board of the *Journal of the American Board of Family Practice,* where I served for 18 years.

In 1978, Merck Sharpe and Dohme (MSD), a big international pharmaceutical company based in the United States, established an independent charity quite separate from the company. It identified general practice as the biggest branch of medicine, and a field that was developing quickly with the RCGP as the centre of intellectual activity. Rather than relating to the College as an organization, it chose to link with its leaders as individuals. When I was approached the Chair was Pat Byrne, and Donald Irvine was centrally involved with Marshall Marinker. The Director was Karl Sabbagh, a Palestinian-British writer and television journalist.

This was a national level think tank focused on general practice development and with substantial resources. I was unpaid but with expenses reimbursed and accommodation in very good hotels. There were some distinguished specialist members like Sir Richard Bayliss (1917–2006) KCVO FRCP, Physician to the Queen. A big bonus was having long discussions over dinner with him and others.

Sabbagh's expertise as a TV producer and the Advisory Committee's interest in analysing the general practice consultations led to the Foundation video-recording GP consultations, with full consent from patients. This was Pat Byrne's strength as his book *Doctors talking to Patients* had become a classic in 1976 (Byrne and Long, 1984). After Byrne died in 1980 and Sabbagh moved on, Irvine was appointed Chair and Marshall Marinker the Director. Marshall then ran GP leadership courses in virtually every region of England and Scotland with great success. After Colin Waine joined, he and I pressed for support for GPs in caring for patients with common chronic diseases. Our work on asthma led to a couple of articles in the *BMJ* (Waine et al., 1981a, b). Eventually, the company closed the Foundation.

The College nominated me as the GP for a team assessing the medical services in Guernsey, led by Sir Douglas Black. This was a pleasant chance to visit general practices outside the NHS and I learned much from Black, a former PRCP and also Chief Scientist. At the final feedback session I was asked for suggestions. I noted that the GPs related distantly to the Wessex Faculty of the RCGP in England and suggested it might be helpful if they similarly linked up with the GPs on Jersey. This went down like a lead balloon! Faces were frozen and I was told afterwards that this suggestion was unacceptable! Context is everything (Black Report, 1985).

By 1984–1985 the quality initiative was running out of steam. The question was how to sustain it. I privately began to believe that it would be necessary to link any College quality initiative with some clear incentive or reward. Donald and I never talked this through, but he came to a similar conclusion that an incentive was needed but he decided a contractual incentive was the solution. He saw the "good practice allowance" as a way of defining quality of good practice and rewarding GPs for providing it. He then led the College in an all-consuming campaign to achieve a "good practice allowance" in the

NHS contract. GPC was dominated by it, considering drafts at every meeting. In his final months in the Chair he focused on the publication *Quality in General Practice* on which he and Sally worked intensively. This analysed general practice and proposed to embed quality in general practice through a "good practice allowance" in a new NHS GP contract. Diplomatically it stated: "…Clearly the GMSC (General Medical Services Committee of the BMA) would need to take the lead in any further development since implementation would involve the doctor's contract." Jill and I published it. This document was aimed at the DH and Government. We arranged distribution to all members as *Policy Statement No 2* (RCGP, 1985a) and the Irvines sent numerous copies to key policy-makers.

The result of the huge effort Irvine and the RCGP had made on the GPA was failure. The GPA idea disappeared. It was a well worked up idea that convinced a department of state and Government, but it was never implemented. Its Achilles heel was that implementation depended on a trade union, the BMA. Irvine led vigorously and did all in his power. Despite great expenditure of College time and resources, the quality of care of general practice probably did not improve in those years. The College's eggs were placed in a single basket that the Conference of LMCs ditched (Chapter 22, Downs and Ups of Institutional Life).

I learned a lesson. If I ever became Chair, I needed to find a College quality programme, entirely within the College's control, which could not be stymied externally. This led to the idea of Fellowship by Assessment (Chapter 24, Fellowship by Assessment story).

The idea of incorporating measures of quality of GP performance was resurrected 16 years later as the NHS Quality and Outcomes Framework in the 2003 GP NHS Contract. Instead of an overall good practice allowance the performance markers were divided into many separate targets, each with specified price tags.

Serving under John Hasler as Chair

In November 1985, John Hasler was installed as the Chair of Council. I had to make the best of it, so I dug in to prepare to re-apply for the chairmanship in 1988. In the event I was in his cabinet for only 14 months because of the unforeseen events described in Chapter 22, The Downs and Ups of Institutional Life.

Elections

To remain on the Executive I had to keep being re-elected. First, it was necessary to be re-elected to the Council and then secondly to the Executive. There were two routes to the Council. One place was available from each faculty and mine sometimes elected me. The second route was an annual vote by all members of the College for six places a year. For the 1991–1994 councils I was in one of these postal ballots with Donald Irvine. We were both comfortably re-elected and I was encouraged to receive a bigger vote than he did.

Some big names were not re-elected. Marshall Marinker had been a leader on the Council and the Executive for years. He spoke in favour of GP fundholding, which was his idea. This did not endear him to the membership, which did not re-elect him to the Council – a collective political punishment. One of the sharpest minds in British medicine, the leader of the most effective GP leadership course, and one of the most able GP eponymous lecturers was removed. Marshall was deeply hurt. He played no further role in the College but became a professor at Guy's Hospital, writing and lecturing persuasively. I saw him over the years for lunches.

Leadership in medicine depends on successive elections by colleagues who vote secretly. This process attracts little attention but deserves more. Even leadership success can be followed by dismissal. I have seen two presidents of medical royal colleges, three royal college editors, and one RCGP Chair of Council being ousted, as well as two chairs of BMA Council and three chairs of BMA committees.

Serving under Colin Waine as Chairman

Colin Waine, succeeded me as the Chair of Council after November 1990. He decided there ought to be a history of the first 40 years of the College and pressed me to write it for 1992. There was no proper budget, and the plan was to finance the book with adverts. The timetable was dire and seriously uncomfortable. A further problem was there was a need for a series of articles and some authors did not deliver so I had to write some of those as well. I was rescued by Margaret Hammond, the College Librarian, who threw herself into the work and was in touch virtually every day. I only just managed it as Jill developed breast cancer at the time. The book was called *Forty Years On: The Story of the First 40 Years of the Royal College of General Practitioners* (DPG, 1992a).

Between 1990 and 1996 the Royal College of Psychiatrists with the RCGP led a national "defeat depression campaign." This was not easy for the RCGP as research showed that the depression was common, was often undiagnosed by GPs, and when diagnosed was often undertreated, according to research. The campaign was led by the RCPsych. Clinical problems are far bigger for GPs who have to diagnose every kind of illness and detect cancer as early as possible, as well as diagnosing depression. GPs were the target and the RCPsych wanted to teach them. I was elected to represent the RCGP with Paul Freeling and was involved in several exchanges reflecting differences between the disciplines. Once I defended the lower doses of antidepressants used by GPs, arguing that a principle of general practice is to use a dose that is enough and which is tolerated by the patient. If a patient gets better on a dose, it is not logical to increase it. Secondly, after some patronising comments about GP prescribing, I pointed out that psychiatrists in many trials had not been able to keep many of their patients taking the drugs, as the published drop-out rates were 25 to 30% (Wells *et al.*, 2013): GPs had to maintain working relationships with their patients for years.

The campaign was a modest success (Rix *et al.*, 1999) and led to the idea of a two College book. This had a bumpy start when the psychiatrists proposed two editors from the RCPsych and one from the RCGP, which we refused. With two Editors from each College then agreed, Alastair Wright and I were elected the GP editors. Each College chose half the chapter authors, and Alastair and I contributed several chapters. The book was published in 1994 by the RCPsych as *Psychiatry and General Practice Today* (Pullen *et al.*, 1994). It was a commercial success for the RCPsych. As far as I know, this is the only textbook to have been co-written by two medical Royal Colleges, which is a pity as the model has great potential.

I was present when Colin Waine made a moving and a ultra-proper resignation from the Chair of Council because a patient had made a complaint about him in circumstances that suggested to many that he had given reasonable care.

Serving under Bill Styles, John Toby, and Michael Pringle as Chairs

Bill Styles succeeded Colin Waine, but was dogged by ill health and he tragically died of cancer in office. My experiences under the chairmanships of Toby and Pringle are in Chapter 29 the JCPTGP story and in Chapter 35, President of the RCGP, 1997–2000.

Summary

I served on the Council for thirty years, December 1970 to November 2000, as observer, member, or Chair for nearly four years. I served under nine other chairs of Council. John Fry and Donald Irvine served longer on the Council but both had much shorter terms on the executive. None of the founding fathers did more than 23 years and Irvine did 15 years on the executive. I am the only GP to have served over a 30-year period on the council executive. I was a member for 27 of those years with a three-year gap after the Chairmanship. Sometimes I was elected by the Council to the GPC, but mostly I was elected to executive posts: Chairmanships of the Communications Division, the Research Division, the Council and GPC, Chairmanship of the JCPTGP and President, with ex-officio membership.

I saw changes over time. In 1970, members were mainly working GPs, like me, mostly principals. I had 3,000 NHS patients and was working nights and weekends with no academic appointment. The College's early links with private practice (three presidents) were still present, with John Hunt, President. There were few professors of general practice in the world and no regional advisers in general practice. There were few researchers or GPs leading institutions. There was no postgraduate GP training and no place for the College on the GMC. However, the leadership was not afraid of controversy and repeatedly achieved innovations.

Thirty years later, members' expertise had much increased. Several members were experts in education or research and often held senior positions in important institutions. However, as the membership grew and resources increased, the College's academic focus weakened and it became more doctor-centred and less patient-centred. The Research Committee was closed. Fostering quality of care by Fellowship by Assessment was abandoned. The College became less ready to challenge national institutions to achieve much needed reforms. After organising *Destination GP* (Medical Schools Council and RCGP, 2017), the College ran away from facing the bad news that it found that only 3% of British medical students saw general practice having intellectual challenge. The library changed from pride of place in Princes Gate to a shrivelled cupboard in Euston Square. An excellent archivist was mismanaged. The Trustee Board cancelled the budget and removed staff for the Heritage Committee, revealing lack of understanding and pride in the College and its history. Some College leaders said general practice was "undo-able" and largely stopped encouraging GPs to do more for their patients.

Membership of the Council Executive was a great privilege. With a dinner the night before and day-long monthly meetings with a two-day 'retreat' annually, I mingled with interesting people with exciting ideas. Long-term membership of this group was one of the privileges of my life as I learned from and made friends with some very talented GPs, who gave me continuing education. They sustained and inspired me.

21

Consultant Adviser to the Chief Medical Officer of the Department of Health and Social Security 1984–1987

Advisers advise: ministers decide.

Margaret Thatcher (1925–2013)

In 1984, I was approached by the Chief Medical Officer (CMO), Sir Donald Acheson (1926–201) who invited me to become his Consultant Adviser for General Practice. This came as a considerable surprise because the only two consultant advisers in general practice whom I knew about had been Pat Byrne and John Horder. Both were much more senior than I was and both had been presidents of the College. I was under fifty and had not held either of the chief posts in the RCGP.

I did not know why I was invited, but I suspected that I had been recommended by either David Ower, the senior GP in the DH, who had stayed in our home in Exeter and with whom I got on very well or by Sir John Reid (1925–1994), CMO Scotland, whom I had got to know when he came to the WHO Seminar in the Exeter Department of General Practice the year before, as described in Chapter, 13 in the Department/Institute of General Practice story.

The CMO said the post would not be onerous. It meant giving him private and confidential advice, whenever he sought it, and attending the meetings of all his consultant advisers whom he called together periodically. The post was unpaid and I was not asked to sign the Official Secrets Act.

Expert Advisory Group on AIDS

Sir Donald also invited me to join the Expert Advisory Group on AIDS, which he and Michael Abrams (Deputy CMO) chaired. It was set up to consider the profound medical implications of what was then a new disease. I attended the first of these in January 1985 where I was the only – token – GP. I hugely admired his initiative as the Thatcher Government was finding this disease difficult to manage and Acheson showed great professional leadership. He was radical in choosing members and invited people who were HIV positive to join the group, the first major patient involvement that I know of in the DH. I was put on one subgroup.

I made only one serious recommendation, which was that general practitioners should no longer be excluded from the management of the treatment of AIDS. I observed that specialists in their mainly London clinics were not informing GPs of the diagnosis and in some cases were engineering patients to sign forms that they did not wish their GPs to be informed. Some patients were frightened that GPs would not maintain strict confidentiality. AIDS then was a very serious disease from which most people died. However, treatments were improving and I foresaw that palliative, and hopefully long-term care, would sooner or later impinge on general practice. I got absolutely nowhere: the specialists

DOI: 10.1201/9781032713601-26

running AIDS clinics were receiving substantial resources for them; it was in their interest to be exclusive and they did not respect general practice (just GPs).

Joe Pilling and the Limited List of Drugs

As the Consultant Adviser, to the DHSS, I was involved in private discussions with Joe (later Sir) Pilling (1945–), then a Grade 3 civil servant developing a limited list of drugs restricting what general practitioners could prescribe. Grade three civil servants are very senior and lead great tracts of policy within departments of state. Pilling was only 38 at the time.

This proposal was an early and very gentle step towards rationing in NHS general practice. Pilling and I had several quite vigorous debates on the rights and wrongs of limited prescribing lists. I was accustomed to winning most such discussions, but I found he had an alpha mind. Although he was about ten years younger than I was, he often defeated me in some of those confidential debates face-to-face, alone in the DH.

I got on with him well and I invited him to visit our practice in Exeter. We had a great day discussing practice data and built a working relationship that lasted for over 20 years. He later became Director General of the Prison Service, was knighted as Permanent Secretary in the Northern Ireland Office and was a guest at my final RCGP council dinner in 2000.

Meetings of the Consultant Advisers to the CMO

I have probably had more experience working in groups that were predominantly composed of medical specialists than any other GP in Britain, starting with these meeting of the CMO's consultant advisers. The CMO held periodic meetings of all his consultant advisers in the DHSS for which he had one for every specialty. I was very much alone at these meetings being the only GP – the token GP – in a room amongst 40–50 leading specialists. My experiences were not comfortable. It was not that I did not know the others, as I did not expect to, but there was something awkward about the way they responded to me. The opening questions were always: "What branch of medicine are you from?" But my reply general practice had a deadening effect on conversation. Some couldn't think of anything to say, many asked what part of the country I came from, and none could talk intelligently about the job. Some even turned away to talk to other more interesting colleagues. I felt very much "just a GP."

I wondered if it was personal, but soon I realised that it was about professional grouping. These specialists, all leaders in their fields, simply did not know anything about general practice, did not rate it, and could not talk even socially about it. In subsequent meetings, I introduced myself saying that I was involved in computerising medical records, partly to give them something to talk about, and partly because this was an aspect of medical practice where general practice was leading hospital practice. Years later I learned that Dame Margaret Booth, when a new female judge also in the early 1980s, encountered fellow male judges "who simply refused to talk to her" (*The Times*, 2021), so this was a cross-professional arrogance by experts. By contrast, the CMO in the chair, was always courteous to me. He never refused my request to speak and he brought me into discussions. He and I were the only two people in the room who thought that there was an important world of medicine outside hospitals.

I was extremely fortunate to have two subsequent opportunities to work in groups with a big majority of specialists: the Exeter Postgraduate Medical School and the Academy of Medical Royal Colleges. In neither setting was I made to feel that I was "just a GP," and in both groups big consultant majorities paid me the ultimate compliment of electing me as their leader. That generation of consultant advisers probably had serious deficiencies in their training and had not been taught properly about general practice. I became an advocate for all doctors, especially career specialists, being given postgraduate training in general practice.

Debate in Exeter

Someone in Exeter discovered that there were two Exeter doctors who were consultant advisers to the CMO, unusual in a small city, Tom Hargreaves, the consultant biochemist and me. I knew him as a very pleasant man, who was always supportive to GPs and their use of his pathology services. I was asked to take part in a debate on the future of pathology services. There was anxiety in the staff group in the Department of General Practice as they thought I was being set up to fail on Tom's subject but I felt I was duty bound to do it.

The lecture theatre was full. Hargreaves went first giving an elegant lecture on quality assurance of biochemical investigations. He described auto-analysers (machines doing multiple chemical tests) and showed how they could process, cost effectively, huge numbers of samples and obtain very greater precision of results than had ever been possible before. All tests should be done by these machines in central district hospital laboratories. There was no future for local equipment used outside the laboratory. He was a national expert on this subject and it showed. I realised mid debate that this was an exercise to discourage GPs from using in-practice tests. My departmental colleagues had been ahead of me in sensing danger.

I said that the main problem with investigations was that they were never available to the patient or the GP when they were needed. GPs were having to take samples, send them to laboratories, and then patients had to come back or telephone for results. What was needed was the result whilst the patient was still with the doctor so that they could discuss it together.

I dared to suggest that quality assurance was not my top priority. For patients with diabetes, the GP has essentially only three decisions to take: to increase the treatment, to keep it the same, or to reduce it. I thought it would now be well worth trading off perhaps half a milli-mole of accuracy in order to get the result available at the time of the initial consultation. I pointed out the huge increase in efficiency if patients could get their GP's advice in one consultation. Suddenly the audience clapped! Hargreaves was horrified. I was throwing doubt on his life's work and his huge experience in quality assurance in pathology laboratories. I doubt if he had ever heard the other side of the argument put so forcefully. There are two different perspectives on quality and that day they got a proper airing.

Resignation

My sudden election to the Chairmanship of the RCGP in 1987 ended this role. I wrote to Sir Donald explaining that I could no longer give him independent advice, as I was now the policy lead for the RCGP and would be recommending college policies. The CMO wrote me a nice reply thanking me for my work and confirming that he thought I had done the right thing by resigning. Boundaries were clearer then as it was generally understood that the head of an institution was the voice of that institution. Nowadays boundaries are blurred as governments often invite the heads of institutions to serve on committees, but then claim that they serve as individuals.

22

The Downs and Ups of Institutional Life: 1982–1987

A week is a long time in politics.

Harold Wilson (1916–1995)

From 1982–1985, Donald Irvine was Chair of Council. His Chairmanship was one of the most political that the College had seen. I had a ring-side seat on the General Purposes Committee (GPC) throughout.

In December 1984, Donald Irvine invited me to dinner with him alone. He told me he was now entering his last year as Chair and one of his duties was to help plan his succession. He understood I would be the choice of the Council in the forthcoming election for the Chair and I should start planning practice arrangements. I was flattered to hear this and we talked over the Chairmanship. We saw no problems if I were to succeed him. He was keen that his idea of the good practice allowance should be supported.

The College electoral system was old-fashioned and similar to the system previously operated by the Conservative party. Names were supposed to 'emerge,' i.e., be nominated by the leader group. If there were two or more names, the Secretary of Council, then Bill Styles, telephoned all members of the Council and sought their views.

In the first half of 1985, I privately worked on the briefing Irvine had given me and thought about the Chairmanship. In the spring I heard that John Hasler's name was also in the ring. He had been a successful Secretary of Council, a post which had been a steppingstone to the Chair with Donald.

There was then a long delay, longer than I had expected and, ominously, no contact from Donald Irvine, the Secretary, or the Treasurer – the three key officers. Then, suddenly, in the summer, Bill Styles the Secretary, rang to say that he had done the ring-round and John Hasler was the choice of the Council for its next Chair. He said I could take it to a vote if I wanted but there was a clear majority for Hasler. Caught on the hop, I had to think quickly and surrendered as gracefully as I could, saying I would serve under Hasler. I was left profoundly upset – more than any other setback in my professional life. It was a big and humiliating rejection by a substantial number of colleagues.

A few weeks later the journal secretary was in Princes Gate and overheard a member of Council saying he felt sorry for Denis, as being beaten by a younger man meant that he had probably lost his chance of the Chairmanship! Alastair Donald, a former Chair of Council, took me aside and said how sorry and surprised he was at what had happened as he had strongly supported me. He had expected me to be elected. He thought the system needed changing as it gave too much power to the Honorary Secretary and officers in post. "Too much power?" Did he mean that some Council members seeking advice could have been discreetly steered to Hasler? What had happened between December when Donald Irvine was so sure I was to be elected and the summer when I wasn't? In the summer of 1985, John Hasler was announced as the choice of the Council for the Chair and he took office in November.

Such a big defeat for a top post made me review my position within the College. Donald Irvine was one of the most intelligent and political College chairs. He had not only expected me to succeed him but had dined me to prepare me for the role. I knew of nothing in the first six months of 1985 that had affected me or changed in the Council. When people vote for colleagues in professional bodies, there

DOI: 10.1201/9781032713601-27

are always two questions: Is the candidate competent to do the job? Can they be trusted? Had I fallen on one of these?

John Hasler had great strengths. He had an MD. He was one of the four leading regional advisers in general practice in the UK. He led a great team in Oxford and he had been a good Secretary of the Council. He had a pleasant personality and was well liked. However, he had had a much shorter College and Council career than I had, having been drafted into the Secretaryship from outside the Council. He had not previously been elected to the Council, had never held a college leadership post like my Editorship. He had not led a university department like the Exeter Department of General Practice. He had written articles but nothing like my output: three eponymous lectures including the James Mackenzie, a widely cited *Occasional Paper*, a College *Report from General Practice* and a successful textbook. Finally, I too was a regional adviser of about equal standing but with a much bigger and more geographically complex area.

As for trust, my writings were being cited a good deal, and at big meetings colleagues were often coming up to me to say that they had advised their children to apply to the Exeter GP training scheme (then getting huge numbers of applicants per place). The College had been generous with prizes and I had received the George Abercombie award, the Foundation Council award (the College's highest honour) and I had been the youngest James Mackenzie lecturer ever. This did not suggest a lack of trust. The unpalatable conclusion was that I had been the better qualified candidate but had still lost. I did not receive letters of commiseration from the four key players: Donald, the Secretary, the Treasurer, or the General Manager with whom the Chair works most closely – significant non-verbal communication.

I approached Douglas Garvie as an officer. He and I got on well and he had a reputation for speaking out. I asked what I had done wrong? "Nothing," he said, "It was just felt that you were too much like Donald Irvine and the College needed a quieter time." This helped. Such analyses were not how many Council members were likely to have thought and sounded an officer view.

With John Hasler in post, the Council held an election for membership of the GPC, as a postal ballot of all the members of the 1985–1986 Council. There was one place for members of Council not holding major committee chairmanships. This vote was only a few months after the Secretary's ring-round on the Chairmanship, so the electorate was virtually the same as the one that had rejected me. This time I not only came top of the ballot but received a vote dwarfing everyone else. I was not sure if this was a sympathy vote, giving me a consolation prize or whether I actually had strong support in Council.

November 1985 – Good Practice Allowance (GPA)

Irvine's main contribution as Chair was developing the idea of a good practice allowance (GPA) to form part of the remuneration of NHS general practitioners. He led endless discussions in the General Purposes Committee (GPC) and Council on this and it was well thought through. The aim was to measure and reward quality of general practitioner care. The Council endorsed the idea. The tensions over the earlier out-of-hours arrangements also meant lines of communication between Irvine and the top of the BMA GP Committee were not warm.

In November 1985, as Irvine left office, the College published *Policy Statement 2*, a powerful document called *Quality in General Practice,* arguing the case for a good practice allowance (RCGP, 1985a). It was formally approved in the College. Jill and I designed the white cover format and published this from our Exeter office and sent it to every member of the College. It was also widely distributed to Government and national institutions (Chapter 10, Exeter RCGP Publishing story).

During 1985–1986, I remained an elected member of the GPC. However, I was active in national events, including the Conference of Regional Advisers and I had contacts who briefed me about reactions in the GMSC. All sources confirmed the leadership of the GMSC, now Michael Wilson, was negative on the good practice allowance and would have none of it.

The two main general practitioner bodies were fundamentally different in the type of doctor each attracted and in the core priories of the two institutions. The GMSC was the medical trade union for general practitioners and the BMA's main role, as defined is: "to uphold the honour and interests of the medical profession." It is therefore by definition doctor-centred. The RCGP by contrast is a registered charity and its central objective, as confirmed in its Royal Charter, is "to encourage foster and maintain the highest standards of general medical practice." It is therefore patient focused. The GMSC is the stronger body in terms of history, numbers of doctors involved, democratic structures, and financial resources but its decisions are made on the basis of majority vote. A majority of one in a vote confers legitimacy.

The RCGP Council, as the governing committee of an academic body, is more concerned about evidence and at times a minority opinion based on evidence determines policy. For example, Clifford Kay told the Council that in the oral contraception study (RCGP, 1974), which he directed, that he had found that women over 35, who were smokers and were obese were at greater risk of developing a thrombosis. He said this group should probably not be prescribed this drug, when he was the only GP in Britain who knew or practised that. Prescribing policy quickly followed him.

Members of the Council of the RCGP usually had more enthusiasm for their job and were much better read. The quality of intellectual debate in the College Council was exceptionally high. In 1986 there was no comparison between the intellectual firepower of the two bodies, the RCGP with Alastair Donald, Donald Irvine, Marshall Marinker, Julian Tudor Hart and three other professors, analysed the place of general practice in society more deeply than their opposite numbers in the GMSC. The key difference was the belief in the RCGP that society had changed, and the status quo could not hold. Consumerism was growing and quality of care was now the name of the game. Good general practice was being undervalued. The Conservative Government was favouring payment for measured performance. These were important differences from the GMSC, which did not accept this analysis.

Irvine's and the College's aim was to think through a good practice allowance and publish a policy arguing the case for quality in general practice and incentivising and rewarding this (what later came to be called pay for performance). The target audience was firmly the Government and the DH.

Primary Health Care: Agenda for Discussion 1986

In April 1986 the Government published its proposals for general practice under the title *Primary Health Care: An Agenda for Discussion* (DHSS, 1986). Crucially it proposed introducing a good practice allowance. Seeing the GPA included in the Thatcher Government's proposal, *Primary Health Care–Agenda for Discussion,* for the future of general practice represented a substantial political success for Irvine and the College.

This document is important as there has been some attempted re-writing of history by those opposed to Mrs Thatcher who have wrongly claimed that she always imposed solutions on the medical profession. She did not do so in April 1986 when her government with this document publicly offered general practice a good practice allowance, just as the RCGP (1985a) had proposed, four months earlier. The title of the document said it all: "...Agenda for *Discussion*" (my emphasis). Government was being reasonable.

Three Articles in the *BMJ*

I was a member of a private lunch club run by Marshall Marinker, which included Julia Cumberledge (1943–; later Baroness), Chair of a Regional Health Authority and later a conservative minister, Alan Maynard (1944–2018), a Professor of Health Economics at York, and Geoffrey Rivett, a civil servant in the DH working on general practice. This group analysed the issues rigorously and with much wider perspectives than from general practice as two of them were not doctors. The group decided to respond in public to what we saw as a serious crisis with the BMA preparing to reject the GPA. Three of us agreed to write as a team with all three of us signing three different articles. Two of us, Marshall Marinker (1930–2019) and I, held no chairmanships in the College, but we were members of the Council and had been members of the GPC that had refined *Quality in Practice*. We were anxious as we believed *Primary Health Care: Agenda for Discussion* offered a real opportunity to general practice.

We also anticipated that a rejection might well provoke the Government into a much less desirable reaction. We cared a great deal about general practice and were both steeped in all the arguments. We wanted the case stated in as public a way as possible so that all GPs were fully informed of the key points. There was also a sense that John Hasler, the new College Chair, was not supporting the GPA as much as had been expected.

Marinker, Maynard, and I agreed to write three articles signed by all three of us, each being first author of one and making the three main points in the case for the GPA. Those three points were: 1. Society had changed and change was coming inevitably to general practice; 2. The GPA was practical and feasible; and 3. (Like it or not) competition in health care was a serious possibility.

The *BMJ* published these articles in three successive weeks in May 1986. I was first author of our first article (DPG *et al.*, 1986), arguing that the status quo for general practice in contractual terms could not hold. Change was essential, indeed desirable, as it offered opportunities, and this should be the backdrop to discussions on the GPA and other policies. This was the key: the central difference between the RCGP Council and the GMSC. The BMA did not agree, and many in the RCGP thought the GMSC was inward looking and complacent.

Our second article (Marinker *et al.*, 1986) argued that the good practice allowance was feasible. Crucially there would have to be agreement upon any such allowance; i.e. it would be negotiated by the BMA and would be based on research evidence of the value of general practice activities to patients which had been increasing in recent years.

Our third article (Maynard *et al.*, 1986) was different. Alan Maynard led on describing the international scene and set out how competition could be introduced in health care and had been introduced internationally. This was topical at the time, as only the year before the Nuffield Trust had invited Professor Alan Entoven (1930–) from the United States, who had produced a monograph on this theme, to give a big lecture at the Trust (Enthoven, 1985).

The articles attracted interest in the College, but from the BMA, which was the target audience, there was no visible reaction. On the grapevine I heard the articles were considered "unhelpful." The advice was not to comment on them as the authors would then get a right of reply. Despite the importance of the subject, no letters on them were published in the *BMJ* in the following weeks.

At that crucial time when all was to play for, Marshall Marinker and I in the GPC and that lunch group had identified the key issues and set them out in public in the journal most read by BMA GPs. We got the key arguments into the open and into the hands of every one of those LMC representatives. We took the political horse(s) to the water, but we could not make them drink. We lost completely, illustrating how professional leadership sometimes means having big, public, defeats.

Conference of Local Medical Committees 1986

The Conference of Local Medical Committees met twice in 1986. In one meeting in July of over 400 GPs, only one or two representatives voted for a good practice allowance. Then a special meeting of the Conference was held in November. The key debate on the GPA was introduced by Michael Wilson, as Committee Chair. He said the proposed BMA response had been prepared by: "practising doctors in day-to-day contact with patients" and he attacked the GPA strongly, alleging it had been produced by: a "think tank of philosophers, privateers and trendy professors" (*BMJ*, 1986)'. 'Trendy professors played deliberately to the anti-College and anti-intellectual elements in the Conference'. In December 1986, the General Medical Services Committee sent its final comment on agenda for discussion to the Secretary of State, Norman Fowler (*BMJ*, 1986). Para 20 read: "A good practice allowance would not be acceptable if based on subjective assessment by peer audit. There are dangers inherent in audit if used for this purpose: excessive rigidity, discouragement to individuality and new ideas, interference in clinical freedom, and disregard for the doctor's duty of confidentiality to the patient." The Chair, Michael Wilson, in point 5 of his accompanying letter wrote: "The concept of good practice allowance as proposed in *Agenda for Discussion* was rejected by the Conference without dissent. It would not improve the quality of general practice and would be divisive, unfair and unworkable."

None of these alleged factors stand up to scrutiny and only 16 years later when the prospect of a big pay rise for quality of care was in sight, the BMA Committee ignored all these factors. In 2002–2003 it pressed for a basic practice allowance-like quality payment, divided into many small components called the quality and outcomes framework, which then entered the GP NHS contract.

This leadership deserves analysis. First, it was a historic misjudgement of the question before that Conference, which was how to respond to a major offer from the Thatcher Government. Second, his wording is an example of a leader stooping to conquer. He knew well that the idea of a GPA had been developed by the RCGP and he had been sent a personal copy of *Quality in Practice* (RCGP, 1985a). The key point was that this was an offer by Government. Ian Bogle, another negotiator (later both Committee Chair and Chair of BMA Council), also opposed it, saying it would not be paid equally to all GPs. The Conference overwhelmingly rejected the idea of a good practice allowance. The idea of the College, Irvine, and, more importantly, the Thatcher Government, idea, was killed.

The profession thus threw away a great opportunity as any such GPA would have maintained a dialogue with Government and an allowance would have had to be negotiated with the BMA GPs. There was virtually no comment in the medical press. To the BMA this was not a big issue, as they never wanted a GPA. To the College, it was a setback but not a central academic issue. To those understanding wider relationships, it was a disaster.

Such big conferences have dozens of motions over several successive days. Most are relatively unimportant. This decision, however, was of exceptional importance and of historic significance. It helped change the relationship between British governments and the medical profession fundamentally, especially when specialist medicine made an equivalent mistake the very next year (described in Chapter 23, the Chair of Council story.

General practice had turned down a major, public offer from the Thatcher Government, one of the strongest governments of the post-war era, led by an exceptionally powerful Prime Minister. The BMA had slammed the door in the face of the DH and rejected the offered discussion on the GPA. Personally, I think this decision must rank as one of the medical profession's greatest mistakes in the twentieth century.

I doubt if Irvine seriously considered the possibility of the GPA being rejected by the BMA, as he did not discuss it. What union would not explore a new pay offer? So it is necessary to analyse the situation in those seven months in 1986 between April, when the Government published its proposal and November when the LMC Conference rejected the GPA. How could this happen?

'Allowance' was a term in the GP NHS contract meaning pay for a specific function. The Government was offering a new form of pay. It seemed inconceivable that any experienced national trade union, whose prime function was to improve the pay and conditions of its members, would not want to explore a new source of pay. Doctors in the NHS faced a virtual monopoly employer and so were particularly constrained. The default negotiating position of most trade unions to any big new offer from the employer would be to talk about it and see what it might mean.

The political background was well known. The Thatcher Government had won a bitter battle against the miners' union strike only the year before. Unions were not flavour of the month with that Government. Furthermore, the new Secretary of State for Health, Kenneth Clarke, had already had confrontations with two other occupational groups and dealt robustly and successfully with both of them. Any union would tangle with him at their peril.

The BMA was bigger, much older (1832 versus 1952), and much richer than the College. Its special experience, honed over the years, lay in responding to governments. It was to be expected it would respond to a government proposal with skill. However, the BMA had had previous tensions with the medical Royal Colleges. In 1948, Lord Moran, as President of the Royal College of Physicians of

London, outmanoeuvred the BMA and dealt directly with Aneurin Bevan (Pater, 1981), securing multiple privileges for specialists. Some in the BMA resented the influence of the medical Royal Colleges. Even 20 years after 1948, when I was on the BMA Council, I heard anger expressed about Moran and the Colleges. Any proposal involving a medical Royal College, even indirectly, was seen by some as tainted.

There was, however, another side of the argument, which the RCGP and Irvine under-rated. As the RCGP Council member most recently also elected a member of the BMA Council, I was sensitive to it. The College was always proclaiming it was centrally concerned with research, education, and standards of care. However, the good practice allowance was about none of these, but proposed radical change in a new GP contract, which was the core business of the GP Committee of the BMA. Such a proposal from the College was bound to irritate the BMA, and it did.

There was in the BMA's collective memory a battle with the government in 1965, which the BMA had won. Some of their leaders and older members of that Conference had (like me, Chapter 8, LMC and BMA story) been involved. As recently as 1973, only 13 years earlier, the same Conference had repeatedly voted against the introduction of GP vocational training and successfully delayed it. Some members of the Conference of Local Medical Committees thought they could stop developments they did not like. They and their leaders were over-confident and complacent.

There is no evidence that in the BMA, there was serious analysis of the risks in breaking off discussions with the DH on the GPA or what counter measures the Government might take. There was no realisation that the Government might impose a new GP contract. It was politically naïve to reject in public an offer from such a government at such a time.

From 1948 to 1988, successive governments always consulted the medical profession and then took the profession's views seriously. Even when the profession's policy was obviously reactionary, its view was not over-ruled. For example, the idea of postgraduate training for GPs was obviously sensible. Yet the DH waited year after year whilst the Conference of LMCs voted against it. The DH acted only after the LMC conference approved the policy in 1974 (and then by only two votes!) (DPG, 1982). The LMC representatives had come to believe they were decision-takers, underestimating the power of the state.

The important last word in the title of the government's offer, Agenda for *Discussion,* escaped them. Most of them failed to realise how public the offer of the GPA had been in a document published by the Government and how rejecting it out of hand and without the offered discussion would be seen by any government at any time as a public snub.

GPs are practical people with good communication skills. The Wanless Committee (2002) found they had the highest level of satisfaction of all the British public services. If asked politely in either a professional or social setting to discuss something, most GPs would agree to do so. The fact that several hundred NHS GPs, albeit strongly encouraged by their leaders, could completely reject a polite, public offer of discussion by the Government of the day, illustrates the negative power of big groups.

Changed Relationship between Government and the Medical Profession

After the LMC Conference rejection, the Secretary of State for Health, Kenneth Clarke, concluded he could not do business with the 'reactionary' BMA.

Provoked by this LMC Conference rejection in 1986 and the three Royal College Presidents' letter (Hoffenberg *et al.,* 1987), which was published the very next year, the whole relationship between the medical profession and the government changed decisively. This is described in detail in Chapter 23, the Chair of Council story.

Personal

In July 1986, I got a letter from the Vice-Chancellor of the University of Exeter informing me that I had been appointed to a personal chair in general practice, with effect from that October. I became the first professor of general practice in the University and the first in the South Western region (Chapter 13, Department/Institute of General Practice story).

That month, I was at a meeting in Princes Gate, and had time before my train. Unexpectedly and unplanned, I received an insight into what became the biggest crisis in the history of the College. It was a lovely summer evening and I wandered onto the terrace at Princes Gate where I found an agitated discussion going on between John Hasler (Chair) Bill Styles (Secretary), Douglas Garvie (Treasurer), and Sally Irvine (General Manager). The subject was Andrew Belton, the Chief Examiner of the College. I knew before this that there were concerns about Belton, as he had written a letter to the press about the examination without clearing it with the officers of the College and there were rumours of prickly relationships. They were discussing Belton's behaviour at a meeting in the College where Sally Irvine, angrily, said he had been very rude to College staff. I sat at the end of a bench, as I was not involved. The three officers: Chair, Secretary, and Treasurer, were discussing if something should be done and if so what.

I said nothing, but Hasler said: "What do you think Denis?" I said I had not been at the meeting they were discussing and was not involved. The discussion went on and focused on the possibility of sacking him. Then Hasler again turned to me and said: "Denis what would you do?" I was on the spot. I did not know Andrew Belton. He had a reputation of being intelligent and hardworking but very much a Yorkshireman, doing his own thing. I asked how long his contract was for and was told until November. I said in that case, as the summer is the quietest period in the College year with many people on holiday, it should be possible to hold on and then consider not renewing his contract. This comment was not welcomed or supported. I then had to leave.

Soon afterwards the General Purposes Committee was informed that the Chair had sacked the Chief Examiner. In September this Committee held a scheduled meeting. The Chair made a statement about several problems he thought the Chief Examiner had created. He had decided these were against the interests of the College and, as the examiner was a paid employee of the College (part-time), he had terminated his contract. By then the news was in the weekly medical press with adverse comments about the College. GPC was unusually subdued and unenthusiastic but there was no overt criticism. The Treasurer, Douglas Garvie, spoke strongly in favour of the decision and said that the executive owed loyalty to the Chair. Marshall Marinker, one of the strong characters on the Committee, said coldly: "I might be more inclined to support if I had been consulted."

We were experiencing classic features of cabinet government. Cabinet (group) decision-making has many advantages as it draws on the brains and experience of a wider group; and if the Chair is skilled at listening and is able to synthesise conclusions, decisions are often better. A second important feature of cabinet discussions is that after proper discussion members feel committed to the group decision, even if it is not what they themselves wanted. Cabinets, through the convention of cabinet responsibility, support the final decision and the chairman of the day. This Chair was now on his own with only two other officers in support: he was dangerously exposed.

The main item on the agenda was the College's draft response to the government's consultation paper *Primary Health Care*: *Agenda for Discussion*. The text for such a major document was traditionally written by the Chair of the day. The draft text was weak, and the Committee said so and referred the text back. It was assumed that the Chair, who was known to be a good draftsman, had been distracted by the examiner issue.

During lunch at the September GPC meeting I told each member that I was to be a professor at Exeter. The reactions varied and were revealing. Most were warm, some regretting it had taken so long. However, one officer of the Council said: "What? You a professor?!" This was a clue to officer thinking.

The September Council meeting was a replay on a bigger scale of the GPC meeting with heightened tension, as examiners were present who supported their chief. Front-page stories were in the medical press. No progress was made.

The annual general meeting was held in November, with the President, Michael Drury (1926–2014), in the Chair. The Chair made his statement. This time, however, Andrew Belton attended and spoke as a member of the College and spoke well. He argued that his sacking was an excessive over-reaction. The meeting had a high attendance with many examiners present. So many people spoke that the meeting hopelessly over-ran. It was held in a London hotel, and the meeting had to be moved to another room. This was the only time this has ever happened at an AGM, and it was a metaphor for confusion. Late in the day some people, like John Fry, sought a compromise, and an amendment was moved. There were frantic discussions on the platform as to whether this was competent. The College's solicitor advised that it was. The motion was carried but it was not clear what it meant! The essential issue was unresolved (*RCGP Members' Reference Book,* 1987c).

The Chief Examiner remained sacked. Without a motion of no confidence in the Chair, he continued in office. The meeting ended very late with general low morale. As I left, the member beside me expostulated: "It's a mess!" During the approximately 15 hours that this subject was discussed in these three meetings I never spoke about the Chief Examiner or the Chairman's action.

General Purposes Committee – December 1986

The next meeting of the GPC followed in December. The Committee had dinner the night before. Going down the stairs, Sally Irvine appeared at my side: "This may be a dinner that I'll have to leave suddenly," she said. She had previously been on the staff of the London County Council and knew about power politics. She was percipiently expecting blood on the carpet that night. Early on there was a sharp serious attack on the Chair by (Professor) John Walker from the Northern region, who had spent years developing the College examination. He sided decisively with Belton. We realised this was about to lead to a call for the Chair to resign. However, Colin Waine, also from the Northern region, intervened and protected the Chair. The group, with Hasler chairing, was stuck. The topic blew over, but raw feelings remained.

The next morning the GPC met with the main item being the latest draft of the College's response to *Primary Health Care: Agenda for Discussion.* This draft attracted severe criticism, especially from Marinker. Then I followed with an equally critical but different contribution. I outlined omissions and gave a long list of points, which I suggested ought to have been included. The Committee signalled its support. The College now was in crisis, as the text was scheduled for final approval by the Council in a few weeks' time.

Suddenly the Chair snapped. "Well," he said, "If the Committee thinks Denis can write this response better, he can write it!" Someone said, "Here here." I was gobsmacked. There was no precedent for this situation. "Do you mean that?" I asked. "Yes," the Chair said. Ever the constitutionalist, I looked round the room. "Is it the wish of GPC that I do a re-draft?" Everyone said "Yes," or nodded. I stood up in the middle of the meeting and called across the room to Sally Irvine that there was no time to lose. I needed a desk, access to computer, and staff support. She said: "Yes of course." And then, for the first and only time in my life, I walked out of an important meeting with her and up to the central offices and started dictating at once.

The timetable was daunting. I thought the previous text was unusable, so I started from scratch, knowing it had to be ready for January Council and there was Christmas in between. I worked by dictating and typing myself a good deal in both London and Exeter. I had the advantage of experience, having been the draftsman four years before for *Healthier Children-Thinking Prevention, Report from General Practice 22* (RCGP, 1982). This time I was on my own. Mercifully, I had light duties on call for the practice over Christmas and spent hours drafting. I completed it in time and it was sent to council members.

Meanwhile in Exeter, the academic medical staff had elected me and then the University appointed me, as the next Director (Dean) of the Exeter Postgraduate Medical School for five years from 1 April 1987 (PGMS story).

Council January 1987

The meeting of Council in January was strange. Chairs normally present such documents, but Hasler in the Chair said I had written the draft document, so I should present it from the back of the room.

It was well received. A serious challenge came from John Ball, a former Chair of the GMSC, now a member of the RCGP Council, with an eye on the presidency. He said he knew about GP funding and strongly attacked my proposal that there should be a million-pound development fund established. He ridiculed this saying it was absurd and so weakened the rest of the response. Nobody else spoke. Should I just let that point go or fight one of the heavy-weight debaters in the Council? On the spur of the moment, I fought. I reminded the Council of the longstanding capital deprivation of British general practice, which had affected my grandfather's and father's careers. There was an obvious need to computerise the service and ensure modern buildings for all practices. The Council responded with applause and voted with a big majority to retain the development fund. The text went straight back to Exeter where Jill and I edited it for publication. This document started and finished in our home. The overwhelming approval of my text by the Council did not go unnoticed.

Men in Grey Suits

Telephones were ringing, but not in Exeter. Then one evening the President rang me. We were going out and I was with Jill changing in our bedroom. He said the Chair of Council had lost the confidence of the GPC. Everyone had been consulted and no one favoured him staying. Half dressed, I said as I had lost an election to this Chair only 18 months before, it was not appropriate for me to be ganging up on him and I might be seen to be motivated by jealousy or revenge. I said I would abstain. "That settles it!" Michael Drury said. Leader groups get to know and understand each other. The President laughed, saying he had foreseen this, and he was ringing me last. One new, young member was uncertain, but the rest were "solid" (so Colin Waine had changed his mind). This was my third abstention in a nationally important vote. Drury ended the call cryptically: "Get ready for more work."

The phrase 'men in grey suits' is a shorthand to describe a situation when the leaders of an institution decide a change of leader is needed and a few leading members go to see the leader to call for resignation. The aim is to avoid the public and humiliating process of a vote of no confidence. In 1986 I thought that this process always worked but I had a different experience in 2001, as described in Chapter 38, the Chair of the Academy of Royal Medical Colleges.

Michael Drury, President, operated the College's 'men in grey suits' process. He and the Vice-Chair of Council, Robin Steel, went to see the Chair at his home. Hasler agreed to resign. An emergency meeting of the GPC was called for Saturday 29 January 1987. The timing could not have been more inconvenient for our family. Penny, our oldest daughter, was a member of the dancing team of the University of Bristol, which had qualified for the finals of the university team dancing championships. Jill and I had already agreed to go to the Winter Garden ballroom in Liverpool to support her that very evening. Then, unusually, I developed influenza. I was running a high temperature and Jill and I conferred anxiously. She knew my view about important meetings – always be there. We were both scarred by the 1985 vote to reject me and there now was a once-in-a-life time chance to reverse it. We agreed I would go to the meeting and then on to Liverpool. Jill went straight to Liverpool.

That meeting of the GPC was held in the common room of Princes Gate, the only formal meeting of its kind held there in my 30 years. It had no table and was furnished with armchairs. I felt awful with a headache and a high temperature. I sat in a corner, swallowing paracetamol, and did not speak.

The President and Vice-Chair of Council summarised their ring-round of the Committee and their visit to Hasler. They confirmed his resignation letter had been received. The questions were how to get a new Chair and how soon it could be done. Constitutionally, it was clear that only the Council could elect a chair. It was quickly agreed the College could not manage without a chair until the next planned Council meeting. The question was how soon could Council be recalled for an emergency meeting? Council members were working GPs who would have surgeries booked. How much notice was reasonable? Eventually a date 12 calendar days ahead but only six working days was agreed upon, but would members of Council object at the short notice?

My name came up as the successor, with Marinker rooting for me. I had the great advantage of not being in office when the sacking decision was taken. There was clear support for me, but the Committee felt it should not be seen to seek to pre-empt the Council. Colin Waine reserved the right to stand. No other name emerged. I left feeling I had the most support, at least in the executive. Harold Wilson (1916–1995) once said: "A week is a long time in politics." This was true me for me for those six working days.

For once, I did not stay for lunch when in doing so I would almost certainly have gained valuable information and been able to cement relationships. Instead, I rushed for a train to Liverpool. I arrived just in time to see Penny dance with her partner Paul Dawson, who came from a leading dancing family and whom she later married. Sadly, they were soon knocked out. Jill took me home while I still had a temperature and I have no memory of the journey.

Emergency Meeting of Council – February 1987

The emergency meeting of the Council was on 10 February. The President and Vice-Chair reported what had happened. With the resignation received, the key business was electing a new Chair. Colin Waine changed his mind about standing and proposed me. I was seconded by Robin Steel, Vice-chair of Council. I was asked to leave the room. I waited in the room opposite, the John Hunt room. I was recalled and told I had been elected to applause. I appreciated the great privilege of unopposed election.

I thanked everyone for coming at short notice and those who had borne the brunt of the events. I promised to do my best. I paid a full tribute to John Hasler and all he had done. The College had been through a constitutional crisis and there was a collective responsibility to resolve it. I hoped everyone would exercise listening and learning skills and said I would be open to any member of the Council telephoning me. I finished, saying I was confident that College members would work together in the future (Martin, 1987). Walking down the stairs, a Council member from Oxford appeared at my side. I hesitated to speak, as he was a colleague of Hasler's, but he smiled at me and said: "Cometh the hour: cometh the man!"

My election in a formal democratic vote by the Council was the first such election of a Chair of Council. It ended the old-fashioned ring-round system. I thus experienced the last of the old and the first new style voting. All elections for the Chairmanship since have been by a formal vote by members of the Council.

I inherited responsibility for the College's response to the Government. Sally Irvine suggested I take the name of the College Chair when this was published, as I had written it. I declined, as constitutionally it had been approved by a Council chaired by Hasler. I did, however, choose the title. I had a strong feeling about the phrase "front line," which I thought had great resonance. I wanted to secure it for general practice – *The Front Line of the NHS, Report from General Practice 25* (RCGP, 1987a). The term was little used until 33 years later in 2020 when it came into use for staff treating corona virus. It was then widely used by both the UK and US governments, but not for general practice.

Later, I analysed my circuitous route to the Chair of the Council and realised that the remarkable exchange between Hasler and me in the December GPC, when he handed over to me the drafting of the RCGP paper, represented an acting out symbolically of the transfer of the chairmanship that followed two months later. Most people think that the Chair's fall was because of the Chief Examiner. Only the executive members appreciated that the inability to deliver a national document to the standard required was also very important.

John Hasler invited me to his home. However, I was more pressed for time than I had ever been in my life. The College was in its biggest ever crisis, having lost its Chief Examiner and its Chair within six months. The press coverage for the College was dreadful. I had had only a fortnight's notice of the Chair, less time than any chair before or since, and I needed time to talk with my practice partners.

I had to give the Chair's speech to a general meeting with hundreds of uneasy members present in Edinburgh the next month.

In addition, I was only weeks away from starting a new big job in Exeter. I regretted not going to see John and his wife Lindsay, both of whom I liked and with whom I had always got on well, but I had no time. I was more pressed for time than at any other stage in my life with the College in its biggest ever crisis. Only seven weeks later, on 1 April 1987, I became Director (Dean) of the Postgraduate Medical School of the University of Exeter (Chapter 27, Postgraduate Medical School).

It was quite a transition from a humiliating rejection by my peers in the Council in the summer of 1985 to a Professorship, the unforeseen Directorship of the Postgraduate Medical School, and the unexpected Chairmanship of the College, all within 20 months. Such are the downs and ups of institutional life.

Section VI

23

Chair of Council: February 1987 to November 1990

The final test of a leader is that he leaves behind him in other men the conviction and the will to carry on

Lippmann W (1945) *New York Herald Tribune*

I was elected Chair of Council unopposed on 10 February 1987. Outside the College I continued as a member of the JCPTGP and became an ex-officio member of the Standing Medical Advisory Committee, chaired by the CMO, Sir Donald Acheson.

In Princes Gate I had the advantage of the use of the Ian Watson suite with a sitting room, bedroom, two beds, and a WC. This was invaluable when I was often arriving late at night. Jill could also come and stay the night on occasions.

I took over with the College in crisis after losing its Chief Examiner and Chair within six months and, for the first time, it was experiencing sustained adverse press publicity. Most new chairs relish publicity and interviews, I did the opposite saying I wanted to listen to colleagues. The press soon lost interest. My first public test was the Spring General Meeting in Edinburgh. This brought together several hundred uneasy members and the crisis was in everyone's mind. My speech had to reassure the members and seemed to do so (DPG, 1987a).

The General Purposes Committee had an annual weekend. At dinner the first night I asked if anyone thought College members were better doctors than non-members? Everyone said "No, of course not." I asked what the prime aim of the College was and they all said that it was to improve the quality of general practice. I then sprang the question: "So, if the College, for 35 years, has spent ever-increasing funds, and if College members are not better, has the College been wasting its time?" This set the tone of intellectual challenge for the weekend.

A stabilising role was played by the Membership Division, with John Lee (Chair), John Ferguson and Philip Tombleson, leading examiners, the College had diplomatic leaders helping to cool things down.

Jill as an Exeter-Based PA

I wanted a base in Exeter as a Chair needs privacy in drafting. The Exeter office was an editing/publishing room, not a base for a national chair. Sally, the General Manager, offered Jill the role of being my Exeter PA, with an honorarium. Jill then helped to co-ordinate the mass of papers now pouring into our home (the Post Office often sent a van) and did this well. She attended meetings of the Council sitting silently, in a corner facing the chair. She developed great skill in analysing the theatre that meetings of a national Council always are. She read between the lines. What is the mood and why? Who is speaking as expected and who is not? She gave me invaluable feedback. We used to go together to an Exeter pub afterwards to debrief.

An important event was the Government's offer to GPs of a good practice allowance in April 1986, *Primary Health Care: Agenda for Discussion* (DHSS, 1986) and its crushing rejection by the

DOI: 10.1201/9781032713601-29

Conference of Local Medical Committees in November, which is described in detail in Chapter 22, the Downs and Ups of Institutional Life. There was virtually no comment in the medical press. To the College it was a setback but not a central academic issue. To those understanding wider relationships, it was a disaster.

Letters in Medical Journals

There were two letters published in the *Lancet* during the 20th century both of which had permanent influence on the medical profession. The first was the Rose-Hunt letter of 1951 (also published in the *BMJ*), which proposed the formation of a new college of general practice. This was a brilliant leadership move by two very different British GPs. Its timing was critical and perfectly judged. It was remarkably successful and achieved all that its authors hoped. I was later fortunate to meet both of them and have a dinner alone with John Hunt. The positive response to that letter led to the formation of the College of General Practitioners and a permanent change in the balance between specialist and generalist medicine in Britain and the English-speaking world.

The second letter was published in the *Lancet* 36 years later in December 1987, while I was Chair. It was written by the Presidents of the oldest three medical Royal Colleges in England. These were Professor Sir Raymond Hoffenberg (1923–2007, President of the Royal College of Physicians of London); Mr (later Sir) Ian Todd (1921–2015, President of the Royal College of Surgeons of England); and Sir George Pinker (1924–2007, President of the Royal College of Obstetricians and Gynaecologists). I knew all three and had meals with each of them.

Since 1948, the NHS had received a lower share of the gross domestic product (GDP) than most developed countries as NHS funding was under strict government control. Many countries had insurance systems, which are a mechanism for adjusting premiums to costs and they operate at arms length from their governments. Such countries mostly spent more per person on health care than the UK.

All the medical Royal Colleges are registered charities and have a duty to act in the public interest, i.e. exist to improve the quality of care for patients. Any professional approach from the Royal Colleges to a government or to a Prime Minister needed five components: a carefully prepared document showing (a) how standards of care for British patients were a problem, (b) how resources or support from Government could improve them, (c) an offer to work in partnership with Government including making changes in the profession to improve quality of care, (d) a solid team of Colleges in support and (e) private, analysis on what responses a Government might make (2, Chess story).

However, no such preparations were made by those Presidents. When invited to see the Prime Minister they went unprepared into the Thatcher den, over-confident that they could tell the PM what to do. A professional approach was needed to draw on the experiences and skills of all the main branches of the medical profession and all the existing Medical Royal Colleges and Faculties.

The investigative specialties, like pathology and radiology, had important insights and strong Colleges. The RCPsych had an important perspective on mental health and the RCGP alone understood medical care outside hospitals. As the RCGP Chair at the time I knew they had neither consulted nor even informed us. The three Presidents acted on their own. They were living in the past: from 1930–1952 there had been just those three medical Royal Colleges in England, but by 1987 there were several other active medical Royal Colleges.

The three authors who signed that letter were each responsible for it, but one of them was the leader. Sir Raymond Hoffenberg, KBE PRCP was a brilliant man, a South African who had valued black people so much, that the apartheid government forced him to leave his country (Humphreys, 2010). He moved to the UK, becoming PRCP, a remarkable achievement. Perhaps his contempt for the South African government rubbed off on the UK government? I was later a Trustee with him at the Nuffield Trust. He was a strong personality and led the other two.

Textual analysis of the letter with my GP perspective and my emphasis, was:

> "Every day we learn of new problems in *the NHS – beds are short, operating rooms are not available. Emergency wards are closed, essential services are shut down* in order to make financial savings. In spite of the efforts of doctors, nurses and other *hospital* staff, patient care is deteriorating. Acute *hospital services* have almost reached breaking point. Morale is depressingly low."

> "It is not only patient care that is suffering. Financial stringencies have hit academic aspects of medicine in particular, because of the additional burden of reduced university grants committee funding. Yet the future of *medicine,* depends on the quality of our clinical teachers and research workers."

> "Face saving initiatives such as the allocation of £30 million for *waiting lists* and an immediate overall review *of acute hospital services* is *mandatory. Additional and alternative funding must be found.* We call on the Government to do something now to save our *Health Service*, once the envy of the world."

In its 158 words, it makes eight references to acute or hospital services which it consistently equates to the 'NHS' and 'medicine.' The authors made no mention of any other branch of medicine, any other Royal College, or health care outside hospital or the health of the population. They offered no evidence for their claims. There was no suggestion that the medical profession should make any changes. The tone is authoritarian: "*must be*" and "*is mandatory*"; i.e. do what we tell you. There was no offer to work with Government. The letter was a spectacular failure of leadership. Writing it so that all the other Royal College leaders were left in the dark, not consulted, and feeling left out and bruised, was poor team leadership.

This second letter also influenced the whole of the medical profession permanently but in a way opposite to the intention of its authors. Its timing was also critical and influenced the response it generated. Margaret Thatcher was not amused, especially as there was then a press campaign about NHS cardiac surgery. She reacted all right – but not as any of those three Presidents foresaw. She soon went on television and I watched her announce a complete review, not just of hospital services but of the whole NHS. She set up a committee of cabinet ministers, *excluding every doctor in the UK, even the Chief Medical Officer* (my emphasis).

In 1988, Hoffenberg had another opportunity. On 3 October Margaret Thatcher went to the Royal College of Physicians for lunch, a critical visit at a critical time. A photograph of her in the RCP shows Hoffenberg (President), David Pyke (Registrar) and Tony (later Sir Anthony) Dawson (Honorary Treasurer). If ever there was time for bridge-building between the medical profession and the Government, this was it. However, Hoffenberg and the College officers got into an argument with her saying that the UK was near the bottom of OECD countries in terms of expenditure on health services. She hit back with accusations of the "exploitation of junior doctors" and the "duplication of services." So bad were the feelings that as Hoffenberg showed her to her car, her parting shot was: "You won't expect a letter of thanks from me for the lunch, will you?!" (Humphreys, 2010).

A policy failure was compounded by a diplomatic failure. Hoffenberg was right about the low level of expenditure on health, but the prime need then was to engage with Margaret Thatcher and try to help her have pride in British medicine and work with the Colleges. I don't underestimate the difficulties. I got nowhere in the two meetings I had with Margaret Thatcher nor my one with the Secretary of State, John Moore, but those three Presidents were in a much stronger position and could have done better.

Changed Relationship between Government and the Medical Profession

The BMA GPs by rejecting the Government's offer to discuss a good practice allowance mainly riled the Secretary of State, Kenneth Clarke (1940–; now Lord Clarke) who was reported as saying that the

BMA was not a union with which he could do business. However, the three specialist Presidents' letter angered Mrs Thatcher personally.

Ever since 1948, when the NHS was established, the medical profession had been seen by successive governments, of both main parties, as a trusted and reliable partner. The mantra was that doctors know about healthcare. So great was the former deference to the medical profession that even when an obviously sensible reform like introducing much-needed vocational training for general practice was persistently opposed year after year by the Conference of Local Medical Committees, the Government did not move to implement it until the Conference of Local Medical Committees finally agreed the policy (in 1974 by two votes!). Successive governments openly respected the doctors' views.

The Conference of Local Medical Committees in November 1986, by rejecting the Government's offer of discussion on a GPA, followed by the three Presidents' letter in December 1987 with its hectoring tone, between them squandered a nearly 40-year precious relationship. The medical profession had previously always been consulted on important policies by successive governments and often had had a decisive say.

However, from Thatcher's decision in December 1987 onwards the mantra became that politicians know best about healthcare. The medical profession was no longer so respected and might not be consulted. This changed relationship became public in Thatcher's white paper *Working for Patients* (DH, 1989), in which she wrote the foreword herself. This White Paper was published only 13 months after the three Presidents' letter and became law in 1990. I was, by an accident of history, the College Chair when the relationship between Government and the medical profession changed radically and probably permanently.

Repercussions occurred in the Conference of Medical Royal Colleges and Faculties. The excluded Colleges saw that the three Presidents' letter had both damaged communication with Government and had relegated them to second division status. It was not only Thatcher who was not amused. The letter had been signed by their Chair (Todd) who had not consulted them, stating in public his relationship with two Colleges was more important than his chairmanship of all the Colleges. The Conference became more sensitive to constitutional changes, much less inclined to follow the lead of the older Royal Colleges, and more sensitive to the interests of other Colleges. I was to be a beneficiary a decade later.

Michael Drury (1926–2014; RCGP President and then sole GP representative in the Conference) and I agreed the RCGP line would be to express deep disappointment that our College had not been consulted, but to avoid a direct challenge or criticism of the three Presidents concerned. We were playing the long game. This matched the reaction of the other excluded colleges. Our College was steadily gaining in stature and influence.

Ian Todd (1921–2015) PRCSEng was succeeded as Chair of the Conference by Margaret Turner-Warwick (PRCP; 1924–2017) in 1990. The leadership by the older three Colleges continued, but only because of her high personal stature and a feeling that it was high time for the first ever woman leader. The reaction to the three Presidents' letter occurred in the next election after that for the Chair of the Conference. A big effort was then made, in which I actively participated, to elect a Chair outside the three older Colleges. Professor (later Sir) Dillwyn Williams (1929–; PRCPath) was elected. He soon became a Professor at Cambridge and was only the second Chair of the Conference from outside the three older Colleges (Academy of Medical Royal Colleges, 2000). The Presidents of the three older Colleges continued private meetings before Conference meetings, which did not endear them to the other Presidents.

All through 1988 I sought to analyse what big changes the Government was likely to make and how best general practice could prepare and respond. One of my responses, stimulated by a loss of confidence in the specialist leadership of the Conference of Medical Royal Colleges and triggered by the launch of the White Paper on 31 January 1989, was to establish a new national Conference for GPs in April 1989. This is described in Chapter 25, Conference of Academic Organisations of General Practice.

Medical historians will ponder why after nearly 40 years of the NHS the relationship between the Government and the medical profession changed radically in a very short period. My understanding is that it was because the Government was twice provoked within only 13 months by the leaders of the two main branches of medicine, by the GPs in 1986 and the specialists in 1987.

As this story has not been told before, my understanding is described in detail since, probably alone in Britain, I knew all the main people involved: the BMA negotiators, all three Presidents of the older Royal Colleges, the Prime Minister and Secretary of State for Health, as well as the CMO and senior officials. I had had meals with seven of them. Many have since died. Why these professional leaders, working quite separately, unwisely provoked one of the strongest British Prime Ministers of the 20th century is an important question. There was no communication between the GPs and the three Presidents but they shared similar attitudes of entitlement, over-confidence, and political naivety. Neither group understood that being consulted by Government is a privilege that has to be earned and is not a right. Both groups learnt the lesson painfully within months when the Government stopped consulting both of them.

A generous amount of influence in the 1948 NHS arrangements gave GPs places and often chairmanships of NHS executive councils and statutory rights of consultation for local medical committees. This was compounded by a political battle with the DHSS, in which I played a small local part, in the mid-1960s, which the BMA won (Chapter 8, LMC and BMA story). The BMA GPs concluded they were politically stronger than they really were – a serious error for a medico-political organisation and trade union, for which such judgements are crucial.

Of the two provocations by each half of the medical profession, that of the GPs in 1986 was the more culpable for four reasons. First, the idea of a good practice allowance, whoever had designed it, was essentially reasonable (paying for performance as in many other walks of life) and later the GPA idea, broken into multiple fractions was introduced with strong BMA support, as the Quality and Outcomes Framework (NHS Confederation and the BMA, 2003). Second, the idea of the GPA was designed and promoted by fellow GPs and its rejection included an element of petty jealousy in trying to do the College down. Third, the case for change (DPG *et al.,* 1986) and the feasibility of the GPA (Marinker *et al.,* 1986) had been set out in three *BMJ* articles published only months earlier. The Conference of Local Medical Committees' GPs had informed analysis from its own College (RCGP, 1985a) and prescient analysis in the most read British medical journal. Fourth, the Government paper (DHSS, 1986) proposing a GPA was eminently reasonable and entitled "Agenda *for Discussion*" (my italics). Slamming the door in the Government's face in public and refusing the requested discussion was provocative, especially as only a year earlier the same Government had seen off the politically strong National Union of Miners. Finally, the LMC GPs had from April to November to respond.

The three Presidents were similarly over-confident and politically naïve. They seemed to think that they had a divine right to tell governments what to do using words like: "must be…it is mandatory." They were arrogant in thinking that they did not need to consult the other medical Royal Colleges, which by 1987 included: the RCGP (founded 1952), the RCPath (1970), the RCPsych (1971) and the RCRadiologists (1975), as well as three Faculties for dental surgery, public health and occupational medicine. Two of the Presidents (Hoffenberg and Todd) had been Chairs of the Conference of Medical Royal Colleges and their Faculties and Todd was in the Chair of that Conference when he signed the letter without consulting and so let his fellow Presidents in the Conference down.

The thinking at the top of the specialist medical colleges was revealed to me after I joined the Conference of Colleges in 1989 as the first RCGP chair to do so. The specialist Presidents were then cushioned by the NHS in ways they did not appreciate. They all had the top-level distinction awards which doubled their incomes (and were more than double mine) and which were pensioned in a system then rare in the public service. One President told me that when he was elected President of his College his hospital then appointed an extra senior registrar to cover his work when he was away on College business, whilst my College was paying, from GPs' subscriptions, the cost of my locums. The NHS subsidised specialist presidents only.

One evening after a dinner, I was engaged in a long discussion with a group of the specialist Presidents quizzing me about the independent contractor status of the NHS GPs, which they saw as an anachronism. In defending it I referred to my article (DPG, 1977b) which none had read, and the involvement of GPs in the service (skin in the game) which it encouraged. I said that consultants were being treated as independent contractors in hospitals whilst in law being salaried servants of the hospital. I suggested that sooner or later that legal relationship would be called in. One President closed me down saying firmly "That's never going to happen," and all the others agreed. However, the 2000 NHS Act made chief executives the boss in NHS hospitals. After I retired, the practice moved to new premises where all consulting rooms were to be painted the same colour. One female GP, as a partner and independent contractor, asked to have her room painted in a different colour. The partnership quickly agreed. No UK consultant could have asked for this or been given a positive answer. The leaders of specialist medicine in the late 1980s had not rigorously analysed their own salaried situation.

Edwina Curry

After meeting Edwina Curry as a Health Minister, she accepted my invitation to dinner with the College Officers. They travelled from around the UK for it, incurring travel and locum costs. I organised flowers so the building looked beautiful. When the doorbell rang, I opened the door myself to welcome her. Standing there was a senior male medical civil servant. He said Mrs Curry was sorry she was unable to come and he had come instead! We assumed she was absent on parliamentary business but later, news of her then unknown relationship with John Major emerged, which provided another possibility.

David Willets

David Willetts (1956–; now Lord), Principal Private Secretary to the Prime Minister (later Minister and member of the House of Lords) contacted me. He was then a 32-year-old highflying civil servant at No 10. We met several times, sometimes in 10 Downing Street and had deep discussions about the role of general practice and its strengths and weaknesses. He was very intelligent, being nicknamed "two brains," and read extensively. He was a superb analyst but did not understand general practice. I saw my role as briefing him, hoping he would then brief Margaret Thatcher (1925–2013). I was able to match him reference with reference and invited him to the practice. That visit is described in Chapter 34: The Practice story, 1987–2000.

"Avalanche of Change" 1988

The Spring General Meeting in April 1988 was in Cheltenham, in my own region and gave me a chance to inform members. I knew that big changes were coming and had jointly written the three *BMJ* articles (DPG *et al.*, 1986, Marinker *et al.*, 1986; Maynard *et al.*, 1986). With hundreds of members present I had to do all I could to puncture complacency and help colleagues prepare for radical changes. Not knowing what the changes would be, the message had to be general. I spent ages seeking a sound bite for my Chair's speech and eventually found one.

> …The message of change can now be clearly seen not just through the mists on the horizon but in print before our eyes. There is now no doubt of the *urgent need* for all of us to read and to think, and to think harder than we have ever done before, about the nature of our discipline….I expect an *avalanche of change* to sweep not just across general practice but across the medical profession as a whole.

(DPG, 1988)

'Avalanche of change' was a brief, alliterative and accurate metaphor. In three words it captured four essential messages. What was coming would be top down, sudden, immensely forceful and irresistible. It resonated with Jack and Gertie Cole, my uncle and aunt living in Cheltenham, who had come to hear my speech. For my large GP audience, however, it did not register at all and was not discussed. Some said it was "OTT." A leader's lot is not a happy one!

John Moore, Secretary of State DHSS

In 1988, at a conference, I spoke immediately after John Moore (1937–2019; later Baron Moore of Lower Marsh), Secretary of State for the DHSS. He announced the Government's acceptance of Project 2000, a reform of nurse education. He walked out when I started speaking – as Ministers often do.

I met him on other occasions and he invited me see him. I was cautious as he appeared to be influenced by the United States, very right wing, and unbriefed about NHS general practice. I went to one of the two least satisfactory meetings I have ever had with a Minister. Whilst we were still standing, he said "You've got to get your GPs to be more like businessmen!" I replied, as any representative of the College would, "Actually the College does not deal with remuneration, we concentrate on standards of care for patients, education and research." He completely ignored this, raised his voice, and impatiently said, "I mean you've got to get GPs to be more business-like and be aware of costs." "Costs," I said. "Do you know what it costs to get a washing machine repaired?" He looked surprised and said: "No, why?" I said: "My wife has just had our washing machine repaired by an engineer on a weekday home visit, so I know the cost and told him. "The point," I said: "is that your Department is paying GPs less than that sum for an average of four face-to-face consultations a year." He looked surprised. I rubbed it in saying "and that includes all home visits and working on bank holidays, including some work on Christmas Day!" We were standing facing each other and as a GP and interested in behaviour, I noted he took a step backwards. He turned to his senior civil servant asking: "Is that true?" I admire the skills of the civil service in finding the right words under pressure. "Well," the civil servant said. "It's one way of putting it!"

After that uncomfortable opening, he sat me down and enquired why GPs were so inefficient in accepting patients who lived at distance when there were other GPs closer? (Just GPs). I explained about patient choice and the importance of trust built up through continuity of care and long-term GP patient relationships. I gave him an example of a family I knew well, although they lived some distance from the practice, where we had recently accepted a granny who had come to live. He was not impressed and soon dismissed me.

Handbagged by Margaret Thatcher, Chequers 1988

In the spring of 1988, Margaret Thatcher was chairing a group of cabinet ministers reviewing the NHS. Consultation in the ordinary way did not take place. She held some consultative meetings at Chequers, the PM's country home: one day for doctors, another for managers etc. I was invited to the doctor one, as the RCGP Chair. The invitation said this was secret. Nevertheless, I consulted the cabinet, who were unanimous that I should go. The meeting was on a Sunday and I took her some Devonshire cream, which I gave her on arrival. She was charming and at a preliminary gathering on the ground floor she was a gracious hostess.

We went up to a meeting room arranged around a long table where she sat at one end. Some cabinet ministers were there. Amongst the doctors whom I knew were: Lord Butterfield, a physician and Vice-Chancellor; Clive Froggatt, a GP from Cheltenham who was active in the Conservative Medical Association; and Cyril (later Sir) Chantler (1939–), a leading medical manager at Guy's Hospital. The seating was awkward for me as it was difficult to make eye contact with the PM. There were no papers.

Thatcher called people round the room, one by one, and spoke one to one, with little discussion. She called me very late. I spoke of the need for general practitioners to have more educational support, as their responsibilities were increasing. I chose this as a broad-brush suggestion that could fit into any new NHS arrangements. In College policy terms it was pretty routine.

I was taken by surprise by her exploding at my suggestion. "Absurd!" she said. "These doctors have already had seven years' training." She made it clear she thought very little of GPs (just GPs). I tried to reply with one or two facts but she raised her voice and simply brushed me aside. She appeared surprised by what I had said, but any civil servant could have predicted that any College Chairman would probably speak about GP education, medical audit, or research. She was not interested in the College or general practice (just GPs).

After the meeting I reeled downstairs, shaken and anxious that I had let the College down. We were given lunch and I was sitting next to John Major, Chief Secretary to the Treasury. He could see I was shaken. He was charming and supportive, pouring me a drink: "Don't worry," he said. "We've all been there!" He chatted in a friendly way and helped me considerably. Lord Butterfield came over: "Outrageous!" he said. "Of course you were right to ask for more training for GPs, they need it. She should never have treated you like that."

I reported back to the GPC, who was surprised and supportive. All agreed that Margaret Thatcher had 'handbagged' me. The conclusion was that she had her own agenda and was not in the least interested in general practice (just GPs). Her response was seen as an 'unforced error.' Why rubbish me? She only had to say some neutral phrase about considering the idea and move on. Margaret Thatcher's (1993) book describes these seminars as being "to brief myself."

North-East Thames Region 1988

In 1988 the JCPTGP, chaired by Dorothy Ward from the BMA, received a report of a visit to the North-East Thames region of an unsatisfactory inspection, the third running. It had found that in several training practices the records were not in order and hospital letters were folded higgledy piggledy. This was one of the most basic national standards for trainers enforced nationally in visits around the country.

The GPC met in April. It decided that, as the JCPTGP was publicly stating the training was not satisfactory, something had to be done. The Committee decided unanimously (including Lotte Newman who came from that area) that, since the trainees were not getting an appropriate training experience, to withdraw the right of trainees in that region to sit the MRCGP examination until the region had a satisfactory report. This was a matter in which the College had sole responsibility. The region was informed.

There was a huge backlash from the region, its trainers, and various organisations. Letters of complaint poured into Princes Gate. The medical press seized on the issue. I was invited to a mass evening meeting of course organisers and trainers in the region. When severe public criticism is mounted, even senior people may stand back. The heat falls on the person in charge. President Truman observed: "the buck stops here!" I went alone. The Regional Adviser in charge of vocational training in the region, Eddie Josse (1933–2020), did not come. The atmosphere was threatening, and the whole room was seething with indignation; the trainers were virtually all male.

The opening speech claimed multiple allegations of high-handed, unreasonable behaviour by the College and the people in the room, already angry, were well worked up. Then it was my turn and I was in a very tight spot. I went through the whole story, slowly and precisely. First, why the policy of having the medical record in order was a logical policy, without this a GP could not see the hospital letters and could not follow hospital advice or know that was going on. Patients were at risk. The standard was essential in a practice that had volunteered to be a teaching practice. I made it clear I was a working GP and that the records had been in order in my own practice for years and it greatly helped the work (my father had done it in the 1950s). This was a standard that applied all over the

UK; trainers had either not been appointed or had lost their trainer status if they did not meet this standard, as had happened in my region. I then detailed the three different visits to the region made by the JCPTGP all of which had found training practices with medical records out of order. Each time the region had been told in writing. There had been fair warnings in writing and plenty of time to put things right. It was not fair that GPs all over the country were working hard to meet this standard which North- East Thames was breaching. I ended on a positive note. This was a temporary decision. Once the region put things right and once the JCPTGP said national minimal standards were in place then the College would allow trainees to take the MRCGP again. This speech shook the room.

Most trainers said they had never heard the facts before and that nobody had told them about any JCPTGP report. Questions arose about the Regional Adviser and what he had not done about standards. Some trainers said their records were in order and felt it was unfair they were tarred with the same brush. I commiserated and explained that the JCPTGP assessed whole regions.

Then the mood swung to being hostile again as the room considered how the decision had been taken by the GPC as the Council Executive not the full Council. I explained that the GPC had 16 democratically elected members and had power to act on behalf of the Council between Council meetings. The matter would come to the next Council. An unmentioned irony was that the region had one of the lowest numbers of MRCGP candidates in the UK.

All the letters of criticism got full replies. Disappointingly, some leading public health physicians accused the College of acting against a socially deprived area. Did they care that deprived people were getting poorer care since their doctors couldn't see hospital letters about their patients?

Such was the pressure that I needed to explain the situation to the whole College membership. I found myself alone. I wrote text for the College *Journal* (*JRCGP*, 1988) setting out the story. I also wrote a detailed paper for the Council giving chapter and verse of exactly what had been done and why. The Council meeting was tense with some criticism of the GPC, and by implication of me, but the GPC decision was formally endorsed. I had the vote taken by roll call. There were six votes against, including John Ball. I learned about the striking indifference of the DHSS to professional standards. The civil servants who knew about this were not interested in quality of care.

Looking back, the College was right to react to recurrent, provocative failure to meet agreed national, minimum standards. However, it would have been more diplomatic for the GPC to recommend the decision to the Council rather than acting itself. As I chaired the GPC, I must take the prime responsibility.

Academic Work outside Princes Gate

I gave the McConaghey Memorial lecture in Lifton to the Tamar Faculty. The room was packed. Sadly, two people whom I hoped would be there were not: Gussie McConaghey (Mac's widow) and Irene Scawn (Journal Business Manager). I had spent hours working out the story as I had multiple aims: I wanted to honour Mac as one of my professional father figures. Secondly, I wanted to tell the story of the founding of the College *Journal,* Mac's greatest professional achievement. I particularly wanted to emphasise that this had been the first general practice journal in the world in 1961 to be included in *Index Medicus* and so recognised as scientific by the National Library of Medicine in Washington, USA.

Going through the early books by GPs, helped by Margaret Hammond, the College Librarian, I found it was 1961 when for the first time two clinical books were published, written by GPs, which could not have been written by any hospital consultant: Clyne's (1961) *Night Calls* and Fry's (1961) *The Catarrhal Child*. The year 1961 was also when the College became debt free; so this was the date when general practice became an independent discipline (DPG, 1989).

I discovered that a group of senior doctors was meeting called the Academic Medicine Group. This had been established by the RCP, it met in the RCP and was chaired by the PRCP. It had 38 members, of whom about half came each time. I found that there was no GP on it. I wrote to the PRCP, whom I knew, suggesting that GP representation was appropriate. I got no answer but was suddenly included in the group and then attended regularly as the sole, token GP. This group had no executive responsibility but brought together key national players in the Colleges, in Oxbridge (both Regius Professors), the deans, and the NHS. It operated as if general practice did not exist, and it was never mentioned unless I did (just GPs). By 1994 I had managed to get a second GP, Michael Pringle, as a member.

By January 1989, there were fears in the GMSC that the College was undermining it and I was keen to establish in the minds of BMA activists that the College was entirely independent, as some of them resented the College making statements or giving advice. Michael Wilson and I signed a concordat which gave us both what we needed. The statement read that the GMSC was the sole negotiating body, and the College was not seeking to become one (we couldn't as a registered charity). I got the statement in that the College was an independent body and could advise whomever it chose.

White Paper – *Working for Patients* 1989

On 31 January 1989 I was invited as Chair, with the leaders of the medical profession, to the launch by the Government of the White Paper on the Health Service called *Working for Patients* (DH, 1989). As I sat in the Cathedral room in the DH, opposite the Cenotaph, I knew it was a historic moment and that the relationship between the state and the medical profession was being changed fundamentally, perhaps for ever. I saw this as an example of pipers and tunes. Government had been paying the NHS piper since 1948, but had previously devolved to the medical profession much influence. New proposals included the 'purchaser provider split,' the idea of 'GP fundholding,' meaning some volunteer general practices would hold an NHS budget and be empowered to buy certain defined services. Most of all it meant, probably permanently, Government control.

The radical change in relationships between Government and the medical profession is encapsulated on the public record in two Government documents published only 34 months apart. In April 1986, the Thatcher Government published a (Green Paper-like) consultation document on the future of general practice entitled *Primary Health Care: an Agenda for Discussion*. By contrast in January 1989 *Working for Patients* was a White Paper indicating planned legislation, which soon followed. It was not for consultation and doctors and health professionals were told how things were now going to be. Some commentators have suggested that Mrs Thatcher was hostile to the medical profession. However, the record is that in April 1986 her Government offered in public the GP branch of the profession a perfectly reasonable proposal. Moreover, the tone of her Government's offer was also reasonable, i.e. "for discussion."

I was able to get Kenneth Clarke to come to dinner with the GPC in early 1989. This was the only time a Secretary of State for Health had come to just a committee, meaning he saw the RCGP as important. He got many questions and responded robustly, pointing out that the NHS then did not know what anything cost (true). Decisions had to be taken on the basis of known costs – if costs were not known, then good management decisions were impossible. Several members of GPCs, aware of the widespread opposition, suggested the White Paper would have to be delayed. "No" said Clarke, "I'll have it in law in 18 months." He was not believed, but I noted the dates, and he did.

Entering the Conference of Medical Royal Colleges 1989

Stuart Carne, President after November 1988, and I worked well together. He was often generous to me, once using a Jewish metaphor that he saw me as one of the 'prophets' in general practice. Stuart had also built a good relationship with Ian Todd, the Conference Chairman, who after the consequences of the three Presidents letter (described in the previous chapter) was ready to make changes.

Stuart, skilfully, broached a second place in the Conference for the College Chair. He persuaded Todd, recently knighted, to come to the RCGP and discuss the possibility. We had lunch as a three at Princes Gate in February, and Todd agreed in principle. With my interest in home visiting, I thought it encouraging that the Conference Chairman had come to the RCGP rather than getting us to go to him. The Conference approved the RCGP Chair coming to meetings, as well as the President, in April 1989.

So I became the first Chair of the RCGP Council to attend the Conference of Medical Royal Colleges, alongside the President. I was however admitted on limited terms. I could attend only those meetings designated as full Conference meetings and not the alternate ones, which were held before meetings of the Joint Consultants Committee called 'briefing meetings.' These meetings formed a continuum, with minuted items flowing across. I kept asking about the other set of minutes. The artificial distinction soon led to my being invited to all meetings.

Council Dinner with Kenneth Clarke April 1989

The Council dinner of 1989 was in April. The College was in the public eye as the White Paper *Working for Patients* had stirred considerable controversy. For the first and only time national television crews attended the dinner.

Kenneth Clarke was seated on my right and was a relaxed and charming dinner companion. He was witty and we had a few laughs. I could understand his reputation of a man who enjoyed a drink in pubs in his constituency. However, when he came to speak there was a transformation. Speaking to the cameras, he delivered a powerful speech for his White Paper. Fair enough, any Minister would have done the same. What was dramatic, however, was that he jibed at GPs saying: "GPs are only interested in feeling for their wallets!" This was particularly inappropriate as he was in the home of a Royal College that did not deal with doctors' remuneration or terms of service. He knew this, as civil servants told me privately later that they had advised him not to say this in our house. Politics is politics. He had his sound-bite and it was quoted extensively. However, he riled the members of Council, who looked at me expectantly.

I had to speak immediately after him. As the toastmaster thundered out my name and title, I rose with a heart rate of about 120 per minute! The cameras swung onto me and a note was passed: "The big camera is *ITN News at Ten*!" not the most reassuring message for an amateur. I thanked the Secretary of State for Health for coming and told a story of a competition between a doctor, a designer and a politician about who represented the oldest profession. The doctor went first and claimed victory as Adam and Eve were the beginning, and the removal of Eve's rib was a medical procedure. "Not so," said the designer, "before there were Adam and Eve there had to be an earth, and it was a designer who created earth out of the chaos. I win." "No," said the politician, "I win, who do you think created the chaos in the first place!" The Council laughed approvingly, *at* Kenneth Clarke. I survived.

Special Council Meeting April 1989

The week before the meeting of Council I was profiled in *Pulse* (Feinmann, 1989) with a big caricature of me and suggestions that the Council might force the officers and me out of office.

The special meeting of the College Council was the day after the dinner. It was unlike any Council meeting before or since. The faculty representatives arrived having, as advised, attended faculty meetings. They were mandated to reject the White Paper. This was a special meeting with just one item on the agenda. The debate was slow to take off as Council considered a lengthy paper I had drafted seeking to show ways in which general practice might achieve various gains. Alastair Donald, highly influential, and a former Chair of Council, led an onslaught against the White Paper. He saw GP fundholding as an abomination. Brian Goss soon to leave the RCGP Council for the GMSC where he became a BMA negotiator, also spoke strongly against.

The Council passed a motion to reject the White Paper out of hand and even insisted on a telegram type summary on the front page to be sent to the DH.

> *"The College rejects the White Paper, Working for Patients, on the grounds that if implemented as proposed it will seriously damage patient care and the doctor–patient relationship."*

This sentence was included three times in the final text (RCGP, 1989a). A few voted against this tidal wave, including Douglas Garvie, Donald Irvine, Marshall Marinker and Colin Waine but only about half a dozen. It was, in a Council of 65, an overwhelming vote reflecting the feelings of the majority of those present and the wider membership. The College for the first time since 1952 had been politicised. Unusually, the Council gave me a standing ovation at the end of the day for my chairmanship, which I did not enjoy. I co-chaired a full press conference indicating the national interest in the College's decision.

The document was quickly sent to every member. It was received with relief and approval. I wrote to Kenneth Clarke and informed him of the decision of the Council. He wrote back quickly telling me he thought I was "particularly weak-kneed! reaction" (Clarke, letter to Chair of Council, personal communication, 1989). The DH then cut the College out of all consultations.

Why did this happen? First, faculty representatives naturally followed the mandate of their faculty meeting. Secondly, the profession was in shock since most people had not seen the White Paper coming and had not noticed the gathering storm (like the BMA's rejection of the good practice allowance two and a half years before). The three articles in the *BMJ* which I had co-authored with Marinker and Maynard not been digested, even though the one I first authored had set out why change was inevitable (DPG *et al.*, 1986). My speech the year earlier, warning of an impending "avalanche of change," had not registered. There was a determination to stand by the GMSC. GPs were always saying "divide and rule," certainly an important political principle, but it became all absorbing.

The College had made its name by disagreeing with the Conference of Local Medical Committees when for years it consistently advocated vocational training. There were some who believed that if they rejected the White Paper they could stop it, as the medical profession, including me in the mid-1960s, had seen BMA GPs winning a big confrontation with the DH (Chapter 8, LMC and BMA story). There was a political group that saw the White Paper as a right-of-centre attack on the NHS and who therefore opposed it. Scottish members were more hostile to competition. Finally, there was no understanding of the balance of power; i.e. what the Government might do.

The summary paragraph was a political not an academic statement. The Council had no evidence that the White Paper would "damage patient care." Nor in the day-long debate did anyone offer such evidence. On the doctor–patient relationship, there was one argument often deployed, that if a doctor

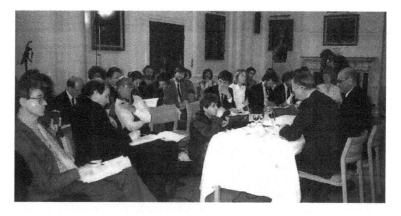

FIGURE 23.1 Press conference with Bill Styles after RCGP decision on White Paper, 1989.

has both responsibility for an individual patient and a budget for a population of patients, there would be a conflict of interest. However, the Cogwheel Report (1988) and the BMA had long campaigned for consultants to take hospital posts as clinical directors and share rationing decisions, and consultants had done so throughout the NHS. Ever since 1948 GPs had been paid on the basis that they would provide care for individual patients who consulted and simultaneously be responsible for a registered list (population) of patients.

Members of Council did not believe what they had resolved, since after the White Paper was implemented, several members enrolled as GP fundholders without concern about their standards of care or their patient relationships. The meeting was an unprecedented outpouring of emotion. The democratic basis of the College's constitution delivered a result that the members and their representatives desired. However, many Council and College members were very surprised when the College was excluded from meetings in the DH and the White Paper was "implemented as proposed." Many members regretted that the College was excluded from consultation by Government.

I was included in a damaging article in *Pulse* (Illman, 1989), which, by describing my visit to Chequers in 1988, implied I was one a group conspiring with politicians behind the profession's back.

The BMA

There was a useful convention that the Chair of the College and the Chair of GP Committee of the BMA met together alone over dinner regularly. The purpose was to build working relationships, to share confidential information and to consider the broader good of general practice. The arrangement worked well.

My opposite number, Michael Wilson, had become a master of the "Red Book," a loose-leaf, red-covered book, on what could be paid to GPs by the NHS. He had no qualms about the rejection of the good practice allowance (DHSS, 1986) weeks before my election. We never argued about it as it was all over when I came into office. We got on well. We were both real GPs and cared about general practice. We came from similar cities, York and Exeter, both well distant from London.

It was in 1989 that things got difficult for Michael. He was always on time for our dinners, as I was, but once he was very late and came immediately after a session of several hours with Kenneth Clarke. He told me about it and kept quoting the *Red Book*. I commented "but Michael, he is tearing up the *Red Book!*" Heresy! He looked taken aback.

The tense meeting of the RCGP Council in April 1989 was mirrored by much angrier meetings in the BMA. Michael had a major debate in the Conference of Local Medical Committees at which he and his negotiating team argued strongly that discussions on the proposed new GP contract should continue. However, the Conference was furious with the White Paper, *Working for Patients* and with Clarke's proposed new GP contract that flowed from it. Some, who were College members, rang me for advice. "Keep lines of communication open," I said. "Really?" some said. Michael spoke strongly to the Conference, but it rejected his advice and rejected the proposed contract.

It is unusual for this to happen in the BMA. The previous crisis had been in the mid-1960s, when a revolt had forced the resignation of the GMSC Chairman. Everyone knows that leaders have access to more information and leaders usually speak well. That Conference thought it knew better. Many members of that Conference in 1990 were the same as those who had so blithely rejected the good practice allowance only 31 months before. They over-estimated their own power and greatly underestimated the power of Government. Some thought if they rejected the contract they would stop it.

After the Conference voted down a proposal from the Chair of the GMSC, Michael to continue talks with the Government, Kenneth Clarke responded in the same way that he had responded to the RCGP and simply cut the BMA out of meetings. He and his civil servants redesigned a new GP contract without negotiation. As in 1986, the Conference of LMCs had not worked out the opponent's next move nor realised how strong it could be (Chapter 2, Chess story). As Kenneth Clarke had a well-known record of being tough with staff in other Departments of State before he came to Health this was an expensive mis-judgement. Michael and I had one of our two-chairs dinners when this was happening and he bemoaned how details of the new GP contract were being sent to the BMA "for information" not "for consultation."

One reason why the 1990 GP contract (DH and Welsh Office, 1989) was vilified by some GPs is that the rules were written by civil servants. That contract was the only one in the 20th century in which the profession had no say. The medical profession had got itself into a strange situation. The Chair of the BMA GPs and the negotiators and the Chair of the College and its officers, had both been simultaneously excluded from all consultations through decisions of their governing bodies. GPs had only one choice: accept the new contract (Department of Health and the Welsh Office, 1989) or resign. The power of Government was starkly revealed. GPs had no stomach for resignation from the NHS, so it was accepted in its entirety. This was a bigger problem for the GMSC than for the College. The College had a big academic agenda whereas the raison d'être for the GMSC was pay and contracts.

Apart from these dramatic medico-political events, Michael Wilson and I collaborated in a campaign to sensitise GPs to a growing problem of drug abuse in Britain and to encourage some GPs to take on their care. We spoke together at a meeting in the BMA council chamber.

The DH consulted the two national GP Chairmen about the regulations governing the body, which considered appeals by trainers. Michael made his comments and was surprised at the time I spent on this and the length of my comments on it. For him it was a minor issue, whereas for a College Chair it was a key standards issue. We had agreed to synchronise our reply as we knew that would increase the likelihood of our advice being accepted. "Is it really worth all this effort?" he said to me. I persisted and generously he supported me. The DH then accepted most of what I had requested.

Michael invited me to the annual dinner of the Conference of LMCs several hundred strong and I was on the top table. When the host Chair speaks it is customary to welcome national guests and he did so elegantly for the others but did not mention me. A College activist said he was sorry the College had been ignored. I said I thought Michael was protecting me, as I knew that John Horder as PRCGP had previously been booed at that conference dinner.

Margaret Turner-Warwick was Chair of the Conference of Colleges when the White Paper was introduced. Most Presidents were hostile and academics feared the purchaser-provider split and GP fundholding would affect academic medicine. Anti-GP feelings were suppressed with two GPs present but were palpable. Jim Johnson (a leading BMA consultant) had previously said (*Hospital Doctor*, 1997) that a primary care led NHS was "an irritating idea…….and absurd." Many Presidents wanted to reject the White Paper but with our GP experience, I advised keeping lines of communication with Government open. Initially, I was isolated but was soon supported by Oscar Craig (1928–2020), President of the Radiologists. We were a minority but an effective one. Margaret Turner-Warwick went to see Margaret Thatcher but returned empty handed.

The College had to get away from the political furore of the April meeting and get back to academic issues, the core business for the College. The agenda that Summer was full with academic topics but we also met international politics.

The College was invited to visit China, which was rethinking its 'barefoot doctors,' who were not doctors at all. The exciting question was whether China, with the biggest world population would back a generalist doctor-based system. The College team was selected including me. However, the Tiananmen Square crisis occurred that June and the visit was reviewed by the Council. Strong arguments were advanced for the visit going ahead. Medicine should be above politics, this was a professional visit to support GPs in China, Chinese GPs needed help and were asking for it, the College had great international experience and was well placed. Chinese people and doctors could benefit from the UK experience. Other countries were sending teams anyway.

Strong opposing arguments were advanced. The Chinese Government would inevitably be involved and at receptions our representatives would be used for Chinese propaganda. Would we have to shake hands with the people who had ordered the guns to be fired? It was a good debate and I did not speak as I had an interest. The Council decided to withdraw. At the end, a member called out: "Within two years, Ministers of the British Government will be shaking hands with the Ministers of the Chinese Government!" He was howled down. However, Li Peng, the Prime Minister who had ordered the massacre of students, continued in office for almost a decade and was indeed later photographed with John Major.

Course organisers were crucial. They were GPs running local vocational training schemes. They were paid by a strange mechanism agreed by the GMSC as the money came from funds for GP remuneration. This gave then them a GP 'trainer's grant,' without the right to take a personal trainee. NHS GPs were paying for the income of GP course organisers. By the late 1980s this job had greatly expanded. Course organisers had to be skilled in running groups, know about curriculum design and be involved with trainer appointments and reviews. They had to negotiate with local consultants the selection of hospital SHO posts in vocational training schemes. They were key middle managers and were greatly underpaid as the trainers also got substantial work in kind from the trainees. It was anomalous that their pay was at the expense of NHS GPs.

Some regions like the South West were exacerbating the problem. We brought all the course organisers and the associate advisers together in the Devon and Cornwall educational group in the annual course organisers and advisers retreat and in the Devon and Cornwall trainers' conference. There they worked alongside associate regional advisers in general practice who were paid at the top point on the consultant clinical scale. Something needed to be done. The course organisers themselves lobbied the GMSC but to no avail. Regional Health Authorities, which paid for the advisers, were not interested. The GMSC was not an educational body and the course organisers became more and more disgruntled. Soon there was talk of a strike or go slow.

I wrote a paper proposing that regional adviser teams should be re-organised, that course organisers and GP clinical tutors (also in an anomalous position) should all be re-branded as associate advisers. Council approved this making it College policy. and it was published in the *College Plan* (RCGP, 1989b). The course organisers were offered a compromise with minimal extra, but the College policy stiffened their resolve and they refused to compromise pressing for the associate adviser scale. However, the GMSC did not understand the consultant scale and messages came asking for briefing. Finally, the course organisers were put on that scale. They had to work their way up it, which was fair. This was a big improvement for them. Crucially, their salaries moved out of the target net income so NHS GPs generally stopped having to bear the cost of all the course organisers (now called programme directors).

I arranged working dinners with the main groups of academic GPs, e.g. the leaders of the university departments in which their officers and the College's officers met. Similarly, we met the regional advisers in general practice. Each event went well, but I was left worried. General practice was fragmenting under our eyes. I fostered cross-communication as much as I could and this encouraged me to establish a new GP Conference (Chapter 25, Conference of Academic Organisations of General Practice).

After the publication of *Healthier Children,* the BMA GPs started talking to the DH about it. John Ball, the GMSC Chairman, wanted a handbook produced by the College which Colin Waine wrote and which we published from the Exeter office. Child health surveillance was included in NHS general practice in 1990 following the College's (1978) policy on child care and *Healthier Children* (RCGP, 1982) The DH informed Family Practitioner Committees (FPCs) but made no comment on standards. The College agreed standards with the British Paediatric Association (later a College) and informed the FPCs. The GMSC took exception seeing this as a regulatory matter but about which it had done nothing. The *BMJ* of 27 January 1990 reported an outpouring of anger at me personally. My letter to Michael Wilson of 15 January was considered and parts of it reproduced (*BMJ*, 1990). The GMSC told Wilson he had been too polite to me! It instructed him to write to me again and sent its policies to the NHS. Within the College this kerfuffle attracted little comment.

Occupying 15 Princes Gate

In the 1970s, as Treasurer, Stuart Carne successfully negotiated with a couple living next door in No 15 Princes Gate. He bought the building for the College with £330,000, a down payment of £150,000 and payments of £15,000 for 12 years. This was a remarkable deal as inflation in the mid-1970s was at times over 20% pa. The College officers' instructions to leading London solicitors were that the objective was to gain possession at the end of the defined time. When that time came I was Chair. The occupier then claimed to be a protected tenant. The legal position was not as clear as we expected. Lengthy discussions with the solicitors led to counsel's opinion. We consulted surveyors, asking for the value of No 15 as it was and what would be the effect on value of owning both properties. The answer was that the two properties together would greatly enhance the overall value by millions of pounds. I called and chaired a working breakfast for all the professional advisers starting at 8 am. I said we needed a conclusion by 9 am. Everyone was being paid hundreds of pounds an hour except Sally Irvine and I (an honorary Chair). We reached a unanimous decision to sue for breach of contract. This was vigorously resisted by occupier's lawyers. At the court case, we were suddenly told that the occupants would leave if we paid £250,000! This had to be balanced by further legal fees if we continued and a small possibility we might lose. It seemed to me that certainty was to be prized and even with such a payment the College was getting a bargain. The Officers all agreed. We paid, "settling on the court room steps." We had discussions with the original lawyers subsequently.

The costs of medical litigation were rising and causing increasing concern. The CMO set up a working party and invited me on to it. Sometimes lawyers' fees exceeded the damages awarded. The biggest costs arise from babies injured at birth as the costs of lifetime care can be awarded at levels of £30 million or more. The working party could not resolve the problems. The logic of the situation is NHS priority for staffing in midwifery and obstetrics. Yet there is a serious shortage of midwives and obstetricians. In 2021, at a time when 80% of general practices were classified by the Care Quality Commission as "good," the same Commission classified 41% of maternity services as "inadequate" or "in need of improvement," a serious failure of NHS management.

Constitutional Issues

Some constitutional issues arose. First, the tenure of the Presidency, which had always been three years, had during Irvine's chairmanship been reduced to one year. I took careful soundings and found the change was not popular. The President, Drury, had great stature, was making superb after-dinner speeches (an important presidential role) and had held the fort during the Hasler Chairmanship. He was the first GP Vice-Chair of the Conference of Medical Royal Colleges in 1987. I led the strongest lobby in the history of the College to get Drury knighted and this happened in 1989, the first academic GP for 21 years with such an honour since Dame Annis Gillie in 1968.

The case for reducing the term was to give more people a chance to hold the office and a view that the presidency should be reduced in status vis-a-vis the chairmanship. I wrote a paper presenting the view that on balance a three-year term was better. This sailed through Council showing that there was no steam behind a one-year term. The term remained at three years (apart from Royal Presidents) until in the 21st century, when it was reduced to two years.

A big question was who should elect the President then being done by the Council. Graham Buckley from Edinburgh proposed election by the whole College membership. Opening the franchise was well argued: more democratic and enfranchising the membership. Against was that Council has much more detailed knowledge of the individuals and their performance. Amongst medical Royal Colleges, only the Psychiatrists, elected their President through the membership. After a good debate, the Council gave the whole membership the franchise. It was too late for the forthcoming election, so I chaired the Council for the last presidential election within the Council. This was a three-way race between Stuart Carne, Paul Freeling and John Fry. All three were Council members, two had CBEs, and all were nationally known. Carne won after his long, successful Honorary Treasurership and the world GP Presidency.

For Fry (1922–1994), it was his third attempt and a great disappointment after an outstanding general practice career. He illustrated the issues of the voting system. He was very able and had put practice-based research on the map. He had written extensively and was internationally known. But John was not clubbable, made no efforts to get on with people, or go to Spring Meetings. He irritated many by dealing with his correspondence during Council meetings. I gave his farewell citation as he left Council in 1990 and he received an exceptionally warm standing ovation. His death in 1994 prevented him standing in the first open voting election by the membership. I contributed to his *Times* obituary (1994), which stated he was "the best known GP in the world." If election by the membership had come sooner he would probably have been a President, as he was receiving big national votes in GMC elections.

A problem taking much time was the representation of the faculties on the Council. Historically, each faculty elected one member. But faculty divisions meant the Council membership was growing, unmanageably. The Council twice rejected papers so I wrote one proposing that faculties with 5% of the College membership could have two places on the Council and all faculties kept one place. Big faculties had to keep growing to keep two places and so were in gentle competition and the Council membership was stabilised. The Council approved it (RCGP *College Plan*, 1989b).

Some challenges arose on the meaning of the certificates the trainers were giving the registrars at the end of the registrar year. It was suggested that there was no quality component. Donald (later Sir) Irvine was Chair of the JCPTGP. Legal advice was that 'satisfactory' meant the trainer making a quality judgement. A three-Chairmen letter (Irvine, Pereira Gray and Bogle, 1990) was published in the *BJGP*. This was much quoted but its existence showed how weak training attitudes were. Ian Bogle became Chair of the GMSC. We were both third-generation GPs in family practices. However, the chemistry differed. Ian was suspicious of the College and was not a member.

The Prince of Wales

The constitution of the RCGP is more flexible than those of the specialist Colleges and allows the occasional election of a Royal President. The Duke of Edinburgh was the College's first Royal President in 1972. When Prince Charles was preparing to be the College's second Royal President, I was invited to lunch with him at Kensington Palace and later in Highgrove. He agreed to speak at our conference. I briefed him whilst being anxious about his well-known support for complementary medicine. However, he was quite fair, saying that orthodox medicine should think about how complementary medicine sought to understand the whole person. I was happy with the final version but just before the conference following an accident, after many members had paid to come, he withdrew. He offered to video his speech if the College paid. The price was high, but colleagues found the funds and the video was shown.

I represented the College at an event celebrating Thatcher's ten years as Prime Minister. I knew no one but spoke with James (Jimmy) Goldsmith (1933–1997), the billionaire. Ten years as PM and three general elections won was a huge achievement. However, for my taste, the speeches were sycophantic.

College dinners were usually a pleasure. However, seating in order of precedence conveys non-verbal signals, which are never voiced. Once at dinner in the Royal College of Surgeons of England, Jill and I were seated with lower precedence than all other Royal Colleges and Faculties and placed amongst College's staff. Two years later at the same dinner, in the same room, in the same College, but now as a knight and a lady, we were seated on the top table.

Margaret Thatcher 1990

In 1990, I represented the College at a reception at 10 Downing Street. I wondered if I would meet anyone I knew and on arrival, several rooms were packed. I had no expectation of meeting Margaret Thatcher (1925–2013). Then suddenly to my surprise, she came into the room right beside me and started talking to me. It was an extraordinary experience. She started a monologue with no introduction. She never asked who I was or why I was there. She talked and talked *at* me with no interest in how I responded. All I could do was to try to show some interest and nod. I never got a word in and it was not a pleasant experience. I concluded she had become insensitive. At home, more prophetically than I could ever know, I said to Jill: "I don't know how the cabinet stands it!" A few months later they didn't stand it anymore.

Clinical Standards Board 1990

A DH proposal for a new Clinical Standards Board came to the Council. Its Royal Charter requires the College: "to encourage, foster and maintain the highest possible standards." However, many speeches were against involvement, as the BMA was not invited. I judged the proposal was going to be rejected. I said I would be deeply disappointed if this invitation was rejected, putting myself on the line and greatly raising tension in the room. Unprecedently, David Murfin publicly rebuked me, saying this was manipulation of the Council. It was clear to all that if the proposal failed that I would in my last meeting as Chair be damaged professionally. The tension was palpable. Council accepted the invitation but by a small majority.

Initiatives That Continued after the Chairmanship

My top priority as Chair was introducing Fellowship of the College by Assessment. I secured this in the summer of 1989. It is described step-by-step in Chapter 24, the Fellowship by Assessment story. In 1990, the CMO, Sir Donald Acheson, invited the leaders of three Medical Royal Colleges to discuss prison medicine; I attended as Chair and this continued for a decade afterwards, as described in Chapter 26, the Prison Medicine story. Having started the campaign to achieve eligibility for salaried academic GPs to be considered for distinction awards I continued it afterwards, as set out in Chapter 39, Distinction/Clinical Excellence Awards.

Retirement

The Council elected Colin Waine as my successor. I was pleased as we shared much, had had hundreds of telephone conversations, and he was a friend. When the DH requested the College's nomination for the Clinical Standards Board, Colin offered me the place. I declined, not wanting any suggestion that my fight in Council was motivated personally. I need not have worried. After launching the Standards Board with the usual fanfare, the DH soon dissolved it.

Jill and I took the officers and senior staff to dinner at the Royal Society of Arts. The Chairmanship ended in November 1990, after three and three-quarter years. The term of office is usually three years, and no chair before or since has served as long. General practice research in universities was secure, but practice-based GP research was fragile, so as left the Chair I made a donation to establish a research fund for the Tamar (Devon and Cornwall) Faculty to support *local* GP research, including involvement with a higher degree.

Jill and I had a get-away-from it-all holiday that December, a rare occasion when I missed a Council meeting. We stayed with Jill's cousin, Rosamund Cameron (1939–2013) and her husband, Malcolm (1932–2021), in the Caribbean. It was a wonderful break with glorious weather, and we both enjoyed sailing with them.

ADDENDUM

In 2022 I was again invited to deliver the McConaghey Memorial Lecture, 34 years after the first time. This time I was able to have Dr Paddy McConaghey PhD (Mac's daughter) and his grandson, also known as Mac present. This was subsequently the basis of an editorial in the *BJGP* (DPG, 2023) "General practice: The integrating discipline."

24

Fellowship of the College by Assessment (FBA)

Some see things as they are and ask why. I dream of things that never were and ask why not?

George Bernard Shaw (1856–1950)

The medical Royal Colleges are all registered charities and not trade unions, which exist for the benefit of a workforce. The privilege of charitable status is accorded to these Colleges to further public interest in medicine and this means improving care for patients. All the Colleges provide education designed to help their members and fellows to develop postgraduate training programmes and professional examinations but in 1987 none measured the care that established doctors in their field provided for patients.

The Royal Charter of the Royal College of General Practitioners (1967) sets out the objective of the College as follows: "to encourage, foster and maintain the highest possible standards of general medical practice." These words are simple and clear but they raise the questions of what are the highest possible standards and how can they be measured?

The RCGP's work in this field was first developed for general practitioner trainers and this authority was exercised through RCGP leaders in office in the JCPTGP, especially the RCGP-nominated secretary. By 1976, Donald Irvine in that post drafted a document setting out guidance for the selection for GP trainers, which was approved by the Joint Committee on Postgraduate Training for General Practice (JCPTGP) (1976) and was influential.

Training practices were the route whereby working standards for general practice emerged through the criteria agreed for the selection of GP trainers. This was a responsibility of Regional General Practice Committees, which used the national JCPTGP guidance plus any regional policies of their own. Trainers had a right of appeal against non-selection. There was considerable variation in the standards and rigour used in the regional selection of trainers. The Northern region, Oxford and Southwestern regions were the three that took trainer standards most seriously (as shown in Chapter 14, Regional Adviser story). The story of failed trainer selection standards in the North East Thames region is described in Chapter 23, Chair of Council story.

Quality Initiatives

Donald Irvine, as Chair of Council, introduced the theme of his term as the 'quality initiative' which called for each general practice to set out its aims and standards and to describe the services the practice provided (Irvine, 1983). This was strong leadership and helped to set the professional scene. This initiative was supported by many members of Council and a few outside, but it was not sustained and ran out of steam.

Quite separate from the JCPTGP, the College developed an interesting quality assurance project involving GPs visiting each other's practices and commenting on arrangements. The report of this was published as *What Sort of Doctor* (RCGP, 1985b). One principle this helped to establish was the importance of visiting a practice to determine quality of care.

DOI: 10.1201/9781032713601-30

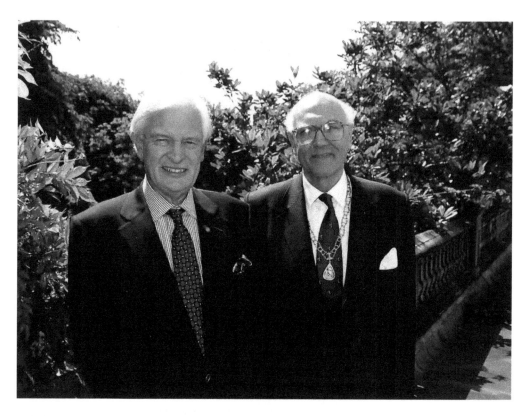

FIGURE 24.1 Sir Donald Irvine the only time the President of the GMC and Chair of the Academy were both GPs, 2000.

Trainer selection in the Southwestern region was my responsibility as Regional Adviser for Devon and Cornwall 1975–1983 and for the region as a whole between 1983–2000. The system we evolved in the Regional General Practice Education Committee is described in Chapter 14, the Regional Adviser story. The principles were that the standards expected must be precisely defined and promulgated widely in advance before any trainer applied. Everything should be public and there should be no surprises. All regional standards were reviewed annually and gradually strengthened. Every practice applying was visited by at least three colleagues who would personally check the standards on site. All decisions were to be the responsibility of the Regional GP Education Committee (RGPEC).

Converting Good Ideas into Practice

As a new Chair of Council in 1987 I had inherited a progressive theme of trying to promote quality of care and the College had tried very hard. However, Donald Irvine's (1983) quality initiative and the *What Sort of Doctor?* (RCGP, 1985a) initiative had both petered out. How then to make quality assurance stick? I eventually drew the following conclusions: First, GPs needed to have a real incentive of some kind but not money, which would devalue any award. Second, the incentive had to be professional status and the level of quality required had to command real respect from working GPs but still be achievable with hard work.

Minimum standards would not be valued and would inevitably become entangled with medico-politics. The system needed to be within the College's control. Trainer approval offered the best working model as GP applicants wanted to be trainers and approval conferred professional status. Only one possibility fitted all these principles and was practical: this was to open a new route to the fellowship of the College (the highest grade of membership) to be awarded through achievement of high standards set by the College, checked in person and in the practice, by college-appointed assessors. So, I made this the top priority for my chairmanship.

It took about nine months for the College to settle down after the upheavals of losing both a Chief Examiner and a Chair of Council within six months and it was soon out of the news. This meant I could then concentrate on the academic agenda. Over Christmas 1987, I wrote the first draft of a policy paper proposing that in future a grade of fellowship of the College should be introduced for those who had passed a rigorous practice assessment on criteria set entirely by the College. This was to be in addition to the traditional route to fellowship by nomination. My allies were a young Vice-chair of Council, Peter Hill, who had come out of the North of England standards stable and Bob Colville, an associate adviser from Glasgow, who was Chair of the Education Division. Young tigers in the Council like Michael Pringle and Jackie Hayden were also calling for this.

However, the policy was radical and there were powerful people in influential positions who did not welcome it. Nor did the more traditional members of Council. I knew one false step and the policy would be lost.

I arranged for the policy paper to be taken through the Education Division on the grounds that FBA was essentially a radical form of continuing education and as an ex-officio member, I went to support it there. It passed, so the paper became an Education Division paper. Then it went to the GPC, where it was also approved. It was now ready to be considered by the Council. This process, which seems bureaucratic, was invaluable; GPC with its expert knowledge and experience often saw flaws in papers and often improved them. It was an effective vetting system. It had another advantage in that it often flushed out opponents and I learnt there that even some of the officers were not enthusiastic about the idea.

The proposal for Fellowship by Assessment came to the Council in June 1988. It was a proposal in principle and had no criteria or details. It was approved easily without any opposition. This set the direction and made a route to Fellowship by Assessment formal College policy. But there was then no means of advancing it. This two-stage process had the substantial disadvantage of being slow; and it was a whole year before a detailed paper was ready. However, the advantage of preparing colleagues and committees by giving them time to adjust to a new idea is a great advantage and a helpful leadership technique, so I chose this route.

Faculty Contributions

There was a further advantage, the approval in principle fired a starting gun for pilots in two of the College's faculties: the Northwest England and Tamar. Both pilots helped, but Tamar, my home faculty, took it very seriously. The organisers arranged test visits to some of their own practices and tested tough criteria from the Southwestern region experimenting with new criteria. Three of five key Tamar GPs were Geoffrey Smerdon, Robert Sibbald, and Richard Parrott. Not only were these three a strong team but they knew and trusted each other as they had run the Plymouth vocational training scheme together. Moreover, they had great experience of serving on the Regional General Practice Education Committee, which set the trainer standards in the Southwest. I knew and trusted them all and I think they trusted me. They understood exactly what I was trying to do.

Two other active GPs in Tamar were respected leaders in Devon and Cornwall; both made a difference individually. Bob Gundry in Cornwall had been a successful GP tutor in Truro, Tony Lewis, was originally from Hayle in Cornwall but had moved to Exmouth in Devon to be involved with the Department of General Practice in Exeter where he later became a senior lecturer. Both these GPs were nominated to be fellows of the College and deservedly so. Then, at this critical time, both declined to accept nomination stating they would accept fellowship only through objective assessment. Their refusals to accept the traditional fellowship for that reason were unprecedented and made a big impression in London. The Tamar Faculty gave me great support in principle and through detailed practical reports on their practice visits. Most of all, it demonstrated strong support for the idea. Rarely has a single faculty played so big a part in the development of central College policy.

FBA Development

An FBA committee was established within the College with the responsibility of devising and reviewing the criteria. I chaired this myself for a short time to get it going and then as soon as possible supported younger colleagues as chairs. Many of the leading younger activists became chairs of this group including: Richard Baker (later professor, Mike Pringle (later professor) and later Alison Kay and John Holden. This Committee's role was to produce criteria, which were demanding but achievable and be possible to obtain in both city and rural general practice. They were also to be, as far as possible, research based and measurable.

One big question was whether to require candidates to submit a video recording of a recent surgery of consultations. By 1988, video recording was accepted in the GP training world as a common and useful way of analysing GP consultations and an exceptionally valuable method for learning about non-verbal communication. But there was not yet any research evidence that video recording improved patient care. A main plank of most criteria was a research basis. Should we enforce video submission without this? I committed strongly to its inclusion, believing that professional judgement mattered. Submitting a video means a GP is putting himself/herself on the line and recognising peer review – values we needed to cultivate in the College's role models. Submission was included as a required condition and attracted minimal criticism.

The GPC retreat in 1989 was hard work, the key item being Fellowship by Assessment. We worked line by line through all the draft criteria, and there were difficulties in principle and arguments in practice. For example, how long was it reasonable to take to respond to an emergency call? The debates were greatly helped by the series of pilot visits carried out by the Tamar Faculty Board and by the proposals from the FBA committee. GPC approved a paper with several amendments, and this cleared its path to the Council.

When the paper came to the Council there was a good debate. Some opposed it on principle, but it had been thoroughly prepared. Having taken a detail-free policy paper to Council the year before proved its worth in spades. It had acclimatised everyone to the fact that the Council had already approved the principle, and this was just the detail for which the Council had asked. The paper was approved in July by a substantial majority. At the November AGM in 1989 four members were awarded Fellowship by Assessment. They included Michael Pringle and Tony Lewis (one of the refuseniks). The principles of Fellowship by Assessment were as in the next subsections:

1. Fulfilling the Royal Charter

The key objective of the College as stated in its Royal Charter was: "to encourage, foster and maintain the highest possible standards of general medical practice." FBA fulfilled this by operationalising working standards at the highest possible level.

2. Highest Possible Standards

The Royal Charter contains the words of "encouraging….the highest possible standards of general practice." But never before had these been defined. There are three fundamental standards in any profession: (a) the basic minimum standard, (b) the usual standard of what the average professional does, and (c) excellent standards. I had worked this out as the Regional Adviser for the Southwest when we introduced a three-category approach to trainer assessment (Chapter 14, Regional Adviser story). Basic minimum standards were not in the College's control and finding a doctor who did not meet them was fraught in terms of doctors losing their livelihood and the need to provide remedial professional education. The College could not do this. Minimum standards in the medical profession were determined by the General Medical Council (GMC). Striking a doctor off the *Medical Register* set the level of unacceptable standards. The GMC had been doing this since 1858, but only for a very few. The aim of FBA was to operationalise the highest possible standards in general practice.

3. What Does Good General Practice Look Like?

Before FBA the RCGP was vulnerable to the question "What does good general practice look like?" It traditionally resorted to naming some well-known GP. But well- known GPs did not always work in practices providing good care. FBA answered this question for the first time. Moreover, it generated general practices in all parts of the UK, which included enthusiastic GPs who were proud of the way they worked. Once patient assessors were included the applicants were literally showing off what good general practice looked like.

4. College Territory and College Control

As I saw it, the College could mount an exercise to determine the average or usual standards in general practice by doing a big survey. But this would be hugely expensive, would have to cover all countries of the UK and all regions. There was no guarantee the funds would be available. Importantly it would soon go out of date. By contrast, determining the highest possible standards would involve dealing with small and manageable numbers and enthusiasts. I had had a ring side seat when the year before the LMC Conference (*BMJ*, 1986) shot down the good practice allowance (Chapter 22, Downs and Ups of Institutional Life). Fellowship of the College was unarguably College territory. No one could gainsay what the Council decided on what was exclusively College business.

5. Profession Not the State

The essence of a profession is that sets its own standards. By 1988 I was fearful the State would take over standard setting for the medical profession. Politically set standards are always vulnerable to political whims and fashions and an excessive focus on minimising costs. FBA was conceived as a bulwark, a precious area of professionalism, where the profession could stand on its own ground that the State could not control. The College could set its own standards for its own fellowship.

6. High Ground

If the College could define a workable high but achievable standard and if reasonable numbers of general practitioners were brave enough to take it, then the College would have taken the high ground in clinical practice in the name of the College.

7. Self-Nomination

The old tradition in the RCGP (and in the other medical Royal Colleges) was that people proposed other people for the award of fellowship. Canvassing was frowned on. FBA allowed self-nomination then a radical idea. It emphasised how continuing professional development required doctors to take responsibility for their own learning and development. This was a big step away from colleague nomination, which often overlooked good but diffident people. This was a modern system with openness and transparency.

8. Open Published Criteria

All systems of nomination tend to have the problem of exactly what criteria are being applied and why. Often there is suspicion of an 'old boys club' or frank discrimination on the grounds of colour, creed, gender, or race. In the old London private clubs sometimes, people would be 'blackballed' for admission with no reason given. FBA by contrast offered precise, open, published, criteria, so there could be no doubt for all applicants about what was required. The principle was that there should be no surprises. Applicants could be sure that they would pass if they could demonstrate that every criterion was met.

9. Compulsory Submission of a Video Recording of Real Consultations with Patients

Another radical feature was the requirement that every applicant was required to submit a video of a set of consultations with real patients in their own practice. This had taken a great deal of negotiation as the theoretical problem was that there were not then any clear criteria of performance of consulting skills which could be applied by assessors. The solution was to insist on the submission of a video as a compulsory criterion without any specified performance skills. I was confident that research on this was proceeding quickly and that criteria for quality would emerge soon. It did. The submission by itself would force self-awareness and a willingness to be assessed clinically by peer review.

10. Every Criterion Required

A core feature of FBA was that every single criterion had to be passed for the award for fellowship of the College. This followed thinking and experience of trainer assessments in the Southwest and eliminated any trading of criteria or leaving out of some important standard for patient care.

11. Annual Review of the Criteria

One problem with any criteria for good professional practice is that new research is always being published and good practice keeps changing. Any set of criteria, however good, will soon go out of date. FBA dealt with this by establishing an FBA committee of the Council charged with reviewing the criteria every year. Every proposed change had to be approved by the Council each year to ensure it was reasonable. Applicants were allowed generous time to apply on previously published criteria so good notice was always given when new criteria came into force.

12. No Age Bar

A new feature was that there was no age bar. All that was required was five years' continuous membership of the College, a rule in the College bye laws of fellowship by nomination tended to produce new fellows in their 50s. FBA made it possible for able younger GPs to achieve it in their early 30s, as happened.

13. Work-Based Setting

FBA moved the setting for assessment away from examination halls into the general practices where the doctors worked and where patients were seen. This was very much in tune with new thinking of the importance of the assessment of performance in the workplace.

14. Three-Person Assessment Team

The assessment system was a three-person visiting team that systematically checked every criterion on site. This followed the trainer assessment system in the Southwest. The leader was appointed centrally and after the first year or two the second assessor was usually a colleague who had passed FBA themselves. One assessor was always from the local faculty of the College, and this ensured that any local feature that affected the delivery of general practice care was properly considered. The second assessor was usually from another faculty to start with but after a few years was increasingly a representative from the College's Patient Liaison Group (later called the Patient Partnership).

15. Patient Assessors

FBA was primarily designed to make quality assurance real in general practice, so it was primarily for patients. The most important development in FBA after it was introduced was the inclusion of a patient representative as one of the visiting assessors. This had seemed a bridge too far when I was writing the policy documents, so I watched with interest as patient inclusion was discussed in the College. The first vote was against a patient representative, but not by a big majority, then within a year or so another vote agreed it. What was happening was important, as the original committee members were people like me who were enthusiasts for the principle of FBA but increasingly members included those who had already achieved it. This group was empowered and much more confident: they positively wanted FBA to be able to demonstrate high-quality general practice to patients and their representatives. They were proud of their practices. The patients concerned were chosen by the College's Patient Liaison Committee. This was the first-time patients became directly and personally involved in assessing doctors for the award of a fellowship to doctors in any British Medical Royal College. The visiting team wrote a report for the central committee. Patients welcomed this new role and often spoke with admiration of some of the practices they saw.

Patients soon became enthusiasts for FBA themselves. Patricia Wilkie (PhD doctor), one of the chairs of the patient group in the College in the 1990s, and later President of the National Association for Patient Participation, went on several FBA visits and spoke of the value of the system. Patient representatives made important contributions to the visits, especially in the non-technical aspects of communication.

16. FBA Registrable with the General Medical Council

Applicants who achieved fellowship of the College by assessment would rank equally with the other route to fellowship and would be awarded at a general meeting of the College. The fellowship would be registrable with the GMC.

17. Geographical Spread

FBA was designed to be available to all members in all parts of the UK, in order to distribute quality around the UK and protect against any London dominance.

18. Empowering College Members

An important reason for FBA was to give ordinary College members all over the country a mid-career aiming point in the hope that it would be an empowering process. I was trying to introduce a further process of professional development, a special form of higher professional education after qualification, to compensate for the unsatisfactorily short period of GP postgraduate training.

After its introduction in 1989, I had a decade on the Council in the 1990s to observing if this process was actually empowering? An encouraging indication was when the partners in a big group practice in Essex where Alastair Mould was a college activist all applied individually and all succeeded. Their group photograph attracted attention in the medical press. In the Eastquay Practice in Somerset all six GPs passed FBA together in 1999, giving me the great pleasure of presenting their certificates and then being photographed with them. In Cornwall, a group of GP educationalists decided to prepare for FBA as a group. It took some time for some members who were lagging but eventually all of them applied and were approved. So great was their enthusiasm that they all came with their wives to London, at their own expense, to have a celebratory meal after the AGM when they were presented with their fellowships. I knew them all as they were heavily involved in GP training. One of that group was Bob Gundry, one of the refuseniks who had rejected fellowship of the College by the traditional route.

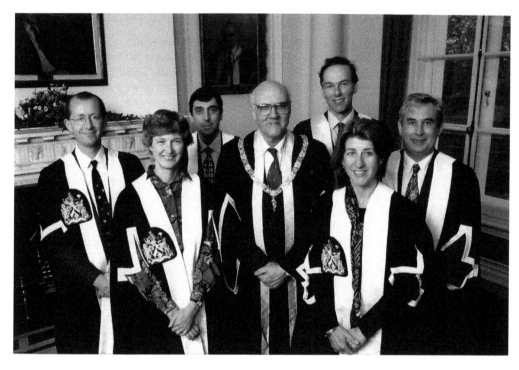

FIGURE 24.2   AGM in 1999. After presenting fellowships to six partners at the East Quay Practice, Somerset, who all took Fellowship by Assessment together.

Sometimes it takes time to see professional empowerment in perspective. I met David Greig unexpectedly at a reunion in St John's College, Cambridge. He was a GP educational leader in the Southwest and a successful course organiser for the Taunton vocational training scheme. We were then both in our seventies and he told me he had obtained two university master's degrees but that the high point of his professional career as a GP had been when he achieved FBA. FBA really was empowering in practice as well as in theory.

Lindsay Smith, an academic GP in Somerset, joined the Exeter Department of General Practice. He obtained FBA and then extended the idea of FBA being an empowering process by having a letter published jointly in the *BMJ* (Selena Gray and Smith, 2000). This noted that an unusual number of GPs applying for research approval status in the Southwestern region in 2000 had FBA or a partner who had obtained it. This was new evidence that FBA gave GPs increased self-confidence and a readiness to take on wider roles. Two GPs in the Tamar area colleagues whom I knew Hayes Dalal from Truro and Chris Clark from Witheridge in Devon, were among the 33 GPs in Devon and Cornwall who achieved FBA. Both subsequently obtained doctoral degrees (one MD, one PhD) from the University of Exeter; they were almost the only service GPs to do so. Both told me they had found FBA empowering and it had helped them to raise their professional horizons. Given how few GPs proceed to doctorates, 2 out of 33 was encouraging.

Writings on FBA

There were several publications on FBA. First, I described it in *Fellowship by Assessment, Occasional Paper 50* (RCGP, 1990). I wrote this but in the older tradition of the College had it published in the name of the College. I had an editorial in the College *Journal* describing FBA as "good general practice" (DPG, 1991a). The *Occasional Paper* went into a second edition, still as *Occasional Paper* 50 in 1995. An article in the *RCGP Members' Reference Book* (Jenkins, 1996) described the experience of a college member going through the FBA process. He was enthusiastic and reported the great educational value of the process to him as he received valuable personal advice. Richard Moore, an RCGP examiner and FBA assessor, wrote a book on the experiences of the *First Hundred Fellows by Assessment*, which reported many of its strengths through the eyes of those who worked for it (Moore, 1998). Finally, there was an academic article using qualitative analysis on professional development for general practitioners through Fellowship by Assessment (Lings and DPG, 2002) in *Medical Education*. This reviewed FBA as an educational process, which was why I had taken it to the Education Division of the College in 1988. Sir Liam Donaldson, CMO, well understood FBA and in 2002 praised it in a DH document. John Holden and Alison Kay (2005) two FBA chairs, wrote an important summary of the achievements of FBA practices and Holden (2013), the last FBA committee Chair wrote "Fellowship by assessment six years on: a personal view" He found visiting FBA practices "inspiring" and often learned valuable new techniques.

The number of members obtaining FBA rose steadily all through the 1990s, and applicants came from all over the UK. They included a GP aged 35, one aged 65 and one in private practice, which underlined that FBA was about professional standards not the NHS necessarily. By the beginning of the 21st century it was still taking about two years to prepare for FBA. GPs with FBA, had on average had three partners (except in a growing number of practices where more than one partner applied) and since many systems operated across the whole practice, over 1,000 working GPs were affected. They had great influence since, although this was a small percentage of the membership, they produced: two Presidents (Pringle and Kemple), two Chairs of Council (Pringle and Marshall), one Treasurer (Hunter), one Chair of the Trustee Board (Hunter), and four Professors (Baker, Holt, Marshall and Pringle). By 2007, 350 GPs had obtained FBA.

Further GP Quality Assurance Programmes

The thinking behind FBA led to two other College quality assurance programmes. One obvious limitation of FBA was that it applied to only a doctor. This rightly led to calls for a quality team award. Scottish members developed this energetically and a quality in practice award, modelled on FBA, soon emerged and proved a great success. I had the pleasure of awarding several of these as President and whole practice teams turned out and were obviously empowered.

Secondly, the principle of objective assessment was also applied to membership of the College to resolve a longstanding problem, unique to general practice, whereby there was a group of practising GPs who had never taken or passed the MRCGP. This did not happen in specialist medicine where in effect passing the membership or fellowship examination of the relevant Royal College is required for a consultant appointment. Taking the MRCGP, which is an examination aimed at young doctors in their 20s, was not seen as appropriate by many, although a few older GPs did take it. Membership by assessment squared this circle.

By the 1990s, the College had four different assessment systems for different categories of doctor or practice. These were: the MRCGP examination for those finishing vocational training, FBA, the quality practice award, and membership by assessment, developed over 30 years after the MRCGP in 1965. As I finished as President in 2000, I was very proud of the College for these four quality assurance systems in British general practice.

Impact outside the College

The greatest impact of FBA was inside the College but there were two effects outside. In the Devon Family Health Services Authority it was noted as an important quality initiative. Julia (later PhD doctor) Neville, a senior manager, made a small payment to defray the expenses in practices, which did it, asking only that she was sent a report. She told me she found these reports uplifting and a helpful reminder of how good general practice could be when part of her job was dealing with the worst of general practice.

Secondly, the Academy of Medical Royal Colleges held a conference on continuing medical education (CME) and as PRCGP I had to speak for general practice; I described FBA as a key new form of continuing professional development. The conference was not usually exciting because all the Colleges reported variations on doctors choosing what education they wanted to do, reporting to their college, and then meeting some arbitrary number of hours and getting them ticked off by their College. This system never interested me much as there was no evidence that the doctors were learning what they needed to learn or were actually learning anything at all. Patient benefit was never demonstrated.

Against this background, my lecture was like throwing a stone into a millpond. College-defined standards of care for established doctors! Objective assessment of standards and performance in the workplace! Compulsory video recordings of consultations with real patients! And patients involved as assessors! Some Presidents could hardly believe their ears. Afterwards, I was pressed to say if this was really true and was it very new? When I said 1989, with a publication in 1990 (RCGP, 1990), over a decade earlier, there was considerable surprise. I noted the asymmetry in the Royal Colleges in which the RCGP kept a close eye on the specialist colleges and what they were doing but the specialist colleges ignored what the RCGP was doing. That was quite a dramatic moment. It was clearly acknowledged that day that FBA of the RCGP meant quality assurance and a good deal for patients. As an officer of the Academy, I had never before seen the other Colleges react like this. In that group of Royal Presidents there was widespread recognition that the RCGP was far in the lead.

FBA Abolished

Then suddenly in the years 2005 to 2007, there was a radical change of thinking at the top of the College. A paper was written stating that the two kinds of fellowship were divisive, although they ranked exactly equally, and proposed that FBA be abolished. The Council, with two presidents actively involved, voted FBA down. The decision was properly done procedurally but as FBA was the jewel in the College's quality assurance crown it was a fundamental reversal of strategy. It decisively changed the trajectory of college policy from the quality assurance course it had been on since it introduced the MRCGP examination in 1965.

There were several threads: a rising role and influence for lay staff in the College made FBA, with its committee needing clinical judgement and assessors visiting practices, hard work for staff to run. There had always been a background tension. One former College officer told me he felt FBA was so impressive it had "devalued" his FRCGP by nomination and others felt this. Furthermore, there was a changing attitude to money, instead of it being a means to an end it was becoming more of an end in itself. The move of the HQ from Princes Gate to Euston Square was necessary and well executed. However, it came at the price of a big mortgage, which needed to be paid annually. FBA was relatively costly to run and did not make a profit, whereas awarding fellowship by nomination to members at around £800 per doctor made the College a great deal of money and made proportionally more members happy. The temptation was great.

The decision to abolish FBA was, I believe, the biggest policy mistake the RCGP has ever made. It took the college off the quality assurance path in general practice, which is the College's central reason for existence: "to encourage, foster and maintain the highest possible standards of general medical practice" (Royal Charter). It stepped backwards away from a measurable clinical commitment to patients, unique in British medicine.

The failure of the College's Patient Partnership to protest when consulted was a serious policy failure of patient representatives. If ever there was a patient issue where the patient group needed to give strong and unequivocal advice to its doctors this was it. Fellowship by nomination is important and proper as Royal Colleges ought to reward those who work hard and go the extra mile. I was proud to accept it for my Honorary Editorship of the College *Journal*. But fellowship by nomination is basically a reward given by doctors to doctors. It was not about the quality of doctoring, nor about good care of patients. FBA was different. It was about meeting high, research-based standards set by the national standard setting body and delivered to patients in local general practices. Fellowship by nomination was for doctors: Fellowship by Assessment was for patients.

Abolishing FBA took away, without replacement, a unique aiming point for mid-career GPs, which was successfully leading many to other achievements. It betrayed over 300 College fellows, around the UK, who had worked hard and paid about £800. Many of them were intensely proud of their achievement. For the 28 years, 1988–2016, the RCGP was the national standard-setting body for general practice, not only examining young doctors, but in addition assessing significant numbers in their practices at a time when work-based assessments had swung into fashion.

Having lost the jewel in the crown, the college a few years later abandoned the quality in practice award too, although it fostered teamwork in general practice and had empowered many practices. Now little is left of work-based assessments and MRCGP by assessment will probably wither away as, since 2007, the MRCGP has become compulsory. The College is no longer practically involved in quality assurance in clinical practice. The state, via the Care Quality Commission has, as predicted, taken over.

Policies reflect culture and values. Such a radical policy change means a radical change in values. The College Council and its leaders in the 1980s held different values from their successors 20 years later.

Professional Symbols in My Presidential Portrait

FBA was the highest policy objective of my Chairmanship. Symbolically, I arranged for *Occasional Paper 50* (RCGP, 1990) which described FBA, to be in my hand for my Presidential portrait as if I was presenting it to the College, as I believed the *Occasional Papers* and FBA were the two most important contributions, I was able to make to the College. Disappointingly, both were later abolished.

25

Conference of Academic Organisations of General Practice

By uniting we stand: by dividing we fall.

John Dickenson (1732–1808)

As Chair of Council I arranged working dinners with the main groups of academic GPs. Each group had an observer on the Council of the College, but I sensed they were drifting apart. Dinners were arranged with each main group, such as the leaders of the university departments of general practice and the regional advisers in general practice. Although each event went well, I was left increasingly worried. General practice was fragmenting under our eyes.

The university staff made snide comments about the regional advisers whom they saw as better resourced but with lower university qualifications. The regional advisers bemoaned the ivory tower attitude of university GP professors who were doing less and less clinical practice. Being a regional adviser at Bristol, a university professor in Exeter and now Chair of the College, I alone stood in all three camps simultaneously – a real privilege. Could these three tribes be brought closer together and become more mutually supportive?

Conference of Academic Organisations of General Practice 1989

My private conclusions were that the fragmentation of general practice made it logical to establish some new bridge-building organisation. I had previously assumed the College would and could be that, but I was increasingly learning that important jealousies existed in some big groups and that the GP course organisers and the GP trainers were feeling left out.

A second and influential strand in my thinking was the three Presidents' letter to the *Lancet* (Hoffenberg *et al.*, 1987; Chapter 23 Chair of Council story). Whilst this letter had been aimed at the Government of the day it also made it clear that the RCGP was not worth consulting and that general practice was not worth mentioning. I privately judged that the Conference of Medical Royal Colleges and its Faculties could not be completely trusted, even though I had just joined it. It was so hospital orientated that there might be some circumstances when we might have to leave it if our position was to not to be compromised.

Thinking this over I realised that if the RCGP were to leave the Conference of Medical Royal Colleges and Faculties its position might, paradoxically become much stronger. This analysis suggested that the existing Conference of Colleges would be greatly weakened and would become in effect a conference only of hospital doctors. Moreover, I thought it was likely that the Government would then have to relate to general practice because it was still the biggest branch of the medical profession and particularly if it was a major player in a new primary care conference. It could end up with a much bigger voice.

DOI: 10.1201/9781032713601-31

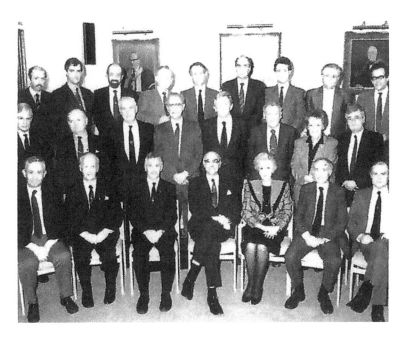

FIGURE 25.1 Inaugural Meeting of the Conference of Academic Organizations, Initially Called the Academic Forum in 1999.

The trigger came in January 1989 with the Government's publication of *Working for Patients* (DH, 1989) that destabilised the existing system in general practice and in the NHS, described in Chapter 23, Chair of Council story.

So in April 1989 I set up a new Conference of Academic Organisations in General Practice across the British Isles. With the College officers I called a meeting in Princes Gate of the College leaders, the officers of the university GPs, the leaders of the regional advisers in general practice, the course organisers and the GP tutors, as well as the officers of the Irish College of General Practitioners with whom I had personal links. The GMSC had observer status.

This was a historic gathering, and a photo commemorates it in the *RCGP Members' Reference Book 1989*. I chaired and spoke about the fraught times we were in and the urgent need for more collaboration between GPs working in different settings.

The first aim of the Conference was therefore to build a new bridge between important groups of general practitioners who had some academic function either in research or teaching; and to try to infuse more academic principles into the GP course organisers and, hopefully, later the GP trainers and to help them both feel involved and recognised.

A second aim was to be able to submit evidence to the Richards Task Force on clinical academic careers, as this was bound to consider the question of distinction awards for salaried GP academics. There was only one GP on that Task Force, Anne-Louise Kinmonth, the GP Professor at Cambridge and I wanted to give her as much evidence and support as possible.

The third aim could not be talked about openly for risk of disturbing the Conference of Medical Royal Colleges but it was to establish a national Conference as an insurance policy if the RCGP ever needed to withdraw from an insensitive specialist-dominated Conference of Medical Royal Colleges.

This meeting brought all these leaders together with officers of the Irish College of General Practitioners of which I was a member. I had hopes of a fruitful partnership between the two Colleges of General Practitioners in the British Isles. However, this was not to be and links did not continue. However, I continued to believe that it was in the interest of both to meet and the RCGP had much to learn from a college that was ahead in achieving specialty status for general practice and which was working in a different relationship within the European Union.

My Chairmanship of the Conference lasted longer than expected as Colin Waine, my successor as Chair of Council, did not have a university post nor was he a regional adviser and so he was less well-placed to chair. He was succeeded by Bill Styles when he was Chair of Council, and under his chairmanship a public call for research general practices was made. However, he developed cancer and died in office prematurely. In this unexpected situation, the Conference re-elected me Chairman.

Publications

This Conference produced two publications. The first was drafted by Nigel Stott, the Professor of General Practice in Wales, whilst Bill Styles was Chair. It was called *Research and General Practice* (CAOGP, 1994) and it was written in accordance with the aim of the Conference to help GPs involved in teaching with the principles of research. Styles (1995) cwrote as conference Chairman to the MRC suggested that the MRC general practice research network be led by a GP and leading GPs be described as such rather than as "epidemiologists" This was not welcomed or implemented but helped to get people thinking.

The second publication was *Developing Primary Care — The Academic Contribution* (CAOGP, 1996), which I wrote. Its aims were: to promote academic general practice in universities where the number of GP academics in medical schools was pitifully small (5% of staff; Just GPs). Secondly, to submit evidence to the Richards Independent Task Force (1997) on clinical academic careers, and in particular to reinforce the need for academic GPs to be admitted for consideration for distinction awards.

However, the consultation draft, which was widely circulated, worked well and identified another aim. There had been a sharp reaction to a publication from the NHS Executive (1994) *Developing NHS Purchasing: Towards a Primary Care-Led NHS*. It was not surprising that many consultants did not welcome this, after all they had been accustomed to being the leaders for 150 years, but we learned that the idea of a primary care-led NHS was not understood by many health authorities. One health authority chairman said: "If only we knew what it was!"

Another aim of the publication was to define and support the principle of a primary care-led NHS. I redrafted the text and included the WHO reversed triangle (Horder, 1983) used in *Planning Primary Care* (DPG, 1992c) as it had attracted positive comment from the Chair of another NHS authority. This model states that the role of secondary care is to support primary care and the test is whether primary care feels supported. We deployed many of the strengths of general practice repeating the phrase it is "the front line of the NHS" (page 6) and pointed out that no health system anywhere offered better access with fewer barriers of care in a service catering for 98% of the population and managing 86% of the problems the population brought to doctors.

Other sections reinforced the need for master's courses in primary care/general practice (200 places nationally) as a form of GP higher professional education; and that there should be 12 research training fellowships in each NHS region. On specialist training, writing that: "It is already embarrassing to find a generation of general geriatricians emerging who have never been trained in the setting where most old people present their illnesses," Priority for postgraduate training for consultants in general practice should be: community paediatricians, geriatricians, psychiatrists, and public health physicians.

Recommendation 29 was that the exclusion of full-time and part-time salaried academic general practitioners from the distinction award be removed. The booklet was published in 1996 and a copy sent to the Richards Independent Task Force (1997), which happily endorsed the policy of including salaried GP academics in the award system. This effort was worth it. When Secretary of State for Health (2000)finally admitted academic salaried GPs to the distinction award scheme, it specifically referred to advice from the Richards Task Force (1997). Both these booklets were published in Exeter by Jill in an A5 format, giving them a distinct and consistent format. I described the Conference (DPG, 1995a) in the *RCGP Members' Reference Book*.

Subsequently, later Chairmen were less enthusiastic about the need for such a Conference and came either from the RCGP or from senior positions in the university world, where the priority of reaching GP course organisers and GP trainers and broadening the academic group in general practice was valued less. The Conference closed down after ten years.

26

Prison Medicine

The mood and temper of the public regarding treatment of crime and criminals is one of the most unfailing tests of the civilisation of any country.

Winston Churchill (1910)

My first contact with prisons was in the 1970s. I was running the Exeter vocational training scheme for general practice and we thought a visit to Dartmoor prison would be educational. It was certainly educational for me as much as the trainees. The prison doctor was cold and remote; the "nurses" were guards with minimal medical training and they sometimes administered drugs as punishments. When discussing prison suicides one guard said to us: "As far as I am concerned every dead prisoner is one less!"

This shocked my young, idealistic, and compassionate doctors. One woman trainee was physically sick in the coach coming home, and others told me later that they did not sleep well that night. I realised that the Prison Medical Service needed radical reform, but it never occurred to me I could do anything.

In the 1980s, the DH approached the Royal College of Physicians of London (RCP) and sought advice on prison medicine. It is not clear why the DH did this, as the Conference of Medical Royal Colleges would have been more logical. However, the prestige of the RCP then, as now, stood high. The President of the RCP was Sir Raymond Hoffenberg, who set up a working party, which he chaired himself. He included a consultant psychiatrist but not a GP, nor did he consult the RCGP (Just GPs), where I was Chair at the time. This was somewhat arrogant as most of the medical work in prisons is general practice. The subsequent report followed the RCP's predilection for subspecialties, proposing a new specialty of prison medicine. The report was published by the DH with a strong dissenting report from the Head of the Prison Service (Hoffenberg Report, 1989).

However, in 1990, the Chief Medical Officer (CMO), Sir Donald Acheson, called the heads of three of the Medical Royal Colleges to see him in the DH. The three Colleges he invited were the RCGP, the RCP and the RCPsych. I attended as Chair of Council. The CMO asked if the three Medical Royal Colleges would together take on the task of finding a way forward for prison medicine. We all agreed. The CMO thus neatly ditched the RCP report!

A Working Party was established with two representatives from each College. It was agreed that the chair would rotate between the Colleges for each meeting and the secretarial support would also rotate. The RCGP Council elected me with Bill Styles, the Secretary; Margaret Burtt was the staff member for the meetings held in Princes Gate. The physicians sent their new President, Professor Dame Margaret Turner-Warwick; the psychiatrists initially sent their President but soon delegated to Professor John Gunn, a forensic psychiatrist. The Prison Medical Service was initially represented by Drs Rosemary Wool and later by Mike Longfield. Various officials attended meetings as well.

The three Colleges started from different positions so the first task was to clarify what the doctor's role in prison was. The RCP had changed presidents and the new president was not locked into the views of the Hoffenberg report. There were useful audits undertaken by Edwin Martin, a GP prison doctor, who had served on the RCGP Council with me (Martin, 1984, 1985, 1986) and some

DOI: 10.1201/9781032713601-32

psychiatric surveys. There were cases from the General Medical Council, documenting mismanagement of diseases like asthma and diabetes.

Gradually it became clear that most of the role was generalist medicine, with a heavy preponderance of mental illness, particularly substance abuse and addiction. The patient–doctor relationship was unusual in prisons since they are run by the Home Office and the custody role had precedence over health. Prisoners have no choice of GP as in the NHS. There were then about 70,000 prisoners which, given an average list for GPs of about 1500 patients, implied that about 50 generalist doctors were needed nationally. We visited some prisons, exploring the medical arrangements. The proposed new specialty in the Hoffenberg report looked increasingly inappropriate and the reasons for its rejection by the DH became clear.

The Role of the Prison Medical Service

Prison doctors (mostly men) were not trained for their job. Worse, they did not even have the bare minimum training that an NHS GP would have. The job was far harder than anyone outside realised and included making life and death decisions. Their working facilities were bad, they were poorly equipped, and unlike most NHS doctors they had no nurses available. Unlike doctors in the NHS, prison doctors did not work in a system primarily orientated to health. The NHS is under the DH and the Secretary of State for Health. However, prisons came under a different department, the Home Office, where the Minister was the Home Secretary. Prison doctors were salaried and accountable to the governor whose first responsibility was security and meeting the demands of the courts. Health and medical care were a lower priority and received few resources.

Many medical conditions were poorly managed. The medical records were primitive and nothing had been done to computerise them even though there were between 50,000 to 80,000 prisoners. If a prison doctor referred a serious medical problem, it was the governor's decision whether to provide resources for the prisoner to go to hospital to see a specialist. Some referrals were refused. Many prisoners were in the wrong institution and should have been in mental hospitals. Many did not receive the psychiatric care they needed. A brilliant insight was published by LS Penrose (1939) that the numbers of people in prison reflected the availability of psychiatric beds. Remarkably Wild *et al* (2022) found this inverse relationship held true in England albeit lagged by several years. Prison doctors had low status and I was often told that they were doctors who could not easily get other work. The parallels with general practice in the 1940s were obvious. General practice had pulled itself up by its bootstraps – could prison doctors be helped to do the same?

Three Medical Royal Colleges' Working Party

I wrote several papers, including one on the patient-doctor relationship and we increasingly pressed for nurses to be employed. Sometimes discussions were sharp. When we discovered a prison doctor might often be faced with a mass of patients all at once as the courts often transferred dozens of strangers on Friday evenings, I said: "I couldn't do it." "But you are a professor of general practice!" a civil servant said. I replied, "I simply could not do it. These patients will all be strangers, there will be no records, many will be on drugs, many will be lying about what doses they are taking, and the doctor's decision of what drugs to prescribe can be fatal and sometimes has been." In 1991, the extent of prisoners with substance abuse was 19% (NAHAT, 1992). Some of these exchanges helped to alter attitudes towards prison doctors.

The business of rotating both the chair and the secretariat from College to College soon proved inefficient, as minutes prepared by a secretary and one chair, were always handled by a different chairman at the next meeting. Margaret Turner-Warwick was much the most senior and experienced member so when she proposed that I should become the permanent Chair of the Working Party this was approved unanimously. I suspect that she had by then privately judged that a likely outcome would be training for generalist doctors. Professor Gunn from the psychiatrists was most helpful. I had substantial advantages having been involved with GP standard-setting as a regional adviser for over 18 years and having been a member of the JCPTGP for 11 years. I drafted several papers for meetings. The Working Party reached agreement but it then took two years before the Home Office published it (Pereira Gray Report; *Three Medical Royal Colleges' Report on Prison Medicine*, 1992). The report outlined the nature of the medical problems in prisons made the case for generalist doctors providing the service and sought to improve their facilities, including nursing support and training.

With the report published, the Working Party engaged in extensive discussions to achieve change. In particular we pressed for computerisation of the medical records. I spent hours with Mike Longfield, the Medical Director of the Prison Health Service, trying to get a working system. There was considerable organisational resistance. However, the Prison Service was much more responsive to our suggestion of appointing nurses to support the doctors. To help get Mike Longfield more orientated to royal Colleges and their roles in a standard setting, I was able to get him made honorary member of the RCGP.

Diploma in Prison Medicine

An ambitious plan was to establish a diploma in prison medicine. This seemed the best way to raise clinical standards in prison medicine. A curriculum was agreed and the Home Office accepted our advice and agreed funding. A proposal was put out to competition. I chaired the tendering committee and we awarded the contract to the University of Nottingham, where Robert Hedley, a former Regional Adviser in General Practice, was leading.

The university did a good job and got the new diploma of prison medicine off the ground in 1996. Prison doctors applied and were selected by the prison service with a quota of 10 for each course. This was the culmination of the work of the Working Party and was the first diploma in prison medicine in the world. It created the need for an examination to determine satisfactory performance on the course. This raised tricky procedural issues, as each College had elaborate policies and principles in relation to examinations in its name. The Working Party established an Examination Board that had representatives from all three Royal Colleges. I nominated Professor Lesley Southgate from the RCGP, as she had led the RCGP membership examination and was a subject expert. Happily, the RCP nominated Professor Brian Kirby, who was one of my close colleagues and Deputy Director of the Exeter Postgraduate Medical School (Postgraduate Medical School story). The Examination Board worked hard and well. We had enough influence to persuade all three Royal Colleges to allow their royal crests to be used on a new diploma certificate. As prison doctors had low status, we wanted to value them by organising a proper ceremony for the presentation of the certificates. The new diplomates were obviously proud of their new diplomas.

It was gratifying to see the enthusiasm of these doctors. The Postgraduate Department at Nottingham, supported by the Examination Board, had all done a good job. These prison doctors had enjoyed the Nottingham course, had learnt a good deal, and in particular they had learned to do medical audits. These are an important key to establishing and improving clinical standards. They spoke to me about their plans to do comparative audits between prisons. Doctors who had previously been characterised by low esteem and lack of professionalism had been professionalised. The reputation of this diploma started to spread and there was talk of applications being allowed from other jurisdictions and possibly other countries paying for their doctors to attend.

I was encouraged by the Chief Medical Officer's 1996 annual report *On the State of the Public Health* (Sir Kenneth Calman, 1997). His section on "Prison Health Care" stated: "In 1992 three Medical Royal Colleges made recommendations about the training of doctors who work in prison health services, which are being implemented by Nottingham University on behalf of the Healthcare Service for Prisoners." He referenced the three Royal College report. Sir Kenneth's section on prisons in his next report for 1997 was even more encouraging (Calman, 1998). Noteworthy developments

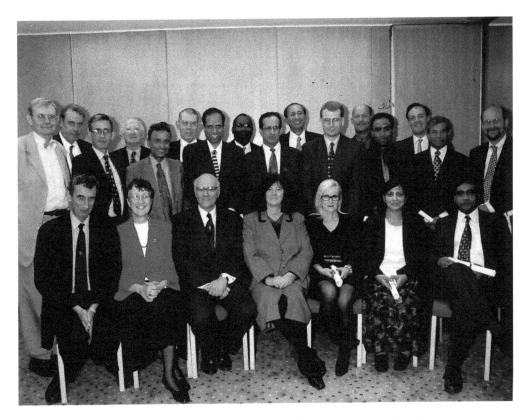

FIGURE 26.1   Presentation of Diplomas in Prison Medicine with Sir George Alberti (left) and Dame Lesley Southgate (centre), 2000.

in prison health care were made during the year. Training for prison doctors in the two-year Diploma in Prison Medicine began in September 1996. The first ten doctors will complete the course in June 1998 and a further ten in 1999. Over the period, the course is being monitored by a committee drawn from members of the Royal College of Physicians of London, General Practitioners and Psychiatrists, who have extended their role to advise the Prison Service on all aspects of training for prison doctors." This all appeared very positive.

We arranged ceremonies to present the certificates, with their three Royal College crests. One- Health Minister pulled out at an hour's notice and I had to make the speech and present the certificates myself.

However, without any consultation, the Home Office cancelled the funding and the course folded. This was a professional tragedy and strangled soon after birth an internationally important initiative that had real potential for raising standards of medical care in prisons. Ten doctors qualifying each year would have soon transformed the standards of prison medicine nationally. Much unpaid work and time had been spent on all this by both the Working Party and the Examination Board. This proved to be one of a series of initiatives with which I was involved that had bloomed initially but were later closed and, as I note in the final chapter, was one of my biggest professional disappointments.

Three Ministers

As Chair of the three Royal Colleges' Working Party, it fell to me to represent the Working Party with three different Cabinet Ministers about prison medicine, with three unsatisfactory results.

The first Minister was the Rt Hon Paul Boetang (1951–) who had the distinction of being the first black cabinet minister in Britain and had a record of taking interest in the underprivileged. The Working Party had identified illiteracy as a key issue on prisons. It wasn't difficult to see. The majority of prisoners at that time were young men and many were illiterate. Adult education was possible and available in several parts of the country. I was referring some patients in Exeter to a local service, which was excellent. Our Working Party had seen a good example of an adult literacy and educational service working in one prison. The argument was that teaching these men to read and write would make it much less likely that they would reoffend after they left. As they were in prison for a substantial period of time, the time was available. I had done my homework, and in the Home Office documentation there was a written aim for prisons to provide rehabilitation.

I met the Minister who was supported by an official in the Home Office. I had high hopes knowing his interest in the underprivileged. We spoke at length. He was charming and positive about the Royal Colleges' Working Party. He agreed the arguments I presented for teaching reading and agreed a young man leaving prison not able to read or write was likely to commit more crimes. He thanked me warmly for coming and I left the room encouraged. However, he had not talked about resources or getting adult learning therapies organised. I made enquiries. There was no ministerial encouragement or instruction to develop literacy services. Crucially there was no budget. Nothing happened: nothing was achieved. The Working Party and I had been skilfully fobbed off.

Lord Williams of Mostyn PC QC (1941–2003) was a Welsh highflyer in the Labour party, who had been awarded the military cross in World War II. He led the House of Lords and died early, aged only 62. I saw him as Parliamentary Undersecretary at the Home Office, and later Minister of State. I had written a paper prison doctors and how they could be better trained and supported, which the Working Party had approved. He sat himself at the end of the table with me beside him and the Director of the Prison Health Service opposite. I made the case for the training for doctors working in prison, based on treating them like GPs for training purposes. The Director of the Prison Health Service said that he had no budget for this and no resources with which to do it. Lord Mostyn was pleasant and friendly and treated me with interest and courtesy. However, he came quickly to the point that I was right to be saying what I did as a professional leader and he thought it was all very reasonable. But there was no money. He looked me in the eye and he said: "Denis, you must understand that there are no votes in prisons!"

After two defeats, I was cautious about further ministerial contacts. I searched to find some ground on which we could stand which was strong. Since Ministers had accepted a diploma on prison medicine, the three Royal College Working Party naturally discussed the desirability of prison doctors being appointed when they held the MRCGP. We enquired and found that very few GP prison doctors had the MRCGP. The two other specialist medical royal colleges saw membership as being of much lesser significance, as in specialist medicine membership examinations are merely a ticket into higher professional training. For example, an MRCP is required to start higher training. My attempt within the RCGP to establish a system matching this process for generalist doctors was fellowship by assessment (Chapter 23, Chair of Council story).

Ironically for someone committed to the RCGP and its examination, I now argued within the Working Party against the MRCGP. This was not because I did not think it was highly desirable but for two different reasons. First, the MRCGP was not then required for entry to general practice in the NHS, so the argument of NHS comparability failed. Second, as virtually no prison doctors held the MRCGP it might seem a bridge too far. By now I had experience of developing summative assessment for general practice in the JCPTGP. I suggested that the Working Party should concentrate on the certificate of satisfactory completion of vocational training, which was a much lower standard but more readily available. The Working Party was not keen, partly because the specialist Medical Royal Colleges had no equivalent of summative assessment and partly because it sounded like a second-class system, which it was. It had, however, two advantages. First, it was a certificate of minimal competence and the lowest possible standard in general practice; so it was an eminently reasonable request. Second, summative assessment was required for entry to NHS general practice, so NHS comparability was clear. I wanted the Working Party, if seeing another Minister, to pitch its tent on exceptionally strong grounds that would be hard to resist. Eventually the Working Party let me have this policy because it was such a strong position to take and we hoped that the MRCGP would later replace it (as it did in 2007 in the NHS). The case was that the Home Office should not allow GPs to work in prisons who were not qualified to work in the NHS. We thought we could win.

I carefully constructed a letter to a third Home Office Minister, then the Rt Hon Jack Straw (1943—) who went on to be a national leader in the Blair Government. Our request was simply that prisoners, when patients, should be entitled to the same level of medical care as if they were outside prison. Since the DH, as another Department of State, had accepted the principle that a GP must hold a certificate of satisfactory completion of vocational training to be allowed to work in general practice in the NHS, we simply requested the same principle for the prison medical service. This was the bare minimum and we sought no more for prison medicine. I knew that departments of state tend to favour consistency between government departments.

However, we were wrong. Jack Straw wrote back to me refusing the Working Party's proposal. It was a brutal decision, flying in the face of professional advice from three Medical Royal Colleges and it meant that he was prepared to have prisoners looked after by doctors who were unemployable as GPs in the NHS and might have no training or qualifications in general practice at all.

Mr Straw was a leading politician who later held two of the three great offices of state. The Labour party and Labour governments make repeated claims to be particularly concerned about the least privileged in the society. Exposing prisoners, who uniquely are unable to choose or change their doctor, to the least qualified and sometimes incompetent doctors denied them this principle.

The Working Party knew the work of Sir David Ramsbottom (1934–2022), later Lord Ramsbottom, the Chief Inspector of Prisons, a post which was established for the first time in the world in Britain as early as 1835. I invited him to lunch in the RCGP, as I admired his work. He was proving effective in raising standards of prisons generally. He was interested in our Working Party as he too was concerned about standards of prison medicine. He approached the problem differently, recommending that prison medicine should be removed from the Home Office and be provided by the NHS. This was far sighted and would solve several problems. The Joint Prison Service and NHS Executive report (1989) agreed. In 2002, the Home Secretary and Secretary of State for Health announced that funding responsibility for prison health services would transfer from the Home Office to the DH from April 2003.

This led to group general practices being contracted to provide prison care with vocationally trained GPs, usually with the MRCGP and nurses and computer systems. Some doctors continued employment in the prison service. Much was still to be done, especially the provision of medical facilities and support within prisons, but more was achieved with this radical change than the three Royal College Working Party could do. Sir David's move was strategically correct and partly worked. He was a good colleague and kindly spoke at the RCGP council dinner in 1990 as I retired as Chair of Council.

Conclusions

This is a story of a relationship between government departments and three Medical Royal Colleges. The Colleges were exploited and between them spent large amounts of college money on the Working Party and supporting College Officers, particularly me as Chair. We did our best to fulfil the remit formally given to us by a Chief Medical Officer, a grade one civil servant. All the professional time in the Colleges was unpaid. The Colleges acted in good faith, and co-operated well, producing a unanimously agreed Pereira Gray (1992) Report. The diploma of prison medicine, which the Working Party and Examination Board devised and implemented was an exciting educational initiative and the first in the world. Had it continued it would have transformed prison medical care but it was cancelled without consultation.

A decade of voluntary work by dozens of doctors in three Royal Colleges did not generate a thank you letter. Government ministers are over confident and sometimes take advantage of doctors. The encounters with three different Ministers, all Labour, revealed hidden values and motives. The interests of prisoners as patients were better served by independent doctors and the Chief Inspector of Prisons than by Government. As I retired, I realised we had failed.

ADDENDUM

In 2019, a pregnant teenage mother in HMP Bronzefield, Ashford, went into labour. She made three calls for help that were not answered and she delivered alone in her cell. The baby died. She received no bereavement care (Summers, 2021). This failure of the Prison Health Service was reported by the Prison Ombudsman. My nine years work with many colleagues in three Medical Royal Colleges seeking to professionalise the prison medical service failed.

27

Directorship of the Postgraduate Medical School of the University of Exeter 1987–1997

A university should be place of light, liberty, and learning.

Benjamin Disraeli (1804–1881)

The University of Exeter received its Charter in 1955 and so became an independent university after being a college of the University of London for years. Soon after this, some farsighted Exeter consultants saw the opportunity of developing a medical department within this new university. The driving force was Clifford Fuller, consultant physician at the Royal Devon and Exeter Hospital, supported by Exeter's best-known doctor, Norman Capener, who had developed the Exeter orthopaedic hospital and became nationally known, as a Vice-President of the Royal College of Surgeons of England and a CBE. In support and coming to meetings in Exeter was RMS McConaghey, a GP in Dartmouth, a foundation member of the Council of the College of General Practitioners and the Editor of its *Journal*. Later FSW (Freddie) Brimblecome, Exeter's first consultant paediatrician, was to become an influential enthusiast.

The Nuffield Provincial Hospitals Trust (NPHT) now the Nuffield Trust (Chapter 44 Nuffield Trust story), founded by Lord Nuffield (1877–1963), was formed in 1940. In 1961 the Trust organised a national conference to review the state of medical education in the country, showing visionary national leadership. Clifford Fuller (1899–1965) was the only provincial consultant who attended and spoke advocating university medicine developing outside the London teaching hospitals, for example, at Exeter. The idea of a new medical postgraduate institute in Exeter received an editorial in the *Lancet* (1962) and Fuller (1963) described a postgraduate teaching unit based on consultants. Fuller applied to the Trust for a grant, which was approved.

Thus the first postgraduate medical department in the British Isles outside London formed in the new University of Exeter, only eight years after the University's formation. It was funded by a five-year grant of £30,000 by the NPHT. David Mattingly was appointed in 1963 as the first Director in the Exeter Postgraduate Medical Institute, starting that October. Brimblecombe (1965) reported on a possible a 'department of social medicine,' and I wrote a paper proposing Britain's first postgraduate department of general practice be developed within the PGMI (Chapter 13, Department/Institute of General Practice story).

Mattingly gradually built up the specialist academic staff, ensured research publications, and ran the biggest course in England preparing overseas doctors to work in the NHS. Five years later when the grant ran out, the University of Exeter took over the financing of this institute, completely unreimbursed, in one of the most imaginative decisions of any British provincial university in the British Isles. In 1973, the Postgraduate Medical Institute was promoted to be the Postgraduate Medical School of the University with Mattingly promoted to professor. He became the first medical professor in Devon and Cornwall.

A Department of General Practice was established within this Institute, and I joined the university staff on 1 December 1973 as Senior Lecturer in-charge of general practice (Chapter 13. Department/Institute of General Practice story).

DOI: 10.1201/9781032713601-33

Mattingly announced his retirement for March 1987. He had a deputy director, another consultant physician named Brian Kirby, who had been appointed as deputy in 1974, so it was generally assumed he would succeed.

However, in the summer of 1986 I received one of the great surprises of my life. One Friday afternoon I was telephoned whilst in the Department of General Practice by the Chair of the Joint Medical Staff Committee of the Royal Devon and Exeter Hospital. He was Robert Hart, a consultant microbacteriologist. I knew him in two ways. First, clinically he was always helpful as a consultant to local GPs. Secondly his wife, Mary, did general practice locums and had helped my father many times. I had seen her often and through her had met Robert socially. I had had no dealings with him as the Chair of the local NHS consultants. He strolled the few hundred yards from the Exeter pathology laboratory to the Department and we had tea together.

He dropped a bombshell of news that the consultant body wanted me to succeed David Mattingly as the Director of the Postgraduate Medical School. I had rarely been so surprised in my life. I stuttered a thank you and quickly pointed out that the staff of the Postgraduate Medical School was 80% specialist consultants with the key votes. These consultants were not the same as the service consultants who formed his Joint Consultants Committee. He was ahead of me and said he understood this but was confident I would have strong support from the consultants with academic appointments in the university. I said I would consult with colleagues and would come back to him.

The following Tuesday I told Keith Bolden, Michael Hall, and Bob Jones in our weekly staff meeting in the GP department. They were as surprised as I was. None of them had sniffed the possibility and there was doubt whether a GP could be elected by predominantly consultant staff. I started private consultations with the consultant academic staff in the medical school and found that they had been briefed and said they would support me.

I saw Freddie Brimblecome (1919–1992), the dynamic Exeter paediatrician and local powerbroker. He was a national medical figure and the country's leading spokesperson for social paediatrics. Later, like Norman Capener, he was appointed CBE. Freddie had a habit of dropping into see me regularly ever since I was appointed as the GP Senior Lecturer, and we had always got on well. For his taste David Mattingly was not being dynamic enough and I suspect he would have loved to have been the Exeter Director himself. He was influential and had been awarded an honorary professorship himself. I thought he might be the kingmaker. He said he had hoped that a paediatrician would be the next director of the Medical School and he had helped bring John Tripp, as Senior Lecturer in child health, to Exeter from Great Ormond Street. He told me frankly that he thought John Tripp was not ready, but hoped he would be in five years' time. I gathered that a five-year term would be all I should expect.

I had numerous discussions with David King, the district administrator in Exeter for the National Health Service (NHS), on whose appointment committee I had served. He was a radical and had closed two mental hospitals in Exeter before most areas in England had closed one. He did not seem to be a great fan of consultants and it gradually became clear that he favoured my appointment. He said he would advise the University to that effect.

The University started the process for the appointment of the new director, which was complicated. It was a university appointment, and the university could appoint whomsoever it thought fit. However, the wave of politics in universities in the 1970s had left a situation where the staff was supposed to elect their leader. The problem of what would happen if the staff elected somebody the university did not want was never clear.

Nominated candidates had to write a manifesto. I ensured that I was proposed and seconded entirely by specialist consultant staff. Brian Kirby was nominated too. We both wrote manifestos. Mine was radical declaring a strong belief in the Postgraduate Medical School but stating that I thought it was threatened and radical developments were needed if it was to survive. I declared experience in the RCGP as Editor and relevantly as a governor of the British Postgraduate Medical Federation, the governing body of the London postgraduate specialist institutes.

Barry Behenna was the administrative officer appointed as returning officer and he reported I had been elected. On 10 November 1986, I was called to the nomination committee of the university, which appointed me Director for a five-year term starting on 1 April 1987. There was then a debate within the PGMS about the most appropriate title. Some reasonably favoured the title of 'Dean,' but there was no strong consensus for change. I was happy to continue with the title of 'Director' as that continued David Mattingly's title.

So on 1 April 1987 I became the second director of the Exeter Postgraduate Medical School. What was little understood in Exeter was that at the very time my election was being arranged, there was the biggest organisational crisis ever in the history of the College of General Practitioners. This led to the resignation of the Chair of Council and me being elected to succeed him on 10 February 1987 (Downs and ups of Institutional Life).

So it was that I entered the director's office in the PGMS in Exeter, only seven weeks after my election in London as Chair of the RCGP. I suddenly held both roles simultaneously, both arriving unexpectedly.

I took stock of the resources available, and they were pathetically limited. The University funded two whole-time equivalent hospital consultant posts with secretarial support and that was it. There was no funding for general practice at all. My manifesto had warned of serious pressures, and I realised I had been elected with the political remit to ensure the survival of the PGMS. It was clear that the University was regretting its long-term commitment to two posts.

The University funded one secretary to support the Director, which was advertised soon after I arrived. The personnel representative advised me to appoint one person and was unhappy when I chose Rosemary Ash instead. She proved to be a great asset to the PGMS, working extra hours and applying a good brain to the many problems. I was lucky to have her.

I had stated in my manifesto that if appointed I would try to build up the corporate identity and cohesion of the PGMS. David Mattingly had made a historic contribution in getting the PGMI established, building a reputation strong enough for the University to grant it the title of Postgraduate Medical School and establish his chair. This was a great achievement starting with only a half-time post and only five-year funding. However, he was not a corporate man and was happiest doing research in his own laboratory. Mattingly had never held staff meetings, never produced an annual report, or any meetings to showcase the PGMS. His leadership style was to appoint the best people he could find and leave them to get on with it.

I immediately initiated regular staff meetings, which brought the academic staff together for the first time to ensure that they had common information about what we were all doing and what was happening in the University. Secondly, I introduced an annual report, printing details of all academic achievements and every publication in the name of everybody on the staff. These reports helped to inform other academics just how much was being achieved with minimal resources. It fostered collaboration, formed a calling card for visitors and for promoting the PGMS within the University (Postgraduate Medical School of the University of Exeter, 1989, 1990 (1989/90 and 1990/91 annual reports). They proved important for complementary medicine.

The third innovation was to hold open evenings, advertised across the University, to showcase the academic work of the PGMS. The format was 10-minute presentations followed by five minutes of questions and I chaired it to ensure the evening ran to time. We provided a buffet supper in the middle. We chose younger staff to help them develop, and every evening always had a representative of the Department of Child Health, from the Department of General Practice, and other hospital academic staff speaking. These evenings drew local colleagues from inside and outside the hospital and one or two VIPs from the University.

Departments within the PGMS

Big hierarchical departments have problems, and I did not want to be become bogged down in administration so I established academic departments within the PGMS and delegated heavily to them. I inherited departments of child health and general practice and established three new ones in complementary medicine, psychiatry and vascular medicine.

A big danger in institutions is bureaucracy and excessive control. Rules tend to proliferate and cramp people's style. The "liberty" in Disraeli's aphorism, above means as much professional freedom as possible and saying yes if possible. Backing juniors is essential. This fits with Disraeli's "light" as young people question the status quo and often bring important new ideas.

Teaching and Research

Teaching and research are the two legs on which universities stand. However, they are not regarded equally within universities where research has always been rated much more highly. Appointments to senior posts, like deans, are usually made on the basis of research not teaching achievements and in many universities teaching income, questionably, is used to support research. This is another example of Snow's (1963) "two cultures." Many teaching staff are poor at research and many leading researchers are poor teachers. It is still common for leading researchers to use cluttered slides that cannot be read at the back of the room and often changing them before the information has been absorbed. Only rarely do researchers when teaching show any interest in their teaching being assessed.

I considered Disraeli's "learning" a core component of scholarship which was best achieved through departments, as they were in regular contact with the greatest numbers of practising health professionals. Throughout my Directorship and ever since I have believed that research and teaching should be regarded as two different but equally important functions.

Finally, I always believed that people who have the privilege of holding senior positions should use their positions to thank. I was often teased about writing so many thank you notes on postcards to colleagues both senior and junior. I spent much energy valuing achievements by whoever made them.

Appointing an Academic Consultant Physician

The first big opportunity was to appoint an academic consultant physician who would have the five consultant sessions a week held by David Mattingly. This was a crucial because those five sessions represented a quarter of all the funded consultant sessions in the medical school. I knew that given the very small size of the PGMS that we were well below the critical mass needed for survival. The strategy had to be attracting doctors of outstanding ability, who could punch well above their academic weight.

The post was advertised as a joint appointment between the hospital and the University of Exeter with the expectation that the consultant appointed would hold the title of senior lecturer in medicine. I was a member of the selection committee as Director and it was chaired by the Chair of the Exeter Health Authority, Murray French. One of the advantages of working in a relatively small city like Exeter is local contacts, and Murray and I knew each other because he had been taught by my mother! This committee was my first consultant appointment committee and produced some tricky points. The first was whether or not David King, the District Administrator would be allowed to attend. It is a measure of the influence that consultants held in the NHS that as late as 1987 the district administrator had no right of access. I was consulted and advised that I thought he should be present as he had overall responsibilities for the NHS in the district and the PGMS was a major asset.

An application was received from John Tooke, which looked very good. He was already a Wellcomed senior lecturer, a prestigious national post and was based in Charing Cross Hospital in London. The first problem in the committee was when the Chair reported that he had received a message from the Joint Medical Staff Committee that the newly appointed consultant would do equal out-of-hours with the other consultant physicians. I reacted briskly and said that this was completely unacceptable. Everyone looked surprised because the consultants' committee at that time wielded great influence. I said simply that this was an improper request and that the procedure was improper as well. First, half this post was being funded by the University of Exeter, which I represented, and this was the academic component which did not include any service out-of-hours. The NHS component was half time, and this doctor should therefore undertake half the out-of-hours duty of a full-time consultant physician. Second, I said the process was improper as the University should have been consulted and this was the first, I had heard about it. I was determined that the university appointed a high-quality, international level, academic that needed all the time possible to undertake research. This double-barrelled argument worked, and the Chair ruled that the doctor appointed should only undertake a half share of out-of-hours work.

The committee proceeded uneventfully, and it looked as if John Tooke would be smoothly appointed. Then, suddenly, the external assessor from the Royal College of Physicians of London intervened destructively: "I think," he said, "this candidate is too good to be appointed to a small unit like Exeter!" I was stunned and whilst gathering my wits a lay member said, "Oh, do you think so!" I faced a crisis and let fly in full debate. Fortunately, I have always been one to read the small print and as this was my first consultant appointment committee, I knew that the external assessor was present only in order to ensure that any candidate was appropriately trained. That man was hopelessly exceeding his brief and his intervention was improper, so I said so.

I then had to weaken the credibility of his argument, so I expanded at length on how Professor Brimblecombe from the PGMS had been appointed the Chair of the National Children's Committee and was a leading exponent of social paediatrics. As for the medical Royal Colleges, one of which he was representing, he needed to know that I too was a member of the Council of one of them and was present at that committee as its Chair. This gave the Chairman the ammunition that he needed, as he was as keen to get John Tooke appointed as I was, so he made a brief reference to the role of external assessors from the Royal College of Physicians and summed up in favour of John Tooke. I was confident that we had brought to Exeter an academic doctor of great ability who would hugely strengthen the PGMS.

John Tooke had a research colleague, Angela Shore, working with him at Charing Cross and when he was appointed to Exeter, she very bravely agreed to follow him. She had completed her PhD and was engaged with John in some exciting, innovative, experimental research. She was taking a considerable personal risk, as there was no funded post for her. When she first arrived, we were only able to offer her about three months' security of income.

John Tooke brought some Wellcome Trust funds with him and hit the ground running with a plan for a diabetic centre that would bring together research staff, patient care and teaching staff. He launched an immediate plan to reform the specialist diabetic services in Exeter. His special research technique was to examine micro-capillary blood vessels and his team was able to do this better than anyone else. This team had an article published in the *New England Journal of Medicine*, the highest ranked general medical journal in the world (Sandeman *et al.*, 1992). They related capillary pressure to metabolic control in diabetes. This was when few British authors were being published by the *New England Journal of Medicine* and was experimental medicine of the highest order. I trumpeted the success everywhere as it was the proof of the Exeter academic pudding – world-class research being done in the PGMS.

One of the research grants in the Department of General Practice was on the subject of depression, which led to numerous contacts in London. I was pleased to meet Rachel Jenkins (later professor), an academic psychiatrist, who was as passionate about developing psychiatry as I was about general practice. She held a staff appointment in the DH, which she used to promote psychiatry skilfully. Our research grant involved having an advisory committee on which she sat, as did Professor Anthony Mann from the Institute of Psychiatry. This led to an introduction to Keith Lloyd, an academic psychiatrist also on the staff of the DH, who suddenly showed an interest in moving to Exeter. He was still working for his MD, but he obviously had the skills. I was able to persuade the mental health authorities to provide honorary academic sessions for him, and eventually we appointed him to the PGMS as a Senior Lecturer in Psychiatry, funded mainly by the mental health trust.

Second Term as Director

My term of office as Director was due to expire on 31 March 1992. I had never expected to serve more than one term having been tipped off to expect that. By 1991, I was looking for successors, but there were few possible candidates. Essentially the challenge of welding the disparate academics into a coherent team had succeeded and many of them, particularly John Tooke in vascular medicine and John Tripp in child health, were busy, both being real consultants in their respective fields as well as being part-time academics. The detailed reporting, I was giving the staff had alerted them all to the pressures the PGMS was under and how difficult it was for me in the University finance committees. Increasingly, the accountancy approach to university governance expected all departments to generate income to cover their costs. The PGMS was not doing so, although it was producing a string of academic successes, including prestigious publications, prizes, and eponymous lectures. The difficulty was that there was no funding stream to support a *postgraduate* academic institution. We had no core funding from the University Grants Committee or the NHS. The Department of General Practice was self-funding, through a heavy teaching programme, which specialist staff could not match.

There was one obvious source of income – Exeter was taking an increasing number of undergraduate medical students from the University of Bristol medical school. Moreover, Exeter had persuaded the University Grants Committee, in David Mattingly's day, to provide student accommodation, so Exeter was offering medical students attractive facilities. Bristol was being funded generously through the special increment for teaching (SIFT) at a rate per student. I argued that for every 52 weeks that Bristol students were in Exeter, we should receive the SIFT payment for one medical student. The Bristol Dean was not interested. The academic staff elected John Tripp to try again to negotiate some payment, but he too came back empty-handed.

One academic, John Tooke, obviously had the ability to lead the Medical School but he was heavily engaged in achieving academic breakthroughs and I was then strongly proposing him for the award of a personal chair. Taking over the Medical School was not right for John at that time. It dawned on me that the staff were not queueing up to succeed me so I made it clear when my term of office would end, taking no other action. As time ran out, the University formally called for candidates and I indicated I would continue to serve if wanted. My reappointment was proposed by John Tripp and John Tooke. I was elected unopposed, which was to be a pattern in my life. The University confirmed me as Director of the Postgraduate Medical School for a further five years.

Chair of Complementary Medicine

In the early 1990s, it became clear that the Laing Foundation was willing to fund a chair in complementary medicine in a British university. Other universities were initially considered, but Exeter was approached through the personal adviser to Sir James Laing (1918–2008), Admiral Sir James Watt, KBE FRCS. Sir James (1914–2009) was a distinguished naval surgeon and historian, who was later President of the Royal Society of Medicine in London. He came to sound me out on the possibility of this chair coming to Exeter.

The background was complex because Exeter had a fairly high-profile presence in complementary medicine, which it was practising and also teaching in a unit in the social science faculty. Contact had been made and the complementary practitioners there were hopeful that a chair would be funded. However, Sir James was not happy. He had a clear view that complementary medicine, if it was ever to be taken seriously by mainstream medicine, had to be underpinned by research that mainstream medicine recognised. He noted that the social science unit was not doing such research and he came to ask me if the PGMS was. We had several meetings. I gave him the annual reports of the PGMS and emphasised we were committed to rigorous research, and we had a fair number of publications across several disciplines to prove it.

I argued that general practice was an interesting analogy, as it too had been regarded with suspicion by traditional specialties and that it was in a now winning acceptance through producing high-quality research. Sir Maurice increasingly took the view that if this chair was to come to Exeter, it had to be based in the science faculty and in the PGMS and not in social sciences. As it became clear he was influential with Sir Maurice Laing. I went to see the Vice-Chancellor as it looked as if two departments and two faculties might be competing for this substantial endowment. The VC, Dr (later Sir) David Harrison (1930–2023) assured me he was neutral and would support any arrangement bringing the funds to Exeter, which was satisfactory to the Laing Foundation.

Potential candidates started arriving in Exeter. None of them were interested in the Centre for Complementary Medicine, and all of them said they wanted to be in a medical unit. This was not surprising and followed the stipulation of the Laing Foundation that the professor must be a doctor. I showed potential applicants round but had to make it clear that it would be a high-level decision of the Laing Foundation where any such chair would be placed. All of them wanted to join the PGMS. A negative factor was that vibes from the Royal Devon and Exeter Hospital, and particularly from its Chair, Professor Dame Margaret Turner-Warwick, indicated that she was not keen on complementary medicine. Once it became clear to complementary medicine and to the Dean of Social Sciences that the Laing Chair might be placed in the PGMS, there was deep resentment. They saw this as their contact, their subject, which they alone practised in the University and saw my efforts as predatory. A letter from the Dean of Social Sciences accused me of "academic piracy!"

The selection committee for the new chair was big and widely representative and I was on it as the Director of the Medical School. An Oxford academic was appointed with the second place going to a German national applying from the medical school in Vienna. The successful candidate came, and we had long discussions but it was not possible to agree arrangements to suit the University and him. The University therefore turned to the second placed candidate, Edzard Ernst, who accepted with alacrity and quickly came to see me. We got on well, and his French wife Danielle was an anglophile. They gave Jill and me dinner and we had another dinner together with Sir Maurice Laing.

I was alert to the problem that Ernst was not going to have a consultant appointment and so would not be eligible for a distinction ward. Therefore, if he was as able and successful as I hoped, some analogue was needed for his remuneration so that he would not fall progressively behind his consultant colleagues. I drafted a unique distinction award equivalent to be externally judged by three national colleagues, including the Chair of the RCGP and the President of the Royal College of Physicians. The Vice-Chancellor approved this unique arrangement and included it in his contract. The first five-year review worked well whilst I was still Director; the second failed, as described in Chapter 39, Distinction/Clinical Excellence Awards story.

Ernst's appointment placed him in both the Centre for Complementary Medicine and in the PGMS simultaneously, which was the University's way of trying to square an impossible circle. His relationships with colleagues in complementary medicine soon broke down as he was committed to researching the subject and not to practising it. He left the Centre and moved entirely into the PGMS. I was able to offer him a room close to mine in the corridor that formed the buildings of the PGMS but did not have the space to offer accommodation for a team. There were continuing negative vibes from the Royal Devon and Exeter Hospital questioning if complementary medicine was an appropriate academic subject. Then Ernst found rented accommodation very close to the PGMS that gave him plenty of space.

My brief to Ernst as his Head of Department was simple: research complementary medicine fearlessly and publish whatever you find. As his Head of Department, I met sustained criticism by those practising complementary medicine who saw the first professor of complementary medicine in the world systematically undermining, as they saw it, their work. However, not all his research was critical of complementary therapies and Ernst wrote a justification of the use of St John's Wort for clinical depression (Ernst, 1995a). He produced a tsunami of publications, many in high ranked journals. He devised interesting investigative techniques including sham acupuncture. Within a few years, he had produced the most impressive body of research on complementary therapies in the world and was recognised internationally for it.

Ernst came to see me to say he had been reviewing the history of the medical school in Vienna from which he had come. This was a big medical school with a substantial international reputation. He had been examining the papers and had unearthed a dreadful story of anti-Semitism when Germany had taken over Austria. He had found that about three-quarters of the academic staff had been Jewish and had been

sacked. Some of them had died in concentration camps. He was a German national who became natu-
ralised British later. German was his first language and he had been on the staff there as a professor, so he
was ideally equipped to research this. I asked if he was Jewish, anticipating later attacks, and he said no.

I encouraged him to check his sources rigorously and then publish. He then came to see me to report
that his article had been rejected by leading European journals including, the *Lancet*. I was concerned
as this sounded like a European problem that ought to be reported in European medical journals.
I advised that he should pursue publication, if necessary, in American journals. He did so and his
article was published in the *Annals of Internal Medicine* in the United States: "A Leading Medical
School seriously damaged, 1938." He reported that as many as 153 of 197 members of the faculty had
been dismissed; moreover, survivors had not been welcomed back after the war (Ernst, 1995b). I have
always been uneasy that European medical journals did not publish this.

When this chair of complementary medicine was established, it was agreed that the Laing
Foundation would contribute £1.5 million and that the University would provide funds over the years
to keep it going. However, the University did not do so.

Charles Seward, an Exeter consultant physician had written a successful textbook, *Bedside
Diagnosis* (Seward, 1947), which described medicine from the point of view of symptoms rather
than diagnoses. Towards retirement, he shared the authorship of later editions with David Mattingly.
As Mattingly retired, I tried hard to persuade him to preserve this Exeter success by including a new
Editor as Seward had done; however, despite 13 editions, I failed and the book sadly died.

When senior staff go to London meetings regularly, tension occurs. What's in it for the unit? I countered this feeling by reporting fully to staff meetings about what was going on in London. They usually

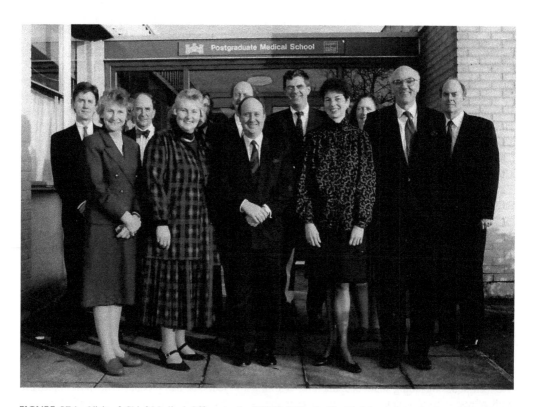

FIGURE 27.1   Visit of Chief Medical Officer to the PGMS 1993. Staff with left to right: Professor John Tooke,
Professor Dame Margaret Turner-Warwick (Chair, Hospital Trust), Dr Brian Kirby, Baroness Fritchie (Chair Regional
Health Authority), Professor Ernst, Sir Kenneth Calman (CMO), Dr John Tripp, Ms Pamela Mason (Regional Manager),
Dr Rita Goble, DPG, Dr Michael Hall.

found this interesting as people like to be in the know. I was able to bring the Chief Medical Officer, Sir Kenneth Calman, to the PGMS to meet staff. Such a visit was unusual, was appreciated, and was visible evidence of some value for Exeter from my London contacts.

Exeter a Model for the Clinician Scientist

The Exeter PGMS emerged as the model of the clinician scientist in the UK. From David Mattingly onwards, many of us sought to be real clinicians in our clinical fields, both general practice and hospital medicine, working part-time, and doing research published in leading journals, as well as teaching.

The Exeter PGMS was the first postgraduate academic unit in a British university outside London with a group of a dozen postgraduate institutes, all in the specialties. Exeter's example was increasingly noted elsewhere. Five other universities approached me, all interested in copying this model. The University of Hull came to visit me and sought advice especially on Exeter's general practice element. The newly appointed Director of a Postgraduate Department at Swansea came to seek advice and I was also given a dinner with the Vice-Chancellor and invited to advise and open a building for the University of Ulster in Northern Ireland. Plymouth colleagues came too.

A Conference of Postgraduate University Medical Departments was formed which moved around the country and held one meeting in Exeter. When years later, bids were invited for new undergraduate medical schools, many of these postgraduate departments, including Exeter, Hull, Keele, Plymouth, Norwich, and Swansea all became new (undergraduate) medical schools.

Two Institutes

John Tooke developed an interesting idea of developing his Department of Vascular Medicine into a multidisciplinary institute. He had the correct idea of seeking to foster multi-professional teamwork and he wanted to build bridges with staff in the natural sciences on the main university campus. He did much work in setting out these plans for what he wanted to call an Institute of Clinical Sciences. Simultaneously, I had realised the need to develop the Department of General Practice, as it was now entirely self-funding down to the cost of the photocopying paper. We had expanded beyond the original remit of developing vocational training for general practice and were doing research, had postgraduate masters' and doctoral degree programmes, and were increasingly advising governments and WHO. I planned for it to become an Institute to reflect its multidisciplinary nature and national role.

There were several eyebrows raised in the upper echelons of the university when, as Director, I proposed two institutes be established. Were they really necessary? Did they matter? I had been on several key university committees for six years and interpersonal relationships with the Vice-Chancellor and policymakers were good. I said: "You're not funding us, so the least you can do is give us the titles we need." Both Institutes were established in 1993.

An exciting development in the mid-1990s occurred when John Tooke said there was a possibility of attracting Andrew Hattersley to the PGMS. He was at Oxford and had had a brilliant career but was attracted by what was being achieved in Exeter, particularly by John Tooke in vascular medicine. He was also an excellent yachtsman and could see sailing opportunities in Exeter.

It was to John Tooke's credit that he was able to persuade him to apply and also persuaded the management in the Royal Devon and Exeter Hospital to construct a suitable consultant post. His arrival marked the third and final step in my campaign to bring academic stars to Exeter, and he would glow the brightest by subsequently being elected a Fellow of the Royal Society (FRS).

Public Orator

Between 1994 and 1996, I was three times appointed by the University to be a public orator. This meant writing and delivering a citation for someone who being awarded an honorary degree. The orators were usually senior professors who were often heads of the schools of the University. The honorary degrees were always awarded as part of the degree giving ceremonies in the great hall of the University, which holds about 1,000 people.

I had the privilege of delivering orations for General Sir Steuart Pringle, KCB, Sir Michael Peckham (1935–2021), and Sir Donald Irvine (1935–2018). Sir Steuart (1928–2013) was much respected as a marine general, who had had a leg blown off. He was a role model for the disabled. I had served with Peckham on the Governing Body of the British Postgraduate Medical Federation and later he was an effective NHS Director of Research and Development. Capital allocation is always problematic in nationalised industries, as they compete for government funds. Day-to-day expenditure often erodes capital planning. Peckham persuaded the Secretary of State for Health, Virginia Bottomley, that the NHS budget reserve 1.5% for research and development. This great idea was not sustained by later governments.

I nominated Irvine (1935–1918), the first GP president of the GMC, for an honorary degree, as it was time Exeter had a GP honorary Doctor of Science. It was strange after working so closely to be together on a university stage, with him the graduand and me the orator. I took him and his wife Sally to visit the Practice.

Dame Margaret Turner-Warwick (1924–2017) was appointed Chair of the Royal Devon and Exeter Hospitals Trust 1992–1995, after retiring as PRCP, so I met her several times alone as Director.

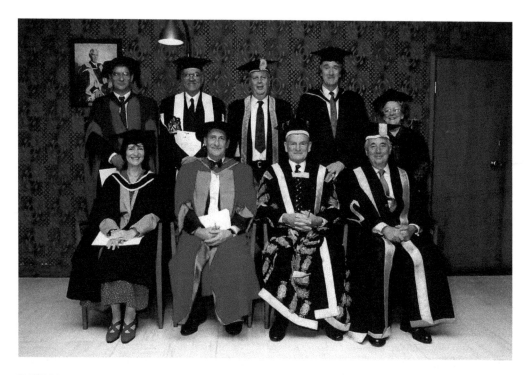

FIGURE 27.2 University of Exeter, 1996. Public Orator for Sir Michael Peckham. With Chancellor Sir Rex Richards, University of Exeter. Public Orator for Sir Michael Peckham (red gown) next to Sir Rex Richards FRS (Chancellor), DPG (second left) in back row next to Sir Geoffrey Holland (Vice-Chancellor).

After seeing her often in London when we were leading the RCP and RCGP and working together it should have been easy. Superficially, all was charming, and Jill and I gave her dinner in our home. However, professionally it was often difficult. She disliked me welcoming a professor of complementary medicine and we had a sticky discussion when I sought an ex-officio place on a local body. I pointed out that in medical schools, as she well knew as a former dean, the dean was always an ex-officio member, but she refused. Once when discussing the future of postgraduate medical centres, we discussed GPs having educational meetings in practices. She said: "I hope they always have a consultant present." Suddenly, I realised that she saw GPs as permanent pupils (Just GPs). In fact, GP-led educational meetings had been happening for over 20 years. "No," I said, "that's not necessary as they are discussing general practice."

National Reviews

In the 1990s, the DH tackled the multiplicity of teaching hospitals in London. These duplicated services but these hospitals had great political power. Teams were established to review several specialties, especially their research. I was seen as a suitable GP as I was a professor, a GP, and a Dean. I was on two of these reviews including the one on renal services and the Maudsley group (Review Advisory Committee of the DH, 1993).

The renal review was led by Professor (later Sir) Netar Mallick (1935–). I saw renal services were being duplicated in hospitals only a few miles apart and how casually our visits were taken. At one teaching hospital, our reception was not welcoming. I said to the team that the training practices in the Westcountry received assessors better. I learned that NHS's restricted funding meant the second lowest rate for dialysis in Europe – estimated to cost 1,000 lives a year, through the rationing that was necessary. I contributed little. Our report recommended rationalisation, ensuring eligible patients up to age 80 were offered treatment and expanding services. The Treasury delayed our report because of the cost (Mallick Report, 1993). I contributed more to other reports where I my editing experience enabled me to spot a serious flaw in some draft wording (Review Advisory Committee, 1993).

The Chief Medical Officer held a conference on continuing professional development in general practice (Calman, 1998). There were 43 people, 13 from DH or NHS, plus two health authority chief executives. The CMO got eight national leaders, including the chief executive of the UKCC. I was one of four postgraduate Dean/GP directors. There were three working groups. I was with John Toby in a group chaired by Janet Grant from the Open University, exposing a problem, as John, Chair of the RCGP was the most influential person present and should have been the chair. The conference decided that all practice education should be multidisciplinary. This is a half-truth and in the St Leonard's Practice away days were whole-team events and multidisciplinary. The Conference ducked the other half-truth that keeping GPs up to date across the whole range of medicine is a huge task. Learning about new tests, treatments, diseases, and consulting techniques is not best learned by GPs with receptionists and secretaries. The conference proposed, managerially, that each practice should have a whole practice professional development plan and was an expensive failure. The multidisciplinary plans never appeared. GPs' real educational needs were missed.

"Star Chamber"

The Academic Policy Committee (APC) was the university body managing the finances of the schools of the University. It was nicknamed the "star chamber" in staff meetings. These meetings were difficult for me as Director. The university's financial formula expected each school to generate funds to cover salaries. Most schools/departments did so with funding for their undergraduate students supplemented with funds from the research assessment exercise (RAE). The *Post*graduate Medical School had no undergraduates and so no such funding. The APC showed the PGMS costing £178,400 for the year ending July 1995. I was expected to cover that. We won many research grants from charities. Both general practice and vascular medicine held grants of over a third of a million (£654,000). But since charities paid no overheads to universities, neither the university nor the PGMS benefited. We had a top ranked research group with John Tooke's team, top graded 5 in the RAE, but RAE funds related to the number of staff and that group was tiny.

The star chamber nickname was all too appropriate, both in relation to power and threat. The PGMS, at least the specialist part of it, faced closure, as the pressure from the top of the University was to cover the costs of our two whole-time equivalent specialist posts. The Institute of General Practice had, particularly through Keith Bolden my deputy there, built up such a big teaching programme that it was self-sufficient financially. Whilst I had developed some good working relationships, the iron fist was always present. One of the other school heads said bluntly the PGMS was taking a share of their money. Others spoke of "subsidising" the PGMS. In 1994, I faced calls for "early retirements or redundancies." The Chair of APC wrote requiring that I should "squarely address the over-funding problem." I was alone in the Committee, on the defensive, fighting for the survival of the PGMS.

I negotiated some early retirements and scoured university and national publications for facts. My long defence paper stated: "The School had doubled the number of academic staff in the last three years all at no cost to the University..." By September 1994, the University was benefiting from five posts funded externally for each of the two FTEs post funded by the University itself. In September 1995, the gearing ratio was over 6:1. In 1994: "...already the PGMS brings in 14% of the all the University's research grants for 0.25% of the university's resource..." (PGMS Academic Plan 1994/5 to 1997/8).

Fearing they might close the PGMS: "Without the PGMS' research income Exeter would fall many places in the national league table...Expressed as research income over whole-time equivalent member of academic staff the PGMS was first among all departments in the University at £271,859 per FTE staff member. ...the average medical school in the UK has a research income of about £80,000 per FTE member of staff" (CVCP, 1994). I fended off threats during my term as Director (DPG, 1995c, 1995d; PGMS submission to APC, 1994).

In 1996 with my term ending, I announced I would not stand again. John Tooke stood and, as the outstanding candidate, he was easily elected and appointed. Once John Tooke was confirmed as my successor, I took him with me to the star chamber where I was harangued about the PGMS finances and the need to generate more income. He was taken aback by the incident, and it helped him realise that some radical new system of funding was needed.

As Director I proposed and actively supported two professorships, both for physicians, John Tooke and Brian Kirby, both were well deserved and were approved. Between 1963 and 2001 the PGMS only ever had five professors and one honorary chair.

Late in my Directorship, I tried to relate to the Plymouth Postgraduate Medical School. There were good working relationships with Plymouth GPs. The two cities are only 42 miles apart but there was an Edinburgh/Glasgow rivalry. I spoke with Mr Wilkinson, a consultant surgeon in Plymouth who was supportive. The Dean of the Plymouth Medical School was repeatedly ill, several appointments were postponed, and no meeting happened. It fell to John Tooke to build the bridge between Exeter and Plymouth Universities.

My term of office ended on 31 March, but I was asked to continue to 31 July 1997, so I was Director for 10.3 years. That April, I was elected PRCGP, for November. I was fortunate because the timing could not have been more convenient.

My knighthood in January 1999 was the first for a member of the academic staff of the University of Exeter and it was a sign of the times that I had always worked part-time for the University.

ADDENDUM

John Tooke as Director closed all the departments in the PGMS, so the Institute of General Practice died when I retired on 30 September 2001. The big financial nest eggs the gang of four had built for their GP successors was spent elsewhere. John Tooke skilfully built a partnership with the University of Plymouth and successfully bid for a new undergraduate medical school jointly between the two universities. The Exeter and Plymouth postgraduate medical schools merged into this, and it opened in 2002 with him as Inaugural Dean. He was elected Head of the Council of Deans of UK medical schools and was knighted. Later, he moved to London and was elected President of the Academy of Medical Sciences. Later still, Exeter and Plymouth universities separated so that in 2013 Exeter again had its own medical school.

Edzard Ernst was awarded many professional honours FRCPEd and FRCPLond, and, notably, Fellowship of the Academy of Medical Sciences (FMedSci). His book *A Scientist in Wonderland* (Ernst, 2015) describing his experiences sold well. Keith Lloyd moved to the Swansea Medical School, becoming Dean. One of our GP trainees, Sarah Purdy, became Dean of the Bristol Medical School.

The staff of the Exeter PGMS never exceeded 20 at senior lecturer/professor level, but produced two knighthoods, two CBEs, two OBEs, Chairs of both the Academy of Medical Royal Colleges, and the Council of Heads of UK Medical Schools, plus four fellows of the Academy of Medical Sciences, including one of its Presidents and an FRS. This was documented in the *Journal of the Royal Society of Medicine* (DPG, 2015) after Professor Baum, from London, wrote of the: "academic backwater like the Exeter Postgraduate Medical School!" Angela Shore's research career blossomed. She was appointed professor and later Vice-Dean of Research in the Exeter Medical School.

Andrew Hattersley's (1958–) research was outstanding. He became a world authority, identified glucokinase as a gene contributing to diabetes and was elected a Fellow of the Royal Society (FRS) in 2010, Britain's highest academic accolade. In 2017, he was the fourth Exeter doctor since the war to be appointed CBE. He was elected FRS through part-time research in Exeter (in the postgraduate school and then the new medical school). Being a skilled and respected consultant physician throughout, he is the ultimate example of Exeter's model of the clinician scientist in a provincial centre.

Section VII

28

Chair of Research 1993–1996

Winning prizes is always a pleasure, especially as they come from colleagues.

Zalatan Ibrahimovic (1981–)

In 1993, with Bill Styles Chair of Council, I was approached by Sally Irvine, who surprised me by asking if I would consider the Chair of the Research Network. It was most unusual for a past Chair of Council to take the chair of a committee. There was also a big obstacle as the Council had already elected a Chair of Research, Ivan Cox of Birmingham who was a hard-working, College activist, much involved in health promotion in Birmingham. However, he did not have a senior university appointment when most serious research had moved to the universities. He was not seen in the university world as a serious researcher.

Two years earlier I had had an article published in the *BMJ:* "Research in general practice: law of inverse opportunity" (DPG, 1991b). This was written from the Exeter Postgraduate Medical School, where I had learned as Director how many obstructions existed to general practice research compared with research in specialist medicine. This had made an impact in the DH. I accepted the proposed role, provided that the Council elected me democratically and that I would in no way be involved in removing Ivan Cox.

The RCGP was on the back foot, having lost a second Chair prematurely within six years. Bill Styles had a distinguished educational record but he was not a researcher. He and Sally Irvine had decided to strengthen the College's research wing. Ivan Cox came under pressure and resigned. I felt sorry for him, as he had done his best, but royal institutions have to protect their central interests. Council elected me unopposed.

GPs with MDs

Once elected, I had to identify priorities within my tiny research budget. A major weakness of general practice is its inadequate postgraduate training, which follows an inadequate undergraduate medical curriculum which, then as now, does little to teach medical students the special features and principles of general practice (Chapter 46, An Unfinished Campaign 2013–2023). Specialist medicine throughout the 20th century had a strategy of ensuring that its future leaders were properly trained, which meant doing a doctoral degree. Working for a doctorate teaches three specific skills: first how to review the literature of some subjects critically; second, how to think clearly, which is a transferable skill for life; and third, to write accurately. General practice was short of colleagues with doctorates and still is.

The early leaders of the College well understood doctorates. In my father's generation keen GPs did MDs. When I arrived in Exeter in 1962, there were three GPs in the area with an MD. John Hunt, when picking the members of the Foundation Council, chose between two Devon GPs, Mac and Laurence Jackson, both with doctorates. Mac required a doctorate amongst GPs for appointments to his early Editorial Boards. By valuing them in 1993, I followed this tradition.

DOI: 10.1201/9781032713601-35

All I could do in the Research Network was to value the acquisition of doctorates by GPs much more and encourage university departments of general practice to supervise GP colleagues in obtaining them. I did manage to identify all new ones for three years but overall I did not do very well and I was disappointed to hear several university departments tell me that there was no status and no money to be made from this activity. The wider objective of developing a profession escaped them. The notable exception was Professor George Irwin at Queen's University Belfast, who led the UK in producing a stream of GPs with MDs. Throughout my three years I valued GP MDs, wrote to many of the people who acquired them and promoted them as best I could. I am afraid I achieved little.

The RCGP Research Network had six-monthly meetings with the Medical Research Council (MRC), which were uncomfortable. They did not see general practice research as a priority. Crucially, they did not recognise general practice as a discipline but as a setting for collecting data. They relied on their GP research framework. I asked what percentage of their funds was spent on general practice and was told they did not know. I repeated the question at subsequent meetings, expressing surprise that their data processing could not answer this. Eventually, I extracted a figure of 7%, which I then argued was too low.

The MRC General Practice Research Framework was a national network of general practices in which the MRC paid nurses to gather data for their studies (The hypertension study, MRC Working Party, 1985). I had several sharp brushes with the MRC leaders in which I stated that such a framework should be developing general practice and encouraging GPs in acquiring research skills, publications and research degrees. I said that the general practices were just being used as collecting vehicles and all the publications came out in the names of specialists. The MRC leaders were irritated. They were not used to criticism. They had no answer to the point that this national network, called "the General Practice Research Framework," had never helped GPs to obtain higher degrees or to develop any research skills. No changes were made. This struggle culminated in a letter along these lines from Bill Styles, to the MRC (Chapter 25, Conference of Academy of Academic Organisations in General Practice), which annoyed the latter. Later this research framework was closed.

RCGP Research General Practices

One new idea was to develop RCGP-appointed research general practices. I wrote a paper seeking to persuade the Council to create such practices. There was opposition in the Council, as not all members wanted to spend membership money on research. However, I got the policy through the Council, with the support of the officers, on a majority vote in 1993. The College provided £20,000 (equivalent to about £53,000 in 2023) for RCGP research practices. The College advertised for four RCGP research general practices each to receive £5,000 a year. This was a pitifully small sum, but I hoped it would be enough to give encouragement to some practices, which might be able to use this title to attract other funds (DPG, 1995b; 1996a).

I chaired the selection committee and we got enough applications to make four good appointments starting in 1994. One was to Jim Cox, a rural GP from Cumbria and a leading member of the Council, who went on to do an MD. Another was to a practice in Honiton in East Devon, led by David Seamark, whom I knew, and who already had a PhD. The research general practices succeeded, and given the tiny investment generated worthwhile returns. The Honiton practice continued to produce publications in peer-reviewed medical journals for 20 years.

Another contribution made by the RCGP practices, however, was in offering a working model to the NHS just when there was an awareness that more needed to be done to help research in general practice. Most dramatically in the South Western region, the new Regional Director of NHS Research and Development was David Mant, who had been an academic GP at Southampton and whom I had met several times. He was later Professor of General Practice at Oxford. As Research Director for the Southwestern region, he teamed with me as the Regional Adviser in General Practice, allocating £1 million in one region for NHS research general practices. He made the practice funding £15,000 a year, which was much more appropriate. We agreed measurable criteria. After advertisements, we appointed about 1% of general practices in the region.

Simultaneously in every NHS region primary care networks were established, on a multidisciplinary basis, to foster staff in primary and community settings, to support research, to build capacity and to learn research skills (Chapter 14, Regional Adviser story). This collaboration between a regional research director and a regional GP education director was unusual and had other benefits. Led by David Mant, we were able to take a regional overview of general practice and map the undergraduate teaching practices, the postgraduate training practices and the research general practices (Gray S *et al.*, 2000). We found that 56% of 1,031 general practices were involved and 15% did both research and teaching.

Four National Committees

The 1990s were the time when the DH and national research institutions at last tried to do something serious about academic general practice, especially research opportunities. Four national committees were established in that decade, and I was invited to serve in some way on all four. Sometimes I represented the Institute of General Practice or the Postgraduate Medical School at Exeter, and at other times was the RCGP Chair of Research. I was not the leader in any of them but I was the only British GP involved with all of them.

The first, the Culyer Committee, was examining the way the NHS handled research funds, particularly in district general hospitals which excluded access for general practitioners (just GPs). Tony Culyer (1942–) was an Exeter graduate and economics lecturer before moving to York where he became an expert health economist. I was not on the main committee but on one of the subgroups, where my sole objective was to open access to these funds to GPs. The Culyer Task Force (1994) recommended the opening of NHS research funding to GPs.

The second committee was a working group within the DH, chaired by Diana Walford (1944–), who later became NHS Medical Director. We had met when she had inspected the Exeter Department of General Practice. Her objective was to reform the so-called Special Increment for Teaching (SIFT), which was a huge sum of NHS money paid to the university medical schools as compensation for the cost of teaching medical students. Funding then for general practice teaching was excluded (just GPs). John Howie, the GP Professor at Edinburgh, was campaigning for reform of the equivalent body, Scotland (Addition for Clinical Teaching, ACT). He wrote good papers and made substantial achievements. I spoke little in this group, and Diana Walford used me to respond to those trying to keep the money for specialist use. Her group contributed to a report: *SIFT into the Future* (Winyard Report, 1995). SIFT was reformed and at last made available to support general practice teaching.

Third, the Medical Research Council reviewed general practice research: a "topic review£". This followed skilled footwork by GP leaders, particularly Nigel Stott (Cardiff) and John Howie (Edinburgh). I played a back-bench role. The final report was very satisfactory for general practice (Medical Research Council, 1997).

The fourth national committee was the Department of Health's review of research in general practice/primary care. I was one of six GPs among 18 members. This was skilfully chaired by David Mant. I contributed more here as I was an unusual member in being a research professor in the University of Exeter and simultaneously a Regional Director of General Practice Education for the Southwestern region. Of the 30 references in the report I wrote seven. David Mant steered the group well to produce a helpful report (Mant Committee, 1997).

House of Lords Select Committee on Science and Technology Session 1994–1995

A Select Committee of the House of Lords was taking evidence. I drafted a paper of about 100 pages as draft evidence from the RCGP. When this came to the Council it was a knockout blow. Few if any committee papers in Council were as long or so fully referenced. It was endorsed unanimously. Godfrey Fowler, the GP Reader at Oxford, was effusive in praise, as the document called specifically for chairs of general practice in both Oxford and Cambridge. The House of Lords almost inevitably decided to take verbal evidence from the RCGP. As Chair of Research, I chose the RCGP team: Bill Styles, Chair of Council and Professor Roger Jones, Head of the Society for Academic Primary Care (then the Association of University Teachers of General Practice) to show solidarity between the GP academic bodies. I invited two young academic GPs so that we could demonstrate that we had able juniors and to give the two political experience which young GPs lack so much. I invited Andrew Farmer from the University of Oxford and Kieran Sweeney from the University of Exeter and our practice. I led this team of five in giving face-to-face evidence in the House of Lords on 24 January 1995.

Professor Sir Keith Peters of the University of Cambridge, was the adviser to the Select Committee and sat beside the Chair (Lord Walton) supplying difficult questions! We made our case for research in general practice. Peters whispered to the Chair, who asked us if there was any general practice research, which was of real importance?! I offered Beale and Nethercott (1988a, b), who had shown that local unemployment led to increased morbidity. The House of Lords published the College's evidence (15 pages) with all the questions and answers (14 pages). It reads like a manifesto of general practice (Select Committee on Science and Technology, 1995). Years later, both Andrew Farmer and Kieran Sweeney were appointed professors. Involving able young members to give them experience was then common in the College. More recently, the RCGP tends to send administrative staff to meetings which I believe is less appropriate: Outsiders need to meet able young GPs who themselves need experience of representation and reporting.

Professors of General Practice at Oxford and Cambridge

In the 1990s, I received an appeal for funds from Cambridge. I scribbled a protest on a postcard saying that I was not prepared to give a penny to Cambridge when it did not have a professor of general practice, whereas the University of Exeter had had one for several years. Surprisingly, a senior University figure replied. This ended with me donating a book prize for the Cambridge GP Department.

The RCGP had to take a national overview. The serious deficiency was the absence of chairs of general practice in both Oxford and Cambridge. This was a status problem; if the two best universities in the UK did not recognise general practice at professorial level it had not made the academic grade. However, colleagues saw no chance of effective action. I was repeatedly reminded that these were independent universities and the most powerful in the land. However, I had had experience in the South West where service GPs, combining together, forced the University of Bristol to establish a department of general practice it did not want as I describe in Chapter 15, South West General Practice Trust story.

At Oxford, Godfrey Fowler (1931–2022) was subjected to some patronising comments about GP professors "diluting the Oxford professoriate!" (Just GPs, Fowler, letter to me, unpublished). I wrote a reference for him for a chair, an important way the RCGP could help. His Chair was confirmed in 1996 during my time in the Research Committee. He was the first GP Professor at Oxford.

To put pressure on Cambridge, Bill Styles skilfully, got Sir Keith Peters (1938–), the Regius Professor of Physic at Cambridge (Dean), to dinner with the Director of Public Health for East Anglia. It was a good dinner and the key moment occurred over coffee. Sir Keith spoke directly to me. I was surprised as Bill was host and in the chair but Sir Keith had identified me as the ringleader. He said:

"There isn't a GP in England fit to hold a chair at Cambridge!" (Just GPs). I had to confront him. We were both Trustees of the Nuffield Trust, where we were having a vigorous debate about medical generalists and he was outrageously claiming he was one. "Not true!" I said, "the tide is running for general practice, the broadest branch of clinical medicine, with the longest relationships with patients, and GPs are the only doctors embedded in communities." Within a year, Ann-Louise Kinmonth was the first ever GP Chair at Cambridge. Sir Keith refused to pay for her post from university funds ("Just a GP"), persuading the NHS to fund the post.

The twin peaks, the GP chairs at Oxford and Cambridge, were both conquered within a year of each other. There were, of course, many different pressures that led to them to appoint professors of general practice in the mid-1990s, but I like to think that the Research Network of the RCGP helped those processes. And it was a special pleasure seeing both happen during my term of office.

The College always held a symposium with the AGM and in 1995 I was able to get this devoted to research in general practice. It went well with high morale.

RCGP Research Paper of the Year

Ruminating about how the Research Network could make a national impact in general practice research, at no cost, I had the idea of the Division offering a national award for the best general practice research publication of the year. This was a new idea and the College staff took it up well. Boots sponsored the award funding an annual dinner for 30 people at Princes Gate, when the prize was awarded. The Research Network invited GP leaders and others so these dinners gave me a chance to promote GP research. The RCGP Research Paper of the Year has developed, now with several variants and is going strong 28 years later.

Developing GP Research

As a GP, Alan Dean invented and developed the VAMP GP recording system so well that it became a national vehicle for data about general practice. He later sold it to the DH. Our practice was using VAMP so I knew its potential for research in general practice. During this chairmanship I met the DH, which now owned the system, and tried hard to gain access to this database for the College. The licence fee was about £500, which was not in the research budget. I tried to persuade the DH that as the College was a charity and the leading Royal College in the field, it should make the database available to RCGP researchers. I was refused, and a great chance was lost. This decision in the mid-1990s marked an increasing concern within the DH about money. So I lost another objective.

The national Research Assessment Exercise (RAE) was introduced to assess research quality in British universities. I got the RCGP to nominate Philip Hannaford and he was appointed to one judging panel.

Bill Styles generously invited me to interesting meals. One lunch with the Prince of Wales at Kensington Palace was very pleasant. Another was dinner with Sir John Laws (1945–2020), a high court (later appeal court) judge. He was charming and spoke about the role of the judiciary, introducing me to "judicial activism." The *Annual Report of the Council* 1995/1996 included five pages reporting the work of the Research Network (*RCGP Members' Reference Book,* 1996).

In 1996 I sought a successor. Among members of Council, Yvonne Carter met all the criteria, but she was hesitant. Fortunately, I was able to persuade her. She became one of the most successful RCGP Chairs of Research, developing masterclasses and excellent booklets on how to do research. She became the first female GP Dean of a Medical School at Warwick and was appointed CBE. I thought she might become Britain's first GP Vice-Chancellor. However, she sadly died in office of breast cancer aged only 50 (1959–2009). Later, I spoke at the naming of the Yvonne Carter building at Bart's, London, where she held her first Chair and where I had introduced her inaugural professorial lecture.

29

Chairmanship of the JCPTGP 1994–1997

The plane of general practice training flies on two wings: the RCGP has set the direction and the GMSC has controlled the pace.

Pereira Gray D (1980a) Gale Memorial Lecture
Journal of the Royal College of General Practitioners

The Joint Committee on Postgraduate Training for General Practice (JCPTGP) was established in 1976 and was recognised by the Secretary of State for Health and Social Security as the governing body for vocational training in UK general practice. It was established when mandatory vocational training was in sight, as it was set up the year before the 1977 *National Health Service Act*. It later became the official UK 'Competent Authority' for general practice training in Europe.

The constitution provided for two 'parent bodies': six places plus a GP trainee nominated by the RCGP and six places plus a trainee nominated by the GP Committee of the BMA. There were three officers: a Chair whose term was three years, with the post rotating alternately between the RCGP and the GMSC; and two Joint Secretaries, one nominated by each parent body. This structure was designed to give control to the two parent bodies.

It had wide representation, which included three places for the Joint Consultants Committee (reflecting its power in the 1970s), a representative of the Postgraduate Medical Deans, the Regional Advisers in General Practice, the University Teachers of General Practice, and the National Association of Clinical Tutors. There were (non-voting) observers from the DH, the Scottish Home and Health Department, the Northern Ireland Council for Postgraduate Medical Education, and the Scottish Council for Postgraduate Medical Education.

In 1976, the College was not yet strong enough to be the controlling body in the way the specialist medical Royal Colleges were. It still had fewer than half the UK GPs as members but more important were the residual anti-RCGP attitudes in the Conference of LMCs. Speakers at that Conference could still get applause by criticising the College. The situation was gradually improving from the College's perspective as more and more GPs passed the MRCGP and grew up proud of the College and their qualification rather than feeling outside it.

In the final compromise to establishing the JCPTGP, both the RCGP and the GMSC made concessions. The RCGP surrendered its control of vocational training via the College's Vocational Training Committee, which then assessed vocational training schemes. The GMSC gave up its LMC control of GP trainers. Equal representation was disputed but finally agreed.

As the College had invented vocational training for general practice and had campaigned for it (CGP, 1965), it took special interest in the JCPTGP. Each year it elected its strongest educational team, always including its Chair of Council, Secretary of Council and Chairman of Education. In addition, it often elected its Secretary of Council as one of the two Secretaries of the JCPTGP: Donald Irvine, John Hasler and Bill Styles all served like this. The JCPTGP was situated in the basement of 14 Princes Gate, then the headquarters of the RCGP.

I first became a member of the JCPTGP in 1981, elected by the College Council as one of its six representatives, every one of whom was a regional adviser. The team included five who would in time

DOI: 10.1201/9781032713601-36

be elected to Chair the College Council and four who would be elected President. Joining the College team for the first time meant serving alongside Sir James Cameron, who was one of the GMSC representatives, a political giant of general practice whom I had got to know in the BMA (LMC and BMA story). John Chisholm was the GP trainee representative. The 1981 elections also illustrated the influence the Exeter Department of General Practice had acquired, as the RCGP trainee representative was Clare Ronalds, and Bob Jones was a deputy member of the GMSC. Bob never deputised, which denied us the unusual pleasure of serving together and representing two parent bodies at once.

The staff was headed by Hilla Gittins. She had previously been a member of the College staff and technically remained so, but she was in effect leading in a separate organisation. Her title, Administrative Secretary, was chosen to match the equivalent title of the Head of the College staff. She had years of valuable experience. She understood the subtle relationship between the two parent bodies and the nuances of the Vocational Training Regulations, which governed the work of the JCPTGP. I always listened to her very carefully indeed.

The staffing was lean and mean. One staff member handled up to 2,000 applications a year for certificates of satisfactory completion of vocational training. The other staff member ran the visiting (inspection) programme in which the JCPTGP visited every region to assess vocational training. I met Catherine Messent there. She stayed with the College and later gave me support in the Awards and Heritage Committee. There was also a Secretary who supported the Chair. An informal arrangement evolved whereby the GMSC-nominated Secretary led on the certificates and the RCGP-nominated Secretary led on professional standards and the visits.

As to how the JCPTGP worked, in my Gale lecture I used the metaphor of an aeroplane: "The plane of general practice training flies with two wings. The RCGP has set the direction and the GMSC has controlled the pace" (DPG, 1980a). Now, 14 years later, I was able to see if that analysis was correct.

Chairmanship 1994

The Chair was due to change in May 1994, after a three-year term held by Idris Humphreys, a GP from Wales, and the GMSC's educational lead. The decision who to choose as the College's nominee for the Chair lay with the Council of the College, usually voting on the advice of its officers. The three criteria for JCPTGP Chairmanship in the College were: being a regional adviser (hence familiar with and responsible for vocational training for general practice in a UK region), substantial experience of membership of the JCPTGP, and, in practice, also having previously been the Chair of the College Council.

In November 1993, Bill Styles was elected Chair of the College Council. Soon afterwards we spoke about the Chairmanship of the JCPTGP. There had then been three previous College-nominated Chairmen: John Lawson, Alastair Donald and Donald Irvine. All three had been regional advisers and all three had been previous Chairs of the Council. By 1993, I had been a regional adviser for 18 years, a member of the JCPTGP for 12 years, and I was the only available former Chair of the College Council. It was inevitable that the College officers would nominate me. The Council duly elected me as the RCGP choice as the next Chairman. The GMSC was informed and in the first four months of 1994 I went to the JCPTGP offices to meet the staff and learn how it all worked.

In May 1994, it was the College's turn to hold the Chair, so I was formally elected by the members of the JCPTGP unopposed as Chairman for a three-year term. I was exceptionally fortunate with the two Secretaries who were also elected. These, throughout my three years, were Justin Allen (RCGP nominated) and Malcom Freeth (GMSC nominated). Justin was an associate adviser in general practice (later a regional adviser) and was a great supporter. He also undertook important educational research on simulated surgeries (Allen *et al.,* 1998). Malcom Freeth was hardworking and scrupulously loyal to the JCPTGP and to me.

The background to what was to be my central agenda in the JCPTGP was that an assessment working party had prioritised the development of assessment. However, the view of my GMSC predecessor was illustrated by a press report in September 1992. Idris Humphreys, was reported in *Pulse* saying that "He doubted if a major change was needed…to weed out a relatively small number of incompetent would-be GPs." This was a classic trade union-type statement, taking no account of the interests of patients. No plans existed to change anything.

The idea of continuing to allow a group of doctors who were incompetent to have unsupervised responsibility for about 1500 patients each in general practice was absurd, but the constitutional structure of the JCPTGP allowed the GMSC a blocking vote. All would depend on the next College-nominated Chair.

Summative Assessment of Vocational Training

I had six months' notice of this chairmanship, unlike the Council chairmanship, so I had proper time to think out priorities. I discussed ideas and possibilities with educational leaders and activists. The big issue in educational and political terms, was the endpoint assessment of vocational training; in other words to define the credibility of the system which decided whether a doctor had satisfactorily completed training and was fit to work as an unsupervised GP. The three Chair letter (Irvine *et al.*, 1990), which I had co-authored, had stated that vocational training meant achieving 'satisfactory competence' and the JCPTGP in 1993 the year before I took the Chair had agreed that an endpoint assessment, independent of the training practice, was needed.

The legal requirement was merely getting a certificate of satisfactory training from any approved general practitioner trainer in the UK. Most trainees chose to take the RCGP examination, the MRCGP, voluntarily, which admitted them as members of the College.

However, this left two problems. Firstly, how competent or safe were those trainees who failed the MRCGP? Secondly, what were the competencies of doctors who never took the examination? Much was known about such trainees through the deaneries in the regions. In the Southwestern region, we had been promoting the MRCGP, systematically telling trainees, even before they were appointed, that all trainees were expected to take and pass the MRCGP. In our deanery's view, the MRCGP was the national external endpoint assessment of vocational training.

We had observed that whilst most trainees did indeed take the MRCGP, there was a small group who declined to take it. It was voluntary and there was no way then of making them take it. The advisers and associate advisers often analysed these doctors and over the years we found that one group of them comprised overseas nationals who saw no point in the MRCGP if they were going to practise in another country, often Ireland. By and large, however, we concluded that the non-takers were weaker clinically, ill, or lazy. Meanwhile, they virtually all got a statement of satisfactory completion from their GP trainer. The RCGP (1985a) *Quality in Practice* document had noted, coldly, that of 7,000 applications by trainees for approval of prescribed training experience only 0.2% were refused. There was no quality check in the system apart from the MRCGP, which was voluntary. Patients were not being protected against incompetent doctors.

There was some other evidence, including a double tragedy when a newly certified GP with a brand new JCPTGP certificate had seriously mishandled a patient with diabetes. The patient died, and the young doctor was struck off the *Medical Register* by the GMC. This doctor had not taken the MRCGP. In a formal enquiry, the trainer said he thought the young doctor was not very good, but just OK. The regional adviser had no quality assurance systems, so the single trainer's signature was enough. A national patient safety problem was revealed.

I concluded that the top priority for both patients and trainees was to introduce a system that actually checked the competence of every single trainee and stopped them practising if they were incompetent. I hoped the JCPTGP would be able to enforce this and it was clear it was the only body in the UK which could.

Professional standards exist at three levels: the minimum acceptable standard, the usual or average standard, and the excellent standard. The need in the JCPTGP was to introduce a minimum standard.

This was the opposite of my aim five years earlier when I had been Chair of the College. Then I had gone for Fellowship by Assessment as the highest achievable standard of general practice.

Standards are described as 'summative' (pass/fail) if they come at the end of a course of training and if failure has bad consequences for the candidate. Examples are GCSEs, A levels, and university degrees, including medical finals, which are all summative. Formative assessment is by contrast not a high stakes process for the learner and information and advice is fed back to the learner for the learner's benefit. I took a plan to establish summative assessment to the other two officers and the Committee and we agreed we would make summative assessment of UK vocational training the top priority for my three-year term of office.

A National Endpoint Assessment

At first, the problem did not seem too big. Most trainees were taking the MRCGP, so if this could be recognised by the JCPTGP as a satisfactory endpoint assessment, everything would be relatively simple. Numbers remaining would then be relatively small, about 15%, and it would not be particularly expensive.

I talked privately to the GMSC leaders, who were members of the JCPTGP. The message was clear. They would not accept the MRCGP as the national endpoint assessment of vocational training nor was this just the view of one or two of their team. Their feeling was that their Conference [of LMCs] would not wear it. I brought the question to the full Committee and the GMSC team confirmed their view 'in public.' This confirmed my analysis in the Gale lecture (DPG, 1980a) that in the JCPTGP the RCGP did set the direction and the GMSC did control the pace.

This was a disappointment but not a surprise. But it was bad news for patients and general practice. As most trainees were already taking the MRCGP, this examination was *de facto* the majority national standard. Adopting it would have brought general practice closer to the systems in the other specialties in the medical profession, although even then the MRCP was an entrance ticket *into* medical training. The point was that all the specialist medical Royal Colleges had evolved a system whereby every future consultant had to pass a Royal College examination testing each individual doctor and eliminating the incompetent.

Using the MRCGP would have made use of an examination then 29 years old and well honed. The rejection looked at first like a body blow as the JCPTGP was not constituted to develop a new endpoint assessment and the College saw nothing to gain from it. However, the GMSC, having shot down the MRCGP, did agree with me to accept an alternative national assessment system if it could be shown to be effective and fair. They made no trouble as this slowly emerged.

The new problem was how to develop and administer a national system. The JCPTGP and the profession were saved by the Regional Adviser in General Practice in the West of Scotland, Professor Stuart Murray. He was one of the more academic regional advisers (with a PhD and MD) in the UK and he was one of the few who did high-quality research with articles published in good journals. He had built up an educational research team, wrote extensively on medical education and he had an interest in developing a new minimum assessment system. I was fortunate that during my chairmanship he was Chair of the UK Regional Advisers.

Stuart Murray was himself a member of the JCPTGP, so he was well informed. The Committee encouraged him, and I particularly encouraged him to publish his results. It was obvious the JCPTGP could not adopt any system which was not in the public domain and valid. Murray and the Glasgow team steamed ahead. A steady flow of articles was published. It was not long before a four-part package emerged: a multiple-choice test of knowledge, a skills test, an analysis of a set of real videoed consultations with patients, and an audit. These were progressively refined by testing on trainees.

A second major management problem was how to roll out any agreed system across the UK. Here the College, to my regret, was not interested and indeed I was getting some flak from colleagues in the College for setting up an alternative national system of GP assessment. Two fears were expressed to me. First, if trainees were offered a free assessment system at the end of their training, perhaps they would not then take the MRCGP examination, which was much more difficult and for which they had to pay substantially. Second, there were several in the College who thought that if summative assessment was made compulsory then trainees would not take two assessments. I found it ironic to be accused inside the College of rocking the College boat. I assured my college colleagues that trainees were generally good and would want to have a proper professional qualification. I thought the MRCGP was safe. I emphasised how the summative assessment would only be a test of *minimum competence*. GP trainees were mixing and sharing junior hospital posts with junior specialists who all sought Royal College memberships. These memberships were the professional norm and gave them letters after their name of which they were proud.

The solution to the problem of managing a national system of assessment lay with the Conference of Regional Advisers. Here it was important that I was present as a regional adviser in my own right. These meetings were held regularly and separately from the JCPTGP.

The Conference had to decide where it stood. It came good. There was acceptance of the importance of the principle that the regional advisers were responsible for vocational training for general practice in each NHS region. More importantly, the Conference accepted the role of managing a national endpoint assessment once the JCPTGP introduced it, even though it was obviously going to mean a great deal of work. David Percy, Regional Adviser for the Wessex region, was elected to take on the national co-ordinating role, which suited his management skills. He went on to do an excellent national job and made the system work UK-wide during my time (Conference of Postgraduate Advisers in General Practice, 1995).

During my three years as Chair, there were a whole series of educational publications documenting and evaluating an emerging system of summative assessment of vocational training. The great majority of the publications came from the West of Scotland's Department of Postgraduate Education, where Stuart Murray was well supported by a team of colleagues including LM Campbell and Murray Lough, as well as by his Postgraduate Medical Dean, Norman McKay, who co-authored some papers. Other centres contributed, like Oxford and Leicester. The theoretical and political importance of the West of Scotland was immense. I was very conscious that to introduce a UK-wide national system of assessment for doctors at any stage of their careers, the system needed to be well documented and tested in the field. The probability of complaints by those who would inevitably fail was high in my mind and, worse, the possibility of judicial review if the processes were not seen to be fair by a judge. Judicial review is essentially a review of process. Judges do not seek to usurp the decision-taking process rather they ensure that the processes are reasonable, clear, transparent and fair. We were an administrative body taking decisions, which would be detrimental to doctors who fell foul of them. I was constantly thinking of judicial review if our methods were not fire-proof.

The series of publications on vocational training from Glasgow (Campbell *et al.*, 1993a; Campbell *et al.*,1995; Campbell and Murray, 1996; Campbell *et al.*, 1996; and a doctoral thesis, Campbell, 1996; Lough *et al.*, 1995a–c; Lough and Murray, 1997.) Stuart Murray co-authored nine of these publications. Their importance was three-fold. They described the process of summative assessment in public and quantified several issues. They formally evaluated, with real GP trainees, the different components proposed. The Oxford region, led by John Hasler, undertook the challenge of systematising the GP trainer's report and did it well (Johnson et al., 1996a,b; Johnson and Hasler, 1997). All these articles were published in good journals like the *BMJ, BJGP*, and *Medical Education*. The dates of publication were critical, 12 of them coming out in my chairmanship. Perhaps never before had a professional medical examination been developed so academically. I watched with pleasure as they all came together into a substantial body of knowledge.

It was a failure of the civil honours system in Scotland that Stuart Murray, who led this team, never received a civil honour, which he much deserved. The West of Scotland built most of the bullets; the JCPTGP fired the gun.

Amongst the previously unknown facts one question stood out. How many GP trainees at the end of their trainee year were incompetent as defined? The whole rationale of summative assessment was that there would be some, but there were big problems if the numbers were very high, and the system might look ridiculous if the number was very small. All we knew was that the failure rate in the MRCGP was then around 15%.

As well, there was a big NHS problem emerging. Assuming summative assessment became compulsory – given the vocational training regulations a doctor who failed would not be allowed by law to work unsupervised in general practice as a principal (partner) in a salaried post, or as a locum – only work under supervision as a trainee would be possible. Furthermore, vocational training posts were limited to 12 months at that time. Where would the failed doctors go, and would the NHS pay their salaries?

These discussions could only begin once we knew the expected figure and it was the West of Scotland group which first produced the failure answer, namely 4–5% This was good news. It was not going to be too frightening for trainees and such numbers were manageable. In the JCPTGP we immediately examined the legal basis of what we decided to call 'remedial training' for a further 6–12 months. We alerted the DH to the probable extra costs, and it reluctantly accepted it would have to pay for extended training for the failures, essentially an additional six months in a training general practice.

Simultaneously, we initiated discussions with the regional advisers through their conference, and individually alerted them to the need to start planning remedial training. Some problems like persuading trainers to take doctors known to be weak, were difficult. If an incompetent trainee damaged a patient, the trainer was at great risk as the trainer, as supervisor, could face an NHS complaint.

Higher Training for Highflyers

I lobbied the DH that, in addition to funding the small number of extended training posts for those trainees who failed summative assessment, it should simultaneously fund some posts for highflyers in general practice. I said that general practice training was too short anyway, and much too short for future leaders in general practice. The same DH was funding several years of postgraduate training in the medical specialties, some as long as seven years.

This request revealed the lack of concern about the development of general practice in the DH at that time and I got nowhere with my requests. The DH did not yet realise that general practice is as important, and in many ways more important, than many hospital specialties. There was one rule (many years of postgraduate training for specialists) and quite another for generalists (just GPs).

Teamwork

Of the JCPTGP officers, I was a full regional adviser and Justin Allen was an associate adviser, so we had two different regions where we could explore practical issues.

With legal, academic, professional, and financial issues involved, this was a time for teamwork and good communication amongst the key players. I was exceptionally fortunate that all the key players were together on the JCPTGP at the same time in those critical years of 1994–97. Stuart Murray was elected by the regional advisers, Jackie Hayden, the first GP to be appointed a Postgraduate Medical Dean, was elected from the College Council, and the Oxford region was also represented through John Toby, elected by the College. All the areas generating the main research on summative assessment were there. The College was led by its Chair, Bill Styles, a strong educationalist, a leading regional adviser, and a William Pickles lecturer. He held a briefing meeting over dinner in the College the night before every JCPTGP meeting, which Justin and I attended. Sadly, Bill Styles developed cancer and became increasingly incapacitated during 1995 eventually being forced to resign his chairmanship of the Council. The Council elected John Toby to succeed him and as he too was already on the JCPTGP he then chaired the pre-JCPTGP College meetings.

The significance was that general practice had got its act together. In the early 1960s it had, through the College, created the MRCGP and lobbied successfully for vocational training. Now, 30 years later, the general practice educational leaders were all working together again to close the hole in the training system, which for years had been allowing one in 20 incompetent trainees to have unsupervised responsibility for patients. I gave many talks to colleagues and trainers and often used the metaphor that "the bucket of general practice training has a hole in it and we are leaking credibility."

I kept reiterating that all the other branches of medicine had had individual medical assessment of their trainees for years and we were late to catch up. Secondly, I said what I had long believed, that one bad GP could attract more publicity than 500 good GPs doing a good job. I gave as an example the new, JCPTGP-approved doctor who had been struck off by the GMC.

This time round, the College could not lead by itself as it had no authority over doctors who were not members. The College, unlike the specialist Colleges, had no locus over weak trainees. The leadership had to be through the JCPTGP, which alone could make a minimum assessment compulsory with legal backing. Of course, all the educational writers and researchers like Stuart Murray, Jackie Hayden, and Neil Johnson were College fellows, as were Justin and I. The JCPTGP at that time was in effect the executive arm of the College.

1995

There were important developments in 1995. In the General Medical Council Donald Irvine, Chairman of the GMC Standards Committee, piloted a new document, *Good Medical Practice,* through the GMC. This was radical. It tore up the old 'blue book,' which was what the GMC had previously issued setting out what doctors should *not* do. Now *Good Medical Practice* set out a list of new patient-centred principles (GMC, 1995; GMC story). As I had been elected to the GMC by the registered medical practitioners in England in 1994, I was fully briefed there and voted for it at the GMC meeting when it was adopted. This development gave a big boost to transparency in medical practice and education.

The same year there was the Medical (Professional Performance) Act which empowered the GMC to assess the performance of doctors – a big development which was in step with our work on measuring trainees' performance.

During the long series of discussions at one point a block occurred as the BMA leaders told me they could not get agreement. We needed a decision by the date of a JCPTGP meeting. With an impasse threatening I called a 'summit' meeting of all the national GP chairs in a private room. Dates and places were very difficult to arrange, and the final extraordinary solution was to meet in a hotel room at Heathrow airport, late in the evening before the Committee met next day. The advantage was that we had the regional advisers and non-RCGP/BMA members present. The RCGP trainee representative was Alex Harding from my own Exeter practice, who later became a partner in the Practice, a University of Exeter sub dean and a co-Chair of the GP undergraduate teachers (HOTS). This was a special one-off meeting, which I had called as JCPTGP Chair, and everyone expected me to chair it. However, I had one more trick up my sleeve, and just before the meeting started, I offered John Chisholm, the BMA leader, the Chair. He was surprised but accepted. This was a logical move, as my soundings beforehand had suggested that Chisholm wanted a deal, and I hoped that the resisting BMA members would be more reassured by the arguments from the wider group if one of their own was in the chair. Chisholm chaired a complex meeting well securing agreement at last, although it took until midnight to do so.

It seemed settled, but when I was chairing the formal JCPTGP meeting the next morning trouble arose. The agenda item, after the previous night's agreement, ought to have received routine approval. Instead, to my horror, the BMA team split in public and had a sharp policy disagreement, arguing vigorously against each other in full Committee. I realised that the BMA had some representatives present, including a negotiator, who had missed the summit. I waited and waited for John Chisholm and Brian Keighley to prevail, but they could not as the dissenting minority dug in. We had a large majority in the JCPTGP and could have voted it through, but I was unsure of the price the BMA would pay.

With the Committee clearly stuck, I suddenly banged the gavel and announced that the Committee would adjourn to give the BMA team a chance to meet alone and to regroup in private. This they did and 20 minutes later I was informed they were ready to return. The agenda item was approved immediately and unanimously! Brian Keighley was generous in thanking me on behalf of the BMA.

Multi-Chairmen Letters to Ministers

The multiplicity of general practice organisations was a potential weakness. I tried to counter this. I drafted a letter to the Secretary of State in November 1994 seeking 50% training for part-time GP trainees instead of the proposed 60%. My signature was joined by those of the Chairs of the RCGP, GMSC, and regional advisers. This formula worked so well that I engineered a letter signed by ten different GPs who were national chairs which we sent to the Secretary of State in 1996 calling for new training regulations (Pereira Gray *et al.,* 1994).

Summative Assessment of Vocational Training

The JCPTGP was progressing well towards making training compulsory in 1995, but the timing of the final date for implementation was exquisitely sensitive. It was important not to rush too soon or to hang back too long. We had to be clear and consistent and allow proper time for the trainees to plan for it.

The package was to be in four parts: a test of factual knowledge, a multiple-choice questionnaire; a test of communication skills with an assessment of a set of videoed consultations with real patients; a test of thinking and writing skills, a research project or more commonly an audit; and lastly, the longstanding signing by the approved trainer was extended to become a structured trainers' report. This package was validated by the research articles, do-able in practice in the regions, and had face validity with both trainers and trainees. There were, of course, concerns that trainers and/or trainees would be put off. An MSc dissertation in the Exeter Institute of General Practice showed that trainers, at least in the Southwest, were not bothered (Grieg D; personal communication).

The College, led by Bill Styles as Chair, having been equivocal about the introduction of summative assessment, moved to recognise it by proposing that some sections of the MRCGP should give exemption from the knowledge test in summative assessment. Moreover, exposed by the absence of an assessment of the trainees' consultations by video in the MRCGP, it introduced videos too.

In August 1995, a good discussion in the Committee led to the adoption of the policy of 'professionally led assessment.' This was a big step. It answered objections from some trainees that there were no regulations requiring them to take summative assessment. It enhanced the profession. It meant a trainee bucking the system could not be sure of getting a reference or even a post. It was a good narrative, and it empowered the profession when encountering difficulties.

After aiming for 1 January 1996, the Committee agreed to a date for implementation of 4 September 1996, for reasons set out in my second position paper (JCPTGP, 1996b). A *BMJ* editorial in September 1996, announcing summative assessment that month, was quite negative but it did make two strong points that a newly qualified trainee had been incompetent and that only 16 GP trainees out of 6,200 completing between 1990–1995 had not obtained a Certificate of Satisfactory Completion of Training from their GP trainer (Carnell, 1996).

September 1995 was a key month. The Minister of Health (Gerald Malone) wrote to me confirming support for the principle of summative assessment but ruling out a change to the regulations in 1996. That same month, the three JCPTGP officers with the Chairs of the RCGP, GMSC, and the regional advisers met the Medical Director (Graham Winyard) and colleagues from the NHS Executive to discuss costs and the changes to the regulations.

In the final run-down, to my concern, I was taken aside by the representative of the Department of Health and told summative assessment could not go ahead as the Department had not agreed to it!

He said it needed parliamentary regulations. As a representative of the DH, he had attended all meetings of the JCPTGP as an observer and he had witnessed every step along the way. I said I well understood it needed regulations, but they were not complicated. The civil servant then leant on me hard by saying that I would be exposed if I went ahead without his say so. Suddenly, I was facing one of the big professional decisions of my life. He was right that I was very exposed. The decisions on summative assessment had been widely promulgated. If I delayed, for whatever the reason, I would as Chair, lose face. Moreover, knowing how slowly government departments move, there was no guarantee how long it would take for the DH to draft the regulations. I was, however, greatly empowered by the huge commitment from GP colleagues across the UK and in particular by the JCPTGP's decision to introduce summative assessment on the basis of it being 'professionally led.'

I judged that if we went ahead the political pressure on the DH would force it to deliver the regulations and I owed much to the big team of professional colleagues who had worked so hard to prepare for summative assessment. "Too late!" I said, "If you had any doubts you should have spoken much earlier." "You're exposed," he repeated. "Yes," I said, "I understand that – but I'm not as exposed as the Secretary of State for Health." What do you mean?" he said. "Well won't it be a tad difficult for him to debate with me on television that he wants incompetent doctors to see patients?" The Department of Health then quickly introduced regulations to underpin it. The hole in the educational bucket of general practice, which had existed since 1948, was closed at last.

During my term, there was full consultation on adopting formal standing orders, which were agreed unanimously.

European Directive – Acquired Rights

In the mid-1990s, a European Council Medical Directive (1995) came into UK law. The background was that the continental countries had been catching up with general practice training. Strong lobbying by the academic GP bodies and the political general practice body (UEMO) had led the European Union to adopt compulsory general practice training, as the UK had done in 1982. This was good news as it stopped doctors without any training entering general practice.

However, the requirement then was minimal: only two years in all and only six months required in general practice. The price for the UK was that any doctor completing this minimum training and certified by any national 'competent authority' in Europe had free right of access to UK general practice under the free movement of people provision. GPs who were already working in 1981 were granted an exemption from training through what came to be called the 'grandfather clause.' A second price was a provision called 'acquired rights,' which was a grandfather deal for doctors who wanted to work in general practice but had not been trained for it and who presented an assortment of previous experience. We found ourselves stuck with an interpretation that meant that even having been a locum in practice for as short a time as ten days could be enough to gain the precious acquired right, which was a ticket to work in NHS general practice for life.

Furthermore, as the JCPTGP had now been designated as the European Competent Authority for General Practice Training in the UK, it had to issue these acquired rights. This was disappointing as someone aged 30 in 1995 might continue to work in general practice until 2030. Thus, I had to preside over the issuing of these rights to doctors who were untrained and whose competence was unknown. This was a distasteful administrative role.

A Problem in Australasia

There were many ramifications of the European Directive and one affected doctors outside the EU, especially those in Australia, Canada and New Zealand. For many years, doctors in the UK had been visiting these countries, especially the latter two, or arranging exchanges in each other's practices.

Now, suddenly, whilst British GPs could continue to go abroad, those coming from outside the EU could no longer enter a UK practice, as they were not EU nationals and had not completed GP training with a certificate from an EU competent authority.

GP training in Australia and New Zealand was long-established and comparable to that in the UK. These doctors spoke English better than many EU nationals. A stream of critical letters came to the JCPTGP from doctors affected, mainly from Australian organisations. The UK Government replied it was the responsibility of the JCPTGP as the designated competent authority for the UK! More letters arrived and we stated that we had no discretion and that the UK Government had agreed the EU arrangements. The Australian High Commission then waded in.

As an internationalist who had visited both Australia and New Zealand, I was unhappy. These doctors brought ideas and energy with them, and these exchanges were educational. Could we do anything? As a compromise, the officers of the JCPTGP drafted a proposal that would allow doctors who had vocational training recognised by Australia and New Zealand to come to UK training practices under a special arrangement. The JCPTGP approved this, and we sent it to the DH, which refused it. I pressed so hard that a meeting was arranged with a (Conservative) Health Minister, Gerald Malone, the Minister of State in the Department of Health. We discussed it fully and he simply said "No." This was disappointing but did at least stop the DH blaming the JCPTGP in public.

Recording Joint Committee Policies

One of the problems the JCPTGP had was a tight budget with no funds to publish its work, so its successes were little known outside the membership. I knew that introducing summative assessment in general practice would be of historic importance and that afterwards the story would be spun to suit the perspective of the storytellers. I therefore wrote a lengthy annual report for 1995, which was formally approved by JCPTGP without comment. I was able to arrange, as Editor of the *RCGP Members' Reference Book*, for it to be published in full in the 1996 book at no cost to the JCPTGP (JCPTGP, 1996a). This ensured that the story was in the public domain permanently and also made it possible to publish as an appendix my long, second position paper (JCPTGP, 1996b), the letter to me from the Minister of Health (Malone, 1996), and the JCPTGP (1995) policy on exchange doctors. By combining my two honorary roles, full transparency was achieved. I marked the JCPTGP's achievement with an editorial (DPG, 1997b) "Summative assessment of vocational training to be required by law."

In the latter part of my chairmanship, Hilla Gittins retired after many years of skilled and loyal service. She had led the small JCPTGP staff for many years and the staff's work had long been underestimated. In 1995 alone the JCPTGP issued 3,067 certificates allowing GPs to practise and dealt with an estimated 19,225 letters and enquiries a year (JCPTGP, 1996a). The Committee gave her a retirement dinner, which let me thank her.

We advertised for a successor, and I chaired the appointment committee when Katie Carter was appointed, and I was pleased to work with her until my own retirement.

My Final Meeting of the JCPTGP

My final meeting as Chair was scheduled for May 1997, and the GMSC had elected Brian Keighley, one of their leading educationalists, to succeed me. The change-over in Chair came early in the agenda. Normally a retiring Chair just sits out the meeting, but I wanted to use the special opportunity of being a member, but not the Chair. So, I had sent in two papers (both unpublished) which I had written, so they had to go on to the agenda.

My first paper proposed that in future the Chair of the JCPTGP should be remunerated for whatever sessions they worked at the rate of an 'A' plus merit/distinction award. The background was

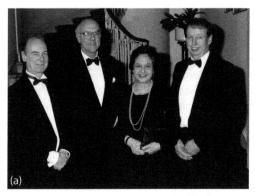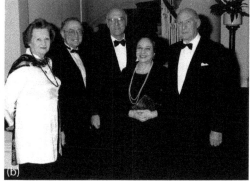

FIGURE 29.1   (a) JCPTGP dinner in 1997. Officers Malcolm Freeth and Justin Allen (Secretaries) with the author and Hilla Gittins. (b) Hilla Gittins and with four Chairs of the JCPTGP. Dorothy Ward Eddie Josse, DPG, Hilla Gittins, and John Lawson, 1997.

that regional advisers in general practice were then paid on the consultant clinical scale, without any possibility of any merit award. All GP advisers were on this scale, as I was. [I took no remuneration for being Chairman of the JCPTGP and did it as an honorary position.] I reckoned that I had enough sessions in the University of Exeter and as regional adviser for the Southwestern region, and any more sessions might have jeopardised my role as a partner in the St Leonard's Practice, my priority. On the other hand, the top group of consultants were receiving an A plus merit award, which approximately doubled their remuneration and was pensionable.

My aim in presenting this paper was to destabilise the national system, which kept GPs in academic positions in both undergraduate medicine and postgraduate medicine on pay scales much worse than specialists in the same jobs. For me, it was not so much the money, but I saw it as a significant status "just a GP" issue.

I started by saying that I had waited until I was no longer in the Chair so that there could be no question of my seeking any personal benefit. I simply made the points that the Chair of the Specialist Training Authority and the President of the General Medical Council (at the time a general practitioner) were both being paid sessions at the consultant scale with an A plus merit award. Was general practice training of lower importance than specialist training? Was it right, fair or appropriate that the Chair of our JCPTGP was paid so much less than the other two regulatory authorities in medicine?

The Committee was thrown into disarray, faced with an issue it had never considered before. The BMA GPs were discomforted: although they lived and breathed GP remuneration, they did not deal with consultant scales and merit awards where they had no locus. A consultant from the Joint Consultants' Committee objected saying that merit awards were for consultants not GPs. The DH observer, Robin Cairncross, said nothing could be done, as there was no budget for this scale. All the Committee could do was to agree to look into it.

My second paper proposed that in training practices patients should normally be offered ten-minute appointments. I had a longstanding interest as I thought the average length of consultation was a key statistic in general practice. In my 1979 Gale Memorial Lecture, I had launched the first attack on the then common five-minute consultation (DPG, 1980a). Now, 18 years later, I was having another go.

I summarised the research evidence, which by 1997 was substantial. It had started in 1986 at the Department of General Practice at St Thomas's Hospital, London, which had shown that patients received more personal preventive medicine in longer consultations (Morrell *et al.*, 1986; Roland *et al.*, 1986). Later research showed increasing benefits for patients from longer GP consultations. A systematic review concluded that longer consultations were better for patients and allowed better care, especially for psychosocial problems (Wilson and Childs, 2002). Unsurprisingly, longer consultations improved patient-doctor communication and also were found to reduce stress for GPs (Howie *et al.*, 1991).

The real punch in my argument was not just that ten-minute consultations were better for patients but that GP trainers had *volunteered* to be trainers and that they had agreed to support trainees, which included being available for interruptions during their surgeries when trainees had problems. Finally, I said that at that time, 1997, in the Southwestern region where I had detailed information, ten-minute consultations in training practices were already the norm. Academically, this was a pretty strong, evidence-based case.

The response was dramatic. The members of the GPC team on the JCPTGP, including all their top negotiators, lambasted my proposal in a carefully pre-planned assault. This was a heavyweight team, led by John Chisholm, Chair and included Laurence Buckman, who succeeded Chisholm as Chair, and Hamish Meldrum who later chaired the BMA Council. These were national union leaders in full flow. I wish it had been recorded as a dramatic incident. The arguments were shared between the GMSC team. One said the proposal was absurd as GPs needed flexibility and not bureaucratic rules. Another said the JCPTGP needed to think of GPs "in the real world" (as opposed to the Exeter ivory tower!). Another ignoring research said that in his experience ten-minute consultations were not necessary. The gentlest comment was: "The paper is very interesting, and merits thought, but it is too soon to adopt." The kiss of death!

All five speeches came in quick succession like machine-gun fire. They were followed by a stunned silence. The RCGP team had not anticipated this attack at the pre-meeting dinner. All present knew the proposal was dead in the water with such opposition from one of the parent bodies, which now held the Chair as well. Interestingly, and ominously, none of the young tigers on the RCGP team, nor any of the large number of academics, spoke. This incident revealed that in practice, not only did the GMSC "control the pace" of the work of the JCPTGP (DPG, 1980a) but that it also wielded a 'blocking vote.' The group of able academic members was not prepared to argue with the trade union. I was left completely isolated.

The new Chair, Brian Keighley, scrupulously asked if I wanted the proposer's right of reply? I said with studied understatement that I did not detect a great deal of enthusiasm for the proposal. I noted that no one had disputed the research. I was disappointed but as many training practices were already routinely providing ten-minute consultations, I was confident that ten-minute consultations for trainers would become the national standard. And that was it. The JCPTGP formally rejected my proposal.

Afterwards colleagues quizzed me why I had done it. They were not used to seeing me lose in committees and I was now their President-Elect. First, I said that in public life it is sometimes necessary to press for what is right, even if unpopular. Second, focusing on the length of consultations was much needed to stimulate further thought. Finally, I said it was good for the College to be seen on the side of patients and trainees through one of its representatives. After all, other eyes were watching, and other minds were thinking. "Other eyes and other minds?" some asked. "Yes," I said. "Leading consultants, a medical postgraduate dean and four health departments were all silent spectators."

Indeed they were. In the Academy of Medical Royal Colleges, which I rejoined as PRCGP five months later, one specialist President said: "I don't know the research you cited but it is blindingly obvious that GPs, especially GP trainers, should provide ten-minute consultations. *It makes you wonder why the BMA is there in such strength or there at all?*" (author's emphasis). A few years later the DH abolished the JCPTGP, forming the Postgraduate Medical Education and Training Board (PMETB).

The reasons for this new body were certainly not just this incident. However, in May 1997 in the JCPTGP those BMA leaders did themselves no favours. They won a battle, but they helped lose the war of BMA GP representation on national educational bodies. The General and Specialist Medical (Education and Training and Qualifications) Order passed in Parliament in October 2003 creating the PMETB (DH, 2000). All BMA GPs were removed. The RCGP Council debated consultation length and I spoke as President. A working party was formed which commissioned a review. In 2004, the Council of the College agreed that the booked duration of consultations in general practice (not just in training practices) should be ten minutes – seven years after my JCPTGP paper.

ADDENDA

In 2007, the MRCGP finally became the endpoint assessment of UK vocational training and a requirement to practise as a GP. This at last brought general practice into line with the other medical specialties. Summative assessment became redundant. Some fourth-year posts were established in general practice training, called specialist training year four (ST4) funded for six months.

In 2016, Chaand Nagpaul, Chairman of the BMA GPs, speaking at a national Conference, railed against 10-minute consultations saying they were much too short.

An article I co-authored with Peter Orton showed longer GP consultations are significantly more patient-centred (Orton and DPG, 2016).

30

Dentistry

Every tooth in a man's head is more valuable than a diamond.

De Cervantes Miguel (1547–1616) Spanish Writer

Our family was fortunate in having a very good dentist in Exeter, Wilfred Selley, whom I had met in the Round Table. He and his successor, Clive Pidgeon, Wilfred's son-in-law, were our dentists for three generations of our family. One daughter for years travelled 100 miles to see him. Good dentists go to great lengths to preserve teeth as long as is possible. Unlike most of my patients, both Jill and I valued being able to keep our teeth into our 80s and as the costs of repairs rose, even in the NHS, our teeth appeared as valuable as diamonds.

After the Exeter Department of General Practice was established, I wanted to make it more multidisciplinary by including Wilfred Selley, because he held the FDS RCSEng (a higher qualification in dentistry) and was interested in research. I proposed him at a staff meeting in the Department, but the suggestion was opposed by others. This created a leadership problem as I was proposing several initiatives at the time, and in all teams a balance has to be struck between the leader and the group. Groups only work well if all members believe they are being listened to and have a reasonable say in decisions. I decided to let this one go for the sake of teamwork, but I long regretted it (Chapter 13, Department/Institute of General Practice story). I continued to see Wilfred Selley and gave him personal encouragement. He succeeded in getting papers published on his innovative treatment with prostheses for patients after a stroke (Selley *et al.,* 1995).

I was able to secure a link with dentistry which did work when Julian Scott, another local dentist, registered for the degree of MPhil by research. I supervised him and he became one of the very few, probably the only, dentist in the Southwestern region to obtain this higher degree. I learnt from his external examiner, a female dental professor, how to approve a dissertation in style. After passing him she produced a bottle of champagne!

Whilst I was Chair of the College, several leaders in general dental practice started the idea of forming an academic institution for general dental practitioners (GDPs). I met them several times and we had meals together. I briefed them fully on how the College of General Practitioners had been founded, had developed and what it had achieved. I warmly encouraged them to form a college for GDPs of their own, as at that time they had no academic home. They secured the name of College of General Dental Practitioners but were daunted about launching a College.

A strange situation arose when the President of the Faculty of Dental Surgery of the Royal College of Surgeons of England became involved. This Faculty represented specialist dentists, most with a higher degree like the FDSRCSEng, and many were doubly qualified in medicine as well. They included maxillary-facial surgeons and were mainly hospital specialists. It was natural that the President of the leading academic organisation for specialist dentists would take an interest; what was curious was that it was Derek Seel, who was the Dental Postgraduate Dean in the Southwestern region. He and I were attending meetings in Bristol, chaired by the Medical Postgraduate Dean, in which he spoke for dentistry and I spoke for general practice. We got on amicably and never had a

DOI: 10.1201/9781032713601-37

cross word within the region, but simultaneously we were both lobbying hard in London on opposite sides. I was recommending the dental leaders should form a College and he was advising that they should form a second Faculty within the RCSEng. Apart from the academic rights and wrongs, forming a second Faculty was easier and less expensive for the dentists than establishing a new College, and Seel skilfully lobbied inside the College of Surgeons to make that process easy and acceptable. In another Exeter link, Julian Scott, one of those GDP leaders, became Editor of their journal. So, the academic journals of both general medical practice and general dental practice were initially edited in Devon.

I kept in touch with the dental leaders after I finished my chairmanship of the College in 1990 and always had good relations with them. In 1992 I lost my campaign, and a new Faculty of General Dental Practice was formed within the Royal College of Surgeons of England.

As Chair of the Academy of Medical Royal Colleges in 2000 I reviewed the constitution and the membership carefully. The Royal Colleges had grown over hundreds of years, the oldest being the Royal College of Surgeons of Edinburgh (founded 1505). The Conference of the Medical Royal Colleges had formed in the 1970s. The structural problem was that the membership was heavily biased towards physicians and surgeons, because of the history of the older Colleges. There were (and still are) no fewer than seven places reserved for them as there are Royal Colleges of Physicians in Edinburgh, Ireland, and London and three separate Royal Colleges of Surgeons in the same cities, each with a place and a vote. In addition, the Royal College in Glasgow includes both physicians and surgeons and elects a President alternately from each.

When constitutions are out of date there are two approaches: revolution or evolution. Revolution is traumatic and in this case was impossible, so the obvious approach was evolution. This meant broadening the membership to achieve a wider perspective outside hospitals and a better generalist/specialist balance. Since the Faculty of General Dental Practice was a full faculty of the Royal College of Surgeons and as it had long had membership on the Academy, one obvious move was to suggest the admission of the new Faculty of General Dental Practitioners, with its new RCSEng recognition, to the Academy.

I therefore approached the President of the Royal College of Surgeons of England, Barry Jackson, and made the suggestion. The response was unexpected and dramatic: he looked slightly shocked and said, "But they are high street people." I did not say anything for a minute or two whilst I digested the significance of these words, which had great narrative power. 'High Street' had the connotation of small shopkeepers and echoes of the 19th century division between the professions and trade. It was a striking expression of attitudes to those who did not work in hospital. The word 'people' was also significant as it did not include the concept of professionalism. This was a comment from the top of a London teaching hospital.

I realised at once that my suggestion was dead in the water with that reaction from the President of the Royal College within which the general practitioner dentists now sat, and the person who was academically responsible for them. I did not argue the case which was obviously unwinnable and simply said, "But Barry, I'm a high street person too; I see unselected patients coming off the street and work entirely in the community." He looked uncomfortable and made no reply. I never brought the suggestion up again. 'High-street people' equates to "Just GPs".

General Dental Council

The General Dental Council (GDC) is the equivalent for the dental profession of the GMC for medicine. Its constitution at the turn of the century provided for one place nominated by the GMC, with a tradition that this member served on the GDC Education Committee as well but did not enter general political debate. A vacancy arose whilst I was on the GMC, which asked if any member was interested in dentistry. I volunteered, explaining that I respected the dental profession, was a satisfied patient of my local dental practice, and had successfully supervised a dentist for a master's degree by research in Exeter. The GMC then nominated me and I became a member of the GDC as well. This was my third national regulatory body. It was chaired by Professor (Late Sir) Nairn Wilson, Dean of Dentistry at King's. I was not on the GDC long as its constitution changed and the medical place was removed.

Two Seminars in the Nuffield Trust

As Chair of the Nuffield Trust, I tried to help dentists by setting up two seminars for them in the Trust. The first was for the Dean and a group of general dental practitioners from the Faculty in which we discussed ways of developing education and research for dentists and raising their status. I was hoping at that time to get a grant for some educational initiatives from the Trust. The evening was pleasant and productive. Behind the scenes I proposed a grant from the Trust to support a GDP educational initiative.

The second seminar was for the dental deans in the schools of dentistry. However, listening to the discussion was uncomfortable as they repeatedly spoke disparagingly about ordinary dentists and regarded them with contempt. This proved to be the most irritating and least successful seminar with which I was involved in the Trust over nine years and the only one in which I summed up negatively. I concluded it by saying that I had been disappointed in the seminar as almost the whole conversation by these deans had been inward-looking and self-congratulatory. They had hardly ever mentioned patients and never discussed any educational initiative to improve dental care for NHS patients. If general dental practitioners were not performing as well as they thought they ought to, then the deans were the people responsible for educating and examining them! Why had there been no mention of helping dental practitioners to do research when I had myself supervised one to do a master's degree? The reputation of dentistry in the country did not depend on a small group of deans: what mattered to the British people was the quality of their local dentist. In dentistry the proportion of generalist dentists to specialists was higher than in medicine and so they should have a high priority. The Deans were taken aback. Looking shaken, they mumbled their thanks and left.

My relationship with the leadership of the general practitioner dentists continued, and in particular with the Dean of the new Faculty; Raj Raja Rayan and I spoke on research to a dental conference. I went to see his impressive educational initiatives in the College of Surgeons. We had lunches together and shared ideas.

Raj Raja Rayan invited me to speak to the Executive Board of the Faculty in 2002. This was in Lincoln's Inn Fields, the home of the Royal College of Surgeons of England. I summarised the history of the formation and subsequent successes of the RCGP. I lauded my own local NHS dentist in Exeter saying he was dentist to three generations of our family and that one of our children was travelling miles to see him. I drew parallels with medicine and thought that dentists had a rich field of clinical practice and research, which would include dentist-patient relationships and family practice. They were, like medical GPs, self-employed independent contractors in the community and different from salaried hospital staff. I thought the status of dentists was too low and they had no place on the Academy of Medical Royal Colleges, whereas the Faculty of Dental Surgery had long been represented.

Their question was status. Could they ever achieve what they deserved through a faculty in a medical specialist college? The words 'high-street people' rang in my ears but I did not use them as their speaker was still around. I finished by saying that as long as general dental practitioners remained in a faculty of a specialist medical college, they would "always be seen as second-class surgeons!" This shocked the room. Over lunch it was clear that I had split the Board: a few came to chat, but the majority avoided me. The Dean was charming.

There were no continuing bad feelings and an unexpected and pleasant event came in 2003 when the Faculty of General Dental Practice elected me an honorary fellow (HonFGDP Appendix 1). This gave me the new experience of wearing the gown of the Royal College of Surgeons of England and speaking in their hall. I was their first medical fellow. My own dentist teases me about this 'qualification.'

A College at Last

I thought that my involvement with the Faculty had been a failure. However, *Primary Dental Care*, the Faculty Journal, reported that the Executive Board decided on its 25th anniversary in 2017 to leave the Royal College of Surgeons of England and to form a new 'autonomous body' for dentistry. I sent a donation at once to indicate my strong support. A College of Dentistry was established in the summer of 2021. I hope it will raise the standards and status of general dental practitioners and will in due course become a royal institution.

31

The General Medical and Dental Councils

The guiding purpose of the government regulator is to prevent something rather than to create something.

Alan Greenspan (1926–), Former Chair of the US Federal Reserve

The General Medical Council (GMC) was established in 1858 after a series of campaigns to reform the medical profession. Its formation was important, as it was a prototype for regulating a major profession. The medical profession, which had many privileges like prescribing, was given considerable autonomy and power to regulate itself. The three main functions of the GMC under the *Medical Act 1858* were first, maintaining the *Medical Register*; i.e. publicising who is recognised as a medical practitioner, second, maintaining the standards of the medical profession with power to 'strike off' a doctor from the register thus stopping the ability to practise medicine, and third, regulating the medical schools.

Its best-known function is disciplinary, which could lead to doctors being struck off the *Register* because the GMC's Conduct Committee met in public with the press present. This meant that stories about doctors disgracing themselves were published, sometimes with salacious details. Initially, the GMC was dominated by the Royal Colleges, which gave it an orientation towards specialist medicine and GPs were weakly represented.

My first involvement with the GMC (apart from registering when I qualified) was in the 1970s, whilst on the Council of the BMA. A political row developed because the GMC, which until then had registered doctors on the payment of a one-off fee now introduced an annual fee. This caused a political uproar, led by the BMA. One BMA GP, John Marks, campaigned vigorously and later became Chair of BMA Council. There were threats of refusal to pay the fee.

The Government established a committee to review the regulation of the medical profession under the Chairmanship of Sir Alec Merrison, Vice-Chancellor at the University of Bristol. Crucially for general practice and for the future of the GMC, a GP member was the young Donald Irvine. The Merrison Committee (1975) produced a skilfully drafted, modernising report that was both acceptable to Government and to the medical profession. The principle was no taxation without representation and the proposal was that there should be a small majority of doctors democratically elected by the whole of the medical profession, from separate constituencies of England, Northern Ireland, Scotland, and Wales. So-called 'appointed places' continued from the medical Royal Colleges but were adjusted in numbers. The Royal College of General Practitioners, then 23 years old, was given a place for the first time. The BMA accepted this in return for a democratic majority of GMC members. The Government legislated with a *Medical Act 1978* based on the Merrison report.

In the cabinet of the RCGP Council (Chapter 11, College Cabinet story) a competition developed for the new place on the GMC starting in 1979. Ekke Kuenssberg thought he was entitled to it, having been both Chair and President. Donald Irvine, having been a member of the Merrison Committee, was determined to have it. I had no vote, but Irvine saw me as influential and rang me repeatedly at home. I was torn, as both were colleagues and friends. I assumed the Council would vote, but Kuenssberg did not press it and was, I think, afraid of losing. A vote might have gone either way. However, Irvine was elected unopposed with big implications for the future of the GMC.

DOI: 10.1201/9781032713601-38

On a night call which I did jointly with my trainees I discussed the GMC with Angela Douglas my then GP trainee. I suggested she stand for election and she agreed. Westcountry GPs then elected her from England in her twenties, the youngest doctor ever elected as described in Chapter 16, The Practice 1976–1986.

Irvine was elected Chair of the Standards Committee and led a big reform of the guidance the GMC gave doctors. Previous guidance was the 'blue book,' which informed doctors that they risked being struck off the *Register* for criminal behaviour, sexual relationships with patients, or conduct deemed damaging to the reputation of the profession. Irvine's Standards Committee turned this upside down and produced a booklet of positive attributes and behaviours called *Good Medical Practice: Duties of a Doctor*. I was never on the Standards Committee with Irvine but voted for *Good Medical Practice* (GMC, 1995) in the full Council. It was the biggest reform of the century and became an international model. It illustrates Greenspan's statement that the function of regulators is "to prevent something not to create something."

In 1994, I stood for election for the first time. I was elected from the constituency of England after multiple rounds of the single transferable vote (STV) system. I finally got in when a consultant in North Devon was squeezed out and a block of votes, obviously from Devon doctors, transferred to me.

The main Council did not meet often but had several committees where much of the work was done. The Professional Conduct Committee was the best known, as it dealt with the disciplinary cases. The problem in serving on it was that one could be stuck with a case that went on for weeks or even months. The unwritten code was that members of Council should serve on disciplinary committees whether or not they were interested in other committees, like the Standards Committee or the Education Committee, which attracted me. With my commitments in the practice (Practice stories), in the region (Chapter 14, Regional Adviser story), and as director of the Exeter PGMS (Chapter 27, PGMS story), I tried to protect myself by not volunteering to serve on the Conduct Committee, applying for the Standards Committee and the Education Committee. That ploy did not work and I was not elected to any committee.

Later I was elected to the Standards Committee. This I enjoyed. It was chaired by Sir Cyril Chantler (1939–), and the work was concerned with both professional standards and ethics. Being a member of the GMC meant being buttonholed at meetings, often by people who disagreed with some GMC action or policy. This was a continuing form of accountability.

Election for the Presidency 1994

Sir Robert (later Lord) Kilpatrick (1926–2015) retired as President and the stage was set for the presidential election of the century. For years presidential elections had been competitive but mainly about personalities. The 1994 election differed as each candidate's manifesto contrasted greatly. This election was about policies. The three candidates were all knights: Sir Herbert Duthie (1929–2015), Sir Anthony Grabham (1930–2015), and Sir Donald Irvine (1935–2018). Irvine stood on a manifesto offering reform. Membership of the GMC was just over a hundred and it was obviously going to be a tight election. Lottie Newman and I were Donald's chief supporters. It mattered to both of us because he was the only reforming candidate, the only GP, and had had great success in leading the Standards Committee. Sir Herbert, the academics' candidate, was a nice man, a distinguished academic, and Provost of the Welsh National School of Medicine. However, he did not seem to have answers to the big problems facing the medical profession. Sir Anthony was an experienced BMA leader, having chaired the BMA Consultants' Committee, the BMA Council, and the Joint Consultants' Committee. He was the medico-political candidate. Many feared confrontations with Government if he was elected.

Lottie and I spoke personally to virtually every member of the Council. I had wondered if people would be prepared to disclose their voting intentions, but people were ready to talk and usually volunteered their reasons. It was a fascinating experience. A block of academic doctors saw Duthie as their representative; they admired him and were going to vote for him. The BMA had a strong block vote committed to Grabham. Unions develop strong voting systems and this one held firmly. Even the leader of the BMA GPs told me he would vote for Grabham. The lay members were almost entirely for Irvine as the most patient-centred candidate. These blocks sometimes cut across GP/consultant differences; one leading, knighted, consultant meritocratically told me he would vote for Irvine "because he is the most able."

I kept in close touch with Donald. We stayed the night before the election at Princes Gate and we went in a taxi together to the GMC. In this memorable journey, I told Donald that I was confident he would win. The vote on the STV system gave Donald a lead after the first round, which increased after the first candidate was squeezed out. He was comfortably elected and became the first GP President in the history of the GMC.

I stood again in the 1999 election, again run on the single transferable vote. The standing of the GMC attracted 297 candidates, six from Devon, five Royal College Presidents, and two current or former Chairs of the BMA Council. National organisations like the BMA and Overseas Doctors Association publicised their slate of candidates. By now I was getting to know an increasing number of specialists. This time I received the 12th highest vote and was then re-elected to the Standards Committee and later to the Education Committee as well. Sadly I was the only GP academic elected.

The General Dental Council (GDC) is the GMC equivalent in the dental profession. The GMC elected me to the GDC in 2001 (Chapter 30, Dentistry), my third national regulatory body.

The Bristol Case

I was on the GMC, when the most high-profile disciplinary case in its history occurred. A baby died after cardiac surgery in Bristol after written complaints had been made about the results from that unit, and when a consultant had recommended against the operation. The GMC issued proceedings for 'serious professional misconduct' (SPM), the gravest charge, against two cardiac surgeons and against the medically qualified radiologist, who was chief executive of the hospital. The death of a baby, action against cardiac surgeons, the publicity, and the drama ensured sustained national publicity. Irvine, as President, chaired the Conduct Committee, as was usual. High-powered QCs acted on both sides. The battle was bitter and the defence even raised issues about one of Irvine's family having had cardiac surgery.

After many weeks the Conduct Committee, with Irvine summing up, found the leading cardiac surgeon guilty of serious professional misconduct, as well as the medical chief executive. The Conduct Committee struck both off the *Medical Register*, awarding a lesser penalty to a second cardiac surgeon, explaining their reasons. A key decision was that the Chief Executive of the hospital as a doctor was held to have had a duty of care to patients, which he had not fulfilled, even though he was not acting clinically. These decisions were open to appeal at law and appealed they were. The legal battle went right up to the Judicial Committee of the House of Lords, then the highest court in the land.

In a historic ruling, the Judicial Committee of the Privy Council (1999) supported the Conduct Committee's and Irvine's decision. A doctor is a doctor is a doctor in whatever role he or she may hold. This created case-law at the highest level in the UK. The Bristol case was a fight for professionalism and its success in 1998 marked a high point of medical professionalism in the UK. Irvine was determined that the medical profession could and should be seen by self-regulation to be able to uphold professional standards.

Revalidation

I played little part in the core business of the GMC in my first few years, but later was involved when the GMC took on the challenge of introducing revalidation for the medical profession. The background was a series of disasters in the medical profession where a small number of doctors had disgraced the profession. These included Harold Shipman, a GP who was the biggest medical murderer of all time, the Bristol case, Rodney Ledward, a gynaecologist, and pathologists who had retained body parts without consent. The question was: what should the medical profession do?

Irvine led the GMC on a policy that he called 'revalidation,' which meant reviewing every registered medical practitioner regularly, probably five yearly, in an attempt to protect the public. The debates on this policy within the GMC were long and hard. The idea was bitterly opposed by some members, notably Sir Sandy Macara (1932–2012), a member of the Council and also Chair of Council of the BMA. He disagreed passionately, being partly influenced by his experience in Bristol, as he believed that what the GMC had done was wrong. Macara and others used every possible technique to block progress. I knew Sandy quite well as in 1972 he had, from the Bristol Medical School, sent me Sheila Townsend, my first undergraduate medical student. Whilst we were on opposite sides in all the revalidation debates in the GMC, he was being very helpful to me personally in BMA house on the problem of the exclusion of academic GPs from distinction awards (Chapter 39, Distinction/Clinical Excellence Awards story). Such are the complexities of relationships in different national bodies.

There was a strong block of GMC members who believed this was the right thing to do, including GPs who were more positive about revalidation as a group than specialists. Crucially, BMA GP leaders like John Chisholm and Brian Keighley supported revalidation against their own Chair of Council. GPs found the policy of the GP regional advisers, who regularly reviewed GP trainers, was acceptable, a view which had been endorsed in a BMA ballot of GPs. This tension between the GPs and specialists within the BMA came to a head dramatically in public in the BMA conferences in 2000, as told in Chapter 37, Three National Meetings story.

By great persuasion and hard work, Irvine in 1998 eventually led the GMC to vote formally that revalidation should be introduced. This was the first profession in Britain to do this and also the first in the world. It was a remarkable example of professional leadership. His achievement was to persuade a Council of over 100 members, with a democratically elected majority of doctors, to vote for revalidation, which would mean more work for all doctors – all in the interests of patients. No profession anywhere in the world in the 20th century did as much for their patients/clients in the public interest. I was able to support this policy personally as an elected member within the GMC, but more importantly through the Academy of Medical Royal Colleges, especially when I became Vice-Chair and later Chair (Chapter 38, Chair of the Academy of Medical Royal Colleges).

Medical Data 2000

At the end of the century, the Standards Committee where I was a member under the chairmanship of Sir Cyril Chantler (1939–) became uneasy about patients' medical information being sent around the NHS, usually without the patients knowing. Hospitals were routinely informing cancer registries of new diagnoses of cancer to support epidemiological research.

The Standards Committee concluded this policy was paternalistic and patients should know how their data were being treated. It took the view that distributing data without the patient's knowledge was improper and ought to be put onto a proper legal basis. It decided to recommend that this practice should cease. This recommendation came to a full meeting of the GMC where I again voted for it and it was approved.

The balloon went up! Doctors started withholding information and staff members in the cancer registries were enraged. A political problem arose which reached Parliament. The legal solution was an Act of Parliament in 2001, which established the Patient Information Advisory Group, described in Chapter 41, PIAG story. This had powers to consider the handling of confidential information and the right to advise the Secretary of State for Health when confidential information could be divulged. I was appointed by the Secretary of State for Health to PIAG at its inception. PIAG soon gave powers under a class mechanism for the cancer registries to receive information, now on a legal basis. However, 20 years on, patients are still not properly informed about who receives their data and why.

Disciplinary Work

In my second term on the GMC I put in some spadework on the disciplinary committees. After retiring clinically from the practice and as a professor, I at last had the time. I served on a disciplinary committee, which gave me the unpleasant experience of jointly striking a GP off the *Medical Register*. I also served on the Interim Orders Committee, which can suspend a practitioner's registration pending a full investigation. Once, I did a whole week on this.

On one case I became isolated from all the other eight panel members. A GP was charged with serious professional misconduct (SPM) because he had sent a young man in his mother's car to a hospital 30 minutes away instead of calling an ambulance and the man had died on the way. This was the most serious charge and, if confirmed, it carried the risk of the doctor being struck off the *Medical Register*. The ambulance service sent evidence that they should have been called. The post-mortem showed a rare cardiac condition. The panel was on the point of agreeing the charge when I said I would have done exactly the same myself. The tension in the room was palpable. I pointed out the GP was alone on call for a substantial population in a rural practice on Sunday evening when the mother had brought her son in by car. The GP had conscientiously done an ECG, had correctly noted abnormalities, and had correctly advised hospital admission. As the ambulance base was 30 minutes away calling one would have taken an hour to get the patient into hospital. Asking the mother to drive her son on to hospital in a rural area was medically logical and common in rural areas. That GP could not possibly have anticipated death and the panel should not attribute blame with the benefit of hindsight. There was a sticky discussion but gradually the panel came round and finally concluded that the GP "was not guilty of serious professional misconduct." I have always believed it is essential in the interests of justice that every GMC panel contained a member of the same specialty as the accused doctor. In particular, this case revealed how difficult it is for hospital-based staff to really understand situations in general practice. It was important that day that the panel had one GP member.

Developments in the GMC

In 1999 the renewal of the Presidency came up. Wendy Savage (1935–) a community-orientated gynaecologist, stood against Irvine, a so-called 'stalking horse.' Irvine won, but only by 30 votes which did not strengthen his position.

In 2001, he allowed Finlay Scott, the Registrar, to propose at the end of a long Council meeting, that the GMC should register as a charity. There would be substantial financial benefits for the GMC. A tired Council approved this without debate. However, several members of the Council felt railroaded. The decision may have been correct but the process was odd, especially for a President who had often allowed long debates. Regulators and charities have different images. Proper debate would have been usual and more appropriate.

Charity rules required clarification of payments to trustees, including Irvine's. The Presidency was a paid post and the obvious yardstick for pay was the A-plus merit award paid to hundreds of NHS consultants. Irvine should have declared this openly from the start. However, the figure had been obscured in the accounts. When it emerged, some lay people thought it high, especially as charity trustees are usually unpaid. Edwin Boorman, a BMA consultant, criticised Irvine over the previous lack of clarity, putting him on the defensive.

In my day, a doctor accused of a serious charge was judged by the criminal standard of proof, i.e. 'beyond all reasonable doubt.' There were calls to lower this to the civil standard, i.e. 'on the balance of probabilities.' For once in my life I opposed patient representatives and argued in a speech in 2000 that since society used the criminal standard for all charges that could lead to serious punishments, like prison, and since the penalty of being struck off was so great, then doctors facing that should be judged on the same standard.

In 2000, a bitter battle about revalidation broke out. Two angry national BMA conferences in 2000 passed a vote of no confidence against the General Medical Council and so effectively Irvine in my presence as reported in detail in Chapter 37, Three National Meetings story.

I was actively involved in the Academy in discussions on the size of a reformed GMC. A professional consensus was reached that the size of the Council should be reduced in an agreement obtained between the Academy, the BMA and the GMC with a membership of 35. I was influential in securing increased patient participation of 40% in 2001, which was reflected in the 2002 legislation.

Irvine retired in January 2001, a year before his seven-year term ended. Seven years is too long for such a post. He achieved his main policy aim in having revalidation approved by the democratically elected 100-strong Council. Such a big Council gave professional legitimacy to the decision as there were some members with whom most minority medical groups could identify. But he had become isolated and must have been very tired. *Hospital Doctor* (2000) had earlier captured his position with a heading "Donald on the defensive." His resignation triggered an election. I was asked by several members, GPs and some specialists notably Graham Catto, if I was standing. I decided not to do so and Catto, Chair of the Education Committee, was elected.

The new leadership significantly softened the proposals on revalidation despite protests from the lay members and some medical members, including me. We lost the vote. The leadership smiled as they won, thinking they were in control. However, this watering down was a historic mistake. The new approach was scrutinised in public by the Judge, Dame Janet Smith, heading the Shipman Inquiry. Sir Donald and Sir Graeme were both witnesses. Dame Janet reported she had been prepared to accept the original proposals for revalidation but that changes made late in the day had weakened the original 'seminal' ideas so that they no longer complied with the evaluation of practice required by the recently amended *Medical Act*. Her damning conclusion was that: "for the majority of GMC members the old culture of protecting the interests of doctors lingers on" (Shipman Inquiry, 2004). The GMC thus lost its credibility. Government stepped in and instructed the Chief Medical Officer to report (Irvine, 2006). The medical profession was in the hands of a single civil servant.

Further changes in the GMC constitution occurred. In the next election, I did not apply and so left the GMC in 2003. I was asked to continue on disciplinary panels but I declined, as I believed that doctors sitting in judgement on other doctors should, on principle, be in clinical practice.

ADDENDUM

In 2006, the Chief Medical Officer, Sir Liam Donaldson, reported. He proposed the abolishment of all elected places recommending that all members of the GMC be appointed instead.

He also proposed ending the application of the criminal standard of proof and the use of the lower civil standard of proof. All this was quickly enacted into law and a new GMC emerged with only six appointed doctors and six lay people. The President was renamed the Chair. Initially, members were appointed by a national appointments committee but after this was abolished, doctors were appointed to the GMC by the DH behind closed doors. In this way the Government took control of the medical profession.

Similarly, in 2015, Government established the Office for Students, a quango with draconian powers over all English universities. Parliament passed this when Oxford and Cambridge were at the top of the world university rankings.

Dahrendorf (1982) admired Britain for the number and autonomy of its institutions. A little discussed development in the 21st century is that Governments, of both the left and right, have progressively taken over many of Britain's leading institutions. I do not welcome this it as it often leads to politicisation.

In 2015, I discovered that the new GMC did not have a GP on it! My letter exposing this was published in the *BMJ* (DPG, 2015b). I also wrote to the Chief Executive of the NHS, Simon (1966–; later Sir, later still Lord) Stevens. He wrote to the Chairman of the GMC, Sir Terence Stephenson, and kindly sent me the reply, which was unconcerned. However, one GP was soon appointed. The position of the GMC changed. Most doctors are now unconnected with it. Medical members are no longer elected. All five consultant members come from big teaching hospitals, so Lord Moran would have been pleased. The decisions they take with lay colleagues are not as well informed about the realities of day-to-day clinical practice in district hospitals and general practice as before. Doctors still pay a substantial annual sum for it.

Irvine (1935–2018) wrote a short history of the GMC in 2006 and two books setting out the principles he had espoused and a memoir of his life. These were: *The Doctors' Tale*: *Professionalism and Public Trust* (Irvine, 2003) and *Medical Professionalism and Public Trust*: *Reflections on a Life in Medicine* (Irvine, 2017). He described how the RCGP greatly influenced him in the 1970s and 1980s, as it did me.

32

The Fetzer Institute, USA

In the USA $427.71 billion dollars were donated in 2019 for charitable purposes.

Giving USA (2019)

As Chairman of Research for the RCGP, I had regular meetings with the Medical Research Council (MRC). I argued the case for carrying out research on topics such as the patient-doctor relationship and continuity of care with complete lack of success (as described in Chapter 28, the Chair of Research story). The MRC leadership was epidemiologically orientated and unsympathetic. However, unknown to me, some of the listening, less senior, MRC staff were more interested.

In the late 1990s, Lynn Underwood of the Fetzer Institute in the USA approached the MRC saying it wanted to promote research on doctor–patient relationships and were seeking a UK name. Someone gave them mine. I was then invited to join a working group being assembled by the Fetzer Institute. Thus began, late in my academic career, a rich, pleasant, and productive interlude, which I greatly enjoyed.

The USA differs from the UK in the way rich people are encouraged to set up foundations (charities) in their name to research some topic that interests the donor. US citizens give generously. By 2018, donations to charity in the United States were as much as $42,771 billion (Giving USA, 2019). The United States has many such foundations, of which the best known in the health world are the Commonwealth Fund, the Kellogg Foundation, the Rockefeller Foundation, and the Robert Wood Johnson Foundation. Of these, apart from the Fetzer Institute, I had dealings with the Commonwealth Fund and its Harkness Fellowships, the RAND Corporation, and the Robert Wood Johnson Foundation. This system gives the United States a big advantage, as in many fields there is a foundation able to fund innovative developments. By contrast, the UK has many fewer such charities, and outside the disease-centred ones there are only four. In order of foundation they are: the King's Fund, the Wellcome Trust, the Nuffield Trust, and the Health Foundation.

The Fetzer Institute

The Fetzer Institute was founded by John E Fetzer (1901–1991) through an endowment and was designed to foster his fascination with human relationships, especially compassion. Its headquarters is in Kalamazoo, USA, where I went for one seminar. It was best known for sponsoring the Pew-Fetzer Task Force (1994) on relationship-centred care. The key figure was Lynn Underwood, the Director, who was UK trained with a PhD in epidemiology and good publications from Northern Ireland on melanoma. When she recruited me she was immersed in studying human relationships.

The Working Group

The academic team she assembled was impressive. It included Professor Moira Stewart from the Medical School at London, Ontario, Canada, who had trained under Professor Ian McWhinney,

DOI: 10.1201/9781032713601-39

the doyen of professors of general practice and probably the broadest thinker and most humane of them all. She was a world-class social scientist and was accompanied by Professor Judith Bell Browne from the same department. From the USA, Fetzer had recruited two top professors of psychology: Harry Reis from the University of Rochester and Margaret Clark, soon to go to Yale. These two knew each other well and both had researched extensively on the psychology of human relationships (Clark and Reis, 1988). I found myself not just the only UK representative, but the only representative from Europe. This was daunting. All the other five (with Lynn Underwood) were better methodologists than I was. I was the only one medically qualified and working as a GP (family physician as generalist doctors are called in Canada and the USA). We started meetings in the USA and by telephone.

Face-to-face meetings were held either at the Fetzer Institute in Kalamazoo or in hotels. Given the other activities in my life, timing was tricky. On one occasion I flew out of Heathrow at 10 am, arriving in Chicago in the evening, stayed in an airport hotel, attended an early morning meeting within the perimeter of the airport (quite usual in the United States), and flew back on a late afternoon plane, without ever having left the airport!

The Study

The good news was that the group agreed that the patient-doctor relationship was best studied in general/family practice. The next decision was critical in that we all agreed that the top research priority was to devise a new instrument by which this important relationship could be measured. A third important group decision was that the work should be from the patient's perspective.

Thus this three-nation, international study got going, with patients being recruited from general/ family practices in Canada, UK, and the United States. I turned to colleagues in the Exeter Institute of General Practice and several general practices associated with it, as well, of course, as recruiting patients from my own practice, St Leonard's. As a team we devised the most searching statements we could, using all our combined knowledge and research. All the patient completed forms were sent to Rochester, USA, and Harry Reis supervised the data entry and led the statistical analyses. When he was in England for a psychology conference, I entertained him in the president's flat at the RCGP at Princes Gate, London.

Placebo/Contextual Healing Effect

Fetzer, led by Lynn Underwood, organised an international seminar in Einsiedeln, Switzerland to study the placebo effect, and I was invited. I was pleased to find that Professor Edzard Ernst, also from the small Exeter Postgraduate Medical School, was there too – a sign of success. I had been heavily involved in his being appointed to the first chair of complementary medicine in the world and he was making an international impact (reported in Chapter 27, the PGMS story).

The placebo effect had long fascinated me and I used to teach on it in the Exeter vocational training scheme. Anything that can provide a 30% benefit for patients with minimum adverse effects and at virtually no cost surely needs to be studied. However, in the 1970s and 1980s no one was interested and indeed some trainees told me that their hospital teachers spoke of the placebo effect either with contempt or saw it as a "form of trickery". It was seen as outside science. I enjoyed the seminar, as it produced good papers and I was not asked to write one. The setting was beautiful and the discussions rich. However, I came away without fully understanding the placebo effect.

Two members of that seminar J Kleijnen and Edzard Ernst forged a working partnership. The outcome was a landmark paper in the *Lancet* (Di Blasi *et al.*, 2001). Their group in a much cited systematic review showed that the effect of many drugs when used in real life was often significantly better for patients than the results of the use of the same drug in rigorous controlled trials. They suggested that there was a missing ingredient that improved the performance of the drug and they called it the "context effect." This was a breakthrough. I realised as soon as I read it that this was a stepping stone to measuring the doctor–patient relationship. I thought that "the context" would be that relationship, which has great power to reduce anxiety, and to give hope and reassurance, all of which can have positive physiological and psychological effects.

Medicine likes to discuss big controversies such as nature versus nurture, which by the 1990s had progressed to genes versus the environment. In that decade it became clear that it was not one or the other, but both. Genes and the environment interact continually, both for good and ill. Generalist doctors, who are always being subjected to one theory after another by subject specialists, particularly like to integrate or reconcile different theories. Grasping that genes and the environment interact, meaning that both are important simultaneously, is intellectually and professionally satisfying. Similarly, realising that a good doctor–patient relationship adds value to a good drug does the same. This stemmed directly from the work of the Fetzer Institute and is a good example of how a little known charity/foundation can tackle an unfashionable and generally disregarded subject and make internationally important progress.

Fetzer Article

The Fetzer team concentrated on 'responsiveness'. Harry Reis and Margaret Clark were international experts in academic psychology (Clark and Reis, 1988). They had been writing together since 1988 were a strong partnership and I liked them both. Responsiveness is a concept in psychology meaning the extent to which a person responds to another person; in our case this meant how much patients think their family doctor (family physician) is responsive to them. I had one advantage in the group that I knew the GP research literature, so I realised we were taking a big intellectual step. The theory on the GP–patient relationship stemming from Balint (1957) had for half a century been doctor centred. We were now looking at this relationship through the patients' eyes. I also knew that in the UK the same change in perspective was being revealed in research by Howie *et al.* (1999) who had found that his enablement instrument (empowering patients so that they are better informed and able to self-care) was significantly associated with "how well the patient knew the doctor."

The analysis in Rochester, New York, linked the answers from patients in Canada, the UK, and the United States to facts about the patients and the practices they were in. We discovered that patients in all three countries answered in the same way. Next, we found that continuity of family physician care was significantly associated with patients perceiving that their family physicians were more responsive. This strengthened the continuity literature. A new finding was that patients with long continuity of family physician care reported higher levels of subjective wellbeing. This needs replication and opened in my mind thoughts of a possible neurophysiological basis for continuity of care. Feelings of wellbeing are known to be associated with endorphin release. Back in Britain I linked with Michael Dixon, a GP near Exeter who had contributed patients to the study, and we sought to consult a UK expert in a teaching hospital but nothing came of it. The neuroscience breakthrough came with Anderson *et al.* (2023), who found that patients with strong trust in their doctors experience less pain than other patients and that the patient centres in their brains are measurably different using magnetic resonance.

We wrote an article and submitted to a leading psychology journal. To our disappointment, it was rejected. Nothing happened for a time and I became anxious that all that time and work might be lost. I rewrote the article in a different format and sent it round, still with Harry Reis as first author. This produced a sharp reaction, not from Harry, but from Judith Belle Browne in Canada, who sharply rejected my draft. However, good came of this as it stimulated Harry to resubmit to the *Journal of Basic and Applied Psychology* (Reis *et al.*, 2008), which accepted it. It was called "Measuring responsiveness in the therapeutic relationship: a patient perspective." It had six authors, supplemented by Fen Fang Psi, who had contributed analysis in Rochester.

This article came out in 2008, some years after the team had disbanded. By 2023, it had 61 citations and a recommendation to use it from the King's Fund (Freeman and Hughes, 2010). We used the questionnaire in the St Leonard's Practice in our Health Foundation project *Continuity Counts*. In 2021, the RCGP in its paper "The power of relationships: what is relationship-based care? and why is it important?" recommended the use of this questionnaire (RCGP, 2021).

From 2008 onwards, I reflected increasingly on the two international research groups in the United States with which I had been so lucky to be involved. The first group was with Arch Mainous from the South, the University of Alabama, whereas the second had four colleagues: two from Canada, and two from the US Northeast. The two research groups had no connection and I was the only member of both. Intriguingly to me was that Mainous *et al.* (2001) had shown that trust by patients in their family physicians was significantly associated with continuity of family physician care, i.e. patients changed over time. Reis *et al.* (2008) showed that in the eyes of the patients, family physicians became more responsive to them with continuity of care, i.e. GPs changed over time. I was the first to be able to put these two findings together and so to glimpse a new understanding of continuity of care as a form of human behaviour in which both patients and GPs change over time. A new understanding of continuity emerged in my mind – a reciprocal phenomenon in which each person influences change in the other.

In 2004, Moira Stewart delivered the RCGP's James Mackenzie Lecture (Stewart, 2005), a considerable honour for a social scientist. I took her and her husband to lunch. Subsequently, Lynn Underwood emailed that she had been offered authorship of a chapter on compassion by Oxford University Press in one of the Oxford book series. Would I co-write it? I spent a fortnight thinking it over and then accepted. She came back saying she had just declined! I had made a big mistake. Later, I was able to have dinner with her when she was in London. She wrote a book on compassion (Fehr *et al.*, 2009).

The last chapter of the Fetzer work was in the Institute of General Practice in Exeter. Harry Reis sent me tapes of fully consented consultations of American family physicians with their patients. Pamela Lings, a qualitative researcher, with Evans and Seamark, did the analysis (Lings *et al.*, 2003). We with two partners Kieran Sweeney and Philip Evans and other colleagues formed a reference group which discussed the doctor–patient relationship and produced our article "Towards a theory of continuity of care" (DPG *et al.*, 2003). Happily, the *Journal of the Royal Society of Medicine* accepted both articles for simultaneous publication. Twenty years later they had acquired 96 and 204 citations, respectively. Two new contributions were made to the theory of general practice. First, that the patient and doctor liking each other matters to their relationship. This simple, social, non-professional feeling counts. Secondly, patients can forgive their GP a moderate mistake if the usual previous care had been good (see an example in Chapter 6, Learning the Craft). As complaints now average one per GP at any one time, this further justifies making good relationships with patients.

I was fortunate to be invited by the Fetzer Institute, as in the late 1990s there was a groupthink in England that doctor–patient relationships and continuity of care were not research priorities. I could not get any grants *in* England to research them. It was American vision, American money, and an American foundation that made this research and these publications possible.

33

Non-Executive Directorships in the NHS

Non-executive directors are like baubles on a Christmas tree, there purely for decoration and respectability.

Tiny Rowland (1917–1998)

Twice I was appointed by the Department of Health to a non-executive directorship of a Devon health authority. These posts lasted between five and eight years and they came about twenty years apart.

Devon Area Health Authority

The Devon Area Health Authority was established in 1974 as a result of a national reorganisation of the NHS. This was the first organisational change since 1948 and led the endless roundabout of organisational changes. On arrival, we were told that previous health authorities had been too small in their geographical areas and that there were great advantages in planning health services on a countywide basis.

The remit of the Devon Area Health Authority was to manage the National Health Service in Devon, apart from those services provided by contractors such as GPs and dentists, who related to a different authority. In practice over 90% of the time was spent on hospitals.

The Chair was Sir Derek Jakeaway KCMG OBE (1915–1993), a British colonial administrator. He seemed to have few views and saw his role as chairing meetings efficiently. The Chief Executive Officer, George Owens, became the key figure. I grew to admire him considerably and think he was one of the outstanding health authority administrators of his time. He always listened to arguments and always took a moderate line.

I was amused to find life following art. A famous television programme "Yes Minister," described a hospital being maintained empty without any patients in it. This situation arose with the new district hospital in Plymouth. The engineers, electricians and other technical workers all advised us that the hospital needed to be run empty for some time to test all the systems.

I had a lesson in responsibility when a fire officer reported that several of the hospitals in Devon were fire risks because they were so old and that it would be difficult, probably impossible, to evacuate ill patients from higher floors since the lifts could not be used in a fire.

Still in my thirties, I innocently enquired who was responsible for this situation and was told: "You as a director are!" This was my first encounter with the ambiguities of responsibility and authority in the NHS.

The two medical members of this authority were David Mattingly and me, both from the new Exeter University Postgraduate Medical School. It was understandable that Mattingly was there as PGMS Director, as universities had long had places on health authorities since 1948, but I was lucky to be there.

The membership also included appointees from local government. This reflected the argument in the 1940s between Aneurin Bevan's vision of a nationally run health service and Herbert Morrison's vision of a health service being run by local government. I initially supported local authority representation. However, I was increasingly disappointed. For many of them the authority meetings were

DOI: 10.1201/9781032713601-40

simply a chance to further their political careers through local press reports. They usually took a line that they thought would be popular in their locality, regardless of the rights and wrongs of the policy issue. So blatant was this that some stopped addressing the Chair and turned round in meetings to speak directly to the press.

I was a member when one of the recurrent financial crises struck. A thoughtful debate ensued about cutting costs and a decision taken to change the reimbursement of car expenses to a fixed rate rather than paying a higher rate for bigger cars. At the end, a trade union representative, who rarely spoke in meetings, said to the Chair "I don't think you can do that!" Soon afterwards we were informed that there was an agreement between the Department of Health and the trade unions that mileage would be reimbursed according to the size of the car engine and that our decision was invalid. This was another lesson to me about the complicated layers of actual responsibility in the NHS. The long debate had been a waste of time. Health authority directors are always told that they are responsible and that they take the decisions, but in reality many decisions are constrained. One NHS trust adopted a policy contrary to the DH policy. Its chairman was removed. The DH keeps a tighter grip on local NHS authorities than is always apparent.

One day we were told that the authority was to be abolished, as it was too big. This was the exact opposite of what we had been told five years previously. I pressed for a reasoned paper with some evidence to justify this decision and was told that there was no such paper: this was a ministerial decision. My confidence in NHS policymaking was correspondingly reduced. The Devon Area Health Authority was abolished in 1982 having existed for eight years.

Devon Family Health Services Authority

Family Health Service Authorities (FHSAs) were established in 1990 to replace executive councils, which had been the original organisations for the contractor professions in 1948. Unlike their predecessors the executive councils, which were accountable to the DH, were made accountable to regional health authorities, so the DH heard less about general practice and the other local health professions. When the new Devon Family Health Services Authority was formed on a county-wide basis in 1995, there was opposition as people in Plymouth wanted to keep a separate Plymouth-based organisation. We were assured that county-wide FHSAs were preferable and would be more efficient, but no evidence was provided.

The constitution of the authority provided for one practising member from each of the so-called 'contractor' professions. These were: chiropodists, dentists, general practitioners and pharmacists. All of these professionals were self-employed and had a contract *for* services with the NHS rather than being salaried and employed. I was offered the place as a practising NHS GP and took the offer to my partnership, which quickly decided that I should do it.

The Chair was the Reverend Miriam Gent, who had much experience in previous organisations. The Chief Executive was Eddie Herbert. One of the other non-executive members was Professor Ruth Hawker, with whom I got on well as a leading representative of the nursing profession. She later became Chair of the Royal Devon and Exeter Hospital Trust and was appointed an OBE.

The work of this authority was more relevant to my clinical practice than the Devon Area Health authority had been. The FHSA was in contract with all the 600 GPs in Devon including my practice and I discovered the amount of its time spent dealing with general practice problems, especially complaints and problem GPs. The authority organised the complaints system. As the medical member I was not involved, but I saw the papers dealing with each complaint. Generally, I was impressed with the trouble taken. Patient complaints were taken seriously. The service committee had a lay majority with a lay chair, a superior system to what was then usual for complaints in the hospital service. The GP being complained against could bring colleagues and was given proper time to provide a detailed response to the complaint. The patients were not belittled, there was no assumption as to whether the doctor was right or wrong and decisions generally seemed reasonable.

As Regional Adviser in General Practice, I had visited virtually every trainer applicant in Devon and Cornwall (Chapter 14, Regional Adviser story). What I had not done was visit the weakest GPs and the Devon FHSA gave me that opportunity. I learnt about the worst side of general medical practice. There were six general practitioners who were big problems but who formed only 1% of the GP contractors. One was a chronic alcoholic, another was organising his practice so incompetently that staff were not being properly paid and bankruptcy was a possibility, and one had a record of clinical problems that was disturbing. I believed that some of these should have been referred to the GMC or had their contracts terminated in the interests of patients and the NHS, but there was a great reluctance to act. The professional protections and the national systems were overcomplicated and inefficient. The discussions about those six GPs damaged the reputation of the other 594 GPs in Devon.

I wrote papers for the Authority to focus attention on good general practice. One proposed that modest grants be made available for innovative ideas from health contractors in Devon, as was often possible in specialist medicine. The authority approved this and advertised some to be judged competitively. Two young GPs were given awards: Philip Evans from my own practice (I was not involved in the award) for his interest in high blood fats, and Clare Seamark from the Honiton practice for her interest in women's health. Both these young GPs were encouraged by quite small awards of a few hundred pounds and both went on to obtain higher university degrees by research later. They obtained two MPhils (Exon), an MD and a professorship between them. Encouraging enthusiastic young practitioners should be a strategic priority, and sadly, such small grants are not available today. In 2004 an evaluation of primary care bursaries was later published and was favourable (Lee and Saunders, 2004).

I also reported on the fellowship by assessment scheme of the RCGP (Chapter 24, Fellowship By Assessment story) which had begun in 1989, and in Devon there were more FBAs than in any other county in England. The director of planning, Julia Neville (later PhD) introduced a system whereby she made a small grant for expenses to the practices doing FBA, in return for them sending a copy of their FBA report. Julia told me she found these interesting and a useful counter to the work she had to do dealing with problem GPs.

The Authority became besieged by a mass of generally critical correspondence from one individual, who bombarded the staff with emotional communications threatening legal action. This became a problem, taking up senior management time. I first heard that such a person could be declared a 'vexatious litigant.' Legal proceedings were started and succeeded.

Clinics in General Practice

The DH started paying GPs extra if they concentrated their patients with nominated diseases into special surgeries, called 'clinics.' This was partly through well-meaning but inappropriate advice from specialists, who often think they can advise about general practice without fully understanding it. To specialists arranging people with common diseases in a 'clinic' is sensible and is usual in hospitals. The word 'clinic' is a hospital rather than a general practice term. It is not so appropriate in general practice when patients frequently attend with several different diseases at once and where one of the great efficiencies of general practice is the ability of generalist doctors to handle several different diseases within a single consultation. I spoke with a Devon LMC leader about these clinics. He replied: "If the DH is silly enough to give us money for old rope, we'll take it!" A classic trade union response.

I was taken aside by the Chair of the Authority, with whom I got on well, and she gently said to me that there was concern that my practice was one of very few that was not receiving any payments for these clinics. She suggested it was embarrassing that the medical member was not providing patients the benefit of these clinics. "What benefits?" I asked her. Could she give any evidence that general practice patients were better treated if they were segregated into clinics rather than seen in ordinary surgeries. She looked surprised but had no evidence. This incident illustrates the difference between managers and leaders. Managers assume a policy and see their job as implementing it, whereas leaders are interested in making and improving policy.

I explained why our practice had not claimed for clinics, as we did not think they were in our patients' interest. If a patient with two chronic diseases was seen, the clinic policy encouraged the GP to send the patient home and to make another appointment to come back to a 'clinic' for the second condition. Clinics had to be organised on a particular day of the week, which might not be convenient for the patient or their carer. This was a burden for the patient and an extra consultation for the GP. Worse, it fragmented care, when good general practice integrates care. GPs integrate more than any other branch of medicine: between physical and psychological medicine, between preventive and therapeutic medicine, and between medical and social factors. Specialist medicine in contrast, advances by fragmentation, creating ever narrower fields. Miriam Gent was concerned: "You've lost a lot of money by this," she said. "Yes," I said: "Four figure sums, but we have kept our professionalism." She did not tell me what she did, but she was conscientious so I expect she reported the problem. Soon afterwards the DH stopped paying for these clinics. I never knew if our practice policy made a difference or not.

My time out of the practice for the FHSA drew criticism from my partners. This had not happened when I did the much bigger job of chairing the RCGP. This was because the FHSA met on Mondays, when I had always worked flat out through to a late evening surgery. I had protected Mondays in the RCGP job. I offered the partners my resignation from the FHSA. In the debate in the partnership, I hardly spoke. People are more affected by losses rather than gains of the same magnitude (Hobfoll *et al.*, 2003). Faced with my leaving the FHSA, the partners analysed what benefits my membership brought the practice. I was interested to hear that they thought my ability to "read the tea leaves" about possible future developments was valuable. They asked me to stay! The Devon FHSA was abolished in 1996 having existed for six years.

The Non-Executive Role

There is a built-in tension in the role of a non-executive director, namely in gaining access to all the relevant information and properly holding the executive directors to account. It is far harder for non-executives to get all the information and what they do see is controlled by the executive directors, especially by the Chief Executive Officer, who may not always want to disclose everything. This is not just an NHS feature; the same tension arises in charities, including Royal Colleges. The executive officers in practice often control the non-executives. In the mid-Staffordshire NHS Foundation Trust, a big NHS scandal occurred. The non-executive directors voted to reduce about 100 nurses, even when the hospital was inundated by patient complaints (Francis, 2013). I understood the comment by Tiny Rowland that non-executive directors can be "like baubles on a Christmas tree, there for decoration and respectability!"

The work in both authorities was interesting but it never enthused me as much as serving on GP or medical professional bodies. I gave my time in clinical retirement to developing general practice through research and teaching as described in Chapter 46, Unfinished Campaign story, and Chapter 49, St Leonard's Research Practice story.

34

The Practice 1987–2000

It is more important to know the patient who has the disease than to know the disease the patient has.

Sir William Osler (1849–1919)

The Americans have watches: we have time.

Taliban Commander

The first two-thirds of my career as a general practitioner are described in Chapters 5 and 16: Practice story, 1962–1975 and Practice story, 1976–1986. The year 1987 was a turning point as we had a vacancy following the retirement of Ann Buxton, and we had interesting applicants. One stood out: Philip Evans had recently completed vocational training in Plymouth and his CV included the Treasurer's prize at Guy's Hospital and obtaining a distinction in the MRCGP examination. The three partners: Russell Steele, Kieran Sweeney, and I, with our wives, invited Philip and his wife, Viv, to dinner.

Trial by dinner was then common and, although strange in hindsight, it created a valuable opportunity to meet wives and husbands. This mattered as at this time, the spouses took it in turn to answer the phone in the evenings, at weekends and on bank holidays when their spouses were on call. It mattered very much to the partnership that the spouses were sensitive and sensible. At least one doctor applying to the practice was turned down because his wife had an obviously patronising attitude to patients. We offered the partnership to Philip Evans, and he accepted immediately and started in October 1987. Philip told me when he arrived that he thought I was the academic in the practice and he had come to do a straightforward service role. I replied that that was fine but that if he ever developed any academic interests, I would do my best to support him.

Practice Management

The first challenge was to build a strong partnership team and if possible, to prevent me from being too dominant in it. I had three generations of Pereira Gray history. I was 14 years more experienced than the next senior partner and I was Chair of the RCGP at the time. I therefore immediately proposed a partnership system in which the chairmanship of the practice would rotate every 12 months. This was to make it clear that, as partners, we were all in it together and the leadership had to be shared. I also suggested, as a means of avoiding unproductive discussions about responsibility that sometimes happen in GP partnerships when big jobs turn up that nobody wants to do, that we divide the main responsibilities for running the practice into four 'ministries': a partner responsible for finances, the 'chancellor of the exchequer'; a partner responsible for staff, the 'minister of labour'; a partner to be responsible for external affairs, the 'foreign secretary'; and a partner to be responsible for the legal requirements and the building, the 'home secretary.' We also created a partnership role for quality assurance and audits and elected Philip to this as the most recently qualified partner. Whenever a

DOI: 10.1201/9781032713601-41

new problem arose, the Practice Manager would be clear about whom to turn to, without discussion. Originally, we planned that all these posts would rotate so that every partner would become familiar in time with all the various aspects of practice organisation.

This system generally worked well, and the rotating chairmanship of the Practice was a great success. So too was the division of responsibilities in the four ministries. However, they did not rotate like the chair. It turned out that some people had a flair for some roles, notably Russell Steele who did an outstanding job with the practice accounts and accountants. Hence, when it came to the annual 'awayday,' partners preferred to stay in their 'ministries.'

We instituted an annual 'retreat' when the partners and practice manager spent a day away together, or at least an evening over dinner, when day-to-day problems were banned from discussion and we concentrated on strategic forward planning. We started producing annual reports for the practice, a key test of leadership and management in a practice that I had previously described in a chapter in the *Medical Annual* (DPG, 1985). We established a regular Friday lunch for the partners when we could be together at the end of the week, with our trainee, to brief each other and share experiences. This became an important time. I was the first generation of GPs to be trained in interactive small groups and during all these 13 years worked quietly to maintain those Friday lunches, which were a precious, informal time, fostering partner relationships.

In the early 1990s, a series of interesting and exciting academic developments occurred in the practice. General practice training continued. I stood down as the trainer in 1981, as did Russell Steele, as his career had developed as an examiner for the RCGP; the trainer baton moved on to Kieran and Philip as shared trainers.

Kieran was awarded a Harkness International Travelling Fellowship. This enabled him and his family to travel to the United States for an academic year and let him meet many leading American academics. The Harkness Fellowships had long been prestigious but had never before been awarded to a GP. Kieran broke through an important glass ceiling for general practice. Because he needed a long locum to cover this fellowship, the Practice employed Sarah Purdy, a former trainee of Philip's who therefore knew the practice well and was excellent. Her academic career blossomed, and she later became a professor of general practice/primary care at Bristol and then the first general practitioner dean at the Bristol Medical School.

Since the 19th century, specialist medicine has been good at creating opportunities for specialists in training to visit the United States. It is striking when reading obituaries of leading specialists how many had that opportunity. General practice has never had the same advantages, so Kieran's experience was important and set an example. Martin Marshall, also from the Exeter vocational training scheme, was also awarded a Harkness soon afterwards. Nevertheless, there is still a serious imbalance in travelling opportunities between the two halves of medicine. Kieran came back fired up from his experience, buzzing with ideas, and highly energised. His career never looked back.

In 1994, the four partners had an editorial published in the *BMJ*: "Generalists in medicine," subtitled "Medicine with a human face." This let us to put into print our practice philosophy as we had thrashed it out together. It gave us an opportunity to describe the term 'living epidemiology,' which I had coined, to capture the idea of general practices analysing and publishing data about living patients, in contrast with much of standard epidemiology, which was about mortality rates. We also reported our commitment to personal lists. We thought this was the first *BMJ* editorial written by four managing partners in a single general practice (DPG *et al.*, 1994). As both Kieran and Philip were developing academically, we signed it from the Institute of General Practice, where we were all on the staff, but we wrote it as four GP partners.

In 1995, Kieran was the first author of two separate articles in the same issue of the *BJGP*, both written from the Practice and both of which made substantial but different impacts. The first was on the use of warfarin in atrial fibrillation to prevent strokes. We discussed this at our Friday lunches when it seemed that this treatment might become standard in the UK. Kieran read the so-called 'landmark' studies. He came back buzzing, as one of them (SPAF, 1991) had excluded 97% of patients from the trial; i.e. most of the patients that general practitioners would be considering for such treatment. He also found striking examples of hospital orientation when serious adverse effects, particularly bleeding, were inappropriately minimised. It was published as "A commentary from general practice" (Sweeney *et al.*, 1995a). I was Chair of Research for the RCGP (Chapter 28, Chair of Research Story) and was speaking at conferences. I poured scorn on the so-called 'landmark' studies and argued strongly that if treatments were to be recommended for use in general practice, they had to be tested on general practice type patients. It was not possible to generalise from trials done on highly selected, atypical, teaching hospital populations. There was no defence to this argument and the DH to its great credit changed the NHS system of undertaking drug trials in the UK and instituted a DH network of recruiting general practices to find general practice patients for studies. Kieran and this one article from a single general practice led to changes to the national system.

His second first authored study, was on patients who do not receive continuity of care within general practice. The idea for this arose even before he joined us as I had suggested it when he was seeking a partnership. He examined the records of 100 patients of mine who had not had continuity of care with me (defined as failing to see me in five consecutive consultations despite the practice operating personal lists) and compared them with 100 of my patients who had received continuity of care with me. The results were interesting, revealing that patients without GP continuity made significantly more use of other open-access medical services and significantly greater use of A&E departments. Moreover, my notes on these patients, often stated "difficult consultation," and "am uneasy here" (Sweeney and DPG, 1995b). In about one-third of the hundred index patients I had made such a note of concern showing I was detecting, in real time, ambiguities in my professional relationships with these patients.

This single practice study was the first report of discontinuity of care. Barbara Starfield, the international guru on general practice/primary care, described this approach in her book *Primary Care* as "interesting" (Starfield, 1998). It triggered much research in the United States on broken continuity (Kahana *et al.*, 1997).

Philip Evans

Philip became interested in patients with hyperlipidaemia, partly as they were common in our practice and because it was unclear how best to manage them in an era before statins. We discussed them often and I helped him apply for small starter research grants, one from the RCGP and one from the Devon FHSA. His research interest grew steadily. A US visiting anthropologist interested in culture linked up and we collaborated using the practice data anonymously with Philip and I becoming co-authors in the resulting publication (Dressler *et al.*, 1992).

A big development occurred in the practice in the early 1990s when Philip said he wanted to do a master's degree by research and asked if I would supervise him. This was doubly encouraging, as it vindicated the strategy of the Institute of General Practice to open opportunities for higher university degrees for able local GPs and it revealed confidence in our personal relationship that he thought we could be equal partners in the practice but be supervised by me in the University. When the Department of General Practice established the first MSc in health care in the University for GPs in 1986, it was a St Leonard's partner, Ann Buxton, who had been one of the first GPs to do it; now seven years later history repeated itself with the Institute's other master's degree, the MPhil by research. The academic issues were easy because of his ability; the relationship needed thought so we did the academic supervisions in my Director's office in the Postgraduate Medical School and I wrote the usual follow-up letters from there.

All went very well and soon it became clear that he had amassed a great deal of information about the readings on a set of tests for patients with hyperlipidaemia, most of which were normal. Textbook teaching, based on hospital practice, recommended that GPs should do multiple tests for every patient with hyperlipidaemia to exclude secondary causes, probably inappropriately. This was published in the *BMJ* (Evans and DPG, 1994). This greatly encouraged him.

The data were taken anonymously from his and my patients in the practice, as this was a technique for making higher research degrees possible for full-time GPs. Philip's MPhil dissertation on hyperlipidaemia in general practice was of high quality. Professor Roger Jones, from King's College London, the external assessor, said it was about MD standard (Evans, 1995). On the day he was awarded the degree, we organised a dinner for him and his wife Viv, and his mother who came from Wales, to celebrate his success. I had learned about celebrating academic success when at the University of Nijmegen, as an external assessor for a GP MD ("Celebrating a thesis the Nijmegen way" (DPG, 1992c).

His research justified the RCGP selecting Philip for a national working party on hyperlipidaemia, chaired by Colin Waine, which brought GPs and national, leading lipid specialists together. There we learnt that coronary lipid plaques could be reversible (Nissen *et al.*, 2005) a new big stimulus to general practitioners to treat high cholesterol. The working party report was published, with Philip and me as co-authors, as *Occasional Paper 55* (Waine Report, 1992).

Kieran Sweeney

Kieran then said he also wanted to do an MPhil and he also asked me to supervise him, so I was supervising two partners simultaneously. He studied patients having miscarriages and minor surgery. It was an interesting experience because their writing was so different. Philip's was precise, ordered and logical, whereas Kieran's writing was imaginative and unpredictable. With Kieran I felt I was riding a tiger as I tried to help him develop his intellect and ideas. Miscarriages are important and a subject that had received too little academic attention. His MPhil dissertation was approved the next year (Sweeney, 1996) and we celebrated with him and his wife Barbara.

Both Philip and Kieran were appointed as research fellows in the Institute of General Practice and after both had gained their master's degrees they were both soon promoted to be lecturers in general practice.

Russell Steele

Russell Steele also developed academically. After being appointed an examiner for the MRCGP, he took the job seriously and went to the examiners' conferences and meetings regularly. In 1989, the Council of the RCGP approved a new route to fellowship of the College, called fellowship by assessment (Chapter 24, Fellowship by Assessment story). This defined detailed criteria for quality of care and the College inspected all the practices that applied. Russell was quick off the mark. Kate Force, a secretary in the practice, gave him much support. He became the ninth GP in the UK to achieve FBA in 1991. The partnership planned for other partners to follow, but both Kieran and Philip became involved with their MPhil degrees and GP training.

Russell too became interested in obtaining an MPhil and he registered for one, choosing Keith Bolden, senior lecturer, as his supervisor. They were close colleagues in the University and often worked together on teaching courses. This worried me. Keith was one of the most hardworking academic members of the institute and a superb teacher but he did not love research as I did, he did not read research articles all the time, and he was not interested in the minutiae of research methodology. Keith and Russell were friends and two of my closest colleagues in my two main Exeter organisations. I was not sure whether to say anything or not, or if so, who to say it to, so I said nothing. A few years later I heard Russell's MPhil had sadly petered out. I wrote to him saying how sorry I was and then carefully added a sentence saying that if he ever wanted to think about it again, I would always be pleased to see him. The message was received. Some years later, Russell came and asked me to supervise his MPhil jointly with an academic in the School of Education. This showed great resilience

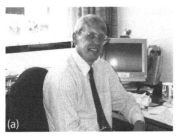 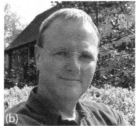 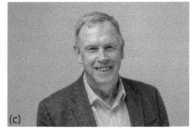

FIGURE 34.1   In 2000, (a) Russell Steele, Partner 1976–2000. (b) Kieran Sweeney, Partner 1986–2000. (c) Philip Evans, Partner 1987– 2000.

on his part and this time all went well and he obtained his MPhil on an educational study (Steele, 2000). Thus, I had the unique privilege of supervising three of my partners in the practice for research master's degrees.

Team Development

We were, as a practice, busy building a multiprofessional team. Other members of the team in other professions, particularly nursing, were encouraged to achieve university degrees, as well as the doctors. During the 1990s, one practice-attached midwife, Teoni McHale, obtained the Exeter MSc as did the Practice Nurse Practitioner in the practice, Dawn Broadhurst from Plymouth. Then the attached district nurse, Deborah Stevens, obtained a bachelor's degree from Plymouth. We do not know of another general practice in which three nurses/midwives all obtained university degrees whilst working in the same practice. The GP partners kept going academically: Helen Keenan obtained the Exeter MSc in 2005 and Alex Harding a doctorate (EdD) in 2017, travelling to London for it, both whilst being managing partners in 2017.

Visitors

Inviting colleagues to visit the practice began in the 1970s (Chapter 16, Practice story, 1976–1986). It was essentially to showcase general practice and to educate us. Leading figures visit hospitals many times more often than general practices and GPs need to think why this is. The sad fact is that there is much less to see in general practice. In particular, there is a dearth of data about what the practice is doing or can do. The challenge is to develop general practices so that national leaders can visit and learn from general practice data (Appendix 10, Practice visitors) and be interested, informed, and sometimes inspired.

The big chance came with computerisation where general practice moved far ahead of the UK hospital service. Bottom-up systems proved superior to top-down ones. Our practice volunteered for the 'Micros for GPs' project, well-run by the Department of Trade and Industry. By 1983 we were experimenting with using a computer. We had some quick wins like repeat prescribing. The real prize, however, was having all diagnoses and consultations recorded and searchable. We took our visitors first to our quality assurance room, showing how we recorded every single consultation in the surgery or at home. Having a room labelled 'quality assurance' on the door made some visitors think.

A notable visitor was Joseph (Joe) Pilling (1945–) who came when he was Grade 3 in the DHSS and he kept in touch as his career progressed. He became Director-General of the Prison Service and his career culminated as Permanent Secretary for Northern Ireland, becoming Sir Joseph Pilling KCB. From the charity world, the Secretary of the Nuffield Provincial Hospitals Trust, Michael

Ashley-Miller (1930–2017) stayed in our home with his wife and it is likely that the demonstration of data in the practice led to my becoming a Trustee of that Trust (Chapter 44, Nuffield Trust story). Andy McKeon first came when he was Principal Private Secretary to Kenneth Clarke as Secretary of State for Health and came back again 30 years later as Chair of the Trustees of the Nuffield Trust. In the private sector, we had the Chief Executive from Merck Sharp and Dohme Ltd. These visitors discussed numerous topics with us and usually met all four partners. We were continually being questioned and informed of new thinking in a special form of continuing education.

Evaluating these visits is not easy, but we had feedback during some of them and afterwards. Joe Pilling who led DH negotiations for one GP contract in the NHS told me in London that he still remembered his visit to my consulting room and the discussions about our figures and said it had changed his perceptions on general practice. Professor Harry Keene came when he was Professor of Medicine at Guy's Hospital and Chair of the British Diabetic Association, dealing with ministers about the care of people with diabetes. We showed him our audits of diabetes care, comparing performance between four partners on the practice computer. We said how we could find every patient with diabetes who had an HbA1c over any figure he chose. He chose 9% and we had the list of patients within a minute. We showed him how we could get the mean HbA1c readings for all our patients with diabetes. There was a long silence as he absorbed this. Then he said: "I can't do that at Guy's!" The future of the care of most people with chronic diseases lay in general practice and he suddenly saw this.

The most high-profile visit was David Willetts, then Principal Private Secretary to the Prime Minister, Mrs Thatcher, whom I had met at 10 Downing Street (Chapter 23, Chair of Council story). He was a highflying civil servant who later switched to politics and acquired the nickname of "two brains." Alone with me in my consulting room, he looked me in the eye over a coffee and said he did not believe the claim GPs were making that they knew their patients. I took him to the office where my paper records were then filed and asked him to pick a dozen records. I explained our coloured star system, which indicates with which partner the patient was registered. I then suggested he simply read out the first name and surname from the front of the envelope. I was able to tell him immediately in ten records whether or not the patient was mine. Sitting on the other side of the room, I was able to give him most of the addresses, usually the family structure and the main medical problems on the summaries. I got them so convincingly right that he stopped after a few and said: "OK, I accept that some GPs know their patients!" This was the only time in my 38 years that I felt the stakes were so high for general practice that I should break some patient confidentiality.

Internal Audits and Continuing Education

We monitored continuity of care received by patients in relation to every partner and displayed the key graphs monthly in our common room. We ran multiple internal audits simultaneously on common chronic diseases with the scores for each partner shown. These were the most important form of continuing education I received. Running a series of comparisons of performance between partners is a test of the personality and strength of mind of those partners. No one likes being shown up as less good than colleagues and a running system of comprehensive audits only works if the partners are committed to quality improvement and the system as a team and are intellectually and emotionally strong enough to live with repeated comparisons. This is not always the case. The running of multiple, internal private audits is for me the essence of medical professionalism.

In 1994, I delivered the Harben lecture to the Royal Institute of Public Health and Hygiene in London (DPG, 1995c). Our series of internal audits were the second leg of our system of using personal lists. It is a powerful tool for quality improvement. Of course, this powerful education was only possible because internal audits by partner relating to defined populations can only be run in general practices using personal lists. We made one interesting and important discovery. Whatever quality criterion we chose, the partners were always scattered with one or other being the best and another being the worst. However, we discovered that with repeated recording two things happened. First, every managing partner improved, and secondly all partners gradually moved to equal the performance of whichever partner was best, all without comment or much discussion. This is one of the most encouraging educational findings I know.

By the mid-1990s, the four partners were working well together as clinicians and academics. We held regular clinical discussions and found we were increasingly identifying women patients who told us they had been sexually abused. We discussed how they presented and their clinical features and found that there was a definite pattern whereby they had high consultation rates and symptoms particularly affecting the urogenital tract. They also seemed to be more likely to suffer from anxiety and depression. The practice had a visitor, Rachel Jenkins, the leading psychiatrist at the DH. She was surprised to find four male GPs identifying as many as 80 of these patients. We decided to write up the syndrome as a four and assembled the evidence of their associated morbidity. We had nearly finished when an article appeared in the *BMJ* reporting many of the same findings as ours (Smith *et al.*, 1995). We wrongly decided to leave the subject as we felt our thunder had been stolen. We should have continued and written it up as four GP partners.

The increasing awareness of this unfortunate syndrome led me to make what was the most difficult diagnosis in my 38 years in practice. One day I saw a woman patient whom I had known since childhood. She was then middle-aged. I suddenly realised that she had almost certainly been sexually abused in childhood and gently put that to her. She burst into tears and said: "How could you know? I have never told anyone at all!" This had been incest, and as a young doctor I had met the abusing father frequently in the home and never suspected anything. Making such a diagnosis correctly in a woman who had never disclosed it is, I believe, an example of the sensitivity that continuity of care and personal lists bring to GPs. The life-course theory is important (Bellis *et al.*, 2017). Its essential message for working GPs is that thinking about patients using a biographical perspective is a privilege and can be exceptionally valuable. This diagnosis illustrates the great power of seeing patients over years, one of the special privileges of general practice, simply not understood by those who have not experienced it. I often wondered how best to teach this feature.

After I retired clinically, I heard a powerful simile from Afghanistan from a Taliban commander: "The Americans have watches: we have time!" This from a developing country which had seen off three wars against the British Empire, forced Russian invaders to withdraw, and was about to do the same to the United States, the richest country on earth. The power of this simile is not only about the concept of time, but it is also of use for general practice in relation to hospital medicine. I was often asked by consultants about what happened to a patient they had seen: it is GPs who over time see what actually happens to patients.

General Practice Fundholding

One big change in the NHS introduced by the 1990 *NHS Act (National Health Service and Community Care Act)* was the option of fundholding for general practitioners. The principle was that selected practices would be allocated a budget for a defined range of NHS services and would have discretion about how it was spent. If they made a saving, the difference could be spent on more services for the practice, but not on the GPs' incomes.

The first year after this was introduced, the practice had numerous discussions but we could not make up our minds. Eventually, I wrote a long policy paper with the tentative conclusion that it would be in the practice's interest to join. This triggered a thorough discussion in the partnership and we decided, unanimously, to apply. A weakness of general practice management is that it is too verbal. In most other walks of life policy papers are usual. We were not big enough to meet the size criterion and we did not see a local Exeter practice with whose values we would be completely happy. We joined with Tony Lewis and Susan Pocklington from Exmouth, with whom we shared professional and academic values. Like Russell, Tony was a Fellow by Assessment of the RCGP (one of the first four in Britain, FBA story, Chapter 24) and was also on the staff of the Department of General Practice. Susan was a committed GP trainer. We were then accepted for fundholding as a combined group.

GP fundholding was controversial. We liked it as it decentralised decisions in an NHS that was overcentralised. It gave more influence to local general practices in relation to the hospital service. We were confident that we could take decisions better, knowing our patients more than middle managers who did not know them. A test case soon arose when the NHS in Devon banned tattoo removal in the NHS. One GP was presented with a young woman with a small tattoo on her face, which she bitterly regretted; she became increasingly upset as she was marrying. The combined group approved the request and it was satisfactorily done by a plastic surgeon when it would not have been considered by a hospital.

The change in attitudes between general practice and the hospital service was most dramatically revealed when a few months after being approved as fundholders, the Chief Executive of the Royal Devon and Exeter Hospital asked to meet us to see how he could best meet our needs. I reflected that my grandfather, my father and I had been sending letters making suggestions to improve care to that same hospital for many years and none of them had been taken up. Many of the letters were not answered. Fundholding changed the practice/hospital relationship significantly for the better.

In our wing of the group, we introduced several innovations to improve the care we could offer our patients. First, we equipped a room to meet the specifications of a physiotherapist and arranged for her to work regularly in the practice. We were influenced by a leading local physiotherapist, Anne Walker, who had completed an excellent MPhil (Walker, 1990) showing that surgery-based physiotherapy was superior to the traditional hospital-based system. This was a big improvement in the service as we could discuss patients face-to-face with the physio, she usually saw them quickly and patients were very satisfied. Second, we negotiated the attachment of a community mental health nurse and agreed a contract so she came weekly to the practice to discuss patients. This worked excellently. Third, we introduced a Liaison Consultant Psychiatrist, Keith Lloyd, Senior Lecturer in the Postgraduate Medical School, who came, sometimes with junior staff, and used my consulting room when I was at the University. He liked this because it was a nicer room than he had in the hospital, and we liked it because communication was better between us. I had some patients who would not go to a psychiatric hospital but were prepared to see a psychiatrist in a consulting room they knew well. Arranging all this took time and the partners held extra meetings, sometimes on Saturday mornings. We invested personal time in the service.

In 1997, a Labour Government was elected. The new Secretary of State for Health, Frank Dobson, was strongly against fundholding and quickly abolished it. The mantra was that it had created unequal arrangements between practices, which indeed it had. However, government policy was to level down by taking away the facilities the fundholders had negotiated so that all general practices would be equal. The alternative policy of leaving the fundholders with the improved arrangements and building other practices up to that level was never considered. To add insult to injury, Tony Blair, as Prime Minister, was later quoted as saying that abolishing fundholding had been a mistake.

The Government paid a price for this policy reversal. Many of the most enthusiastic general practices had invested considerable time and emotional effort in supporting the DH's fundholding system. When it was all reversed after demonstrating many improvements in care some GPs felt let down and distrustful of NHS management.

Once a man arrived at the reception desk with a gun and said he had come to kill one of the GPs! The receptionist was experienced and was superb under pressure. She started talking to the man who said he was annoyed about a decision my partner had taken; she raised her voice enough to alert secretaries working behind a screen, out of sight, but within hearing. They listened carefully and one rang 999. The police arrived quickly. They arrested the man but he was bailed, so my poor partner was left knowing a man was free in the city wanting to kill him.

Mistake by a Regulator

In 1995, the Committee on the Safety of Medicines issued a warning about the oral contraceptive Pill. This induced a media storm. We had large numbers of women on it and GPs had numerous consultations about it. We read it up carefully. My line was "You are taking the Pill to avoid pregnancy, but if you had a normal pregnancy your risk of thrombosis would be greater than the risk of taking this Pill." There were some unusual consultations as when I saw a nurse who came seeking an abortion. We had a good patient-doctor relationship, so I asked her why she had not come to discuss the Pill. She said that it would not have made any difference as: "My husband panicked about the Pill and could not bear seeing me taking them." As I said in my Mackenzie lecture, the role of the GP is to "understand what the patient is feeling at home" (DPG, 1978). The price of this over-cautious medical regulation was tragic: about 26,000 additional conceptions, about 13,000 additional abortions with extra NHS costs of £67 million (Furedi, 1999). Interestingly, patients being prescribed the Pill by GPs seemed to react less anxiously than women on the same Pill prescribed by family planning clinics.

Complaints by Patients

Most of my experience of complaints in the practice were by my patients against the hospital. I usually knew the circumstances well and my sympathies usually lay with the patient. The system was that complainants got a verbose letter from "a quality assurance officer," which was often an elaborate fob-off. What patients needed, in my view, was a meeting with, or at least a letter signed by, the consultant in whose care they had been. Sometimes, the initial response from the hospital triggered litigation, which could have been avoided.

By contrast, a model example of consultant intervention was when a patient complained to me about having been told by one hospital doctor that they should never have a lumbar puncture because of structural abnormalities in the back but was then given one. I wrote to a consultant anaesthetist colleague who saw the family and explained the situation at great length and to their satisfaction.

There were some instances when patients complained against the practice. On one occasion this was because of a rare cancer when one of my partner's notes were, I thought, impeccable, and referral had been appropriate, but the outcome was bad for the patient. I spent much time giving support to this partner, checking the textbook description of the tumour, which stated it was difficult to predict outcomes from it, and offered to go and support him at any NHS hearing. The complaint fizzled out but only after giving my colleague over a year's worry. Another complaint alleged bizarre behaviour by a partner and even involved allegations about his wife, who rarely came to the practice. This complaint was pursued vigorously and we tried hard to clarify it. Eventually, we offered the complainant an hour-long meeting, which I chaired, whilst the partner concerned took notes. After a thick file of papers had been created, the Health Authority eventually dismissed the complaint. The cost was many hours of partner time.

A complaint made against me was that I had continued to prescribe hormone replacement therapy after a patient had been diagnosed with breast cancer. This was easy to deal with as the computer records were clear that I had stopped the treatment once I knew the diagnosis. I was, however, upset as this was a family I knew well and had done dozens of home visits to them.

My experience in the GMC of seeing how practices often mishandled complaints led us to evolve a protocol in the practice whereby an unhappy or angry patient was classified as a 'social emergency.' The receptionists were asked to inform the duty doctor and our protocol was that the duty GP would normally do an immediate home visit in order to discuss the problem on the patient's own territory. One afternoon, when I was on duty, this happened so I visited. I found an angry family steaming because one of the partners had not made a referral he said he would. I sat down and discussed the problem. I was puzzled because the medical problem was not acute or severe, so why was there such tension? I apologised on behalf of the practice, and said they had a right to change practices or, since we operated personal lists, they could change to a different partner within the practice. I said that as they had been registered for some time, the practice would be sorry to lose them. After about half an hour the anger abated and I was offered a cup of tea, which I was pleased to accept. They said that their long relationship with the practice had generally been very satisfactory but explained that they had private medical insurance which was about to run out. If the referral was not made quickly they would lose their cover. I said the referral would be made the next day and they started smiling. As I got up to go, the wife said: "There's no need to send the letter now." "What letter?" I asked. She pointed to one already stamped, making an official complaint. Had it been posted the Practice would have had to spend much time responding formally.

One tricky complaint was against an attached health visitor who had breached confidentiality. She had made a serious mistake and I thought she would be in trouble if investigated. I offered to take her on a home visit to the family. She was unsure, but we were working well together and she trusted me. There was a complex social background and the family was living in poor accommodation. I had known them for many years. We sat in their home together and let them pour out their hurt for a long time. When the steam had gone out of the conversation, I looked the couple straight in the eye and said that modern family doctors worked in teams. Health visitors were important, and I was very pleased to be working with this one and thought she was a good health visitor. The Health Visitor then burst into tears. I said, as gently as I could, that she might want to say how sorry she was and how this would never happen again. She did so, movingly, speaking from the heart. The young couple were shaken by her tears. They said how important our practice was to them. I said I was confident that my colleague would never do that again and I hoped that they could now accept her apology and leave it at that. They agreed. Most complaints by patients are to ensure the professional regrets the mistake and are intended to prevent repetition. Working class families do not welcome paperwork, so I suggested they shook hands with the Health Visitor. The verbal agreement was sealed non-verbally.

In the past, the complaints system was tilted against the patient, particularly in hospitals. Today patients have a fairer say but sometimes at the cost of great expense, time and worry for doctors and staff. There needs to be a review of complaint procedures to ensure they are dealt with more expeditiously. Perhaps arbitration? It is absurd that, in some cases averaging over a year, that the NHS can pay lawyers more than it pays the patient in damages.

During my Presidency I was concerned about receiving a complaint after the Waine precedent (Chapter 20, Experiences in the Executive). Might I have to resign? Nowadays the RCGP must think more about complaints as the average NHS GP has a current complaint to deal with at any one time. When I retired, I was pleased that three generations of GPs in my family had completed 105 consecutive years in our practice without a formal complaint being sustained against any of us.

Hormone Replacement Therapy (HRT) 1995–1996

When HRT arrived, it was warmly welcomed by patients and doctors as it offered better relief from menopausal symptoms than anything else. It was used by increasing numbers of women. Then one day my subscription to the *New England Journal of Medicine* enabled me to read Colditz *et al.* (1995), who reported a significant increase in breast cancer in women taking HRT. We discussed this in the partnership where we were all prescribing HRT increasingly. That week we started warning patients that there was a small but definite risk of breast cancer and were careful to record this in the notes. About half of my own patients decided not to take it, depending mainly on how bad their menopausal symptoms were. We wrote it up as a partnership to alert other GPs "HRT prescribing – a paradigm for the complexity of prescribing in general practice?" (DPG *et al.*, 1996c). The reaction from some women's groups was strongly negative; however, several GPs spoke to us and followed our lead.

Beral *et al.* (2019), 23 years later, summarised the evidence, including randomised trials. The *Lancet's* (Kotsopoulos, 2019) editorial title was "Menopausal hormones: *Definitive* evidence for breast cancer" (author's italics). HRT does cause breast cancer and British women run a 6.3% general risk, women on HRT have an 8.3% risk. For every 50 women taking it one extra breast cancer will occur. I read this with mixed feelings: pleased that our partners' meeting in the practice and our four-GP partner article had been vindicated and that our practice with 250 patients taking HRT, and with the other practices which asked us, would probably have saved several breast cancers. However, I regretted how slow academic medicine had been to tackle this risk. The reason is caution about observational studies; i.e. research not based on randomised trials. Some observational studies have been proved wrong but, as this story shows, some are early warnings. British academic medicine, for the 23 years after our article made a type-2 error, missing an important truth. Whilst research bodies should follow trials, professional bodies should write more about the state of the art and offer judgements on the 'balance of probabilities.' There is a bias towards HRT. Sung *et al.'s* (2022) report that it is significantly associated with a risk of dementia is rarely discussed.

Home Visiting

Throughout my career home visits were a core part of the job. I would sometimes go on one without a request when a family was in trouble. However, each successive generation of GPs valued them less. For me a visit provides special information and understanding about the patient as a person and how they live. Patients divulge more at home and doing visits builds relationships (DPG, 1978). If general practice abandons visits, it will weaken relationships with patients, GPs' understanding of patients, and will exaggerate a physical orientation to care.

Distributed Leadership – Other Awards

Following the quality initiatives led by the doctors, Tim Smith, the Practice Manager, proposed applying for an Investor in People award. The partners welcomed this and he then led us systematically. Investors in People is a quality award for organisations that can demonstrate good organisational systems regardless of their field. A plaque is displayed by the organisation when an award is made. Tim led well and the practice passed easily. A celebration photograph includes Gillian (later Dame) Morgan, Chief Executive of the Health Authority.

In the late 1990s, the NHS advertised for research-active general practices. Philip led the practice bid, which involved us both working until midnight to meet the deadline and this too was successful in 1995. Funds received enabled us to employ a research staff member and rent research premises close to the practice premises. At this time Philip also led us to become a 'Beacon' NHS general practice, so receiving some funds to demonstrate agreed services to other practices. By the late 1990s leadership in the practice had become distributed.

The Academic Triad of Service, Teaching, and Research

British teaching hospitals have long proclaimed the strength of combining service, teaching, and research. Teaching hospitals like the term 'centres of excellence,' and they provide better care for patients than other hospitals (Ayanian and Weissman, 2002). Medical schools are funded on the basis that medical students should learn in a 'research-rich environment.' For 200 years, a strategic challenge for general practice has been how to replicate this triad in general practice. The GP NHS contract has always, sadly, been research free. Professional teaching only developed in general practice in the second half of the 20th century (Chapter 14, Regional Adviser story) but within 40 years became the best in the medical profession (Lamberts *et al.,* 2006; Goldacre *et al.,* 2008; Paice and Smith, 2009;

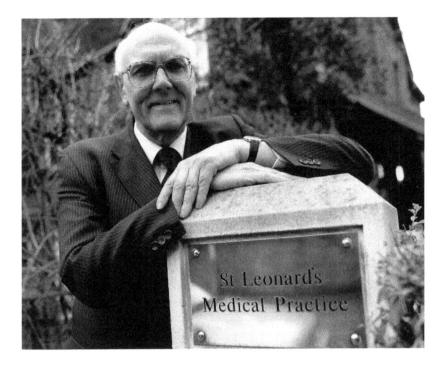

FIGURE 34.2   At the Practice the day the Knighthood was announced. *Express and Echo, Exeter.*

GMC, 2018). Getting serious research done in general practice is a problem as GP academics research in universities and not in their practices. This means designing and conducting research, not just finding patients for other people's studies.

Philip's success in funding a research general practice completed the triad. With an award for clinical service (FBA), higher education awards (seven master's degrees from the Practice) and an organisational award (Investor in People), the academic triad was established in general practice.

My knighthood was announced on 31 December 1998 when I was 63. The press took photographs at the entrance to the practice where I had worked all my life. I became the only medical knight working as an NHS GP in the UK. My patients were hugely enthusiastic, but some were worried about how to address me and I said "Keep it as before...Dr Denis."

Retirement 2000

In 2000, I was retiring as College President in November. I planned to work half-time in the Practice until I was 70 and I was looking forward to having more time with my patients. However, in June the Academy suddenly elected me Chair (Chapter 36; Vice-Chairman, Academy of Medical Royal Colleges). This top leadership position in the medical profession is parallel to the Presidency of the GMC. I gave three months' notice to retire on 30 September, virtually on my 65th birthday. Kieran resigned the same day, to work with the Commission for Health Improvement, a new NHS regulator in London.

My last three months in the practice were unlike anything I had experienced. Patients booked to see me without any problem to discuss, but simply to thank me and say goodbye. I was fascinated by how these patients had obviously prepared what they wanted to say and were able in a few minutes to encapsulate the essence of our professional relationship, often over 30 years. Only a few referred to diagnoses I had made; the great majority referred to care, about my taking a lot of trouble, coming out at night, and "going the extra mile."

I had always been formal at work, wearing a jacket and tie when consulting. Now I was in numerous consultations with women patients, many of whom I knew well, who stood up and came round the side of my desk and kissed me goodbye. It was intensely moving and I was often left in tears. I described those three months to my family as my 'wet' finale. The experience was unexpected and immensely empowering. This was an unexpected evaluation of the real job, which is what matters most. Whatever the academic work in the practice, those patients were saying that the ordinary GP's job was of great value and that they had really appreciated it.

ADDENDA

Kieran Sweeney soon left the NHS regulator and returned to Exeter. His writings were outstanding and he was appointed an honorary professor in 2008, for scholarship. This was just before his tragic death in 2009 from mesothelioma, when he was only in his 50s.

We had a letter, co-signed with two students, reporting the academic triad being achieved in general practice published in the *BJG*P (DPG *et al.,* 2021).

Section VIII

35

President of the RCGP 1997–2000

The ballot is stronger than the bullet.

Abraham Lincoln (1809–1865)

I had been approached in 1993 about the Presidency of the College when John Ball had rung me and asked if I was going to stand in the 1994 election. I was 58 and thought I was too young and with too many jobs I was enjoying, so I said: "No." He then stood himself. Next, Lotte Newman asked me to be one of her nominators. I agreed knowing full well it might be difficult if John Ball won, as I had previously got on well with him. But Lotte had been one of my vice-chairs when I was Chair of Council and she had won BMA elections to its Council in highly competitive elections. I thought it was high time the College had a woman President as there had been none since Annis Gillie in the 1960s. The Presidency was then a tight contest between these two.

John Ball was a big BMA man, a former Chair of the GMSC, and a Consultant Adviser to the DH. He was physically tall and imposing and was an unusually good speaker with great wit. When chairing the publishing section of the College he had taken Jill and me out to dinner. Lotte Newman had served much longer in the College and was a big figure in international general practice on the continent, where she had been President of both the European organisations of general practice: SIMG and European WONCA, and had been influential in helping them to merge. She had delivered her James Mackenzie lecture on women's issues (Newman, 1992), a dignified feminist perspective. It was to be a close election and reading the body language and hearing all the discussion, I thought John would win. Lotte was anxious, especially about getting the vote in from the overseas members, who would support her.

Then, by chance, the GMC circulated its voting papers for its 1994 election to every registered doctor in England. I was standing for the first time in this election. I got several questions at meetings and telephone calls at home, asking me what I thought of John Ball's manifesto for the GMC, which did not mention his College fellowship. Many noted that Sandy Macara, another BMA leader and another candidate, had included his HonFRCGP in his statement.

The doctors who rang me saw an inconsistency between Ball omitting his FRCGP and standing to be PRCGP. As one of them put it to me, if a candidate for the Presidency of the College could not list his RCGP fellowship in the GMC world, there was a problem.

Then came the dramatic news that Lotte had won by only 19 votes across the whole College membership. This meant that if only ten doctors had voted the other way she would have lost. I reckon John Ball had lost more than ten votes amongst those who contacted me, perhaps many more across the UK. This was the closest vote since the election had gone to the whole RCGP membership. It made Lotte Newman President from November 1994 to November 1997 and the second female President after Annis Gillie.

In 1996, Jill and I had discussed whether I should run for the Presidency the next time round. We agreed this was the optimum time and I gathered the necessary supporters to represent all the major constituencies. As soon as the list opened in July 1996, I sent my entry in. Jill said she thought I would be elected unopposed, but I didn't believe her and I thought John Ball might stand again.

I was tense as the days ran out in the closing date for applications of 31 March 1997, as there is a pattern of names emerging late. However, Jill was proved right when Sarah Thewlis, General Manager, rang us at home to say no other candidate had emerged. I was elected, as with the chairmanship ten years earlier, unopposed. This gave me eight months to prepare.

Inauguration as President

My inauguration as President was at the AGM of the College in London in November 1997. The meeting ran very late and sadly some of those who had come from the South West, especially to support me, had to leave before it. In my speech I thanked all those electing me, especially for the honour of being unopposed and for the privilege of serving when the new century came in.

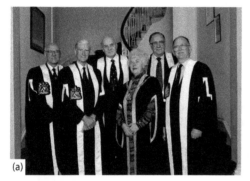
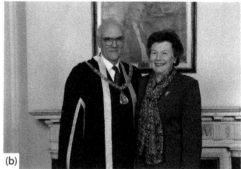

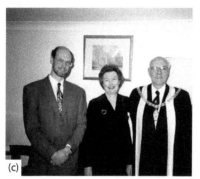
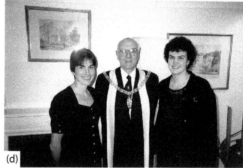

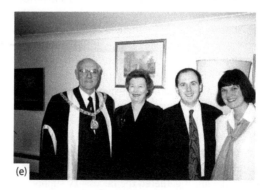

FIGURE 35.1 In 1997: (a) The day before my installation. With five former PRCGPs: Alastair Donald, John Horder, Lotte Newman, Stuart Carne, and Michael Drury. (b) Newly installed as President with Jill. (c) Newly installed as President with Peter (son). (d) Newly installed as President with two daughters Penelope and Jennifer. (e) Newly installed as President with Jill, Elizabeth (daughter), and Graham (husband).

Elections are the mechanism by which people are given power and influence, and a democratic election by thousands of colleagues is empowering. I was particularly empowered by being elected unopposed, which is unusual in the RCGP. Votes are made privately, and in this sense, in Abraham Lincoln's words: "the ballot is stronger than the bullet."

The night before the ceremony I was with five former presidents; and soon after installation I was photographed with Jill; my son Peter; my two daughters Penelope and Jennifer together; and daughter Elizabeth with her husband Graham.

From November 1997, I again became a member of the Conference of Medical Royal Colleges and Faculties, now renamed the Academy of Medical Royal Colleges. As the RCGP was the only College with two members and as I had been the first RCGP Chair of Council to be allowed in (Chapter 23, Chair of Council story), so I became the first British doctor to be a member twice, albeit seven years apart.

I thus had personal experience of six Chairs: two PRCPaths, and one PRCP, one PRCS, one PRCOG. When I returned, Sir Naren (Later Lord) Patel PRCOG (1938–) was Chair. I was serving with John Toby, now Chair of Council, with whom I got on well. The BMA invited me, as President, to be an observer on the Council of the BMA, which met frequently. Thus in 1998 I was, as I had been in 1971, getting the papers for meetings of the Councils of both the BMA and the RCGP.

The President of the College traditionally visits as many of the faculties of the College (regional branches) as possible, of which there were 33, including one in Northern Ireland, one in the Republic of Ireland, and five in Scotland. Some of these faculties had as many as 900 members. I really enjoyed these visits. They were a chance for local members to talk in friendly and informal settings. Some were of outings of various kinds; most were evening receptions. Several times I was asked to present membership certificates to new members. Jill came with me on several visits and always if she was specifically invited. No other member of the College gets the chance to meet so many members and I could feedback to the officers the issues causing concern to the membership. This system is one of the important advantages of the RCGP constitution, as the College Chair would never have the time for so many visits.

I attended the meetings of the officers of the College who met regularly over breakfast, chaired by the Chair. The others present were the Secretary, Treasurer, one or two Vice-Chairs, and the General Manager/Chief Executive. Information was exchanged, tricky topics aired, and action not needing a committee despatched.

The Council Executive met between Council meetings, usually for a whole day, and these were usually preceded by dinner in house the night before. Frequency varied over the years, but there were typically six or seven meetings a year. I remained on the Council.

Honours

In 1997 I delivered the annual address to the Royal Society of Health. This was especially pleasing for someone of my generation, as I was the first GP to be invited since the address of 1962 in which Sir Arthur Thompson's title had been: "Is general practice outmoded?" (Thompson, 1963). I documented the amount of personal preventive medicine in my practice, the first time this had been done (DPG, 1997c). I was elected an Honorary Fellow of the Royal Society of Health.

That year I was awarded an HonDSc at De Montfort University. Jill was invited with me to the ceremony, and I gave a lecture for staff the evening before the ceremony at which Ali Rashid and David Haslam, College colleagues, were present; I then gave an address to the students and parents in the ceremony. At another award ceremony at Harrogate when Jill came with me, on opening the certificate, it read: Professor Sir George Alberti! We did a swap later.

As President, I was fortunate to be invited to give several eponymous lectures, a privilege I always appreciated and enjoyed (Appendix 2) They included the Haliburton Hume in the North of England (1998), the Albert Wander lecture to the Royal Society of Medicine (1998), the Andrew Smith in the North of England Faculty of the College (1998), and the Bruce lecture for the Armed Forces (1999).

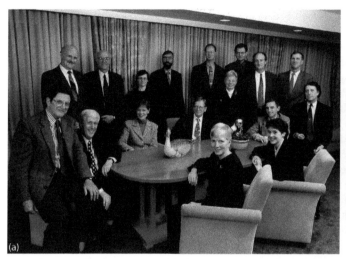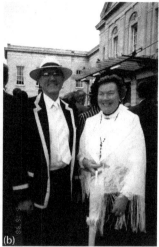

FIGURE 35.2   In 1998: (a) The Netherlands Conference on Dietary Advice. Chris van Weel on the right, wearing his Hon FRCGP tie, Bennelux Press. (b) London party with Jill where I am wearing my Cambridge half blue blazer and tie.

In the latter I took the chance to state that generalist doctors should receive equal pay with specialists at any rank, which was very much not the case at the time (Just GPs). At one summer party with Jill I wore my Cambridge half-blue blazer and tie, which I had never worn at Cambridge.

Knighthood

At the College awards dinner in November 1998, Jill was sitting next to Alastair Donald (1926–2005), President from 1992 to 1994 and had been appointed CBE. Over dinner he said quietly to Jill: "I think Denis might get a knighthood at the end of his Presidency!" which Jill was intrigued to hear. I went home after the College AGM that same weekend to find a big pile of letters waiting. Several of these were asking me if I would write a reference, which was then quite common. I opened a letter without looking at the envelope. "Good heavens!" I said to Jill: "someone is asking me to write a reference for a knighthood!" I realised how ridiculous it sounded and then read the letter carefully. It was from No 10 Downing Street saying that they had me in mind to recommend for a knighthood. Was I prepared to accept? I turned to Jill and asked her how she felt about becoming a Lady? It was a requirement that it was all kept confidential, so we did not know for certain until the press started ringing for interviews on 31 December 1998. The published citation stated: "For services to quality assurance in general practice and the Presidency of the RCGP." I was the only working NHS GP then knighted so I wanted to be photographed at the entrance to the Practice in which I had worked all my life.

The invitation to the investiture at Buckingham Palace stipulated no more than two guests, a problem for a family with four children. However, Jill and I had taken Peter and Penelope to the OBE investiture, so we took Elizabeth and Jennifer for this second ceremony. We felt very fortunate to have had a second bite of the cherry and to be able to involve all our four children.

Coming out of Buckingham Palace, the rest of the family were all there to greet us at the gates and we went to have a big family lunch at the Savoy. Subsequently, the RCGP laid on a party for me to celebrate, as the first RCGP President to be knighted in office, and only the third among 18 RCGP Presidents.

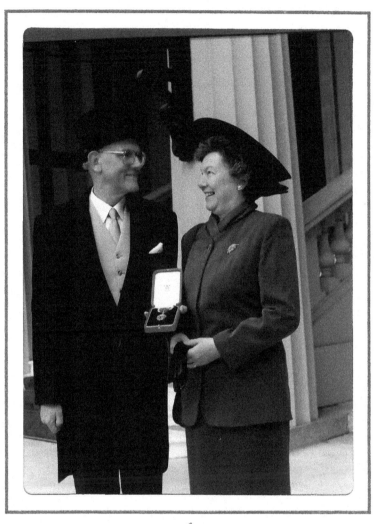

INVESTITURE AT BUCKINGHAM PALACE

FIGURE 35.3   With Jill at Buckingham Palace after being knighted, 1999.

Academy of Medical Royal Colleges

In the election for officers of the Academy at the end of Sir Naren (later Lord) Patel's (1938–) Chairmanship, Roddy MacSween (1935–2015; PRCPath) was elected the next Chair and Leo Strunin (1937–2020) President of the Anaesthetists and I were elected the two Vice-Chairs, to my great surprise (Chapter 36, Vice-Chair Academy story).

This election changed my Presidency as I then had regular officer meetings in the Academy and was an active, working officer which included writing several papers for the Academy. In addition, being an officer of the Academy made me ex-officio a member of the Joint Consultants' Committee and ex officio a member of two national BMA Conferences (Chapter 36, Vice-Chair Academy story; Chapter 37, Three National Meetings story).

I spoke at some wider Academy meetings. At a big conference on continuing medical education, co-hosted by the Academy of Medical Colleges, I presented the radical idea of Fellowship by Assessment which the RCGP had developed, then and now unique amongst the Royal Colleges. This caused quite a stir as described in Chapter 24, the Fellowship by Assessment story, as no other Royal College had anything like it.

On another occasion, it was agreed that the Presidents would present their disciplines to each other. Most of the Presidents gave pot boilers in their field. I tackled the issue of whether general practitioners were clinically inferior to specialists, with numerous references. This showed that in several fields, GPs performed well in direct, head-to-head comparison with specialists (Scott and Freeman, 1992; Carey *et al.*, 1995). Two Presidents said to me: "You were the only one of us to take that session seriously."

As either President of the RCGP or Vice-Chair of the Academy of Medical Royal Colleges, I was invited to a string of meetings organised by the DH. The sites of the meetings varied but several were in the Cathedral Room at Richmond House or, if larger, at the Queen Elizabeth Conference Centre, opposite the Houses of Parliament. I attended the launch by Frank Dobson, then Secretary of State for Health, of the National Institute for Clinical Excellence [later renamed the National Institute for Health and Care Excellence]. It was to be headed by Michael Rawlins, a Professor of Clinical Pharmacology, who had been knighted on the same day as I had been. I was interested in how the profession varied in its responses. Many colleagues like me, saw this as the first systematic Government rationing body, others clearly did not foresee it would soon limit prescribing by specialists. For the first time, I began to wonder if the profession needed to establish leadership training programmes for future College leaders which would teach political awareness.

I disliked the use of the word 'excellence' in the title of NICE, a classic New Labour language technique. It offended my editorial interest in the precise use of words, as whatever this body was to be about, it was not going to be an organisation promoting excellence in clinical care. The word was really loved by the spin doctors with its positive connotations. It was used again later, inappropriately in my view, in the title Committee for Excellence in Health Care Regulators. Later, in a seminar at the Nuffield Trust under Chatham House rules, I was asked for any example of the manipulation of language by DH officials. I raised a laugh by saying that NICE was NASTY! An even worse example of misuse of words came for PCTs when, charged with commissioning health care, in all conscience a difficult enough task, they were burdened with the task of achieving 'world-class' commissioning. Never once did I see the DH, which used this term endlessly, provide a robust comparison of health commissioning in different countries.

Ceremonial dinners by national institutions like Royal Colleges are not well understood outside leadership circles and they are undervalued as a mechanism for networking and allowing ideas to be presented in safe surroundings. In this context, politicians often understand them better than some of their hosts, who are conscious of their costs.

I benefited from a stream of invitations for over eleven and a half years (3.75 years as Chair of RCGP Council, three years as President of the RCGP, 1.75 years more in the Academy, and three years as Chair of the Nuffield Trust), perhaps more than any other British doctor. I found the contacts, the subtleties of status, the informal information and the gossip, invaluable, quite apart from enjoying some very good meals, some in majestic surroundings like the Guildhall in the City of London, and often accompanied by Jill.

In these relaxed surroundings of dinners, leaders meet and mix and exchange news and ideas, which spread quickly. The dinners give cabinet ministers a chance to set out their policies and if they are skilled, they can reach key leader groups in the profession as these dinners in medicine are mainly attended by members of the Councils of the Colleges. Meanwhile, the Presidents may get a rare chance of a private talk with the Secretary of State. Dinners have a cultural significance in fostering relationship building and being a setting where confidential information is exchanged between leaders, off the record.

Spring General Meeting, Exeter 1998

By coincidence, the Spring General Meeting of the College was held in Exeter during my Presidency. I had been involved in the 1977 Exeter meeting (Chapter 13, Department/Institute of General Practice story) when the College had a single faculty across the Southwestern region. Now twenty odd years later it had come round again, but now it was the Tamar Faculty, founded in 1980, which was host.

It was a special event as I was to be on home ground and I knew all the local Tamar organisers and everyone in the Institute of General Practice and I was the only Professor of General Practice in the two counties of Devon and Cornwall. I was interested in patient participation and suggested that there should be an after-dinner speech at the dinner by a patient. Professor Robert Snowden of the University of Exeter, a sociologist who had led a nationally successful Institute in the University,

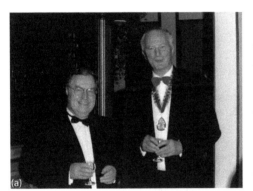
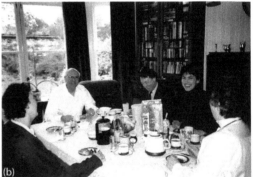
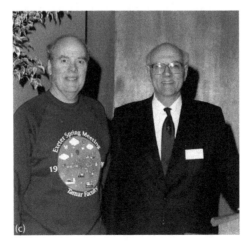

FIGURE 35.4 In 1998: (a) Keith Bolden, Provost, Tamar Faculty at RCGP Spring Meeting with Professor Stuart Murray. Quay Studios. (b) Breakfast at home with Jennifer, Chris van Weel (the Netherlands) Penelope and Jill. (c) RCGP Spring Meeting. Michael Hall, organiser.

was invited. Bob Snowden did us proud, teasing me gently, and describing how I had been the family doctor for many years for his wife and him and their children. He described how I had diagnosed his type two diabetes and how I had arranged a long Saturday morning appointment to take him through the implications and to prepare him to take control of his illness for life.

History of General Practice 1998

John Horder (1919–2012) was crucial in linking with Irvine Loudon and Charles Webster to edit jointly a history of general practice 1948–1997. Webster was a leading historian at All Souls College Oxford, the official historian of the NHS, and he invited me to lead a seminar there subsequently. Loudon (1924–2015) was a GP who left medicine to become a medical historian and had written *Medical Care and the General Practitioner, 1750–1850* (Loudon and Loudon, 1986). Anne Digby was writing a book on general practice for the period 1850–1948, so the challenge was to write the history of general practice in the 50 years after the NHS, completing an historical trilogy. Work on our volume began in 1991 and I was a member of the steering committee. Horder chaired it and gave me chapter 8 on postgraduate training and continuing education. OUP edited rigorously and produced the book *General Practice under the NHS 1948–1997* in hardback (Loudon, Horder and Webster, Eds, 1998). Digby's (1999) book *The Evolution of British General Practice 1850–1948* was published the year after ours. General practice thus has its history covering 200 years covered in these three books.

Honorary Awards

I was elected a fellow of the RCP in 1999. This, the oldest of the English medical Royal Colleges (founded 1518) has long had a tradition of conferring fellowships on medical leaders in many disciplines. In fact, these are honorary fellowships but are not called that. In my ceremony, I was admitted alongside several very distinguished colleagues. However, Jill and I were disappointed with my bland citation, which must have left many in the room wondering why I was there.

There were two ceremonies at Queen Mary College first when I introduced Yvonne Carter's professorial lecture,and then a few years later when I received an Honorary Fellowship of Queen Mary College in the University of London). The Warden there (Dean, Sandy McNeish, 1938–2021) was masterly in capturing me as a person, as well as my achievements and did so with great wit. We are fortunate to have that one on a video. Unlike all the other honorary awards in other faculties and colleges, I used my membership of the Physicians' College regularly. I often went to the Harveian lecture, one of that College's big annual events where the dress code is dinner jacket with decorations. As one leaves the lecture theatre one is given a printed copy of the lecture. This is followed by a formal dinner. I heard both the two, rare, Harveian lectures delivered by GPs: Brian Jarman (2000) and Iona Heath. The latter was outstanding and has influenced several students subsequently (Heath, 2011). I was invited to deliver the citation for fellowship of the RCP for David Haslam, an RCGP President after me and was careful to do it as well as a I could to avoid another GP having my experience.

I never knew who they were, or why I had supporters in the Royal Institute for Public Health and Hygiene. This was a worthy 19th-century body promoting public health. It had a long and honourable tradition of holding an annual lecture, and I was surprised to be invited to deliver it in 1994. The list of previous lecturers was truly world class, including Pasteur, Koch and Alexander Fleming. My brother and sister-in-law, Jonathan and Gay, came with Peter, as did Hilla Gittins and other staff of the JCPTGP, where I was Chair at the time. I made much of thanking the Institution for inviting the first GP, but this revealed my ignorance as Koch (of Koch's postulates) had done his work as a GP in Germany. I should have said 'British GP.' My title was "Primary care and the public health" and I used the lecture to present data from the Practice, including evidence of how inter-partner comparisons of

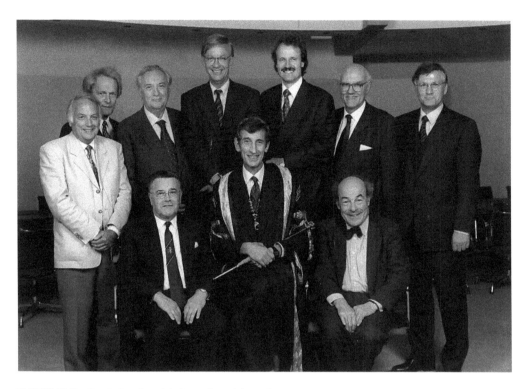

FIGURE 35.5 Hon Fellow Royal College of Physicians of London. Centre, President Sir George Alberti, Front left, Roddy MacSween, 1999.

performance within a group practice using personal lists (DPG, 1979a) were effective in improving performance (DPG, 1995c). This is an exciting educational phenomenon, as we had found not only that every GP improved but also that the group of partners settled at the level of the best of us.

I finished with a strong claim for medical generalists, who alone straddled the dimensions of physical ills and also reached out into families and communities. I also showed how very few adult smokers there were among the elderly. (The computer clerk when searching in our quality assurance room in

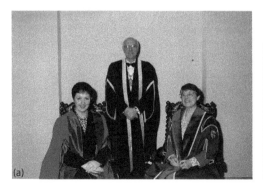
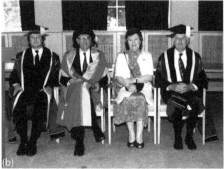

FIGURE 35.6 (a) Queen Mary College. Introducing Yvonne Carter's inaugural professorial lecture, 1988. (b) Honorary Fellowship, Queen Mary College. With Jill, Sir Adrian Smith, later President of the Royal Society (left), and Sir Christopher France (right), 2000.

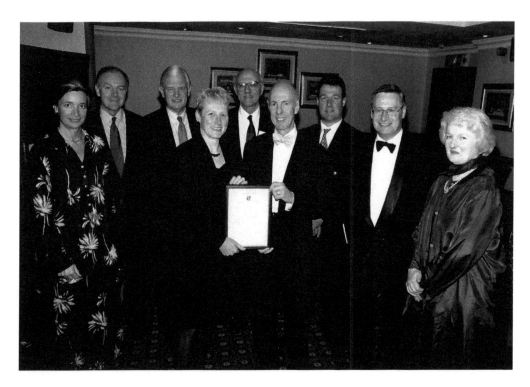

FIGURE 35.7 Judge of the MSD Foundation Prize, with Sir Donad Irvine (third left), Trish Greenhalgh (winner), Sir Denis Pereira Gray, Professor Marshall Marinker, Professor Mike Pringle, Sir Cyril Chantler, and Baroness Neuberger, 2000.

the practice had come anxiously to me to say that she couldn't find more than five in that age group.) The gold medal of the Institute was presented to Sir David Weatherall (1933–2018), Regius Professor of Medicine at Oxford.

Five years later, in 1999, whilst President, the RSPHH awarded me this gold medal and it was presented in London by their President, Sir Donald Acheson (1926–2010). I had to make the after-dinner speech. Donald Irvine delivered the Harben Lecture that year so we were Lecturer and Medallist in the same ceremonies. Our intertwining careers, led some people inadvertently to call me "Sir Donald!" Some years later, this Institute merged with the Royal Society of Health, to become the Royal Society for Public Health and my Honorary Fellowship transferred to that.

I was one of the Judges for the MSD Foundation award won by Trish Greenhalgh, later professor at Oxford.

I was elected to Honorary Fellowship of the Institute of Health Service Managers (IHSM) after it merged with the Association of Practice Managers and Rosey Foster became Deputy Director. They developed a Fellowship by Assessment programme for practice managers modelled on the RCGP FBA (Chapter 24, Fellowship by Assessment story) to which she had contributed. Ali Rashid initiated me being awarded an Honorary Doctor of Science (HonDSc) at deMontfort University and later Michael Pringle was supportive in getting me awarded a second Honorary Doctorate (Hon DM) by the University of Nottingham. Jill and I stayed with him and his wife Nikki in their home and I spoke at the graduation ceremony.

The College bought premises in Edinburgh to provide a college home in Scotland, a beautiful Georgian building. I was involved in the opening and met a young Health Minister, who later became first Minister of Scotland – Nicola Sturgeon.

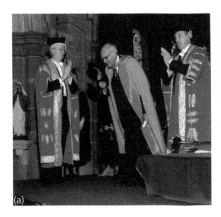 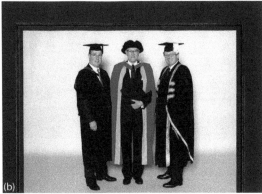

FIGURE 35.8 (a) Honorary DSc De Montfort University, 2000. (b) University of Nottingham. Honorary Doctor of Medicine, with Professor Mike Pringle and the Vice-Chancellor, 2003.

In the Glasgow College at a big dinner, Jill and I were introduced to Mary McAleese, a former President of Ireland. At AGMs in the RCGP I had the pleasure of presenting Honorary Fellowships to Barbara Starfield and Liam Donaldson.

King Charles, then HRH Prince of Wales, came to the College twice (photo) once elegantly supporting a group of people with special needs.

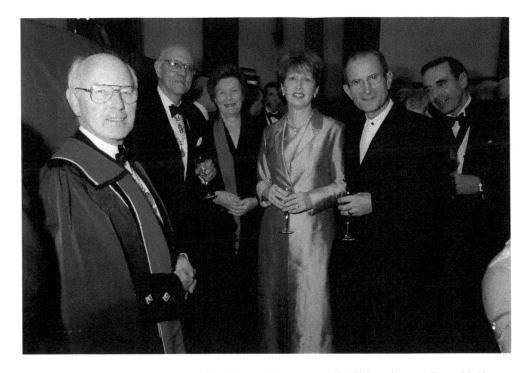

FIGURE 35.9 Glasgow Royal College of Physicians and Surgeons at their 400th anniversary dinner, Mr Norman Mackay (Host President), DPG (as PRCGP), Jill, Mary McAleese, former president of Ireland, her husband Jim McEwen (President Faculty of Public Health) in 1999.

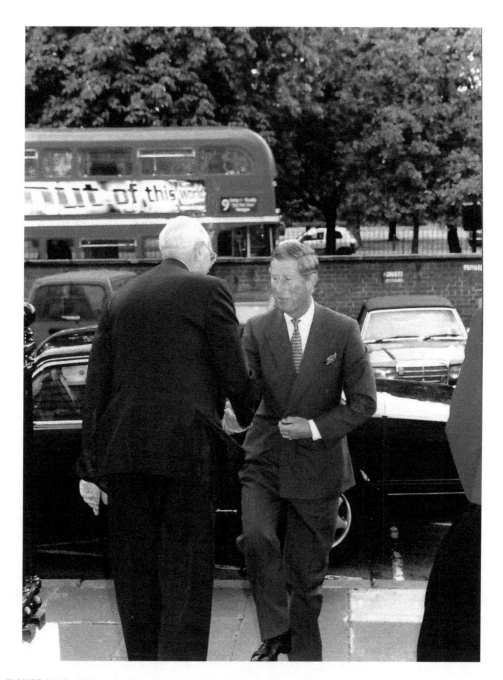

FIGURE 35.10   Welcoming King Charles, as Prince of Wales, to the RCGP, 1999.

Edgar Hope-Simpson (1908–2003)

Edgar Hope-Simpson was one of the most outstanding GPs of the 20th century and, in my opinion, made the single most important GP research discovery of the century. Of special importance is that he did it from an ordinary service general practice and not from a university. When I was a medical

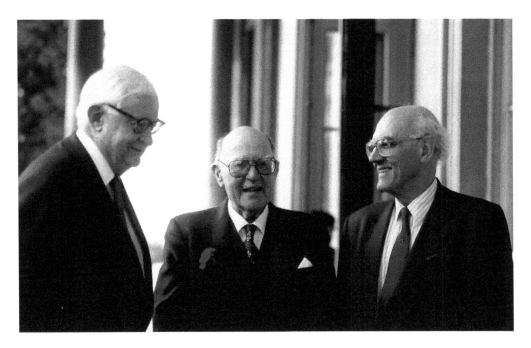

FIGURE 35.11   Gloucester. Presenting the George Abercrombie Award to Edgar Hope-Simpson (centre) in his home. The Cheltenham Newspaper Ltd. 1999.

student it was known that chickenpox and shingles had some sort of relationship but some thought that they were two diseases. Hope-Simpson's brilliance was to grasp that they are two manifestations of infection with a single virus. To make sense of the clinical phenomena he postulated that, after infecting young people, the virus could then lie dormant for many years and be reactivated as shingles. When I qualified in 1960 that seemed ridiculous. However, Hope-Simpson proved it and reported this in the Albert Wander lecture (Hope-Simpson, 1965). This was the nearest any GP got to a Nobel Prize in the 20th century. The researchers who followed up his work and isolated the virus did receive a Nobel Prize, as did other researchers who later found a treatment for shingles. Hope-Simpson was appointed OBE.

In the RCGP, the President is the ex-officio Chair of the Awards Committee. I wrote the proposal for a high award for Hope-Simpson and the Awards Committee recommended the George Abercrombie Award. Council endorsed this and I immediately got in touch with him. However, he was then over 90 and said he could not come to London so I said I would go to him. I went to Cirencester for the only major award I presented on behalf of the College in a GP's home. He was a delightful man, a committed Quaker with a rare tranquillity that I had previously seen only in some nuns after a lifetime's Christian service. His wife, Julia, was very supportive and understood his work. They gave me a lovely tea and then we chatted for some time with him as alert as ever. I stood to read his citation and presented him with the attractive silver award. He had received several honours, but he was a College loyalist and was absolutely delighted. This unusual event gave me great pleasure.

Cuba 2000

In the spring of 2000, Jill and I spent a week in Cuba. We were invited by Patrick Pietroni, whom I had known for years. He was one of the radicals in British general practice who had set up an innovative general practice in the crypt of Marylebone Church in London with an orthodox NHS general practice working alongside a whole range of complementary practitioners. I had gone to see this in action and spent a day with him there. We had met over the years as he had been an associate adviser in general practice and had also served with me on the RCGP Council. Later, he was appointed Professor at the University of Westminster and invited me to his inaugural lecture. He had a rare ability to generate new ideas and put them into practice. In 2000, his main concern was Cuba and building better relationships between Cuba and the UK.

The visit was designed to show us the Cuban medical system, and the UK team would provide a set of lectures at a conference. I was keen to go, not just because Cuba was somewhere Jill and I had never been, but also because its health system was of great international interest. I had read its results, which had been discussed in some WHO seminars where I had been. Cuba was reporting excellent health statistics in the developing world on minimal investment. How was it done?

The whole visit was a great pleasure. We had wonderful weather, and the Cubans have a rare ability to make music everywhere. We were given many interesting talks and taken to several health care facilities. The background political fact was the sustained hostility to Cuba of the United States which relatively speaking was quite close. There were no Americans about. This was a communist state that broke all trade conventions, breaking copyright for drugs and making its own. It was obviously very poor, yet we were told it was overproducing doctors and deliberately sending them to many other developing countries.

For me, an intriguing fact was that the whole system was built on family doctors with a doctor-patient ratio of one doctor to only 500 patients. Was this the key? I knew of no other country with so few patients per GP. We visited some of these doctors: they worked with a very limited formulary of drugs, had constrained referral arrangements, and poor consulting facilities. However, they did many home visits and were very heavily orientated to providing personal preventive medicine. They knew their patients better than did most UK GPs.

We visited a maternity unit where large numbers of women were kept for weeks on end when pregnant (Jill was horrified!). We heard how elderly people turned out to do group exercises every day (for which there is a very strong evidence base). However, I remained puzzled, not because the statistics were so good, but I could not understand why these patients were so compliant. Why were the elderly exercising regularly when Western doctors had such difficulty getting the same advice accepted? Late one evening on the tour I pressed this point with one of our guides. It emerged that these family doctors were linked with the state machine with commissars placed on every estate. The patients comply, I was told, as they don't want to lose their accommodation! Doctors' orders! The conference at the end of the week went well. Patrick Pietroni and I and others gave our lectures, and he and I were elected honorary members of the Cuban Association of Family Physicians.

Royal College of Physicians of Ireland

During the Presidency, I was informed that I had been elected an Honorary Fellow of the Royal College of Physicians of Ireland. For various reasons, I was invited to the ceremony in Dublin the following year in 2001. Jill was not able to come so I went alone. Among the various honorary degrees and fellowships I was fortunate to receive, this one had a family connection. It was an ancient institution, founded in 1654 and I had heard about it all my life from my aunt Gladys, my mother's cousin who lived in Dublin and was the College librarian. The afternoon I arrived, Ireland beat England at rugby at Lansdowne Road. I missed a trick in not asking if the College could get me a ticket. I watched the match on television. Dublin was elated.

The ceremony was held in the College, and the President was Desmond Canavan MD PRCPI (1938–2004) who worked in the NHS in Northern Ireland. He and I were both the sons of GPs and both of us had been elected to our Presidencies unopposed. The saddest aspect of my visit was that my aunt, Gladys Gardner, having given a lifetime's service as Librarian to that College, had died. However, I met several of the fellows who had worked with her and they described a quiet, loyal and hard-working member of staff. I was given a history of the College that mentions her (Mitchell, 1992). The Royal Colleges of Physicians in London and Dublin have St Luke as their Patron Saint so there is an annual St Luke's day dinner in both Colleges each year. St Luke's feast day is 18 October and so that was the week when my ceremony was held, followed as usual by the St Luke's day dinner. I was interested to hear that Gladys often helped with the preparations for that dinner. She would have been delighted if we could have met there.

I had been invited to give the after-dinner speech, which surprised me as my fellow Honorary Graduand was John Hume (1938–2020). He was an experienced Northern Irish politician who had founded the Social Democratic and Labour Party and had been jointly awarded the Nobel Peace Prize three years earlier in 1998. He was the second Nobel Laureate whom I'd met. I later learned he had health problems. When it was time to speak, I knew no one in the room apart from the President. I had an easy opening speaking about England's defeat at rugby that afternoon. This went down well as of all their sporting opponents it is England whom the Irish most want to beat. I thanked the College profusely for the honour as I understood I was the first GP from England to be elected an Honorary Fellow since 1654. The main thrust of my speech was the changing relationship in medicine and how much I appreciated being the first GP Chair of the Academy of Medical Royal Colleges (which was why I was there) and hoped that this would be seen as an integrating role bringing the branches of medicine inside and outside the hospital closer together. In that vein, I hoped that now there was an active College of General Practitioners in Ireland (of which I was a member) that it would be possible to build a good co-operative working relationship between the Royal College and its younger sister College, also in Dublin. My speech failed. It was not welcomed apart from some social courtesies, and Irish colleagues later confirmed that nothing happened.

RCGP Triennial Dinner 2000

The RCGP in my day hosted a triennial dinner to repay hospitality from other institutions and as an occasion to which it can invite VIPs. This fell in my final year and was held in Princes Gate. I pressed hard for an invitation to be sent to another partner to represent the practice as they had supported me throughout. However, coming would have cost a return rail fare from Exeter and a night in London so the invitation was declined. It is different in London and if I had been a London GP I expect my practice would have been more easily able to attend. There was a big turn out from College Presidents as for the first time the PRCGP was Chair of the Academy.

We had invited the Secretary of State for Health a year earlier and when the date came it was Alan Milburn in office; he was seated beside me and gave an after-dinner speech. I welcomed the guests and the traditional third speech for the guests was given by General Sir (later Lord) David Ramsbottom (1934–) Chief Inspector of Prisons, who did it elegantly.

I was conscious of how this dinner with a Secretary of State as my guest of honour was purely social and the opposite to the College dinner 11 years before when I had had another Secretary of State for Health, Kenneth Clarke, as guest of honour and his speech there had made it a political event. My relaxed conversation with Milburn did have one political point but not about health care. We were chatting about devolution as the *Scotland Act* 1998 was then recent. I said I thought the *Act* would have profound implications for the UK and alter attitudes in England as well as in Scotland. He expressed surprise and I said for example, for the first time in my life I was thinking of answering the question about my nationality as being 'English' rather than 'British'. He said that was the first time he had heard this said. Among the guests was Sir Joseph Pilling KCB (1945–; Chapter 16, Practice story 1975–1986). When thanking him as he held the exceptionally complex post as Permanent Secretary for Northern Ireland, he said he wanted to see David Ramsbottom and me together.

There was a big turnout from the DH (three ministers). As I thanked Gisele Stuart (1955–, later Baroness) a Birmingham MP and Parliamentary Undersecretary of State for Health, at the door as she left, for being the third health minister there, she joked with me that ministers were like London buses: "You never see one when you want one and then three come along together!"

Institute of Medicine (National Academy of Medicine) Washington

During my term I was told I had been elected an Overseas Associate of the Institute of Medicine of Washington, USA. I knew of this Institute well and regularly read its influential reports. The election process is based on the circulation of an abbreviated CV to the thousand or so members and by private postal vote. I felt honoured to have survived this process. There were very few GPs who had been elected and I was the first GP from the UK, and so broke a glass ceiling. Then there were 24 doctors elected outside the United States.

The admission ceremony fell at the end of 2000 and Jill and I flew to Washington for it. There were accompanying academic and social events where I saw Don Detmer, a fellow trustee at the Nuffield Trust. I was particularly pleased to meet Rosemary Stevens, an American historian who had influenced me greatly as a young GP through her book *Medical Practice in Modern England* (Stevens, 1966). She had illuminated medical relationships in the mid-20th century and had summarised some of the conflicts between GPs and specialists with her perceptive conclusion that: "Consultants won the battle for hospital beds and the GPs won the patients." A few years later the Institute changed its name to the National Academy of Medicine and I became an 'international member' of that.

Successor

The election for my successor took place in my final year and was a contest between Lesley Southgate and Colin Waine. Lesley won with her multiple achievements in medical education, her professorship and damehood, with about two-thirds of the vote. Colin's one-third of the votes reflected the affection

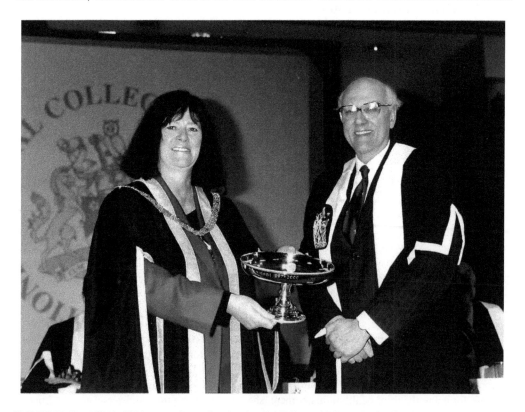

FIGURE 35.12   AGM in 2000, presenting a silver bowl to the College with Dame Lesley Southgate.

in which he was widely held and sympathy for his substantial experience as a working GP. Lesley Southgate therefore took over from me at the AGM 2000. My farewell present to the College was an engraved silver cake stand.

As in many national institutions the RCGP has a portrait of each President unveiled at the AGM at which that President retires. I searched hard for a portrait painter and was anxious about it as Annis Gillie's had been a problem. As a believer in professional peer review, I hoped for a member of the Royal Society of Portrait Painters (RSPP). I found Carlos Luis Sancha who was an Honorary Treasurer and member of the hanging committee of the RSPP. He was very experienced, and had done portraits of Prince Charles, the Duke of Edinburgh, Edward Heath, and the Presidents of two other medical Royal Colleges (Sapper, 2008) He was an expert and required fewer sittings than many other portrait painters and used photographs to support his sittings. The Tamar Faculty raised a large sum towards the cost for which I was most grateful and which I supplemented. As Jill had given me a lifetime's support, I asked for her to appear in the portrait. The solution was to paint her picture on a table beside me. I was painted in the robes and chain of office of the College wearing two decorations (Kt and OBE) as the knighthood citation had specifically referred to the RCGP Presidency. I am shown holding *Occasional Paper 50,* which described Fellowship by Assessment,

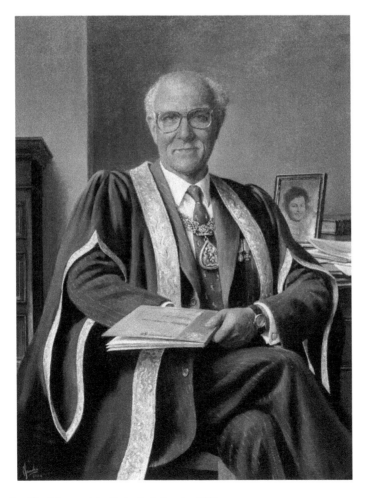

FIGURE 35.13 Presidential portrait by Carlos Luis Sancha, 2000.

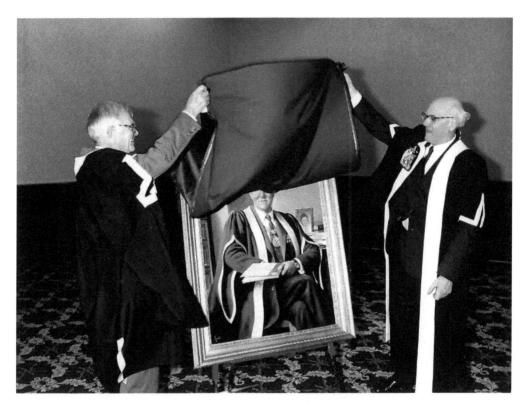

FIGURE 35.14   AGM in 2000, unveiling of the portrait with Dymoke Jowett, Provost, Tamar Faculty.

and symbolically giving it to the College, as FBA and the *Occasional Papers* were two of my main contributions.

I was anxious about Sancha's health and said so to Jill as I feared he might not complete the portrait. There was nothing obvious but there was no reserve if he did not. However, he did so on schedule and it was unveiled, as was customary, at the College's AGM in November 2000 by Dymoke Jowett Provost of the Tamar Faculty. Jill and the family were pleased with it and I was mainlyso but would have preferred it if he had painted Jill's face a bit better. My clinical sense of danger about Sancha (1920–2001) was justified and he sadly died the next year. Mine was one of his last portraits.

36

Vice-Chair, Academy of Medical Royal Colleges 1998–2000

Man is a political animal.

Aristotle

I took office as PRCGP in November 1997 thus becoming a member of the Academy. The other GP was the Chair of Council, John Toby. My arrival in the Academy was a first. I was the first British doctor to serve a second term, as the Presidents of the specialist Royal Colleges serve for a single term. In 1989, I had become the first RCGP Chair of Council to be a member of the Conference, now, eight years later I had the other GP place in the renamed Academy.

Academy Officers 1998

In 1998 the time came for the election of officers. I had seen this before with the election of Dillwyn Williams PRCPath as Chair when I had actively lobbied for him. Naren Patel said his term was ending and asked for ideas. In March, I wrote to him saying the RCGP had been disappointed about its previous share of officer posts. Naren Patel (1938–; knighted in office as PRCOG and later Lord) was finishing his term of office as PRCOG (1995–1998) and Chair of the Academy (1996–1998).

He said he had thought about how to balance the Colleges. He then proposed that all three officers be elected together as a group. He proposed from the Chair that Roddy MacSween (1935–2015; PRCPath) be the next Chair and that Leo Strunin (PRC Anaesthetists (1937–2020) and me be the two new Vice-Chairs. I did not know how much consultation had preceded this as I had not been involved. I suspect influential colleagues had been sounded out about Roddy MacSween (1935–2015) who was popular and had recently chaired the Scottish Academy of the Colleges, which Naren had also done (1994–1995). MacSween was a distinguished histopathologist and co-author of a big textbook of histopathology. I happened to know this, as his co-author was Peter Anthony from Exeter, who had shown me a copy. Roddy had made no enemies and would threaten no one.

Patel's triple proposal was approved en bloc. His trio was balanced but surprised me. There had only ever been two GP officers in the history of the Conference of Colleges/Academy – John Horder as Secretary and Michael Drury as the first GP Vice-Chair. Now I was the second GP Vice-Chair. Naren Patel was a radical. The three new officers of the Academy were all outside the three older English Royal Colleges that had ruled the College roost since World War II. This was probably the first time that the RCPLondon, the RCSEng, and the RCOG did not have an officer of the Academy between them.

The role of the Vice-Chair of the Academy was primarily to support the Chair and share with the other two officers the day-to-day running of the Academy. The three officers met, with Diana Garrett the Administrator, regularly, sometimes more than once a month to deal with day-to-day business. The Academy needed to field a representative at the many meetings to which it was invited. If the Chair was not available this was a natural role for the two Vice-Chairs. Another job was to prepare for meetings of the Academy.

DOI: 10.1201/9781032713601-44

The Chairs I had served under had different leadership styles. MacSween's varied radically from that of Margaret Turner-Warwick who saw herself as a professional leader and led from the front. MacSween rarely initiated policies and saw his role as presiding over Academy meetings. He never wrote a policy paper in his two years as Chair. I had not met Leo Strunin before we became joint Vice-Chairs. We got on well. He was the only colleague I knew who loved dog racing. I met him often in his Presidential office where he had a plaque for John Snow on his desk, as the father of anaesthetists. I teased him about having a GP on his desk. I feared the Academy was under-resourced for its considerable national responsibilities, but I realised that I could help by writing papers when appropriate.

Policy Papers

One Sunday the press carried a piece of investigative journalism reporting that MacSween had participated in a committee taking decisions about a drug, when he had a shareholding in the company that made it. He had apparently not declared an interest. This was embarrassing for Roddy but raised a question about the Academy as its Chair. He was a man of integrity and none of us thought he would have been swayed in his decision-making by his shares, if he had even remembered them. However, I saw this as part of the changing culture in society and thought that doctors would see more of this. I had long been concerned about conflicts of interest. I wrote a paper suggesting that senior doctors holding positions of responsibility should always declare conflicts of interest and before the business started. The paper was tricky because it meant dealing with the size of the shareholding (were some small holdings not worth reporting?) and there was also the problem of shares owned by the doctor's spouse. My paper made people uncomfortable about the details but there was strong agreement that the Academy needed a policy and the paper was approved.

The Academy inherited the 'first-past-the-post' voting method, as used in British national elections. However, I believed that first past the post was not best for professional organisations. The single transferable vote (STV) was the process recommended by the Electoral Reform Society. A problem with the national system is 'spoiler candidates' who can alter the result. In one BMA election there was a consensus that it was time to have a GP in a key post. He was opposed by a specialist. At the last minute another GP entered, with no chance of winning but who took enough votes from the first GP so that the specialist won.

The Academy was particularly open to 'spoiler' candidates because Colleges might want to hold an office and some Presidents can have big egos. In the STV system the voter numbers the candidates in order of preference and if the first-choice candidate is eliminated, the vote moves to the next preferred candidate. Any vote is more effective and less likely to be wasted. Spoilers are avoided as their votes move on. My paper in the RCGP had been approved and was RCGP policy. I had been elected to the GMC in 1994 by the STV system. I therefore sought to replicate the process and wrote a paper proposing the Academy should adopt the STV. This was agreed as policy.

By the time I rejoined the Academy in 1997, I had been trying for eight years to reform the distinction award system in the NHS to overcome the exclusion of salaried academic GPs from eligibility. I had started in the RCGP in 1989 as Chair of Council and in 1990 had secured a unanimous motion in favour of the reform from the Conference of Medical Royal Colleges and their Faculties, the antecedent body of the Academy (Williams, 1990; Chapter 39, Distinction/Clinical Excellence Awards story).

Now in the Academy, I sensed a new chance to make a difference, mainly through being an officer of the Academy, and partly because I had a longstanding working relationship with several BMA leaders, especially Sandy Macara, now Chair of BMA Council. I wrote a policy paper and started discussions in my capacity as Vice-Chair of the Academy. I was constitutionally doing my job as an officer seeking to implement existing Academy policy as I had myself got it agreed in 1990 as is described in Chapter 39, Distinction/Clinical Excellence Awards story.

Joint Consultants' Committee

Both Vice-Chairs of the Academy are ex-officio members of the Joint Consultants' Committee (JCC), the Conference of Senior Hospital Doctors and the BMA's Annual Representative Meeting (ARM). I attended the JCC regularly and was present when Jim Johnson was elected Chair following Sir Norman Browse (1931–2019). I had served briefly alongside Browse in the Academy, as he was JCC Chair. He was a former PRCSEng and held the JCC Chair when it had been the College's turn to nominate. He was a powerbroker and the last JCC Chair knighted. Now it was the BMA's turn to nominate the Chair and the timing was right for Jim Johnson (1946–) as he had previously been Chair of the BMA junior doctors and the BMA consultants.

For its first 40 years, the JCC was a power in the medico-political land. It is a committee almost unknown in the GP world with few GPs knowing about it let alone sitting on it. Its prestige meant that its meetings were attended by the Chief Medical Officer (CMO). I was embarrassed to see how the CMO was treated. Robust debate is one thing but some of what I witnessed was 'bear baiting.'

Election for the Chair of the Academy

In 2000, one President told me that I was the nearest to a prime minister he had met! He proposed I should be the next Chair of the Academy. I knew the history that often a Vice-Chair had been elected but I also knew that no GP had ever been elected Chair. I spoke with Leo Strunin who said he was not standing and supported me by signing as my seconder. I went to see other Presidents, including Barry Jackson PRCSEng, whom I saw in his Presidential office in the RCSEng. He signed a form supporting me. One President asked me if I was standing "to stop the 'Prince of Regent's Park'?!" (The RCP is in Regents Park.) James (Jim) McEwen (1940–), Public Health, was encouraging; he had worked with me in the RCGP 16 years earlier. The chairmanship seemed possible.

Then suddenly the support collapsed like a pack of cards. Late on, Barry Jackson came to see me in my President's flat. He withdrew his support for me and told me he was applying for the Chair himself. He said he had substantial support and hoped to win. My supporters said they thought Barry was being steered by George Alberti (PRCP) and that he did have other support. The Colleges of Physicians and Surgeons had worked together from 1800 to 1929. The older Colleges were allied again.

I spent the evening alone in the College offices writing a paper proposing that Barry and I should job-share the chairmanship (unpublished). I thought half a loaf would be better than no bread. I arranged to see him to discuss this. He rejected the idea out of hand, said it would not work, and that he now expected to be elected. As there were a block of votes – seven places for Physicians and Surgeons alone in the Academy – it did not look good.

The week before the vote I was in a GMC meeting. Arnie Moran, President of the RCSEd waved me over and said: "I am going to vote for you next week!" meaning he was going to vote against a President of another College of Surgeons. I was surprised and asked why? "The other two are prima donnas! You are a team player and you won't do deals without telling us." This suggested a close vote. I wrote to the Electoral Reform Society asking what to do if an STV vote was tied.

The officers met before the main meeting. On the item of the election of the Chair Roddy said that in a tie he would make a casting vote as Chairman. I said I did not think that was correct in an STV election and produced the letter from the Electoral Reform Society, which described their procedure in the event of a tie. Roddy was not best pleased but agreed the recommended process. The Academy meeting followed. In the election for the Chair I received 10 votes, Barry Jackson PRCS six, and Robert Shaw PRCOG, three. Barry was then elected Vice-Chair.

An Academy dinner had been arranged that night and the previously invited guest was Donald Irvine. It was quite a moment when I welcomed him at the door, as we were two GPs together in the two highest offices in British medicine. I made the welcome speech, thanked Roddy for his chairmanship, and presented him with a piece of silver to which all the Presidents had contributed.

Soon afterwards I invited Barry Jackson to a private one-to-one dinner at the RCGP to try to forge a working partnership. We discussed the state of medicine amicably and at the end of the evening he said he would be a loyal Vice-Chair. I thanked him.

37

Three National Meetings 2000

The majority has the might, the more is the pity, but it hasn't the right.

Herik Ibsen (1828–1906)

The year 2000 was a turning point in the political history of the medical profession in the UK. Three national meetings were held which changed relationships forever. I was fortunate to be the only British doctor present at all three meetings.

1. Conference of Senior Hospital Doctors

In May 2000, the annual conference of senior hospital doctors was held. As Vice-Chair of the Academy I was an ex-officio member. Dutifully I registered thinking I could brief myself on hospital issues. I little knew what I was walking into. The conference was held in the Royal College of Physicians of London – an irony that such a meeting occurred in a prestigious academic home.

The press was reporting that consultants were angry at the policy of revalidation that the GMC had approved. Senior hospital doctors, mostly consultants, realised that revalidation was going to apply to them and they didn't like it. I had been in the big BMA conferences in the mid-1960s when doctors had been seething with anger and in 1965 had almost voted to leave the NHS (Chapter 8, Local Medical Committee and BMA). Then, I was 29 and those were GP conferences. Now, I was 64 and in a conference for hospital specialists. I saw only two other GPs in the room: Ian Bogle, Chair of BMA Council and the Chair of the Overseas Doctors' Association. One other College President had come, John Lilleyman, newly elected PRCPath, also to brief himself. The PRCP did not attend.

The conference motion on revalidation was mob rule with a string of angry speeches all criticising it with no attempt made to consider why the GMC had introduced it. If the conference had just been letting off steam no harm would have occurred. However, I was alerted to an impending crisis when a motion of no confidence in the GMC was moved. In all walks of life a no-confidence motion is the most serious motion possible and calls for resignation(s).

An important speech was made by Ed Borman, an able young consultant anaesthetist, whom I had got to know. He had previously written a paper against revalidation. Despite being an active member of the GMC, he spoke strongly against it. I thought the key speech would be by Jim Johnson in his capacity as Chair of the Joint Consultants' Committee. However, he went along with the mood of the conference and never mentioned the position of the medical Royal Colleges. The size of the problem hit me as this speech pandered to the audience and ignored half his role, as the JCC and its Chair represent both the BMA and the medical Royal Colleges. As Vice-Chair, I knew he had not consulted the Academy. I studied Ian Bogle as he was the policy lead for the BMA and realised he was metaphorically burying his head in the sand. He never spoke. The tone of the conference was quite nasty with personal attacks on Donald Irvine.

I never thought when I went that I would speak but it dawned on me that I was a member of the GMC and the most senior representative of the Academy present. Grimly, I realised that I had a duty

DOI: 10.1201/9781032713601-45

to speak and walked down to collect a yellow slip of paper requesting permission. The conference chair was a female psychiatrist who called me quickly as she had no-one else opposing the motion. The situation was ugly and I knew I was up against it.

I began by declaring my interest as a former member of both the BMA Council and of the BMA Representative Body, that I was a Vice-Chair of the Academy of Medical Royal Colleges and a member of the dreaded GMC. I reported the main arguments for revalidation. I was under pressure because BMA conferences work to strict time limits. Their system of coloured lights means a yellow light is a warning that there is one minute left and the red light means stop at once.

I argued that the motion was fundamentally misjudged, that the GMC was still in the process of consulting the medical profession, that revalidation was in the public interest, that a no confidence motion is the most serious possible, and that the press were present. Then my red light came on, and with my experience of seven years of BMA conferences, I knew I would be booed off the stage if I continued. I stopped dead and took two steps back from the podium, signalling non-verbally to the Chair and the room that I was requesting permission to continue. One of the great silences of my life followed. The Chair was uncertain given the anger in the room, and she hesitated. Then from the back of the room came a lone voice: "Let the b….r finish!" The Chair turned to me and said firmly: "Please continue, Sir Denis, I will give you three more minutes only!"

Reprieved, I waded on and presented the rest of the argument that it was not logical to pass such a motion when the conference had no alternative proposal before it. Then realising that the room was relentlessly against me and 400 consultants were about to vote me down, I raised the emotional temperature and in a dramatic finale said: "This motion is crass! If passed it will be the biggest mistake the BMA has made since 1832!" [When the BMA was founded.] I climbed down from the platform back to my seat in stony silence, without even the customary desultory clap usually given to dissenting minorities.

The end came quickly. The Chair asked the Chair of Council, the BMA's policy lead, if he wished to exercise his right to speak. Bogle, in a failure of professional leadership, shook his head. Standing orders gave the Chair of the Consultants' Committee, the last word. Peter Hawker, a consultant gastroenterologist, didn't take long. He smiled at the room, said he had listened to the debate and would do his best to implement the wishes of the conference.

The vote revealed that senior hospital doctors overwhelmingly supported the motion of no confidence. Voting against, I raised my hand firmly in the air; John Lilleyman joined me with the GP from the overseas doctors. There were about 400 votes for and five votes against. Mob rule prevailed. As Ibsen said: "the majority had the might, but they did not have the right." The press next day gave headline news that this conference had passed a vote of no confidence in the GMC. My speech was accurately reported in the *Independent*.

---

2. Meeting of the Academy

The second of the three national meetings was a meeting of the Academy of Medical Royal Colleges. This had been pre-arranged months beforehand and was the meeting when elections were held. By chance it was only a few days after the hospital doctors' conference. That meeting in June 2000 was one of the most important of my life since the election for the chairmanship was the first item on the agenda and I was elected Chair, the first GP (Chapter 36, Vice-Chair, Academy of Medical Royal Colleges).

As soon as the election was concluded, George Alberti left. It had been previously agreed that regardless of who was to be elected as the next Chair, Roddy MacSween would chair this meeting and retire immediately it finished. Although I had been elected at the beginning of the meeting, I was effectively continuing as Vice-Chair with Roddy MacSween in the chair throughout.

An early item was the conference of senior hospital doctors. The Chair asked John Lilleyman and me to report, as we had been the only two College Presidents who had attended. Lilleyman spoke first and said that the meeting had been a great surprise to him, both in terms of the strong feelings expressed against revalidation but most particularly the anger and emotion in the room. He said he had found this "distasteful." He made generous comments about my speech, saying that the position of the Academy had been clearly set out and he thought I had been "brave." He didn't think that anyone could have spoken in that setting and altered the outcome. I then summarised my speech on behalf of the Academy, which was easy as it was seared into my memory.

What was interesting, and politically important, was that several Presidents then reflected on attitudes to revalidation within their own Colleges. Not one of them reported that the mood was like that of the BMA conference. All of them said that in their College there was general, if reluctant, support for revalidation. This was crucial for the officers of the Academy, who were preparing a pro-revalidation line. It was clear, as there were so many Colleges represented, that the conference of hospital doctors was not representing all the views of senior hospital doctors. Doctors aligned with the Colleges were much more moderate.

The Academy focused on the speech Jim Johnson had made at the conference, because he was Chair of the Joint Consultants' Committee, a constitutional bridge between the specialist medical Royal Colleges and the consultants of the BMA. Members of the Academy were clear that they had expected Johnson to make sure the Academy position was both reported and supported and they pressed John Lilleyman and me to report precisely on what exactly he had said. We both did so. There was then considerable irritation, turning to anger amongst many, who felt the Academy had been let down in an important setting. By coincidence, on the same agenda, was what was usually the routine item of co-opting observers to meetings of the Academy, and Jim Johnson was an observer. This was an annual event at the June meeting. Suddenly members of the Academy realised they were being asked to re-co-opt as an observer the person with whom they had become angry. Jim Johnson was waiting outside the meeting to be co-opted and come in. A proposal was made that he should *not* be co-opted and that he should be informed why by the Chair, Roddy MacSween.

This proposal was adopted with one abstention (Faculty of Dentistry). Johnson was invited in. Roddy MacSween explained that the Academy had had a report from two Presidents who had attended the conference of senior hospital doctors and who had reported on his speech there. The Academy was seriously disappointed with the speech he had made as it had ignored the public position of the Academy. As Chair of the JCC he had had a responsibility to represent that view. They were therefore not prepared to re-co-opt him as an observer. Jim Johnson was shattered. It had obviously not crossed his mind that this could happen. He simply had to turn tail and limp away – a wounded man. There was no precedent. This event was a striking demonstration of the two opposing views, for and against revalidation, reflected at the very top of British medicine. Afterwards, as Chair, I went to see the Chief Medical Officer to explain what had happened and to confirm that the Academy's policies remained in place.

---

3. BMA Annual Representative Meeting July 2000

The BMA constitution is elaborate: the democratic, policy-making body is the Annual Representative Meeting (ARM), which brings together all branches of the medical profession. There are preliminary annual conferences of the GPs, the senior hospital doctors, the junior doctors, and the public health physicians, which are followed by the ARM for about a week in July. This is the BMA's parliament and governing body and it sets policy and resolves differences between groups. It was the third key meeting that summer.

As Chair of the Academy I was also ex-officio a member of the BMA's ARM so I attended this conference with foreboding. Although this was my 11th national BMA conference, it was like no other I had attended. On entering it, one BMA GP leader, Brian Keighley, said, "There will be no need for you to speak this time."

The conference that then followed can claim to be one of the most dramatic ever held by the BMA. First, as a national trade union it has enormous experience and is extremely adept at holding the different branches of the medical profession together, at least in public. BMA House works hard to avoid groups of doctors squabbling in public and to smooth over differences behind the scenes. On this occasion, however, one of the biggest splits in history between the BMA GPs and the BMA consultants took place in public and in front of the national press.

The senior hospital doctors presented their case well and formally proposed endorsement of their no-confidence motion on the GMC. But this conference was different. The GP leaders spoke strongly on exactly the opposite side. They used the speaking-as-a-team technique, which they had so destructively applied to me in the JCPTGP three years before (Chapter 29, the JCPTGP story). Because of the time limits for speakers, they divided up the main arguments against the motion of no confidence and the BMA GP leaders spoke one after the other hammering home their case. They did so well that I had no reason to speak.

John Chisholm, the GP BMA Chair was one of the best BMA GP leaders. It is never easy for trade union leaders to split their organisation in public. But on this important occasion he led his team to do just that. He is one of a small minority of BMA GP chairs to be appointed CBE. During that conference and the public clash between the two biggest branches of the medical profession, a speaker at the back of the room cried out: "This motion is a suicide note by a great profession!"

The debate was unbalanced intellectually because those favouring the motion of no confidence spoke emotionally, whereas the senior GPs had all the intellectual arguments: that the vote was not necessary, that the BMA had put forward no alternative plan, that there was a respectable case for revalidation in the public interest, that the GMC was still consulting the profession, that any major change to the GMC would probably be less sensitive to the medical profession, that a no confidence vote is the most serious motion possible, and that it was impossible to foresee the political consequences. The general practitioner branch of the profession led the medical profession that day.

The Chair of Council, Ian Bogle, the policy lead for the BMA, again stayed silent on this critical occasion. It was his predecessor, Sandy Macara, the past Chair of Council, who spoke with passionate advocacy, on behalf of the public health conference for the motion of no confidence, making a bitter attack on the GMC of which he was a member. All then depended on the junior doctors, who are independent within the BMA and they followed their seniors. When the vote came, because the big voting blocks in the BMA are roughly one-third senior hospital doctors, one-third junior doctors and one-third GPs, the motion of no confidence was adopted by the BMA as policy by approximately a two-thirds majority. Self-regulation of the medical profession was doomed that day.

Those three meetings in 2000 in London revealed unprecedented intra-professional conflict. Unusually, the differences were revealed played out in front of the press. Despite the BMA's great experience in papering over cracks between different branches of the profession, it was the BMA's own meetings which exposed one of the biggest ever disagreements between GPs and specialists. The GPs understood the world better. The BMA GP committee had previously held a national ballot that approved the GP trainer system, run by the regional advisers in general practice, which re-accredited GP trainers every three to five years (Electoral Reform Ballot Services, 1992). This was revalidation for GP trainers, and it worked.

Self-Regulation of the Medical Profession

In 2000, the medical profession, through the GMC, operated by professional self-regulation. The two BMA conferences killed professional self-regulation in British medicine and after that July it was only a matter of time before it ended. There were several ironies. First, the BMA's policy was to support self-regulation and second, that all this effort failed and revalidation was introduced. Although the GMC was an independent regulator, it was weakened by the vote of no confidence from the national trade union. A paradox was that senior hospital doctors shouted that they did not have a strong enough voice on the GMC (where there were many consultant members) but passing the no-confidence motion lost them all democratic representation. Within seven years the Government took control. The old GMC was abolished, a new, smaller one established and all democratically elected medical places removed. The cry that that motion was a "suicide note" was prophetic for medical self-regulation.

Despite its cumbersome size, under Irvine's leadership the GMC was sensitive to the public interest and ahead of its time. It adopted revalidation for all UK doctors voluntarily, by formal vote, as a commitment to patients. No other profession has come near such a system. Even 23 years later most professional bodies rely for quality assurance only on members attending educational events with no evidence of learning taking place. No other profession reviews the performance of established practitioners regularly. At the beginning of 2000, the GMC was the established regulator of the medical profession, as it had been since 1858. The accepted principle was professional self-regulation. The ARM decision fatally undermined the GMC and split the medical profession publicly in two. I was the only British doctor who attended all three meetings and so witnessed in person a historic turning point.

38

Chair of the Academy of Medical Royal Colleges, 2000–2002

As for our majority, one is enough.

Benjamin Disraeli (1804–1881, 1880)

The notice of my election as Chair of the Academy in June 2000, was in *The Times* almost immediately and the Government and national organisations were informed. I needed a personal secretary and an Exeter office. I was lucky that I had an excellent PA as Director of GP Education, Jane Eastman, whose job was ending on 30 September 2000. She had always been discreet and efficient, and I had been lucky to have her, so I asked if she would do two more years in a very different role. When she agreed, to follow proper process, we arranged that she would go to London to be interviewed by Barry Jackson, Vice-Chair, and Diana Garrett as administrator. They both warmly supported her appointment.

In June 2000, I was no longer Director of the Exeter Postgraduate Medical School but was still Professor/Head of the Institute of General Practice. I controlled Jane's office only until my retirement on 30 September 2001, whereas my term as Chair of the Academy, and her job, meant June 2002. I negotiated with the University, which was supportive, and the Academy paid the University rent.

Brush with the Department of Health

My first test as Chair of the Academy came quickly and was unexpected and unpleasant. Chris (later Sir) Ham working in the DH, telephoned me in Exeter to say that the Government was about to publish a white paper, as indeed I knew. I was told this was going to give the medical profession a great deal that it had been seeking. The Presidents of the other Royal Colleges were all signing a preface in support of it. They were going to be given a special opportunity to read it in a closed room in the DH on a confidential basis, just before publication. I said that I was interested in principle and how quickly could he get the document to me. Chris Ham then said that the Government was not prepared to release it until it was published. There was a long silence whilst I digested this problem. I said that I had written a great many prefaces for books and publications but in all cases I had either read in full or at least skimmed through the document in question. I did not see how I could sign a preface without knowing what was in the white paper. There was a brief discussion about whether the preface was or was not an endorsement of the text and I said that it was always an implied endorsement, which was why the Government was seeking support from all the presidents. I regretted that I could not sign a text I had not seen. I was told that I was the only President resisting and all the others were happy to sign, but I said I did not sign blank cheques. I was then quickly rung by the Minister of Health, John Denham (1953–) where upon the conversation was then repeated. I explained again that I could not sign a preface for a document I had not seen. After going back to Chris Ham, I asked him when this private viewing

DOI: 10.1201/9781032713601-46

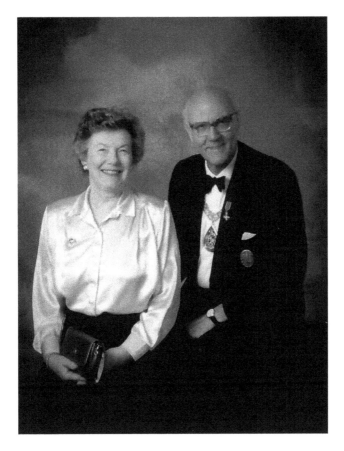

FIGURE 38.1   First GP Chair of the Academy of Medical Royal Colleges with Jill, July 2000.

was to take place and he said: "Oh no you can't go see it now if you're not signing!" In effect I had abstained, neither supporting nor criticising a text I had not read. Other big abstentions are described in Chapter 8, Local Medical Committee and BMA story and Chapter 22, Downs and Ups of Institutional Life.

When the white paper came out: *The NHS Plan: Plan for Investment; Plan for Reform* (Secretary of State for Health, 2000) on 1 July 2000, there was a preface with the names of many Presidents of the medical Royal Colleges. To add insult to injury, Michael Pringle, who was the Chair of Council of the RCGP and who had every right to sign for himself in that role was listed as the PRCGP.

So once again, as in the council chamber of the BMA 30 years before, I was completely isolated at the top of the medical profession. The incident is an interesting reflection of relationships between Government and the leaders of the medical Royal Colleges. The Presidents saw this incident as of little matter: I saw it as improper manipulation.

A Favour Owed?

John Lilleyman was elected President of the College of Pathologists to succeed Roddy MacSween. Soon after his election he asked me if I would make an after-dinner speech at his college's formal dinner. This was the second time I had been invited to do an after-dinner speech at a specialist college dinner, as the psychiatrists had asked me some years earlier. There is not much fun in making such speeches, but he was a new colleague, with whom I got on well, so I agreed.

The guest of honour at the dinner was Alan Milburn, Secretary of State for Health, and he came wearing a lounge suit when the dress requested was dinner jackets. This was common at that time, and Gordon Brown went to a big dinner in the city of London dressed the same way. The Labour Government was trying to make a point. I had an interesting discussion with one of his aides who also wore a lounge suit. After Milburn finished his speech and as I was beginning mine, he walked out. Ministers who do this seem oblivious to the bad impression that they make. My speech went all right and at the end of the dinner John Lilleyman was warm in his thanks saying: "I owe you a favour."

Policy on Revalidation

An immediate question was the Academy's policy on revalidation. Most of us doubted if revalidation would stop all scandals, but it seemed reasonable to hope it would lead to a new focus on quality of care and reduce the likelihood of so many medical horrors. I had supported revalidation as a member of the GMC and had voted for it in the crucial debate there two years earlier.

I consulted on where the Royal Colleges stood and had already been involved in debates as Vice-Chair. The Colleges were split: some strongly in favour and some against, with the majority in favour. However, the BMA was firmly against, with its Chair of Council, Sandy (later Sir) Macara, leading the opposition both inside and outside the GMC. Just before taking office in the Academy, I had personally experienced a bruising national conference of the BMA culminating in a vote of no confidence in the GMC (described in Chapter 37, the Three National Meetings.)

In the national arena, there was a triangle of three big national institutions: the GMC for revalidation, the BMA against, with the Academy perhaps holding the balance. I thought that this was a major issue of standards of care for patients and all their doctors, so started trying to build a consensus within the Academy. The first step was taking on the Chair of the Academy's liaison team with the GMC for several meetings, with Donald Irvine chairing the GMC side.

Leadership in such situations depends on sapiential authority, not on executive authority, as the Academy has no direct authority over the Colleges. I was accustomed to this working relationship as a regional adviser in general practice where there was no executive authority over general practices. The first step is to identify those who are successfully implementing the desired policy and to give them all possible encouragement and recognition. The second step is setting out in writing the reasons and evidence for the policy. The third step is a need to challenge and firmly, but courteously, confront those who oppose the policy.

Leadership is an intellectual challenge, especially when choosing the time and place to fight and winning intellectual exchanges. Often it becomes an interpersonal issue between key people.

I was fortunate that two of the Colleges seized the moment. One of these was the RCGP, which mattered as my credibility depended partly on what line my own College was taking. The RCGP led the medical profession with outstanding leadership from the Chair of Council, Mike Pringle, who before built a partnership with the BMA's General Practitioners' Committee. Here much depended on its Chair, John Chisholm. He shared the vision and a truly co-operative venture emerged. A shared group, which included some leading academic GPs, and where I was an observer, designed a series of measurable criteria and these, unlike any of those other Colleges, defined performance that was not acceptable, in other words failure criteria.

Another key step, which was not attempted in any other branch of the medical profession, was to consult the whole of the practising profession. This the two organisations did jointly and, to their and the profession's eternal credit, obtained majority support from working NHS GPs (RCGP and the GPC of the BMA, 2001). This was outstanding professional leadership. The agreed report was a working model of standard setting in the medical profession and showed how revalidation could be put into operation and introduced, with the consent of working doctors in the biggest branch of the medical profession. This was a high point in the history of medical professionalism.

The RCGP gave the GMC great encouragement and as a college it gave the Academy a powerful example, which I used. The second College to move decisively was the Royal College of Ophthalmologists. This College was led by Paul Hunter, its President, who had been a loyal supporter of the Academy, as its secretary and who gave me much personal support. This was important in the Academy, as it was a college of mainly specialists delivering a revalidation model.

On the other hand, there were Colleges, including the RCPLond, which showed no great enthusiasm. Their Presidents usually blamed their Councils, which were the governing bodies in all the Colleges. I therefore decided to do what I could in my two years in office to lead the Academy and its constituent Colleges into support for the principle of revalidation.

I judged that if the BMA's opposing view was to prevail then a form of revalidation would come anyway, driven by the Government, but in a form which would be insensitive to practising doctors.

Having eventually built a majority in favour of revalidation the next step was to produce a formal policy document. Over Christmas 2000, I wrote a lengthy one, fully referenced, and then circulated it to all members for the January 2001 meeting. It was made clear that this was to be the Academy's evidence to the GMC. The theme was the importance of professionalism in medicine. We spent virtually all morning on this and had a very good debate. Some Presidents, such as John Cox for the RCPsych, were enthusiastic. Others, like Peter Armstrong President of the College of Radiologists, took the trouble to write saying how much they liked it. The usual editing changes were agreed, but the trouble came when one or two Presidents, including Barry Jackson from the RCSEng, said they could not support it. With a clear majority, I ruled that the document was agreed by majority vote. Then it became clear that the older English Colleges seemed to think they had a veto and that if they did not agree a document, it could not become policy.

If true, this would mean that the Academy would always function at the level of the lowest common denominator. I defended the majority in the debate. With Barry discomforted, I said we would respect the small number of dissenting Colleges by printing on the front page that the document had been agreed by a majority vote with the Royal College of Surgeons of England and a few other Colleges dissenting.

The document therefore went to the GMC in that form, and I presented it in person there (Academy of Medical Royal Colleges, 2001). In this way, the Academy matured. It had agreed a major policy for the first time and established decision-making by majority vote, as in other national organisations. However, I paid a high price personally, particularly with the two older English Royal Colleges.

GMC Constitution

The GMC published a proposal to reduce its Council to 25 members. The Academy disagreed and thought halving to 50 would be better to ensure proper representation, including the Colleges. *Hospital Doctor* reported this on 11 January 2001 with George Alberti and Barry Jackson publicly disagreeing with all the other Royal College presidents. The older two Colleges did not think they needed to support the Academy if it did not do what they wanted. The BMA disagreed too. Eventually the GMC, Academy, and BMA all agreed on a new membership with me contributing to increased lay representation.

Building a Team

The constitution of the Academy of Medical Royal Colleges has built-in structural problems. Its great strength is that it includes the President of every Medical Royal College, not just in England but in Scotland and the Republic of Ireland as well. It is a rare example of a professional body across the

British Isles. It also has two faculties as full voting members: the Faculty of Dental Surgery and the Faculty of Public Health. General practice has always been in a small minority position, usually outnumbered about ten to one by specialists. General practice since 1989, when I joined the former body (then called the Conference of Medical Royal Colleges and their Faculties) as a second member in addition to the RCGP President had two members, both with voting rights (Academy of Medical Royal Colleges, Annual Report, 1998/2000).

The first constitutional problem was the membership, as each President served only whilst in office, which in most Colleges was three years. Thus, the membership was continually changing as each new President arrived and others left. This made team-building a considerable challenge. I had some advantages. I was the first British doctor who had ever served in the Conference/Academy in two different terms: 1989–1990 as Chair of RCGP Council and then 1997 onwards as PRCGP. I had served under five different chairs, including a woman, from four different medical Royal Colleges: the surgeons, the pathologists, the physicians of London, and the obstetricians, all with different personalities and leadership styles. I alone had served on the BMA Council for four years. Other advantages were being an elected member of the GMC and having served on a Medical Research Council grant-awarding committee.

I learned that there were two groups of Royal Colleges. First, there was a power group that included the RCPLondon, the RCSEngland, the RCOG, and the RCGP, which were big and relatively well-off in terms of resources, and all of whom had considerable influence. Second, there was a much bigger group of colleges that were less well-informed, had fewer resources, and relatively less influence. I supported the weaker group by providing information and opportunities.

The first group of colleges was generally less supportive of the Academy. They needed it less and, although they never said so, many of them felt that more influence for the Academy meant less influence for their (relatively strong) Colleges. I later encountered this ambiguity personally.

As a first step in building a more coherent and better informed team, I established a newsletter for the Academy, which I wrote, and which Jane Eastman in the Exeter office put together. It was distributed to all members of the Academy. This included public news relevant to the Colleges and information that came my way that was not confidential. I read voraciously and picked up much background information. We sent it out regularly and it was most appreciated by the second group of colleges.

As well, I started inviting VIPs to come for a working seminar with all the Presidents. The VIPs were as keen to come as the Presidents were to meet them. The format was always the same: a visitor spoke for about 10 or 15 minutes and then there was a wide-ranging discussion with all the Presidents. I chaired these seminars, making sure that the big hitters did not dominate. Two of the most successful seminars were with a Minister of Health, John Hutton (1955–; later Lord Hutton) and the Chief Medical Officer, Sir Liam Donaldson. These seminars were held in a room close to the Academy offices and were generally a success.

Sometimes I invited leaders to come to the Academy meetings themselves, for example, Alastair Scotland who was leading the new DH-established alternative system for assessing doctors. This did not work so well because of the problems of timing the agenda meant there was less chance for questions.

Finally, I instituted a series of working dinners for all the Presidents, with some VIPs coming as our guests. One interesting one was when Alan Milburn (1958–) came as Secretary of State for Health, bringing Simon (later Sir, later still Lord) Stevens (1966–), then his health adviser, but who soon moved to 10 Downing Street as health adviser to Tony Blair. This dinner had two points of interest. The first was when Milburn did not know the answer to a question and asked Simon Stevens what DH policy was. The second arose over statements by the DH that cataract surgery was done in Africa by less qualified staff than consultant ophthalmologists. This had irritated the College of Ophthalmologists, which believed, but could not prove, that this story had been fed by another College President, George Alberti, who was personally close to Milburn.

I took these issues seriously and had asked the PRCOphth for a written brief on the risks of cataract surgery in the UK, which he supplied. The complications were significant. I thought the Academy should support the smaller specialties and Royal Colleges and this was a test case. The analogy with Africa was not strong as there were no comparable complaints and litigation systems there and the price of errors was much lower. I was in the Chair when Milburn asked if we had any questions; I said that the Academy had read that his officials had spoken about cataract surgery being done by non-doctors, as in Africa?

Non-verbal communication revealed much. The Secretary of State looked straight at George Alberti who was silent. Milburn hesitated and said he wasn't briefed. I said that fortunately the Academy represented all the main branches of medicine and the President of the Royal College of Ophthalmologists, Paul Hunter, was present. I invited him to speak. He summarised the issue succinctly and made the risks clear. There were no further comments from the DH about cataract surgery in the NHS not needing to be done by doctors.

One feature within the Academy was that the PRCPLond, George Alberti, had a personal relationship with the Secretary of State for Health, Alan Milburn. They both came from the North-east of England and shared many ideas and principles. Alberti spoke a good deal at DH meetings. Once in a meeting with the Secretary of State he embarrassed some Presidents by appearing obsequious. No one felt able to say anything in front of a Minister, but Milburn himself unexpectedly reacted: "Oh George!" he said: "You are speaking like a junior minister!" Later, Alberti was appointed by the DH as the National Director for Accident and Emergency Medicine (the so-called czar), although he had worked clinically in internal medicine with a specialist interest in diabetes.

Visiting Other Leaders and Other Organisations

One advantage of being a GP was having much experience of doing home visits to patients. I had learnt from personal experience that people behave differently on their home ground and often talk more freely than elsewhere (DPG, 1978). I now applied these understandings to colleagues in other institutions at the top of British medicine. I made it clear that I welcomed invitations from other Royal Colleges, and I took many opportunities to visit other Presidents in their own Colleges and Faculties. Once, I made it clear to the Chair of the Junior Doctors' Committee of the BMA, Trevor Pickersgill, that I would be willing to come to his committee. He was surprised but duly invited me and I went, the first Academy Chair to do so. In that Committee I made it clear that I thought medical education had to be a partnership between those who were learning and those who were teaching, I wanted to build as strong a partnership on the academic criteria as possible, but of course the medical Royal Colleges, as registered charities, could not become involved with the topics of remuneration or terms and conditions of service. This experience followed from the relationships that had been built in Exeter. In my *System of Training for General Practice* (DPG, 1977a) a key meeting with complaining GP trainees had been in their mess, symbolising home visiting.

Paul Hunter as President, invited me to be the guest of honour at the graduation ceremony of the Royal College of Ophthalmologists and this meant giving an address. I said to these newly qualified ophthalmologists that they would be faced with several organisations seeking fees. They would have to pay the GMC to be able to practise. They would have to pay bigger sums to a defence body as well. However, the BMA was optional. I hoped they would all join the BMA as medicine needed a strong union to face a monopoly employer, but then they would meet a request from the College they were joining for yet another annual cost. I hoped they would start to think hard about the medical Royal Colleges in Britain and what their memberships and fellowships meant. They should be proud to have passed their examinations and they would see how many doctors in many different branches of medicine used their college letters with pride. They would get no great pleasure from being revalidated when that came in. I hoped they would get recurring inspiration from their college as I had done with mine. I finished by suggesting that the medical Royal Colleges were collectively becoming the conscience of the medical profession.

Writing

As Chair I wrote two articles about the business of the Academy. The first arose after a long debate on the proposal to introduce a new crime of corporate manslaughter. The Presidents were concerned this would have damaging effects in the NHS where many deaths occur. I wrote an article approved by all, which was published in the *BJGP* (DPG, 2001). This contributed to the delay in introducing manslaughter law, but it was introduced later and is the law today. Looking back, I think the Academy was probably over-defensive and too sensitive to the real problems that such a law creates for doctors. However, the problems of charging doctors with manslaughter have not yet been fully explored.

The second article arose when the Secretary of State for Health, Alan Milburn, established a new national organisation, the Postgraduate Medical Education Training Board (PMETB). Its purpose was to reduce the powers of the medical Royal Colleges. This was most unwelcome in the Academy, but that Labour Government had a strong parliamentary majority and used it. The question was where to draw the line and on what territory could the Academy reasonably stand?

The proposal was to merge the Joint Committee on Postgraduate Training for General Practice (Chapter 29, JCPTGP story), which I knew a good deal about having served on it for 17 years and chaired it for three, with the Specialist Training Authority. This gave the GPs special problems because they were afraid that the great expertise that the JCPTGP had built up over 25 years would be diluted in a body that would be principally specialist orientated. The RCGP was therefore lobbying hard for substantial GP representation on the new body.

Since there was no way of stopping the Government and no evidence of strong professional resistance, I reluctantly concluded that the best that could be done in these difficult circumstances would be to fight for the ability of the new body to elect its own Chair. This was a very modest request. However, after taking soundings, I realised to my concern that Alan Milburn was not minded granting even this.

I therefore wrote a short article raising the stakes by suggesting that this was approaching a process of deprofessionalising the medical profession. I took the text to a meeting of the Academy, which approved it without comment, and it was then published as an editorial in the *BMJ* in 2002. I signed it as Chair of the Academy of Medical Royal Colleges. Even the striking title "Deprofessionalising doctors?" (DPG, 2002) did not raise a general alarm and drew only one or two letters. We had hoped that putting the case for electing the Chair to the public arena would achieve more than the usual courteous behind-the-scenes requests. However, it did not, and Milburn insisted on appointing an NHS manager as Chair. This was about power and control and not about trying to make the new organisation work effectively. Dropping an NHS manager into the Chair of the body responsible for the training of all doctors in all branches of medicine was taking a big risk, as no NHS manager would have the knowledge and background of what is a particularly complicated national system. The manager concerned was not seen as a success and a medical Chair, a former dean of a medical school, was then appointed.

My editorial must be seen as a failure in terms of its prime purpose of seeking the right of PMETB to elect its own Chair. It did, however, document for the profession, and for historians, the 21st century governing process by the Blair/Milburn Government. That Government was not concerned with consultation even with the highest elected medical advisory group in the UK. Doctors were seen as the problem rather than as the solution and the planned action was managerial control of them.

Reception at 10 Downing Street 2001

An invitation was received for the Presidents to attend a reception in 10 Downing Street. Then it was discovered that only the Presidents of the English Colleges were included. I got on to No 10 and pointed out that the Presidents of the Scottish and Irish Colleges were full voting members.

I had thought this would be a routine administrative process, but it became quite sticky. Those I was dealing with simply saw the devolution law as operating with health as a devolved function. I pressed hard as I fought for the three Scottish and two Irish Presidents (as they both worked in the NHS in Belfast) to be included. Eventually they were invited. At the reception I had a long talk with Cherie Blair about the GMC. In my thank you letter to Tony Blair (February, 2001) I thanked him for including the two Irish Presidents for the first time since the Republic of Ireland formed. I finished by offering to advise him on anything in "British medicine," but as I did so I knew the world had changed. Government was eschewing consulting the Academy even though many College leaders had a track record and passion for improving the quality of care in their fields. Instead, Government was consulting hand-picked enthusiasts who were likely to say what Government wanted to hear. There are problems in the governance of Government.

NHS University

The DH launched a plan to establish an NHS university, following an idea at a Labour party conference. An official who was a BEE (Bright, Enthusiastic and Eager to serve the Minister) booked a long appointment with me to discuss this. I asked what definition was to be used. Did it include research? "Ah, that is difficult!" "…not necessarily!" I said, leading universities do research but was told that teaching was to be important. Trying to be positive, I said I thought there was great potential for an NHS teaching unit. I thought manual workers in the NHS got a poor deal. Planned education with the opportunity for qualifications and with time available could be transforming. Also, better opportunities for non-graduate nurses (the great majority) were needed and would be welcome.

This went down well until I said that degrees should be awarded only by recognised universities, when the temperature fell sharply. It cooled even further when I explored the proposed line of accountability, which was to the Secretary of State for Health, which the official had assumed and saw as natural. I suggested this was unwise and that no British university was accountable to a serving minister. The official found ideas of intellectual and institutional independence very difficult. The meeting ended with a stalemate. It did not make any difference. The Academy was important enough to be 'consulted' but not influential enough to affect any change. Ministers were set on this idea.

I happened to know that a substantial budget had been allocated as two colleagues in the NHS in the Southwest were moving their jobs to this project. One was Tony Lawrence, the senior administrator in the Southwest NHS Management Executive and the other was David Percy, the former regional adviser and one of my external assessors (Chapter 14, Regional adviser story). These two high salaries from just one region meant big sums were committed.

An important clue was that the man appointed to lead the project came from further, not higher, education. Criticism of the idea of an NHS university grew steadily and the DH started to refer to NHSU, i.e., not using the word 'university'. Behind the scenes, the big university guns were pointing out the legal procedures for calling an institution a university and what university charters meant.

A year after I left the Academy, in 2003, the NHSU was launched with the usual staff, costs and publicity, as a new special health authority. It did not last long and only two years later, in 2005, it was abolished by John Reed, Secretary of State for Health, in one of the periodic 'quango culls.' This story, although it hardly affected me personally, taught me how much government money gets wasted.

Partnership with Nursing?

We had always had good working relationships with nurses in the practice and two of the district nurses attached to the practice, Rosemary Clement and Debbie Stevens, were both clinically superb. In the Exeter Institute of General Practice there were occupational therapists, nurses and doctors working well together.

As Chair of the RCGP in the 1980s I had tried to build a working partnership with the Health Visitors Association. The officers of the RCGP had invited their officers to a dinner to discuss ways of working together. The key figure was Shirley Goodwin and it soon emerged she was not interested. We never discovered why. Some colleagues suggested that perhaps a dinner was OTT.

The headquarters of the Royal College of Nursing (RCN) backed on to the Royal Society of Medicine, where the Academy was based, so 14 years later I tried again. The General Secretary of the RCN was an American, Dr Beverly Malone (PhD), who had previously been in a senior position in nursing in the United States. I met her often as we were both routinely being invited to numerous DH meetings. I invited her to come next door for a coffee. We met alone. After the usual pleasantries I asked her if she had any ideas, she would like to tell me about. She said that nurses were not well enough regarded or paid.

I explained that in the UK, medicine had separated academic research education into bodies that were registered charities, and standard setting from the trade union functions; in medicine it was the BMA that was a registered trade union. I was therefore representing only the academic side but thought there was a great potential for partnership. Perhaps it was an omen that our two homes were neighbours?! I suggested there was great scope for the Academy to work with the RCN, especially in ethics, research, and in multiprofessional teamwork. I went so far, perhaps too far, to suggest that a 'grand alliance' between nursing and medicine might be possible. She responded by saying that what I had to understand was that nurses were not paid enough. My heart sank. She soon left and there was no follow-up note or any suggestion that we might meet again. I had had another complete failure with institutional nursing.

This incident raises the role of the RCN being both a Royal College and a trade union. It was founded in 1916, receiving its Royal Charter in 1928. I have for years thought that nursing is limited by this dual role of the RCN. First, if there is an income or pensions topic then it will tend to dominate internal discussions. Second, when the RCN proposes policies, they risk being perceived as being of self-interest. This is a problem for the medical Royal Colleges, even with their separation of functions, and it is much more difficult for the nurses. It may hinder the status of nursing, which as it represents the largest number of health care workers, ought to be higher than it is. In 2013, the Francis Report (2013) suggested the dual function of the RCN be reconsidered. The RCN did so but decided not to change.

I was invited to the annual conference of the RCN and attended. I was told doctors rarely came and I did not see another doctor there. I was pleased to see Professor Linda Aiken of the United States being awarded an honour. I had been following her outstanding research, which had been the first to show that the mortality rate in US hospitals was significantly associated with the number and proportion of graduate nurses on the wards (Kendall-Gallagher *et al.*, 2011). She had collaborated with Anne Marie Rafferty (1958–), whom I had often met at the Nuffield Trust, which had funded some of her earlier research. I identified with her, as she was isolated and trying to do for nursing what I was trying to do for general practice. She received a Harkness Fellowship to visit the United States, where she met Linda Aiken. She was later Dean of the Florence Nightingale School of Nursing at King's College. In 2018 she was elected President of the RCN and appointed a Dame.

This research influenced me considerably and I thought academic nursing, through Aiken and Rafferty, had moved ahead of academic medicine by showing both that nurses saved lives but that nurse education and qualifications (RGNs, qualified nurses) were the key to this, not nursing assistants, i.e. they showed that nurse education mattered. Their research was a skilled academic response to the management principle of always trying to replace qualified professional staff with less qualified ones. Seeing the power of relating professional activity to mortality was a factor in my mind when, 14 years later, I steered the St Leonard's Practice into doing the first systematic review of continuity of doctor care and mortality (Chapter 49, St Leonard's Research Practice story, DPG *et al.*, 2018).

The Alderhay scandal broke in 2001 when it became clear that body parts in Liverpool had been retained without consent. Patients and their families expressed great concern and there was a debate in parliament. The Secretary of State for Health, Alan Milburn, took a strong line and the CMO arranged a big conference for patients to which the Academy was invited. I was caught with a clash of dates with a long-prepared dinner in Belfast, which I decided to keep. John Lilleyman, as one of the two Vice-Chairs of the Academy, attended, which was appropriate as he was PRCPath and one of the doctors involved was a professor of pathology. It was a difficult and at times harrowing experience for him and he handled it well.

Dinner in Belfast

I had wanted to visit Ireland as Academy Chair as a team-building exercise. The Academy was unusual in having, as two constituent members, two Irish institutions in a different country. Suddenly my childhood background of having an Irish mother and having had many talks with family members about Irish politics was a great help. I saw the two Irish Colleges as a great asset, as their presence supported the unity of medicine across national and political boundaries, and they spoke from an EU perspective within a very different health system. I was concerned that they might be feeling left out as so much Academy discussion referred to the NHS. Both these institutions had been very keen to retain their Royal title after the Republic of Ireland was established. There was good cooperation in examinations especially between the Colleges of physicians.

I discovered that for the first time the Presidents of the Royal College of Physicians of Ireland and the Royal College of Surgeons in Ireland, both Dublin-based institutions in a European country, were both working in Northern Ireland, and so in the NHS. Believing in the power of the home visit (DPG, 1978), I said I would visit Belfast and hoped to see them both. They invited me to dinner and treated me well with an excellent dinner in lovely surroundings.

I talked about my holidays in Sligo, my Irish mother and how my uncle, Jack Cole, had taken me to watch Sir Stirling Moss (1929–2020) racing at the Dundrod circuit in County Antrim. I did a lot of listening. This was the first time a Chair of the Academy had travelled to either the north or south of Ireland to meet the two Irish Presidents and it was appreciated. I outlined my hope for more teamwork in the Academy. We finished with better mutual understanding. I used to say to our children that sometimes in life one is rewarded in unexpected ways for doing the right thing. This dinner helped prove the point. The good working relationships built that night helped save my career in the Academy when, a few weeks later, I faced an attempted ousting that I knew nothing about that night.

Proposed Ousting

The office accommodation for the Academy comprised two rooms rented in the Royal Society of Medicine in Wimpole Street, London. The first room was a secretarial office where Diana Garrett, Administrator, was based, usually with one or two junior secretarial staff. There was another office in the same building, which worked very well for holding small meetings for officers. Off this was a small office with a desk used just by the Chair, which was ideal for me as I could leave papers on the desk and work comfortably from it.

In April 2001, I was working there when Barry Jackson came in. He dropped what was for me one of the bombshells of my life, as he told me that the Presidents had decided that my term of office would not be renewed in June and that they wanted a new Chair! I was completely taken by surprise and asked who this was to be and was told it was John Lilleyman, the other Vice-Chair of the Academy. I said that I had been elected on a two-year term and asked what the problem was, but Barry would tell me nothing.

There followed several of the most difficult weeks of my life as I faced this unexpectedly proposed ousting. The situation was very serious, as the other two officers of the Academy had obviously ganged up against me and were working closely in concert. The first of the other Presidents whom I met was Paul Hunter, the Honorary Secretary of the Academy. He was as surprised as I was as he had not been consulted. This implied that this was a plot concocted by the older medical Royal Colleges in England.

I did some serious analysis on the situation, and it looked grim. This was a classic case of the 'men in grey suits' being sent by a leadership group to oust an established leader. I had read several political biographies and every time, whenever the men in grey suits had called on the leader, that leader had fallen. Moreover, my own experience in the RCGP in 1987 confirmed this, when GP 'men in grey suits' had called on the Chair of Council, he had immediately resigned (Chapter 22, Downs and Ups of Institutional Life). I did not know of a single example when this process had not led to an ousting.

The vote for the chairmanship had previously been set for the first week of June 2002 at the Academy AGM, so I suffered seven of the most difficult weeks of my life in the run up to that date. During it I met one of the other Presidents in the Academy who had told me he had previously supported me as Chair but when asked where he now stood, "I am afraid", he said, "the tide has turned."

Meanwhile Paul Hunter had taken it on himself to act as my campaign manager and was talking with the other Presidents. He came to see me with what he called "good news and bad news". The good news was that there were several Presidents who were also surprised about this proposal and did not agree with it. Some thought I was doing a good job. It was a fact that I had been elected for two years and some thought this plan smacked of an ancient Royal College plot.

The bad news was that I was told the two RCGP representatives in the Academy, Lesley Southgate, President and Michael Pringle, Chair of Council "were not doing anything to help you." This was more than disappointing. I knew them both as we had all shared many years on the RCGP Council. I was never close to Lesley, but knew Mike Pringle well, had nominated him as one of my Vice-Chairs of Council, and he was one of the two Chairs of Council in my Presidency. Jill, Nikki his wife, and the two of us had been to dozens of dinners and social events as a four together. I learnt the hard way the truth of Aristotle's statement 2000 years ago, that "man is a political animal."

I went to see John Lilleyman as Vice-Chair, as I felt that he should at least give me a reason for opposing me even if he felt no loyalty to me. I had always got on well with him, but he was absolutely firm in not giving any reason why I should only serve for one year. He did say that it was not his idea, he had been put up to it, but he had been told that he would be welcome as Chair. One day when walking down Wimpole Street with Barry Jackson, he said he thought it best if I announced that I did not want to stand for a second year. "That way", he said, "you will not have to lose the vote". I said I would think about it.

It was now clear that the campaign to oust me was being led by Barry. Some people suggested that he was being steered by George Alberti, President of the RCP. It looked as if the Presidents of the Faculties in these two older English Colleges had already been approached as it became clear that the President of the Faculty of Occupational Medicine of the RCP, and the Faculty of Dental Surgery of the RCSEng had been nobbled. The arithmetic was most unpromising because with the London PRCP and the English PRCS leading the attack, there were five other votes in the Academy, all in the hands of physicians and surgeons.

I reviewed the situation as rigorously as I could. John Lilleyman was a very strong candidate and the plotters had done well to choose him as the proposed alternative Chair. He was a distinguished academic, a professor in paediatric oncology and was widely respected clinically and academically. He had a pleasant personality and no obvious enemies. He was the strongest possible candidate and was already a Vice-Chair of the Academy.

Then in May 2002 came another problem. I was told that the *Health Service Journal (HSJ)*, the main medical newspaper for UK hospitals, had the story that my chairmanship was in danger. As the first GP Chair I could see that this would make a juicy story and it was clear that the journal had been tipped off from within the Academy. The story would have been damaging for me, so it was clear the tip-off had come from those involved with the plot. It was a standard political move and smacked of a politicised precedent. It was suggested to me that it might have come from the RCPLondon.

John Lilleyman told me about the *HSJ* and seemed upset about this development. I concluded that he had not instigated this, that he genuinely regretted it, and that he thought this was not the way business should be done in a professional body. He said he would get in touch with the *HSJ* and try to stop the story. He later told me that he had done this, and they had agreed to hold the story until after the election. I had no way of telling whether any of this was true or not, but I believed him. Just before the closing date for nominations I informed Barry Jackson that I would be seeking re-election. He was surprised.

Preparing for the meeting, I wrote several papers and was careful to ensure the agenda and the supporting papers gave no indication that I was planning to step down. Several of my papers proposed future action by the Academy.

As the date of the election approached, I was increasingly anxious about the two RCGP representatives. I was twice told they were not doing anything to support me although they had been told what was afoot. The non-verbal communication was ominous as I heard nothing from either of them and got no message wishing me luck. A few days before the vote I wrote a hand-written letter to each of them. I explained that I thought the vote was going to be close, that there was an issue for the RCGP and the College, in that if the only GP Chair who had ever been elected was tipped out after only a year, both general practice and the RCGP would be damaged as it was widely known I had been elected for a two-year term. I said I would appreciate their support. Neither Lesley Southgate nor Mike Pringle responded. I hoped to have done enough at least to stop them voting against me or abstaining. This was the first time in the history of the Academy when GPs would have three votes and each one was crucial.

At no stage had my critics identified any mistake I had made. There were some Presidents who disliked the proposed coup, and I had some loyal supporters. My private judgement was it would hinge on a single vote. I then had the distasteful task of preparing a surrender speech if I was ousted.

On the election day there was the usual pre-meeting of the three officers of the Academy which was not the most relaxed occasion as the two Vice-Chairs were up to their necks trying to remove the Chair. Barry Jackson said to me that he would appreciate the opportunity to say a few words at the end of the day. I agreed, expecting that this would be an unctuous statement of how well I had done after I had been removed. His confidence was ominous.

The item to elect the Chair was high on the agenda of the main meeting, held in the RCPath, ironically the College home of John Lilleyman, not a reassuring omen. It meant that if he won, he would be at home in his own College.

We then received messages that the flights of the two Irish Presidents had been delayed and that they were stacked over Heathrow. However, the PRCSI made it in time. The procedure was simple, as Diana Garrett had prepared voting slips with just Lilleyman's and my name on them. Paul Hunter as the Secretary of the Academy had previously been agreed upon as the returning officer and was supported by the Administrative Secretary. There were only 19 votes, so it didn't take long. Paul Hunter announced that the Academy had re-elected me as its Chair. As I looked at the group, I saw the room split into two in front of my eyes, with half the Presidents clapping and the other half looking stunned. In that moment I knew how everybody had voted, as those clapping were my supporters.

In such a sophisticated group, the others quickly joined in, but in that brief moment I discovered in a dramatic way, where each President stood – a memory frozen permanently in my mind. I had to speak but knew Churchill's maxim: "magnanimous in victory." In the briefest speech of my life, I simply thanked them for their support and said I would do my best for the Academy in the year ahead.

Over the usual buffet lunch several supporters quietly congratulated me, and Paul Hunter told me that I had had a majority of one vote. I smiled and responded with Disraeli's maxim that "one vote is enough!" Actually, I would have had a majority of two because Desmond Canavan, the President of the Royal College of Physicians of Ireland, who a few months before had installed me as an honorary fellow of that College (HonFRCPI), arrived late and missed the vote. He told me he was going to vote for me.

During the afternoon, Barry Jackson sitting on my right as the senior Vice-Chair whispered that he no longer needed time after the meeting to speak to me. I said I understood. Neither of the two RCGP representatives wrote to me afterwards so, as so often, non-verbal communication revealed their ambiguity. I was grateful that they had at least both voted for me. I sent a crate of good wine afterwards to both Paul Hunter who had done more than anyone to get me re-elected and another to the President of the Royal College of Surgeons in Ireland in Belfast, who had stood up for me and voted against the strong advice from a President of another Royal College of Surgeons.

Despite taking a keen interest in professional and political careers in the next 20 years, I have not come across any other example when 'the men in grey suits' failed to depose a leader they had targeted. In my time, I know of 11 medical leaders who had to resign, six in the BMA, including two chairs of BMA Council and five in the Medical Royal Colleges, including two Presidents.

Liaison Committee with the Deans

I was able, with their Chair, Robert Boyd (1938–; later Sir), to establish a new standing liaison group with the Deans of the Medical Schools. He had as Principal of St Georges Medical School invited me to be guest of honour at their graduation ceremony in 2001 (six years after Jennifer qualified there.) This Liaison group usually consisted of three or four on each side and brought two of the main strands of academic medicine together. As it had been my idea, the chair rotated and this group undertook some useful liaison work, usually over dinner. It was whilst listening to the Deans talking about general practice with Presidents of the Academy that I had an important insight. They all saw general practice as "hospital medicine outside hospital." This was important and reasonable for very senior hospital-based specialists to believe. After all, they had mostly not been GP trained, they had little, usually no, experience of general practice, and they had not read about recent advances in the literature of general practice, which had established it as an independent distinct specialty. Furthermore, all the other clinical specialties in medicine were able to learn what they needed essentially within hospitals. Why not general practice? Crucially, they did not see general practice as a discipline.

However, this misunderstanding has serious implications for general practice. Of course, it explained the view of the College President who had said he could not vote for me as Chair of the Academy as: "General practice does not have a discipline" (Chapter 36, DPG, 2023). This discovery set the scene for the academic work I did in Exeter after I finished my term as Chair of the Academy, described in Chapter 46, the Unfinished Campaign story.

Since the start of the NHS, the award of merit/distinction awards and later clinical excellence awards, were a core feature of consultant remuneration. All the specialist Royal Colleges are influential in giving advice and the Academy particularly so. Once a year the Academy seeks recommendations from the Colleges and then runs a special meeting to evaluate all the names. Each specialist college makes its own proposals but endorsement from the Academy as a whole is influential. I chaired this meeting in 2001 and 2002.

Separately, as Chair, I was ex-officio for these two years on the DH top distinction award committee. This is responsible for making the top-level awards then called the A Plus awards (now called Platinum awards). I was the only GP who ever had this privilege (Chapter 39, Distinction/Clinical Excellence Awards).

Joint Consultants' Committee

The Joint Consultants' Committee (JCC) is a long-established liaison committee between the Medical Royal Colleges and the BMA's senior hospital doctors. It was previously a force in the land and was consulted by government on all important policies. The JCC is little known in the GP world. However, the JCC was losing influence, partly because it sometimes mishandled business and I witnessed discourteous behaviour towards the Chief Medical Officer, reminding me of bear baiting. Paddy Ross was the first JCC Chair not to be knighted and I was present when Jim Johnson was elected Chair and he also did not receive a high honour. I was ex officio a member of the JCC as an officer of the Academy and attended every meeting for two years, usually reporting on the work of the Academy.

NHS

The Chief Medical Officer (CMO) set up a task force on litigation in the NHS seeking ways of reducing it and I was appointed to this. The background was that litigation costs were rising steadily and were a charge on the NHS. Costs were predicted to reach a billion pounds a year. The task force had strong legal representation and several experts. I found it interesting. Litigation costs were disproportionately often involved with midwifery, being strikingly expensive. Although midwifery has the highest proportion of healthy patients having a normal baby, when a baby is seriously damaged in labour the child may require expensive care for years or life. By 2007, there were about 100 cases a year being settled at several million pounds each. Subsequently sums of over £30 million a patient occurred. Cases took several years to settle. The CMO tried hard but the task force petered out as reform probably meant changing the law. My view was that there was a need to approach the problem differently. Outside the UK a different system like 'no fault compensation' as in New Zealand looks better.

Some medical mistakes cannot be prevented but many can. The problems can surely best be tackled by quality improvement. This means first ensuring a full complement of staff of both obstetricians and midwives and more rigorous education for both. Much more is needed as the UK maternal mortality rate is amongst the worst in Europe and is five times worse for black rather than white women. This is a national crisis. However, almost the opposite policy has been implemented. There is a shortage of about 2,500 midwives who often work 12-hour shifts, which can be associated with stress. The Royal College of Midwives reports low morale often because of understaffing. There is also a shortage of consultant obstetricians needed for the recommendations of their medical Royal College. The obvious NHS management priority, with risks running in the tens of millions of pounds, is to prioritise maternity services for staffing and training. It has not happened. In 2013, the Health Service Ombudsman, Dame Julie Mellor, called for an "overhaul of midwifery regulation (Ford and Barnes, 2013). In 2021 when 80% of general practices were rated by the Care Quality Commission as "Good," the same Commission rated 39% of maternity services as "In need of improvement" or worse, and 10% "Inadequate" (Care Quality Commission, 2022). Major failures of maternity care occurred in Cumbria, and a bigger failure in Shropshire was reported in 2022. This is failed national management.

I was at a national meeting when the recruitment of nurses was discussed. I argued the UK should train enough nurses for the NHS and that it was unethical to continue to draw nurses away from developing countries who badly needed them. At the time, almost half of new nurses in Britain were from abroad. I was elegantly fobbed off by a senior civil servant and 20 years later 45% of all new British nurses and midwives were still being recruited from abroad (UK Nursing and Midwifery Council, 2022). The UK needs to rethink its responsibility to train most of its NHS staff.

Meeting Tony Blair

The Academy received an invitation to meet the Prime Minister and the meeting was arranged in the cabinet room at 10 Downing Street. As Chair, I led the Academy team into the cabinet room and was received by Tony Blair with whom I was alone for a few minutes. He immediately said: "Denis, I want you to know that my Government is not trying to control doctors." I am fortunate in being able to think on my feet in most situations, but, in that special setting and alone with the Prime Minister, I was speechless. Did he know what his government was actually doing (controlling doctors more than any government had done before)? Did he take me for a fool? Was he trying to ingratiate himself? I was spared replying, as the Presidents started entering the room. I never knew what that extraordinary opening remark was about.

The meeting in the cabinet room was a brief exchange of views and left me searching for a way of getting a more meaningful discussion. Perhaps the Academy team had been too big? There were increasing reports of Blair seeing other groups, most of them with less legitimacy. Since there is a tradition of diplomacy over dinner I began to wonder about a dinner. Obviously, there was no way I could influence an invitation from a PM so I started to think how one could be initiated. I had got to know the Director of the Wellcome Trust, Michael (later Sir) Dexter FRS (1945–) and had several dinners with him. We agreed he would put out feelers about a private dinner with Tony Blair and that it would be best if the Wellcome co-hosted this with the Academy. I hoped this might work as the Trust had a high reputation as the biggest charity in Europe. However, we were told the PM was not interested. Even the combination of the Wellcome Trust and the Academy was not enough. No 10 preferred to see handpicked groups.

I tried a direct approach and wrote to Tony Blair as PM, inviting him to dinner with the Academy. The invitation was declined and instead No 10 proposed that Simon Stevens, the PM's health adviser, would come and see me. It is interesting that the substitution was with an official and not with a minister. So, Simon Stevens (1966–) had dinner with me at the Royal Society of Medicine. He seemed young (aged 36) and I had retired clinically. It was a free-ranging discussion. He was the best-read civil servant I had ever met, and even with my love of reading he analysed as an equal. He was a rare official who wrote articles in academic journals himself, e.g., in the US *Health Affairs* to which I subscribed (Stevens, 2004).

Being Rapped on the Knuckles

In 2001, the CMO sent the Academy a paper stating that it was confidential. It was not controversial and contained a favourable reference to the RCGP's fellowship by assessment. Why the CMO made it confidential I never knew. I heard that it had also gone to the Joint Consultants' Committee and the RCP and that both had replied with their support. Overly conscious of the confidentiality requested, I replied supporting it too. A few weeks later I had lunch with Mike Pringle as part of my regular meals with the various leaders of the Colleges. He seemed more distant than usual but gave no indication of concern. However, in September 2001, at the next meeting of the Academy, he launched a powerful attack on me for not consulting all the Colleges before replying to the CMO. He argued with skill, playing to the other Colleges. These differences of opinion are common in big organisations but what was unusual was the tone, with needle in his words. I explained the CMO had stated this was confidential, that the paper was uncontentious, and that I knew before replying that both the JCC and the RCP had indicated their support. Only one person, Peter Hutton, supported me and it became clear that most thought I should have circulated the paper. The Academy voted that there should be fuller consultation in the future, thus rapping my knuckles. One of the Irish Presidents said he was fascinated at the way leading GPs knock "chunks out of each other!"

I had made a mistake and was wrong to respect the CMO's call for confidentiality. Had I circulated it, majority support would virtually certainly have been received. The question is why Mike Pringle needed to attack me so strongly. We never spoke about it. The favourable mention of FBA may have been a trigger. Mike Pringle had been an enthusiastic supporter and a very early success in Fellowship by Assessment in 1989 but later became critical of it believing it was divisive. (Chapter 24, Fellowship by Assessment story).

Private Finance Initiative (PFI)

The Academy had a ringside seat on health policy by being involved in endless meetings, consultations and public relation launches. I attended the launch of NICE by Frank Dobson when he was Secretary of State in 1999.

One big public policy during my four years as an officer of the Academy was the private finance initiative (PFI). This system was developed under the Conservative Government of John Major, but it was little used. It meant government departments placing big, long-term building contracts with private companies (so-called 'special purpose vehicles') to build schools, hospitals and motorways. The private sector did the work and maintenance over about 30 years.

The background was many examples of poor management of public contracts with cost over-runs and late delivery. It was thought that private sector management would be better in delivering on time and keeping maintenance costs down. An advantage for Government was that accounting conventions strangely allowed this borrowing not to show as debt in the nation's accounts. Ministers could proudly open new buildings without increasing the national debt. The price was the big debt repayments paid by public services for generations. Several academic articles by Allyson Pollock (Gaffney and Pollock, 1999) showed that PFIs in the NHS were expensive, reduced bed numbers and restricted staff.

The Government no longer provided capital for new hospitals, and we heard this separately from health ministers and leading NHS managers. The phrase was: "PFI is the only game in town." There have been attempts to rewrite history and it was said on *Question Time* in January 2018 that the Treasury was always against PFI. It wasn't. Gordon Brown as Chancellor of HM Treasury imposed the policy that PFI was "the only game in town." I heard the phrase myself from Ministers. The Bart's hospital PFI reached one billion pounds and when it opened the managers could not afford to use one floor. Ironically, in 2015, the Care Quality Commission put Bart's into special measures (Merrifield, 2015).

The National Audit Office (2018) found the PFI process cost the state more, and that there were about 700 PFI schemes in existence costing the public about £7 billion pa. In the future, more transparency will be needed with less use of the 'commercial in confidence' veil of secrecy when public money is involved. The comparator should be more like those used on the continent and not the UK system, which makes PFI look artificially cheap. Open contracts would allow evaluation and comparisons. Some hospitals should have been built by the government as yardsticks. The failing was that everyone knew at the time that these were expensive contracts, but no one could do anything about them. Perhaps some new independent body like the Office for Budget Responsibility, separate from Government could evaluate at least the bigger contracts?

House of Lords

A new system made it possible to apply for membership of the House of Lords. Only one GP, the personal GP to Harold Wilson had gone there (and Lord Rea, 1928–2020, a hereditary peer) since John Hunt in the 1973. Donald Irvine had not gone there, unlike all his predecessors. As two recent Chairs of the Academy (Turnberg and Patel) went to the Lords I applied but was not appointed.

A Patient Group in the Academy

All through my second year I made it clear that I particularly wanted to establish a patient group within the Academy. Numerous discussions prepared the ground before I wrote a proposal paper. Presidents were split with a small number thinking this was a good idea, a good many not really concerned, but the RCPLondon and the surgical colleges did not want it. Although 20 years later than the similar proposal in the RCGP, this proposal was trickier. Even three months before I finished, I was not sure if it would pass. A proposal to add another new member of the Academy appeared. It had a good case but there were those who were concerned that the membership was getting too big. An agreement was made to admit emergency medicine and establish a patient group.

I called a meeting of all the patient representatives of the Royal Colleges. Some groups were active and working well. The RCSEng had a consultant surgeon, Charles Collins from Taunton, whom

I knew, who was the Chair of its patient group. I said to him that respect for patients meant facilitating them to elect their own Chair. One Scottish Royal College had no patient group at all. I made it clear that the Academy was now committed to a patient group and its Chair should be elected by the Chairs of the Colleges that had patient groups. Diana, from the Academy, ran the election. Patricia Wilkie, to my pleasure, was elected. She was the outstanding candidate having chaired the patient group in three different Royal Colleges. Her experience was needed as some Presidents were not used to an informed patient voice. She did well and established the group.

Dinners

I arranged a dinner for Donald Irvine as he retired as President of the GMC with all the leading GPs in in the UK: Ian Bogle (Chair of BMA Council), John Chisholm (Chair of the BMA GPs), Peter Hill (Chair of the Postgraduate Medical Deans, a former GP and RCGP officer), Mike Pringle (Chair of RCGP Council), and me. We met in a room at the Royal Overseas League. This was a unique and happy occasion. I made a serious mistake in not organising a photo.

Academy dinners rotated around the Colleges, and I wanted one in the RCGP but the first one there was my retirement dinner. To my great regret we could not use the Long Room at Princes Gate, an elegant Georgian room where RCGP formal dinners were held, and we had to use the much less attractive dining room.

In my speech I described three ways professional leaders spoke. The first was giving the best possible presentation and linking favourable facts persuasively. I suggested this was normal for politicians and professional leaders. The second way was presenting facts in support of a policy but deliberately concealing other key facts, throwing a different light on the conclusion. This is essentially misleading. The third category was lying. I suggested that lying by professional leaders is never acceptable but that the second category was not either. Doctors, when I spoke, were the most trusted occupational group in the UK, a huge privilege needing to be preserved. My warning was timely; doctors later lost their most trusted position and nurses took the top spot (Ipsos Mori, 2019).

Peter Hutton, one of the Vice-Chairs, who had been elected Chair to succeed me, responded graciously. After discovering my interest in history, he presented me, on behalf of the Academy, with a picture of an old barn in Exeter in the exact area where my practice was. This now hangs in our home.

A few days after the dinner, John Lilleyman was knighted.

39

Distinction/Clinical Excellence Awards for Senior Academic General Practitioners

The labourer is worthy of his hire.

The Bible, **St Luke 7**

In 1948 the remuneration systems in the NHS of the two main kind of doctors, consultants and general practitioners, was very different. Consultants were previously unpaid when working at the voluntary hospitals as 'honoraries.' Their income came from the private practice, which followed from their hospital roles. General practitioners were paid by a fixed sum per patient, the capitation fee.

The consultants were happy about being salaried and many were attracted by a regular income. However, their leaders, many of whom commanded high private practice fees, feared that if they were to work for most of their time in the NHS, their income would fall. Their numbers were few but their influence was high and they had a strong network in the three English Medical Royal Colleges.

The circumstances for GPs were quite different. They had much lower social standing, no Royal College, and had no training for their role. In 1948, doctors entered unsupervised general practice with only a qualifying degree. When the NHS came, GPs had no academic clout. There was no GP professor in the world.

GPs thought that they had to stick together. They were hostile to entering a salaried service. Many commentators, usually salaried themselves, criticised this as reactionary. It was, however, logical. General practice, more than any other branch of the medical profession, had always valued the patient-doctor relationship, and since 1911 GPs had campaigned for patients to have a choice of doctor. GPs thought then, and many still think now, that in salaried services many staff look to their superiors rather than to their clients. Salaried bureaucracies do not usually allow patients/clients a choice of salaried professionals. It is extremely difficult for a client to change a hospital consultant, social worker, or teacher.

GPs feared that the control inherent in a salaried system would be used perhaps to post them around the country (the capital value of their practices was being nationalised at the time) by a cadre of external leaders, such as medical officers of health or specialists, who might be unaware of the realities of clinical general practice. GPs saw themselves offering a *local* professional service. Virtually all other professionals working locally in the community were self-employed professionals, e.g. accountants, architects, barristers, dentists, solicitors and surveyors. GPs across Australasia, Europe and North America were at the time self-employed. Crucially, GPs had worked as independent contractors under a capitation fee system since 1913, which they had then chosen to do. It had its faults, but it was seen as the best of the various possibilities. This analysis led to struggles not about the principle of a capitation fee, but the price. The BMA sought to push the capitation fee as high as possible.

The policy of GPs on joining the NHS swung to and fro in a chaotic series of meetings of the BMA's representative body. The BMA's leadership was outflanked by some political moves. First, Aneurin Bevan, the Health Minister in the Attlee Government decreed that capitation fees could be used in the new NHS; essentially this maintained the status quo and extended it to the whole population. Second, he did a deal with the President of the Royal College of Physicians of London, Lord Moran. He allowed consultants to have private practice if they worked 9 out of 11 notional half days per week

DOI: 10.1201/9781032713601-47

for the NHS. In addition he gave an option for consultants, expected to include virtually all the leaders, of substantial additional payments called 'merit' or 'distinction' awards. These would be payable for life, pensionable, and awarded by a professional committee. Consultants swung in favour of the NHS. Aneurin Bevan is reputed to have said: "I stuffed their mouths with gold!" Nowhere else in the British public service was such a deal made.

Merit awards consisted of financial payments at four levels. The grades were usually called C, B, A, and A plus. At any one time, about one-third of consultants held an award at one level or another. After the establishment of the Review Body on Doctors' and Dentists' Remuneration in the early 1960s, the number and value of the awards were determined by this Body. As a broad simplification, they were intended to reward superior performance at the local level (C award), regional level (B award), national (A) and international (A plus) levels of performance. At the international level, the award doubled the consultant's salary at its highest point and was pensionable. From 1948 onwards, distinction awards were an integral part of consultant remuneration in the NHS, as confirmed by the Review Body on Doctors' and Dentists Remuneration. Awards were limited to those appointed as consultants or equivalent in the NHS. Their central importance to consultant pay was confirmed by Sir Stanley Clayton (1982; 1911–1986) when Chairman of the Advisory Committee on Distinction Awards, who reported that by 1982 "two-thirds of consultants retired with an award."

Attempt to Introduce Merit/Distinction Awards for GPs

The College of General Practitioners had had many successes and gained in confidence. It proposed in its early days that GPs should have a merit award scheme of their own. The BMA GPs strongly opposed the idea. The Government offered a significant sum, about £2.5 million of additional money to fund the proposal. However, the annual conferences of NHS general practitioners voted strongly against by about 80 to 20, even though additional funds had been offered and the scheme could have been introduced at no extra cost to GPs. This was because the general feeling was that distinction awards would be divisive, would weaken the solidarity between GPs, and could be used to control them. The rejection of £2.5 million extra on the table is good evidence of the strong egalitarian feeling amongst GPs. The idea of a merit/distinction award system in NHS general practice never arose again in relation to service NHS GPs. Outside the medical profession, payments for good performance became increasingly common over the years and were later introduced in the public services, including the civil service.

After accepting the report of the Royal Commission on Medical Education (1968) the DH had to develop postgraduate (vocational) training programmes for young doctors choosing a career in general practice. In 1972, a DHSS circular instructed regional health boards (later regional health authorities) to establish posts called 'regional advisers in general practice,' one per region (Chapter 14, Regional Adviser story). These were half-time salaried positions. Eligibility for distinction awards was specifically debarred for all regional advisers in general practice. The RCGP essentially professionalised GP teaching by leading and providing many of the regional advisers. Professionalisation meant training the GP trainer to teach and paying the trainer to do so. Selecting GP trainers and giving them only a limited term of appointment as teachers all followed (DPG, 1984a).

Instead of a salary, trainers received a 'trainers' grant,' set by the Review Body each year. But the trainers' grants collectively came out of the 'pool' of national GP remuneration, so GPs were collectively paying for their trainers themselves at no cost to the DHSS. Meanwhile, in the hospital service, consultants doing good teaching received points contributing towards distinction awards separate from and in addition to their basic consultant remuneration.

MSD Foundation 1980s

In the 1980s, Merck Sharp and Dohme, an international pharmaceutical company, identified the importance of general practice. It established a charitable foundation, the MSD Foundation, to develop education for general practice. The charity was independent and not connected with the parent company for policy. The trustees were major figures in the medical profession including Sir Richard Bayliss (1917–2006; KCVO FRCP, a former Physician to the Queen. At the core of the Foundation were its GP members, chaired by Pat Byrne an RCGP President, and including the next generation of RCGP activists such as Donald Irvine, a former Honorary Secretary, David Metcalfe, a College Chair of Education, Colin Waine, and me. The Foundation was generously funded and produced much educational material and some publications (Waine *et al.*, 1981a, b).

The second director was a GP, Marshall Marinker, so the question arose about how he should be paid. It was agreed that he was at the top of the medical profession, having been a foundation professor at the Leicester Medical School. The decision was taken to pay him at the level of the A-plus distinction award for NHS consultants. This was a declaration of intent and was the first example of a GP in the UK being deliberately paid at this rate, albeit not by the NHS.

RCGP Policy 1989

During my Chairmanship of the RCGP Council, I was approached by the Dean of one of the London medical schools. He told me that the salaried professor of general practice in his medical school was outstanding, and was performing better than some of his other senior academic staff. He had therefore recommended him for a distinction award but had been told that it was not possible for a GP academic, however distinguished, to receive an award. Could the College help? I checked but he was right and there was no way. The Dean later told me that he had made funds available from other sources for an *ex gratia* payment to the professor, but was not as much as he would have received in any other branch of medicine. General medical practice as a clinical discipline was disadvantaged and was in effect being discriminated against, especially for its most distinguished members. This sharpened my understanding about the exclusion being wrong in principle and unfair in practice.

As Chair, I wrote an academic plan for general practice that was approved by the Council in December 1989. This included a paragraph stating: "That arrangements should be made to ensure that senior university staff in general practice, postgraduate and undergraduate, full-time and part-time, are no worse off financially than their colleagues of comparable ability in other branches of the medical profession" (RCGP, 1989b, *Academic Plan for General Practice;* Recommendation 27). This was now RCGP policy. The attack on the discrimination against academic GPs being eligible for consideration for awards had begun.

Conference of Royal Colleges and Faculties 1990

In 1989, I became the first Chair of Council of the College to attend the Conference of Medical Royal Colleges and Faculties in the UK (Chapter 23, Chair of Council). I worked my way into the Conference. The next Chair of the Conference was Professor Dame Margaret Turner-Warwick. After we had got to know each other, we set up exchange dinners in each other's Colleges.

Armed with a clear policy position for the College, I asked Dame Margaret about distinction awards for salaried academic general practitioners. She was strongly supportive, so we agreed I would propose this policy to the Conference of Medical Royal Colleges and their Faculties. I did so gingerly in February 1990, and it was approved unanimously. This was now the policy of all the Medical Royal Colleges. I then drafted a letter for the Chair of the Conference to sign knowing it was a once-in-a-lifetime opportunity. By then the new Chair of the Conference was Professor (later Sir) Dillwyn Williams (1929–), President of the Royal College of Pathologists. I knew him reasonably well, having lobbied hard for his election as Chair. He signed it and sent it to Kenneth Clarke, Secretary of State for Health on 12 March 1990 (Williams, 1990; addendum). Although Kenneth Clarke did not respond and showed no interest, I was encouraged. It now looked as if the reform would come, even if I did not live to see it.

The challenge then was to publicise the point. With College policy on awards established and with the Conference of Colleges now in support, it was possible to go public. In June 1991 I wrote in the *BMJ* that: "...The result is that the best academics from general practice are paid almost exactly half what they would earn in any other branch of the profession" (DPG, 1991b). The question was now in the public domain: was the salaried GP academic labourer worthy of his hire?

Some Individual Doctors

Near the end of my Chairmanship of the Council, a new opportunity arose. An editor of the College *Journal* was to be appointed. It had been agreed that the job required paid sessions and I priced these sessions at the B grade distinction award level. I met resistance within the College, as this had never been done before. GPs can sometimes be their own worst enemies. Senior colleagues argued seriously that the rate was too high. I pointed out that in any other branch of the profession I would be receiving an A plus award as Chair of a Royal College. I supplied the critics with the published figures of the numbers of specialists getting A plus, A, B, and C awards. It proved educational. Even at the top of the RCGP, little was known about the award system. The B level distinction rate for the Editor was paid to Alastair Wright, so another GP precedent was achieved.

In 1992, thanks to a donation from the Laing Foundation, the University of Exeter appointed a new professor of complementary medicine, who was medically qualified. I was Director of the Postgraduate Medical School (Chapter 27, Postgraduate Medical School story). However, there was a problem. Complementary medicine was not a recognised specialty and this was the first chair in this subject in the world. The University's non-medical professorial pay scale was well below the rate for medical professors as so many of them received distinction awards.

How could we bridge the gap? The Vice-Chancellor of the University looked to me for ideas. I invented a distinction award equivalent system to be paid to the appointed professor on merit, if judged appropriate, by a trio of external people: the Chair of Council of the RCGP, the President of the Royal College of Physicians, and the Chair of the Southwestern Regional Health Authority. This was agreed with the University, the Laing Foundation and Professor Edzard Ernst who was appointed. This unique system was put into the professor's contract.

After Ernst had been a few years in post, and whilst I was still Director of the Medical School, this review process was activated. I briefed the trio and it worked smoothly. Ernst's academic publications were superb, numerous (the most in the Exeter Medical School) and published in high-ranking journals. The trio of experts recommended that he should receive the equivalent of a B distinction award, paid from the Laing funds. He was surprised and pleased.

After five more years, another review was due but when I was no longer Director. Then Ernst's publications were at international level and he was the leading professor of complementary medicine in the world. However, a different trio of experts got into a tangle about whether he was equivalent to a hospital consultant. Clearly he was not, as he did not see patients, but the point of the system was to provide in his formal contract an external judgement of his performance in relation to equivalent medical *academic staff*. He was not recommended for a higher award. I was disappointed by this, particularly since the RCGP Chair had agreed to it. He, representing the RCGP, should of all organisations have understood the problem of doctors excluded from the distinction award system, and he should have said so, if necessary being outvoted. However, he missed the point.

Donald Irvine, a regional adviser in general practice, was elected President of the General Medical Council in 1994, the first GP to be elected in 137 years. Although never eligible for a merit award as a GP regional adviser the Presidency was a paid post by the GMC itself. The only possible level for one of the two leaders of the medical profession was the A plus distinction award rate then paid to over 100 top consultants. Another key precedent for a GP was established that year.

Research Experience in Exeter

During the same period, another experience in Exeter added to my understanding of the growing need to get academic GPs into the distinction award system. The Institute of General Practice had a research interest in depression. General practitioners and academic psychiatrists were working productively together. My highest cited research publication (Kessler *et al.,* 1999, which later attracted 593 citations) was written by two academic GPs and two academic psychiatrists. David Kessler, a Bristol GP (now a professor) whom I had recruited as research fellow, had previously obtained the membership by examination of the Royal College of Psychiatrists (MRCPsych), but had gone into general practice. Subjects such as depression, which we were researching, were of academic interest to both academic GPs and academic psychiatrists.

I realised that if distinction awards were to be available only to academic psychiatrists and not to academic GPs, there would be a big and continuing incentive for all those interested and capable of such research to move to psychiatry or indeed any relevant hospital-based specialty where they could do the same work and possibly double their incomes over a career. I started to point this perverse incentive out to senior colleagues in the DH.

JCPTGP

My three-year period of office (1994–1997) as Honorary Chair of the Joint Committee on Postgraduate Training for General Practice ended in May 1997. I submitted a paper for discussion at my final meeting proposing that the Chair of the JCPTGP be paid sessions at the rate of an A plus distinction award. I would be out of the chair by the time it was discussed, so I could not benefit personally (Chapter 29, JCPTGP story). The President of the GMC was being paid at the rate of an A plus distinction award and the Chairman of the Specialist Training Authority (the specialist equivalent to the JCPTGP) was always a consultant on the A or A plus level. The debate was lively, as described in Chapter 29, JCPTGP story. The JCPTGP decided to explore the proposal. However, the DH representative was quick to say that there was no budget for this. He told me that the DH would not pay (and it would not happen if it did not). The DH took no action. A few years later, the JCPTGP and the SHA were merged into the Postgraduate Medical Education and Training Board. My initiative failed but raised the differential in peoples' minds.

Vice-Chair of the Academy

In 1998 I was elected by the Presidents of the Colleges as Vice-Chair of the Academy of Medical Royal Colleges, and in 2000 was elected Chair (Chapter 38, Chair of the Academy of Medical Royal Colleges), whilst always being excluded from any distinction award as a GP. I twice chaired, in 2001 and 2002, the all-day meeting where the Academy co-ordinates the recommendations for distinction awards from the various Royal Colleges and specialist faculties.

I was appointed ex officio to the DH top Committee for the award of A plus distinction awards, the first ever GP and the first doctor to do so without being the recipient of an award. The Chief Executive was Professor Sir Netar Mallick, with whom I had served in the 1990s on the renal review of London's teaching hospitals. All this called increasingly into question the bar on academic salaried GPs being eligible for NHS distinction awards.

Trends 1980s–2000

There were several trends in the last two decades of the 20th century that supported the inclusion of academic GPs in a national distinction award scheme. First, a small but growing number of GPs were appointed with consultant contracts. These were mostly academics and their university/medical school agreed consultant contracts with an NHS authority as part of their employment conditions. These arrangements were directly analogous to the arrangements for medical consultants who held academic appointments, most commonly as senior lecturer or professor. I had an NHS consultant contract myself with the Southwestern Regional Health Authority. Holding a contract with an NHS authority was a condition for receiving an NHS distinction award, so as this arrangement became steadily more common it reduced a longstanding hurdle. Some academic posts in university departments of general practice from the 1990s were titled 'consultant' senior lecturer, as in my region at Bristol. Each appointment was a step forward and empowered the next group of academics to seek similar arrangements.

There remained another serious obstacle. Distinction awards were awarded for service only in one defined clinical field and general practice was not one of them. This was a severe disincentive for any doctor working clinically as a generalist. This obstacle started to be overcome as some medical schools presented leading academic GPs for awards in other disciplines, for example, in public health. This solved the short-term problem of getting proper recognition for an individual, but created new anomalies. Clinical generalists were being forced to deny their discipline and some other specialty was being denied one of its awards. This was serious for public health as a small specialty. Some clinical generalists eventually achieved A distinction awards, but only at the expense of each one not being available to a public health doctor. I used the example of a GP professor who was obviously a GP, whose research was all on general practice, who received an A distinction award in public health as a powerful example.

Postgraduate medical deans had been left out of the early form of the distinction award system. They were later included but in such a way that associate postgraduate deans, some of whom were GPs but, however successful, were excluded. All these nooks and byways in the system looked as if they had been designed to preserve a status quo rather than implementing a logical pay for performance system. Later, a GP Medical Postgraduate Dean received the highest award.

Another development was the appointment of a small number of GPs to knighthoods. Although few in number (I was the fifteenth GP knight or dame in the 20th century, of whom only five were academics), these appointments had a disproportionate impact on opinion leaders. The background was a slow change in how society saw GPs, reflected as always by the honours system. In the 19th century and first half of the 20th, GPs were awarded knighthoods only for personal service to the Royal Family or a Prime Minister, or for exceptional distinguished service to the BMA. GPs knighted in the 20th century, through the Chair of the BMA Council, included Sir Henry Brackenbury, Sir Guy Dain, Sir Ronald Gibson, Sir James Cameron. I was on the BMA Council with the last two.

The first academic GP to achieve a civil honour at the knighthood/dame level was Dame Annis Gillie in 1968. She had been both Chair of the Council and President of the College. She was the first College President so honoured. Unusually she had been appointed by the Government to chair a committee on general practice, which produced a successful report: *The Field of Work of the Family Doctor* (*Gillie Report*, 1963). There was then a gap of 21 years before the next GP knighthood/damehood. In 1989, Michael Drury was knighted for his work after finishing as PRCGP and being the first GP Vice-Chair of the Conference of Royal Colleges. In addition to the strongest lobby ever mounted by the RCGP, which I led, he had strong support from the University of Birmingham (then with four Royal College Presidents) and from the Conference of Medical Royal Colleges.

In the 1990s came a trio of GP knighthoods, which set the scene for discrete ridicule of the distinction award system. Sir Donald Irvine (1994), Professor Sir Brian Jarman (1998) and I (1999) were knighted. Irvine had been a successful Chair of Council of the RCGP but his main achievement was his chairing the GMC Standards Committee. Jarman had been a successful GP academic and had developed the 'Underprivileged Practice Area' (Jarman, 1983). Later he was in the team, chaired by Sir Leslie (later Lord) Turnberg, which produced a report reforming the duplication of the London medical schools. He also played a big part in the Bristol Inquiry (Kennedy Report, 2001).

These three knighthoods within five years came to GPs, two of whom had been regional advisers (DI and DPG), and two of whom had been professors (BJ and DPG), but none of whom had been eligible for a distinction award. I started to play, on behalf of general practice, the ridicule card. At various times and when in appropriate company, for example, influential opinion formers in the DH, we used to say that in Britain it was easier for a GP to get a knighthood than an NHS distinction award! Senior policy makers squirmed or smiled ruefully as the anomaly was underlined. Ridicule in Britain is a powerful weapon and hated by those responsible for the arrangements.

External Support for the Principle

In 1995, the University Funding Council's Medical Advisory Committee recommended the end of the exclusion of salaried academic GPs from the distinction awards system. This was an important first from a body outside general practice.

The Richards Independent Task Force (1997) was chaired by Sir Rex Richards FRS (1922–2019). It was particularly important as it was established by the Committee of Vice-Chancellors and Principals to review medical academic careers. I made sure it received as evidence the booklet *Academic Primary Care: The Academic Contribution* from the Conference of Academic Organisations (1996) where I was Chair and draftsman at the time. This policy booklet recommended the inclusion of academic GPs in the distinction award system. I set up a private dinner with Sir Rex Richards as I had met him on the governing body of the British Postgraduate Medical Federation in London and took advantage of him being, like me, a Devonian. Crucially, he was Chancellor of the University of Exeter, with me being Director of the Exeter Postgraduate Medical School. Over dinner I said how important and serious I thought the exclusion of GP academics from the distinction system was and that I hoped he would consider changing that.

This task force had strong GP representation as its one GP member was Ann Louise Kinmonth, the Professor at Cambridge, who I am sure was strong on this issue. The Richards Task Force met in 1996 and 1997 and delivered as hoped: its recommendation 5.34 was "The Department of Health should consult with the appropriate academic bodies in general practice to establish mechanisms to ensure that the terms and conditions of senior clinical academic general practitioners who are full or part-time salaried employees of universities or medical schools match those of their academic colleagues in hospital practice."

Vice-Chair of the Academy

In 1998, I was PRCGP and Vice-Chair of the Academy of Medical Royal Colleges. I then had the right and duty to implement established academy policy as agreed in 1990 and confirmed in the Williams letter (addendum). I was also Professor of General Practice at Exeter and Director of GP Education (formerly Regional Adviser) for the Southwestern region at Bristol, and a nationally elected member of the GMC. Alone in the Academy, I had been for seven years a member of the representative body of the BMA and for four years a member of the BMA Council. I had an unusually wide range of contacts in British medicine and amongst GPs a rare understanding of the organisation and political issues at the top of specialist medicine. These advantages were supplemented by several longstanding personal contacts with the BMA leaders. At this point the problem of eligibility for academic GPs was stuck.

I therefore had the opportunity, as Vice-Chair of the Academy, to initiate discussions on the problem of salaried academic GPs being debarred from receiving distinction awards simply because they were medical generalists. First, it was necessary to forge a coherent, intellectually logical position that could be sustained in high-level discussions. It had to take account of the medico-political history and political realities at the time. My starting position was a passionate belief in the role of general practice. I believed it was as valuable as any other branch of medicine and indeed more valuable than most. Starfield *et al.* (2005) were soon to demonstrate this. This was not essentially an issue of money, but of status, as the continuing exclusion of GPs for 50 years (1948–1998) was unreasonable and discriminatory. The exclusion was based on several different factors, all somehow had to be countered.

My Proposal

There was no question of seeking entry for all NHS GPs into the existing distinction award scheme or similar award scheme. The big vote of NHS GPs to reject merit awards had to be respected. Any contrary suggestion would be opposed by the GPC of the BMA (formerly the GMSC). The case was therefore made only for a small subset of GPs who could be easily identified, who were *demonstrably different* from most GPs, particularly through their contracts of employment. Junior GP lecturers, like junior specialist lecturers, would like specialists not be eligible. Only GP academics holding university appointments of senior lecturer or above would be eligible because in specialist medicine that was the norm. Academic general practitioners in these posts had given up their independent contractor status in whole or in part and had accepted a salaried contract of employment, whole-time or part-time. The salaries had been negotiated by the BMA and the salaries on which academic general practitioners were appointed were those of the universities with medical schools and related to the NHS consultant scale. There was an agreement between the departments of state responsible for the NHS and the universities. This avoided difficulties, as medical professors and senior lecturers worked clinically in the NHS: they had to do so to be eligible for distinction awards, which are NHS awards for NHS service.

The group of doctors involved was small, which helped when proposing funding; and they could easily be identified by virtue of their university/medical school contracts. A substantial group was part-time in their academic role anyway, so any awards would be payable only in relation to the academic sessions actually contracted, as in specialist medicine. Hence costs, if distinction awards were implemented, would be lower still. There would be no skin off the nose of the powerful GPC, which had no locus in terms of these salaries and NHS GPs would not lose anything. This analysis played the BMA GP committee offside but brought the Medical Academic Staff Committee (MASC) of the BMA into play. It had had the same Chair, Colin Smith, for many years and he had never shown any interest in merit/distinction awards for salaried, academic GPs, even though the Committee had had a GP, John Ferguson, as Vice-Chair for many years. I had had much contact with John in the RCGP and he was unusually experienced. Although I was a member briefly of their conference, in 1992. I judged that despite its GP Vice-Chair, this Committee was unlikely to help much.

There was an obvious problem that consultants would oppose the inclusion of any new group if the pool of their funding was to be diluted. This meant that some specialists would lose awards to academic GPs. To counter this, I always insisted that the inclusion of academic general practitioners in a merit award scheme must be accompanied by additional funding.

A big decision was whether it would be better to seek to join the existing specialist system or to devise a new, separate system for GPs. There were pros and cons. A new system would avoid delicate discussions with the specialists and would ensure that awards for generalists would not be seen as taking funds away from them (any new scheme would come with its own funding). It would be flexible and might be more sensitive to general practice. However, a contrary argument was the advantage of adding a small group of doctors to a well-established UK-wide scheme. Of course, including academic GPs in a national scheme meant that for the first time in the UK, leading GPs would compete head to head with leading specialists on the same criteria. I never worried about this as I knew how much unrecognised talent existed in general practice.

There were two parties to discussions between the Government and the medical profession about pay: the DH and the BMA (the sole recognised medical trade union). Most of the gains over the years made by general practice under the NHS had come from pressure on the DH, for example the new contract of the mid-1960s. However, this approach could not be mounted through the College, as a charity, and the College had been trying to crack the problem for 25 years without success. Could an approach through the leadership of the BMA succeed?

Private Discussions with BMA Leaders

I started a series of one-to-one meetings with the key players. I had advantages over all the other GP academics. I was too old to benefit from an award and so was acting without any possibility of personal gain. I knew the history, it was my campaign, and I was now Vice-Chair of the Academy with membership of five national bodies: the Academy of Medical Royal Colleges, the Joint Consultants' Committee, the Conference of Senior Hospital Doctors, the BMA's Representative Body and the DH's top national distinction awards committee. No GP had ever held these posts before or knew their way around specialist organisations better.

John Chisholm was the Chair of the General Practitioners Committee (GPC) of the BMA. Had we first met at the Fourth National Trainee Conference in my Department in Exeter in 1980 (Ronalds *et al.,* 1981), where he was a BMA trainee leader. When I was Chair of the JCPTGP (1994–7) he was a member. We had therefore had many contacts. In 1995, I had given him the chair of a special meeting at Heathrow Airport and the next day when the BMA team was in severe difficulties, I had suspended a JCPTGP meeting to allow his team to regroup (Chapter 29, JCPTGP story). We were used to working together. Chisholm was the first of a new breed of GPC chairs, being the first to have been vocationally trained and to have obtained the MRCGP as a registrar. He grew up with academic general practice, took a broad view, and unlike many colleagues never made anti-College speeches.

The GPC had no locus, but the medico-political reality was that Chisholm effectively held a veto. If he was against the proposal, there were numerous ways he could stop or delay anything happening. However, our talk went well. John carefully clarified that the proposal would refer only to those GPs who were salaried and on the staff of medical schools. He would not publicly support the proposal but was sympathetic to the idea that GP academics should be paid the rate for the job and should not be disadvantaged just because they were generalists. He was big enough to take the wider view.

There were three favourable features about Sandy (later Sir) Macara (1932–2012) being Chair of the BMA where the Chair of Council is the policy leader. His judgement was therefore critical. He too held a veto. First, it was unusual for a public health physician to reach the Chair of BMA Council, as only about 3% of BMA members were public health physicians (Kent, 1986). Public health physicians had not been part of the distinction award scheme when it started and had negotiated their way into it. Macara had been active in achieving this, so he had experience of his discipline being excluded and practical experience of reforming the system. We were contemporaries having been junior members (under age 40) of the BMA in the 1960s and had attended the same BMA junior doctor conferences. There were also westcountry links. He administered attachments for medical students at Bristol, and in 1972 sent me my first medical student. Later, both of us were WHO consultants. I went to BMA House to see him, armed with the 1990 letter from the Chair of the Conference of Medical Royal Colleges to the Secretary of State for Health calling for the inclusion of general practitioners in the merit award scheme (Williams, 1990). Sandy recognised this was policy of all the Medical Royal Colleges.

One strength of the BMA, for which it gets little credit, is long-term and effective support for doctors in minority roles. Would Sandy Macara see academic GPs as such a minority? He did. He saw a direct parallel with the previous exclusion of public health doctors from the NHS merit award scheme. He swiftly grasped the problem and said he would do all he could as long as "GP academic" was clearly defined for eligibility. However, the responsibility on the BMA side for such negotiations lay with the Joint Consultants' Committee (JCC).

Macara followed up with a meeting on 12 May 1998. The Chair of the JCC was then Sir Norman Browse and Johnson attended as the consultant leader. No direct opposition was expressed but a whole series of concerns were voiced: setting a precedent, definitions, part-time eligibility, GPs working as principals, etc.

All these balls fell into my court. I wrote a 13-page, point-by-point response carefully relating most responses to existing consultant arrangements, which I had learned about as Director of the Exeter Postgraduate Medical School. I did not know it at the time but this unpublished paper did the trick.

The Joint Consultants' Committee (JCC) is a hybrid organisation. It was formed after the establishment of the NHS to integrate the academic and political wings of consultant/specialist medicine. Its two parent bodies are the Academy of Medical Royal Colleges and the BMA. It is serviced by the BMA and is consulted by the DH on matters affecting consultants other than pay, which is negotiated by the BMA consultants and specialists committee. It has no GP equivalent.

For many years the chairmen of the JCC had had high status, signalled by most being knighted. I knew Sir Anthony Grabham (1930–2015) from the battle for the GMC Presidency in 1994 and later served with him on the BMA Council, and also Sir Norman Browse (1931–2019) with whom I also served in the Academy. The JCC was going downhill in the 1990s but it still had huge clout. The Chair at the time was James (Jim) Johnson (1947–) who had followed a career in the BMA having previously chaired both the BMA Junior Doctors' Committee and the BMA Consultants' Committee. He was later elected Chair of the BMA Council.

Most GPs know little of the JCC and I may have been the first GP to attend it. I was a member ex-officio, as Vice-Chair of the Academy of Medical Royal Colleges in 1998. I attended its meetings regularly as well as the annual conference of senior hospital doctors, and was present when Jim Johnson was elected its Chair. This attendance gave me insight into its thinking. Jim Johnson was an experienced BMA politician. He had two particular strengths: first a desire to make things happen, perhaps from his work as a vascular surgeon; and secondly a greater readiness to act on his own than many professional leaders. He was quick to seize a point in argument and spoke clearly. On my proposal Johnson not only held a veto but would, if he agreed, have to argue the case himself. He was the single most important player.

Johnson confirmed that the crucial arena on admitting GP academics to the distinction award scheme was the meetings between the JCC and the DH, as far away from most GPs as it is possible to get in the medical world and a setting where no GP had previously ever been influential. He discussed the issues crisply and succinctly. He wanted clear boundaries and was rightly concerned that there were numerous GP academics with various titles, terms and conditions of service, some on only one session per week with multiple pay scales. A definition was needed and my paper proposed senior lecturer in a university was the logical point with its common association with consultant status. In the Exeter Postgraduate Medical School the academic consultants were mostly senior lecturers and the pay scales were equivalent. On that basis he was prepared to proceed.

Special Private Meeting

I was invited to a private meeting of Chief Officers in BMA House with the Chair of Council in the chair. The Chairs of the JCC, the GPC and MASC were present. I presented my proposal again and it was carefully considered. Agreement was privately reached that the BMA would support the proposal through the JCC. There were no administrative staff present, no notes and no minutes. This was a top level, private meeting. No one was to be compromised.

The JCC was as good as its word and the DH was doubtless pleased to see the proposal coming from the professional side. The proposal was formally agreed. The public confirmation was a statement in the Secretary of State for Health's (2000) *The NHS Plan*. Happily, I was Chair of the Academy when the announcement was made. For the JCC and Jim Johnson, Chair, this was a small byway in the medical world. His skilled negotiation and support for a small and politically weak group of doctors who were not the senior hospital doctors for whom the JCC exists was impressive and will always be much appreciated.

In 2001, the DH after consulting on the distinction award scheme, introduced a newly named Clinical Excellence Scheme on 1 August 2003. Documentation specifically referred to the advice from the Richards Task Force (1997). All the effort put into advising it (COAG, 1996) and to Sir Rex personally had been justified. It was at last stated that academic general practitioners were eligible for consideration for awards.

Conclusion

This campaign started in my home when I drafted for the RCGP Council a proposal for salaried academic GPs to be eligible for distinction awards. Turning points were the adoption of the policy by the RCGP Council in December 1989 (*A College Plan,* 1989b) and its formal endorsement by the Conference of Medical Royal Colleges and Faculties in 1990, confirmed in the letter sent to the Secretary of State for Health (Williams, 1990; Appendix). Success depended on my being elected an officer of the Academy of Medical Royal Colleges on BMA leaders outside general practice, like Sandy Macara, Chair of BMA Council, whom I had known for 26 years, and Jim Johnson, Chair of the Joint Consultants' Committee. They rose to the occasion, stretching boundaries, rescuing a small, politically weak, group of GP colleagues. The campaign took 11 years.

ADDENDA

12th March 1990

Dear Secretary of State

The Conference of Medical Royal Colleges and their Faculties in the UK met on 26 February 1990 at the Royal College of Physicians of London. The Conference was very concerned that a small group of doctors, some with full-time and some with part-time contracts with universities/medical schools are severely disadvantaged, simply because their clinical discipline is general practice. This problem does not affect any other main branch of medicine. This group of doctors is especially important since it greatly influences quality of care, research and education and includes many of the academic leaders of the subject.

The Conference of Medical Royal Colleges unanimously recommends to you that they should no longer be financially disadvantaged in comparison with their colleagues of comparable ability and responsibility in other branches of the medical profession. Since there is urgency about this problem which is about to get worse as a result of new responsibilities which you have recently introduced, we very much hope you will be able to resolve this soon.

Yours sincerely,
Dillwyn Williams
Chairman, Conference of Medical Royal Colleges and their Faculties

ST LEONARD'S PRACTICE, EXETER

By 2018 there were three GPs working in the St Leonard's Practice, Professors Philip Evans, Alex Harding, and Jose Valderas. All three had been awarded bronze clinical excellence awards for their university work.

Section IX

40

Patient Participation

Yet the professional contract is at heart not with government but with patients.

Margaret McCartney (2020)

In 1974, I wrote an editorial "Patient power" (*JRCGP,* 1974) which started my involvement with this subject. It was fairly amateur, merely calling for the patient to be a member of the primary healthcare team. In 1977, Wilson described a patient group in general practice and a year later, the National Association for Patient Participation formed, led by Tim Paine, a Bristol GP and associate adviser in general practice with me in the Southwestern region. I wrote an article in a medical newspaper supporting patient participation within the RCGP (DPG, 1980) which stating what I hoped the College would do.

Patient participation and trainee participation in education are linked. I pushed student involvement, and we were early in having two GP trainee representatives on the Southwestern Regional GP Education Committee, both with voting rights on trainer selection. General practice was gradually making leadership moves in the medical profession in relation to both students and patients.

First Patient Group

As Chair of the RCGP Communications Division I set up several new subgroups within the Division (as described in Chapter 19, Chair of the Communications Division). The first was for a patients' group called the Patient Liaison Group. The topic had arisen when an Oxford GP Peter Pritchard (1918–2019), led an influential conference on patient participation. Michael Hall represented the Exeter Department. I published it as *Occasional Paper* 17 (Pritchard, 1981). My proposal for a new Patient Group to be an integral part of the College was approved by the Communications Division in December 1981. This was historically important as the first patient group in a British medical institution.

I selected the chairmen of all these groups carefully and invited John Hasler to Chair the Patient Group, with advice to pass the chair on to a lay; i.e. patient chair as soon as possible. He led the Group well and the Patient Liaison Group (PLG) flourished. He arranged for Nancy Dennis to be the first lay Chair. Soon it was seen as so important that it was taken out of the Communications Division to become, quite properly, a committee reporting direct to the Council.

The RCGP Patient Group, under a later Chair of Council faced a crisis when the GPC (when I was not on it, 1990–1993) proposed its abolishment. To the credit of the Council, of which I was still a vocal member this was rejected. The PLG, later renamed the Patient Partnership, continued as a model for other Colleges.

Theory of Patient Participation

The theory of patient participation was only emerging in 1981. Most patients and most doctors enjoy good working relationships within their consultations. There is good research evidence that active patient involvement improves outcomes in medical care (Kaplan *et al.,* 1989). However, the relationship

DOI: 10.1201/9781032713601-49

between patients and doctors at group level was absent. Whilst there were long-established patient charities, like the British Diabetes Association (BDA), later renamed Diabetes UK, dating from the 1930s, these were primarily concerned with developing research and care for single diseases. What was missing was a collective relationship, at an organisational level, between patients across the board on one hand and GPs on the other, across the whole range of conditions which patients experience. Patient groups have much to contribute to medical care. Patients working together can see collectively what may be difficult for a single patient to see. As well, it is easier for patients to communicate some messages to doctors at group level rather than through a single patient.

Sometimes patient groups can be more effective than doctors. An example was when the RCGP Patient Liaison Group formulated a policy on the difficult issue of doctors putting patients off the list. This is always controversial and sometimes seen as an outmoded privilege. Once, when this became nationally controversial with statements being made in Parliament calling for this right to be abolished, the Patient Liaison Group in the RCGP came into its own. It constructed a valuable document, drafted by Patricia Wilkie, soon to become the Chair, which fairly balanced the rights and duties of both parties (*Removal of patients from GPs' lists: guidance to college members*; RCGP, 1997). The Group called for proper courtesies like patients being given notice and proper reasons by the GPs. They documented two key insights. First, that if a patient becomes violent and hits a nurse then the core patient-practice relationship has broken down and the practice may no longer be able to provide care with compassion. Second, they contrasted the rights of different patients. If an aggressive man, drunk or on drugs, terrorises a waiting room with mothers and children, this is not acceptable. It is not just the man who should have rights. The Patient Group won and the issue blew over. The right of general practitioners to remove patients remained. Patients can speak for themselves and should do so more often.

Patient Group in the Academy of Medical Royal Colleges

In my last year as Chair of the Academy formed a Patient Group in the Academy. This was more difficult than doing so in the RCGP as described in Chapter 19, Chair of Communications Division.

National Association for Patient Participation

The National Association for Patient Participation (NAPP) approached me. In 2003, Tim Paine the GP founder was retiring as President. Roger Battye, the Chief Executive, asked me to facilitate a meeting of Trustees, which went well. The Trustees elected me Patron (non-executive). I tried to get Tim Paine a civil honour for his national leadership and 25 years' commitment and sadly failed. Some epidemiologists, people who have chosen numbers over relationships, undervalue patients' views as 'subjective'. One grade 1 civil servant once told me: "The trouble with patient choice is it can undermine policy!" It took a decade before Patricia Wilkie broke the glass ceiling for patients receiving an OBE in 2013.

Graham Box, Chief Executive of NAPP, negotiated an event at the RCGP. The RCGP Chair, the GPC Chair and the Department of Health (DH) all supported patient groups in general practice. I attended and it went well but it had little impact in the field. After Patricia Wilkie finished as the first Chair of the Patient Group in the Academy, where she worked hard, she was elected President of NAPP, so I had the pleasure of working with her again. NAPP held annual conferences attracting about 100 people. The Trustees invited me to pre-conference dinners and I often lectured or chaired parts of the conference, usually giving a summary. I attended 16 conferences giving me valuable experience of patients' views. I was never a Trustee so all the credit for NAPP's achievements goes to them.

The relationship between NAPP and the RCGP Patient Group was never as good as I had hoped, although they were natural allies. Patricia, who had led both sides, sought to bridge the gap and as I too had been involved with both parties, I gave support. I drafted a memorandum on the relationship, which was amended and eventually agreed by the RCGP and NAPP and I attended one joint meeting, on the NAPP team, which was unproductive. NAPP invited RCGP leaders to speak at its national conferences, including Gerada and Baker (Council Chairs) and Haslam, Kemple and Lakhani (Presidents). Maureen Baker offered NAPP a partnership in the RCGP campaign "Putting patients first." This sought more resources for general practice. Patricia Wilkie took a risk for NAPP and joined in. It gave NAPP more publicity than ever before and entry to 10 Downing Street.

The ESTEEM study, led by John Campbell *et al.* (2014) my successor at Exeter, was in the *Lancet*. This was a multiprofessorial team and was the world's biggest research study on telephone triage for patients requesting new consultations in general practice. It was well conducted. The authors were cautiously optimistic.

I saw in the tables the use of out-of-hours services after telephone triage was significantly increased. Patricia Wilkie and I wrote a letter to the *Lancet* as Patron and President of NAPP (DPG and Wilkie, 2015). "GPs without visual cues and unable to examine patients were unlikely to be as good clinically as GPs who could see patients and examine them". Campbell *et al.* (with a statistician; 2015) criticised our statistics (the chi-square test). They reported a more sophisticated statistical calculation but it was still significant, 22.2%, increased use of GP out-of-hours and A&E services after GP triage, compared to usual GP care. This was not in the original ESTEEM report and questions its conclusion. After GP triage, 20% of patients were so worried that they sought medical care out of hours.

Newbould *et al.* (2017) analysed the "doctor first" system which requires patients to telephone and wait for a GP to ring back. The DH pushed this, claiming it reduced GP work and saved hospital use. Patricia Wilkie and I noted that patient ratings were statistically significantly reduced compared with usual care and many face-to-face consultations became telephone consultations, which were shorter and less satisfactory (Hewitt *et al.*, 2010). GP workload rose on average by 8%. Hospital admissions for ambulatory care-sensitive conditions (ACSC; where general practice can help) rose by 4%, and hospital costs rose by over £1 per GP patient (about £50 million if extrapolated nationally; DPG and Wilkie, 2017). Even statistically significant patient satisfaction is consistently undervalued, although service industries value client satisfaction.

Patient participation is one of the big issues in medicine, albeit not yet fully recognised. NAPP and many PPGs do good work. As a small registered charity NAPP speaks for a big policy. It punches above its weight so I continue to support it as best I can.

41

The Patient Information Advisory Group/Ethics and Confidentiality Committee 2001–2011

Confidential information is what the patient does not want the neighbour to know.

Journal of the Royal College of General Practitioners (*JRCGP*, 1973b) Editorial

By 1972 I had done over 50,000 consultations, built some strong patient-doctor relationships and was receiving many personal confidences. In the *Journal of the Royal College General Practitioners* (*JRCGP*, 1973b), I wrote an editorial defining confidential information as what "a patient does not want the neighbour to know."

Decision by the GMC 2000

In the late 1990s, the Standards Committee of the GMC, chaired by Sir Cyril Chantler, noted the transfer of information about patients in the NHS without them knowing or consenting. This happened when pathology laboratories made diagnoses of cancer and informed the cancer registries. In 2000, the Standards Committee withdrew its approval on the grounds that patients should know and consent. This decision was confirmed by the full GMC. I voted for the change in both settings (Chapter 31, The General Medical and Dental Councils).

This was a patient-centred policy which precipitated a national furore. Doctors began withholding such information and the cancer registries objected as they were doing valuable work and needed the information. In the Academy, those Presidents whose specialties were concerned with cancer diagnosis thought the GMC's decision was a mistake.

The Nuffield Trust, with great foresight, had studied patient consent and commissioned a consultant long before this issue arose. The Trust held several seminars inviting leading players, including Philip Walker, the DH civil servant with responsibility, whom I saw often. The Trust held a conference including representatives of the cancer registries and leading epidemiologists who were particularly hostile to the GMC. Cyril Chantler spoke, and for the first time I saw him under heavy attack from angry epidemiologists. He held his ground.

Two Perspectives

These meetings clarified the division between those whose professional interests were in data analysis, i.e. epidemiologists, and those who saw confidentiality as a matter of trust since patients were disclosing sensitive information to their doctors. The balance of power lay with the epidemiologists, with many influential doctors, whereas those seeing the patient's point of view were less well represented. The doctors who most appreciated the confidential nature of the disclosures they received tended to be GPs, who were not well represented.

DOI: 10.1201/9781032713601-50

Patient Information Advisory Group

The problem was so important that new legislation was needed and the 2001 Health and Social Care Act was passed. This established a new body, the Patient Information Advisory Group (PIAG), which would examine applications to use patient information without consent and would balance the public interest against the loss of patient confidentiality. The Secretary of State for Health was required to consider the advice of the Group but was not in law required to follow it. This new Committee had to balance the conflicts, case by case. PIAG did not cover Scotland or Northern Ireland.

The Government appointed Sir Cyril Chantler (1939–) and me to this group and Professor Andrew (later Sir) Haines (1947–), a former GP who was Director of the London School of Hygiene and Tropical Medicine, but he soon resigned. Philip Walker often attended. The Chair was Professor (later Dame) Joan Higgins, a professor of management. She had little experience and allowed a real consensus to emerge.

The core business of PIAG was to consider a series of applications, mainly from big research studies. There were some extreme situations, for example paediatricians wanted to video-record parents whom they suspected of injuring or even trying to murder their children. Expecting patient consent was unreasonable.

PIAG soon approved a group or 'class' exemption for the cancer registries, solving the political problem, which had led to its establishment. It charged these registries with the responsibility of developing relationships with patients to obtain their consent in the long run. This was a responsibility they did little or nothing to fulfil. These registries have little contact with patients. It is numbers that fascinate them. Ironically after many years, patient information was still transferred, albeit now legally, in the NHS but still without patients' full knowledge or consent.

Another group of studies were those where data had been gathered many years before without consent and where it was impossible or unreasonable to expect researchers to try to track people down and obtain written consent. We called these 'legacy' studies, and usually granted approval as they would run out in time.

Another gain was in policy development. PIAG published all its minutes on the Internet, including a full list of all the research studies approved. There were no secret meetings, as was common in health authorities. Our system published the reasons for all our decisions, which was recommended good practice for executive bodies. Quango (devolved) legislation can be administratively more transparent than the often secret workings of central government.

This open process bolstered the Committee's independence and inhibited arbitrary political decisions, which were common. A minister faced with a decision they did not like, had to deal with written, public reasons from the Committee couched usually in scientific terms. The minister then ran a risk of being exposed in public if they countermanded these, as they were empowered to do.

Two situations recurred. The first was when data were available from very small groups of patients throughout the country, so that missing data about even a few patients could damage the researchers' ability to identify an important finding. Over the years, the PIAG tended to support access to information, even breaching patient confidentiality for rare diseases, providing the disease was very serious and there was no other obvious way of researching it.

The other situation was when informing the patient properly might worry them. Here the Committee usually took the view that patients had a right to be fully informed about their condition in order to be able to give informed consent.

At a big meeting at the Royal College of Physicians, a patient representative spoke. His medical record was clear. He was quite happy for any researcher to see his record and, given how valuable medical research was, he could not see what all the fuss was about! He received loud applause. I put my hand up. It was 1 pm. The Chair hesitated but he knew me and called me. I declared my membership of PIAG, saying I was glad that our colleague did not have sexually transmitted disease on his medical record, and I presumed he had not confided any marital infidelities to his GP either.

I presumed he had not been in prison or attempted suicide, or had an abortion, as patients with these facts on their records are very keen to keep such information confidential. I noted how often patients with depression, when they held a senior position, tried hard not to reveal this. I quoted the Wellcome Trust (2009) survey, that 8%; i.e. 1 in 12 people, reported that there was some information on their GP record, which they considered stigmatising. My contribution was received in stony silence.

Personal Clash

One day a visitor appeared at PIAG who was a distinguished professorial epidemiologist. He had made patronising comments at the Nuffield Trust conference. He described his work, which he thought was of the highest importance and saved lives. He said the GMC decision to withdraw approval for data transfer had been a spectacular blunder and it had simply not understood the situation. It had generated unnecessary bureaucracy (i.e. PIAG!) and had hindered the valuable work of the cancer registries and epidemiologists like him.

My hackles rose and I sensed it did in other members in PIAG. He was exhibiting the worst features of some senior doctors; i.e. arrogance that they knew best and that their interests were superior to the interests of patients. I explained that medicine existed to serve patients, not the other way round. All information imparted by patients, most commonly to GPs was done under a bond of confidentiality going back 2,000 years to Hippocrates. It was epidemiologists who did not understand. They did not see patients, they sat behind computer screens and were not legally allowed to do general practice. They did not understand the emotion of some GP consultations when patients in distress divulged embarrassing confidences to personal doctors they trusted. I was very proud to have been elected to the GMC by all the registered doctors in England (this epidemiologist would never have been elected). Of the decisions I had taken with colleagues on the GMC, I was particularly proud of two, one of which was stopping patients' data being shipped around the NHS without them knowing. The Chair quietly thanked me and asked the professor if he wished to respond. However, looking shaken, he shook his head and left.

Vice-Chair

Soon afterwards in 2009, PIAG elected a Vice-Chair and I was elected *nem con*. I suspect my riposte assisted my election. In 2007, Joan Higgins was appointed a Dame to the pleasure of the committee. This was not only substantial personal recognition but also professional recognition that PIAG had succeeded. However, she soon resigned to take up the Chair of the bigger NHS Litigation Authority. We dined her out, with it falling to me, as Vice-Chair, to thank her.

Committee Process

I analysed the committee process. The two legally qualified members and the six doctor members became dominant. This was because of technical knowledge as a strong legal point usually prevailed. None of the doctors was aggressive or sought dominance but their understanding of research made the difference in spotting weaknesses in proposals and seeing how changes could be made.

Ethics and Confidentiality Committee

In 2008 the Government established a new organisation to be called the National Information Governance Board (NIGB). PIAG was to be a subcommittee of this. Disruption was averted as the Chair of the NIGB, Harry Clayton (whom I knew in the patient participation world as the Patients'

Czar), wanted to preserve PIAG. I never understood why the DH used the word 'czar' for the national directors in the various specialties and for patients. The 'czars' were Russian emperors with a reputation for autocratic and often brutal behaviour.

PIAG was preserved by renaming it the Ethics and Confidentiality Committee (ECC) and keeping the members the same. The statutory instruments changed, and the governance framework became Section 251. Andrew Harris (1951–) was appointed Chair, having been a GP, a paediatrician, and a public health physician. He held an MSc, the MRCP, and a law degree, and so was dually qualified in medicine and the law. He brought new legal skills to the ECC; showing that provision of personal information by a patient to a doctor was protected in common law and did not depend on the medical profession's ethical code. Exceptions were when a parliamentary statute required disclosure.

Andrew Harris treated me differently as his Vice-Chair, consulting me regularly, giving me lunch at one of the legal inns, and inviting me several times to stay with him and his wife Lucinda at their home. He also invited me to accompany him to several meetings with other bodies. As a senior doctor, he was able to set up meetings with national directors and with some NHS audit groups.

However, he was appointed as Coroner in Southwark, a big area. This fulfilled a career ambition but took much time. He started to delegate to me. First, as the ECC streamlined its applications, many more came to me. He sent apologies for some ECC meetings, which I then chaired. Then he opted out of the meetings of the NIGB where he had an ex-officio place, so I went as his deputy. This lasted about a year, with Harry Clayton as Chair, who was followed by Dame Fiona Caldicott (1941–2021), a former Trustee with me at the Nuffield Trust.

The work of the ECC became gradually more complex for several reasons. First, the power of computing was continually extending, and so was the interest of big, private business organisations. We were receiving ever more complicated applications, some of which sought to bring together vast datasets that had never previously been linked and applicants were often private companies.

The Committee was free from cliques, nor were there many interpersonal clashes, which frequently attracted favourable comments from the staff who served the ECC well. Claire Thomson, Natasha Dunkley and Claire Jackson were all well informed, conscientious and had high interpersonal skills. I felt well supported.

I caused tension twice. First, I said that I thought a member might be wise not to speak in favour of an application when she was working for the submitting organisation. The member was furious and she complained about me to the Chair. However, he understood conflicts of interest. Another time, I suggested the Chair should himself abstain, because of a conflict. The Chair was fine, but a civil servant was annoyed and tried to terminate my period of office, which I heard about later. This would have succeeded but the Chair said he wanted me to stay. This led to an ECC code on declaring potential conflicts of interest.

NIGB

The NIGB produced the NHS constitution (NIGB, 2009) which it published with a similar document in the social work field. One of the few arguments I had had with Joan Higgins was failing to convince her that there ought to be an appeal body against ECC decisions. NIGB soon established one. Happily, the appeals to it were all judged in favour of the ECC, so our processes withstood scrutiny. We never had a judicial review of a PIAG/ECC decision in my ten years, although we had several angry academics whose applications we had rejected.

Two Powerful Lobbies

The pharmaceutical industry campaigned hard, establishing a link with the Prime Minister, Tony Blair. It had a strong case because in the early years of the 21st century Britain had few industries that were truly world-class: banking, aero-engines, the life sciences, universities, and entertainment. Pharmaceuticals were one of the few such industries and invested substantially in research facilities. This industry had a strong threat, to move abroad. This threat was credible, as Sir Richard Sykes, when running GlaxoSmithKline, once told me at a dinner that the whole NHS market was worth only 5% to his company. Tony Blair agreed the NHS should be geared to supporting world-class research in the NHS. This decision was reasonable but had negative effects on regional general practice research.

An influential lobby came from the Academy of Medical Sciences (AcMedSciS). Professor Carol Dezateux, a member of the ECC, took me to lunch in her university department describing the obstacles she faced. Applying to every hospital trust caused delay, or worse it might lead to a call for modifications, adding hugely to the work and expense. This was unreasonable: reform was needed.

The AcMedSci set up a working party with Sir Michael Rawlins as Chair. Its report (AMS, 2011) proposed substantial changes in the research approval process. The Government accepted the recommendations and established a new research health authority to streamline approvals. The NIGB, although only five years old, was abolished. ECC became a subcommittee of the new research authority, with a new name, the Research Ethics Committee. Its Chair was to be accountable to the Chair of the Health Research Authority, a changed relationship.

Retirement

I retired from the ECC in December 2011. It is unusual to serve on public bodies for ten years, but the conversion of PIAG to ECC made it possible. It is usual to thank long-serving members, but Andrew surprised me by delivering a eulogy and presenting me, on behalf of the Committee, with a beautiful silver jug engraved with my name and the words: *The Patients' Champion*! I was overwhelmed, never having seen this before in a public committee. I am afraid my response was inadequate.

42

RCGP Heritage Committee 2006–2012

Time future contained in time past.

TS Eliot (1988–1965)

I had been a member of the Heritage Committee since 1994, when the Chair of the Committee was traditionally a President, so Alastair Donald and Lottie Newman had chaired successively. The main recent achievement of the Committee and of Lottie Newman had been the establishment of the Rose Prize, jointly with the Society of Apothecaries, for an academic essay on medical history in relation to general practice. When Lottie retired there were two names for the Chair: David McKinley and me. David and I shared much: We both loved the history of medicine. He was an expert on historical books and had a good collection. We had both been regional advisers in general practice and on the Council. The Committee voted for me as Chair and I said to David he would also be a worthy Chair and hoped he would succeed me.

Managing the Archives

At first my main effort was in getting as many of the archives catalogued as possible. This sorting, analysing, and assessing process is what archivists do. Claire Jackson, the College archivist, had this in hand and knew the archives well. There were small sums of money available for part-time support staff. Institutions vary in their attitude to their archives, and this measures the maturity of the organisation. The Royal College of Physicians of London has marvellous archives of which it is proud. The Royal College of Surgeons of England has the famous Hunterian museum. Sadly, the RCGP, in my time on the Heritage Committee, was relatively immature, allocating only a tiny budget with many senior officers taking little interest. There was no general awareness that history explains the present and may at times points to the future, as the quotation from TS Eliot elegantly describes. I tried to raise the profile and wrote papers explaining how our archives were unique, documenting not just the development of the College but also many of the great reforms in medicine and medical education. In one lengthy report that went to the Council, I envisaged these archives being a core resource for academic study outside general practice, for example by PhD students. I hoped to get the archives on microfiche but funds were not available.

I made links with the Wellcome Trust, the biggest charity in Europe, which had an important commitment to medical history. The Trust had a staff member for outside relations and I was able to persuade Carol Reeves to join the Committee. I also proposed John Ford as a member of the College and he was then able to join the Heritage Committee. He was a GP historian who had done an MD in medical history (at Exeter) and had been a President of the faculty dealing with history in the Society of Apothecaries. I tried to keep Margaret Hammond, the former College librarian, now an HonFRCGP, on the Committee as long as I was there and she gave me much advice. The archives were an important repository and answered many hundreds of queries. There were also important historical books. A Culpeper microscope was often displayed. Lord Brain's (1951) letter trying to block the formation of a College of GPs has been preserved.

DOI: 10.1201/9781032713601-51

Heritage Plaques

I wanted to create new ideas but was constrained by the small budget. Eventually I thought of RCGP presentation plaques. First, they would honour a GP, usually an RCGP person. Second, they would decentralise the College, as these people would come from around the country. Third, I hoped it would enthuse the College faculties and active local members. I hoped to value general practice and GPs. I wrote a paper and the idea was approved so that the Committee could choose the names. I proposed the first – RMS McConaghey (Mac).

RMS McConaghey OBE

I knew McConaghey's general practice in Dartmouth, having been there with Mac when I was on his Editorial Board. I also knew the practice's current senior partner, Andrew Eynon-Lewis, who was an enthusiast and had completed both FBA and a master's degree. The Dartmouth Practice welcomed the idea. I wrote a long piece for the plaque, lest people would forget Mac's achievement in establishing the College journal in his home in Dartmouth and first calling it a journal (Chapter 9, Journal story). The College *Journal* started as a private research newsletter under the Editorship of Robin Pinsent, and McConaghey (Mac; 1907–1975) had taken it over when Pinsent developed laryngeal cancer. He developed the newsletter into a *Journal* in 1958 and did it so well that in 1961 the National Library of Medicine in Washington included it in *Index Medicus,* thus making it the first scientific journal of general practice in the world (Chapter 9, The Journal 1968–1980).

Paddy McConaghey PhD, Mac's daughter, lived in Dartmouth and she got one of Mac's grandsons to come. Furthermore, Miss Irene Scawn MBE, the *Journal's* first business manager, aged 90, was living in Dartmouth and came with Giles Keane, one of Mac's partners in the practice and a member of an early Editorial Board of the *Journal* who had retired locally. The Tamar Faculty was represented by its Provost, Steve Watkins. Jill and I were pleased that the President, David Haslam, stayed with us the night before, the fourth RCGP president who had stayed in our home. He spoke well at the ceremony. Andrew Eynon-Lewis welcomed everyone and I then summarised Mac's achievements. The plaque was unveiled in the practice waiting room as there were difficulties in placing it on an outside wall. Photos included were of Mac's family and Irene Scawn. The partners kindly provided lunch, and there was a good report in the local newspaper.

Fraser Rose OBE

The second Heritage Committee plaque was masterminded by David McKinley. Fraser Rose (1897–1962) had co-founded the College and had brought much needed NHS input to the founding of the College, which was crucial. Fraser Rose's old surgery still stood, now a pub in Preston. David persuaded the local Faculty Board to pay for the plaque and succeeded in getting the Mayor of Preston to speak. The new President of the College could not come so it fell to me to give the speech for the College, which was a pleasure as I greatly admired Fraser Rose. He had started his career in the BMA and then been both Chair of Council and President. The pub kindly provided drinks. The Fraser Rose family came in strength with one son and a family group coming from Canada for the occasion and one of his sons spoke at the ceremony. The Mayor's speech ensured good publicity in the local press.

Annis Gillie OBE

I was keen to install a plaque for Dame Annis Gillie (1900–1985), the first female Chair and first female President of the College. I thought it would be attractive to hold the ceremony when the College had both a female President, Iona Heath, and a female Chair of Council, Claire Gerada. Annis Gillie was the first GP to chair a government committee (*Gillie Report*, 1963) and the first academic GP to be appointed a dame/knight. I visited her practice in Connaught Square twice and obtained permission in principle and explored positions for a plaque. However, there were difficulties in obtaining permissions and sadly I ran out of time. I hope the College will complete that idea. I was hopeful that these plaques provided at an affordable cost an event valuing a GP, often encouraging family members and the local faculty.

Oral History of General Practice

I inherited a good system whereby the Heritage Committee video-interviewed leading GPs and College leaders. This captured images of key people whilst alive and often added insights to important events. The College had been early with the idea, but the problem was funding. In the Nuffield Trust, I had been able to facilitate a grant of £10,000 to the College to support this programme. As Chair I wrote a paper trying to rationalise the choice of subjects, did some interviews, and was interviewed myself.

My term was dominated by extraneous factors. First, the College moved its headquarters, leaving Princes Gate after over 40 years. This had big implications for the archives, which were extensive, occupying much space. The archivist reported the shelf length but got little feedback. Secondly, plans for the new building showed no space for the archives. I invited the Architect to the Committee. She came several times making helpful presentations but said she had not been asked for any space for the archives. I was worried for the future of these precious documents.

I wrote a long paper to draw attention to the archives. The College set up a committee on the archives which I sat on with Philip Evans, who was on both the planning and the heritage committees. The committee included some staff who were becoming increasingly influential. One seemed to think that "history was bunk" and sharply questioned storage costs. She sought a major cull. After three meetings, one of which I left a holiday to attend, a decision was made to put the archives into store, unculled, whilst the architect explored space. Claire Jackson, the archivist, resigned despite my trying to support her. Her retirement present was a piece of silver with the Exeter hallmark. The College then appointed Sharon Messenger PhD, who became one of the best archivists the College has had.

I was keen to compile a list of local GPs who had been honoured by their local communities with a statue or a plaque valuing their core work as a GP. We found several lovely memorials with moving descriptions of thanks for years of compassionate GP care. Herbert Nicholas Chilcote MRCS 1840–1886, a Torbay GP, died aged 46 and a substantial obelisk was built by *public subscription* (my italics): "from all classes in affectionate remembrance of a noble and unselfish life generously spent and prematurely sacrificed in the service of the sick and suffering" (Hawgood D, 2012). Some early GPs provided a great service.

Last Lecture in Princes Gate

The College held a symposium, chaired by the President, Iona Heath, as it left Princes Gate. I was asked to review the College's achievements while in that building. This was a sentimental occasion being held in the Long Room, a beautiful Georgian room on the first floor. This was where I had chaired the Editorial Board, the Publications Committee, the Communications Division, the GPC, Council, the Research Committee, JCPTGP and the Fellowship and Awards Committees; and where I had hosted HRH the Prince of Wales and been involved in some of the big council debates. I was lucky to be the last College lecturer in that lovely room.

At my last meeting of the Heritage Committee after I had served 18 years on it, Philip Evans presented me with a cheque from members. It was far bigger than was usual for retiring committee chairs and I was very grateful.

ADDENDA

Later plaques were well developed by the next Chair, Bill Reith, and archivist, Sharon Messenger. The third plaque in Edinburgh commemorated Richard Scott (1914–1963), the GP who in 1963 became the first Professor of General Practice in the world. Another plaque was for AJ Cronin (1896–1981), whose book *The Citadel* (Cronin, 1937) is a classic. His biographer spoke. At the unveiling of the plaque for Michael Balint (1896–1970) Marshall Marinker, who had been in Balint's original group, spoke elegantly, shortly before his own death. In 2022 a plaque for Donald Irvine (1935–2018) was installed at his former surgery. The RCGP heritage plaques became established.

DOWNGRADING THE HERITAGE COMMITTEE

However, a governance review suddenly proposed changing the status of the Heritage Committee and the Trustee Board in 2022, without proper consultation, approved this. The staff support and budget were removed and it was decreed to be only a "membership interest group". The RCGP thus took another big academic step backwards. A national organisation not prepared to provide any staff support or any budget for members to develop its history and heritage lacks pride and self-confidence and loses a deep understanding of its place in the current world.

43

What About The Children? (WATCh?)

The Child is Father of the Man.

William Wordsworth (1770–1850)

After I had finished my main jobs, Elizabeth, our middle daughter, said to me, as only daughters can: "Why don't you get involved with a really important charity like What About the Children?!" I had not heard of this but enquired and duly joined as a member. A circular arrived asking members if they had any useful experiences. I ticked a box that I had experience of chairing medical conferences. The Chair of WATCh? Christine Ponsford, rang me and quizzed me. She then invited me to chair the WATCh? annual conference.

Diana Dean, a Trustee and the Research Director of the charity had developed an interesting policy of summarising for WATCh? the main scientific articles appearing on the emotional development of the under-threes. She organised a small team of science writers to do these and displayed them at the conferences and on the WATCh? website. I met Christine and Diana together and they invited me to form a scientific advisory board for WATCh? to strengthen the charity's scientific credentials with Diana as Vice-Chair.

I believed in what they were doing; Jill had stayed at home with all our children and had only gone back to work when our youngest was six. Scientific articles were emerging showing that when very small children were separated from their parents, usually the mother, increased levels of cortisol could be detected in their bodies, and I knew that such cortisol levels indicated stress.

However, society was pushing mothers to go out to work even with small children. This was a big political issue. WATCh? was in a David and Goliath situation with all the big guns, like the Daycare Trust, and most politicians working to get mothers out to work. The key argument of the Treasury was that if a mother went out to paid work her taxable income raised the GDP and if she paid a child carer or nursery that second income did so as well. One estimate was that on average after four years this meant about £20,000 p.a. was added to the national GDP. The child's interest was not considered, and there was an assumption that daycare was as good as care from the biological mother. Of course, most women, including mothers, want to go out to work so there were criss-cross tensions about parental care in the feminist world.

Like many small charities, WATCh? was run by a handful of enthusiasts. All the work was done voluntarily by unpaid trustees, friends, and supporters working from home without paid staff. I greatly admired their work, and the charity was run on minimal expenditure and has existed for 30 years.

The annual conference usually drew a thoughtful attendance of about 80 and was an opportunity to inform this group about new ideas. They provided high-quality lectures to promote the organisation and to supply the research reports. My job was to advise the Trustees, chair some conferences and sum up at the end. After a while they elected me a Vice-President. In later years I chaired less, playing other roles: sometimes lecturing and usually summing up.

As Chair of the Nuffield Trust I organised a seminar in Cavendish Street, London on child rearing. This gave the WATCh? Trustees a chance to invite, through the Trust, influential players on the national scene. These included Professor Edward Melhuish, who was undertaking the national review

DOI: 10.1201/9781032713601-52

of the Surestart centres, Professor Sarah Stewart-Brown, Robin Balbernie, Naomi Eisentadt, director of Surestart, and Penelope Leech. I was able to chair a useful discussion and then hosted a dinner where relationships were built.

With Diana we established a strong Scientific Advisory Board with international level skills. I was able to recruit Professor J Belsky, then at Birkbeck College, London, who was an internationally known behavioural psychologist. He was an American who had written extensively. He was a leading critic of children spending more than 30 hours a week in child care outside the home which he found was associated with 'externalising,' i.e. aggressive behaviour (Belsky and Rovine, 1988; Belsky *et al.*, 2007). I took him to lunch and we agreed a basis for working. I also took Professor Sarah Stewart-Brown out for a meal. She was a leading public health physician who had written about parenting persuasively (Barlow *et al.*, 2005). Finally, I was able to persuade Professor Brenda Almond, author of an important book *The Fragmenting Family* (Almond, 2006) to join the Board.

The Trustees funded one meeting a year in London, so it was important to make that work. I wrote a paper proposing that the Board, plus invited others, would write a book on the subject of child care of the under-threes with emphasis on the science as it was known. It was clear that the other members would not have enough time to write much, and a great deal of work would fall on Diana and me. We got a good attendance, but despite my chairmanship experience, I could not achieve agreement on a book. I much regretted this failure. I had got the membership that I had hoped but failed to build a consensus. After this setback, I spent time working how I could help in other ways. Then Belsky returned to the United States, another member fell ill, and the Board never met again.

The Trustees agreed to give evidence to the Duncan Smith Commission. Ian Duncan Smith (1954–) was a former leader of the Conservative party, then in opposition, and was now devoting his time to understanding the sociology of underprivilege (Centre for Social Justice, 2008). I was invited to join the team to give evidence for WATCh? at Portcullis House, London. This Commission was supportive of family values with a 'Breakthrough Britain' report entitled: 'The next generation.' WATCh? held a tea party at the House of Commons and Ian Duncan Smith attended. I was introduced to him there and also met one my fellow Vice-Presidents, Michael (later Sir) Morpurgo (1943–), the distinguished children's author.

The Trustees later elected me, President. I was never a Trustee, and this post was honorary and non-executive. I attended a dozen of their conferences.

Goodman Lecture

The charity had established a biennial eponymous lecture, called after Doreen Goodman, who had been one of the founders of the charity in 1993. She had written a far-sighted letter in the *Guardian* in 1992, after the Bulger tragedy and murder when two small boys had murdered this toddler. She had pointed out perceptively that there were three child victims not just one. The many respondents formed the early membership of WATCh? The Trustees invited me to deliver the 2013 Goodman Lecture in London and Jill came. I wavered over the title. The obvious choice was to use Wordsworth's famous statement that: "The child is father of the man," which summarised my message. In the end I chose a more dramatic title "It's the relationships, stupid!" playing on Bill Clinton's campaign strategy. This wasn't my usual style but attracted attention. I prepared an academic analysis of the research that separating very young from parental care of children is associated with a rise in cortisol levels and discussed the adverse implications of this (DPG, 2013). We got the lecture printed in Exeter and donated it to the charity giving them numerous copies. They also put a text on the charity's website.

Commission for Social Capital

In 2014, several MPs interested in social justice formed the Commission for Social Capital. This was supported by the Relationship Foundation, another charity with which I had been connected. I was asked to give evidence on behalf of WATCh? at a meeting in the House of Commons, chaired by Fiona Bruce MP (1957–). Jeremy Lefroy MP (1959–) was actively involved. This was the same session at which Sir Paul Coleridge (1949–) gave evidence for the Marriage Foundation. He went first and stayed for my contribution. I concentrated on one single point which was to try to persuade them that they should call for more research on raised cortisol levels in small children in all the different settings: at home, nurseries, with child-minders, and in grandparental care. The Commission on Social Capital reported in 2014: *Holding the Centre: Stability and Social Justice* (Lefroy J *et al.*, 2014). The Commission recommended that cortisol levels should be measured in small children in different settings and that this should be a research priority. This seemed to be a small but tangible achievement for WATCh? However, nine years later there was no evidence of any government statement that this was a research priority. Was the effort a waste of time?

Peer-Reviewed Literature

I knew that to make real progress, WATCh? had to convince the medical profession of their cause and this meant articles in good medical journals. This was the policy that Admiral Sir James Watt had used with me when establishing the first university chair of complementary medicine in Exeter, as described in Chapter 27, the Postgraduate Medical School story. Time had vindicated his view. As President of WATCh? I felt responsible for trying to achieve this.

Diana Dean needed to be a co-author of any scientific article since as Trustee of WATCh? she had for years organised the production of summaries of relevant scientific research, enrolling scientists to write the summaries. I greatly admired this initiative and had found many of her summaries interesting and important.

Epigenetics had emerged as yet another powerful strand of argument. Essentially genes and the environment are not static as previously thought but interact so that the environment can affect the activity of human genes. These can then be passed on through future generations. Since the changes in gene activity could be either beneficial or harmful, we needed a co-author who could handle the epigenetic section. Philip Dean PhD, Diana's husband, was a former Wellcome Principal Research Fellow at the University of Cambridge before becoming Chief Scientific Officer of a Cambridge spin-out company, De Novo Pharmaceuticals. He was already summarising peer-reviewed research for WATCh?, so he was a natural co-author. We had an article published by the *Journal of the Royal Society of Medicine* in April (DPG *et al.*, 2020a). The title was "Child care outside the family for the under threes: Cause for concern?" The Royal Society of Medicine issued a sharp press release, but it attracted no media interest as the corona virus dominated attention. However, one consultant paediatrician got the message emailing me: "This could be bigger than the corona virus!"

I was invited by the Editor of the US journal *Epigenomics* to write an editorial. This would be published free to access. I had heard from a leading academic of political pressure against reporting adverse effects of daycare, which made me determined this subject should be evaluated objectively. This would give it a new opportunity to be picked up by medical and lay commentators. Philip Evans and I were supervising a final-year medical student in the St Leonard's practice, Molly Dineen, who was doing an intercalated master's degree. Her subject was family history in general practice, so I offered her involvement. She contributed considerably and soon the two Deans and I offered her co-authorship. She produced the three words: "Science versus society," alliteratively capturing the clash between scientific findings and what society does. Philip Dean led on the key epigenomic section, which we lengthened for *Epigenomics* (DPG *et al.*, 2020b).

About a thousand research studies in medical journal reported four findings: that cortisol levels rise when babies and small children are separated from their mothers, that cortisol is toxic to the brain in several mammals, that cortisol can be toxic to human brains, and that stress (through the cortisol release) can be associated with changes to genes. The biological process is DNA methylation. The big issue of passing genes to the next generation has been live since the 1990s.

There was a striking absence of academic analysis in leading general medical journals. We thought this was the first editorial on this subject, so we suggested that a taboo exists in discussing negative effects of out-of-home child care. The title this time was "Science versus society: is child care for the under threes a taboo subject?" (DPG *et al.,* 2020b) and the editorial was published in *Epigenomics* in July 2020.

WATCh? issued a supportive press release but again there was no press response. Nor, although *Epigenomics* has an impact factor of over 4, after 12 months was there even a single citation. The taboo continues.

44

The Nuffield Trust, 1993–2006

The family doctors' role is a difficult one: if it is to be sustained they must become the most comprehensively educated doctors in the NHS.

Professor Sir Denis Hill (1913–1982) Rock Carling Lecture, 1969

The UK has relatively few big medical charities. The King's Fund is the oldest, founded in 1897 with objectives to focus on London. The second was the Wellcome Trust established by Sir Henry Wellcome (1853–1936), through a legacy of pharmaceutical shares. This is now the biggest British charity. William Morris GBE, later Viscount Nuffield (1877–1963), built a car company near Oxford making Morris cars, earning him a fortune. He made the third big British endowment through a group of medical charities. The original endowment was one million Morris motor shares (McLachlan, 1992). The Nuffield Provincial Hospital Trust's (NPHT) trust deed was signed in June 1940 which, considering the World War, indicated Lord Nuffield's optimism.

In 1954, a Nuffield Health and Social Services Fund was established as a separate charity to give more flexibility for donations and in particular to develop general practice premises in the new town of Harlow. The Trust paid Stephen Taylor (later Lord Taylor, 1910–1988) for this initiative, which involved all 102 general practice buildings there. I chaired this charity later.

A key word in the title of the NPHT was *provincial*. This avoided potential conflict with the King's Fund which was focused on London, and in addition, gave the NPHT the whole of the UK to work on.

Lord Nuffield selected distinguished Trustees, many from the University of Oxford close by. Sir William Goodenough (1899–1951) was the first Chair, and his reforming Goodenough Committee Report (1944) not only ensured that GPs did a year's pre-registration hospital experience (opening the door to postgraduate training), but also broke the discrimination against women medical students in some medical schools like Bart's. This report was written from a committee where both the Chair and the Administrator (Lesley Farrar-Brown) had been hand-picked by Lord Nuffield for his charities.

Other Trustees included three regius professors of medicine at Oxford or Cambridge. One was Sir John (later Lord) Butterfield (1920–2000), who was multitalented with Oxford blues for cricket, hockey and rugby and who became Vice-Chancellor of both the Universities of Nottingham and Cambridge. In 1988 as a Trustee of the NPHT he comforted me after Mrs Thatcher hand bagged me (Chapter 23, Chair of Council story). John Fry was chosen as a Trustee as early as 1957, as a GP who had the most data about general practice and wrote about it thoughtfully. It was then rare for a national organisation to have a GP governor. None of the Chairs of the Trustees were doctors.

The Nuffield Trustees in the mid-20th century were an elite, intellectual group analysing the new NHS. They were rigorously independent. In the late-1940s the NPHT was the first national body to realise that most people receive most of their medical care from GPs not hospitals, so the quality of GP care was crucial. The Trust commissioned a review of general practice and Joseph Collings, an academic Australian GP who had worked at Harvard, undertook it, visiting several UK general practices. His lengthy report (Collings, 1950) in the *Lancet* contained serious criticisms of the quality of many general practices.

DOI: 10.1201/9781032713601-53

A medico-political storm ensued. John Hunt, a leading London GP, used Collings' report to argue that general practice needed a standard-setting body and an academic voice of its own. The next year, the famous Rose-Hunt (1951) letter appeared calling for a GP College. The Collings report increased the urgency, encouraging Fraser Rose and John Hunt to write their letter and also influenced the many GPs who responded positively to them. The College of General Practitioners had to be formed in secret in November 1952 because of specialist opposition (DPG, 1992a) and this occurred within 17 months of the publication of the Collings report.

The NPHT was concerned about the storm it had caused. It commissioned Stephen Taylor (1910–1988) who wrote *Good General Practice* (Taylor, 1954). I have an autographed copy. This demonstrated positive examples of good general practice. Later, Taylor became an MP and Labour Minister before going to the Lords, choosing Harlow in his title.

The capital of the NHPT was still in Morris motor shares when Lord Nuffield died in 1963. The Chair of the Trustees (1951–1966) was the Hon Sir Geoffrey Gibbs KCMG, a banker. He and his Trustees were slow to diversify so that the capital and income fell as the British motor industry ran into difficulties. The motor industry shares were not sold until "a considerable time after Lord Nuffield's death." The income of the Trust had been over £500,000 p.a. three years running in the mid-1960s, but fell to under £200,000 in 1971, before "reasonable stability of income" was achieved (McLachlan, 1992).

This unfortunate experience influenced the Wellcome Trust when Sir Geoffrey's son, Sir Roger Gibbs (1934 to 2018), was Chair of the Trustees. He persuaded those Trustees to sell shares between 1986 and 1995, so achieving diversification. Previously, Wellcome supported medical research with about £50 million a year. Afterwards, the Wellcome Trust became the biggest charity in Europe. This Charity now funds research worth about £1 billion a year helping the UK punch above its research weight.

Medical Education in Britain

The Trust instigated national discussions on medical education in Britain. In a brilliant leadership move, steered by the Trust's Secretary (Chief Executive) Gordon McLachlan, it organised a national conference which was held in Christchurch, Oxford in 1961 (Pickering, 1962). Most of the leaders in British medical education attended the conference, which was a huge success, triggering several reforms in British medical education. General practice was absent. Only one consultant attended that conference who did not come from a teaching hospital. This was Clifford Fuller, physician from Exeter, whom I knew, having been a patient of his. He and his wife were friends of my parents. At a time when London dominated medical teaching, with half of all the medical schools in England and all the postgraduate medical institutes there, he spoke of the need to establish medical education in the provinces. After the Conference he led a bid to the NPHT to fund a Postgraduate Medical Institute within the then new (by charter in 1955) University of Exeter. This was approved by the Trustees for a five-year, time-limited grant. Thus, the first Postgraduate Medical Institute in the British Isles outside London was established in Exeter in 1963 (Chapter 27, Postgraduate Medical School story).

For me, born in, living in, and working in Exeter, it was wonderfully fortunate that Exeter, through a small number of far-seeing hospital consultants was the first place in Britain outside London to develop postgraduate medicine in a university. It was this Medical Institute, which I proposed should expand to include the first postgraduate University Department of General Practice in Europe (Chapter 13, Department/Institute of General Practice story). Through many initiatives, including funding the Manchester university GP department building Darbishire House, and funding the first regional adviser post. This Trust gave more practical support to general practice than did any other body.

Nuffield Trust Lectures

Eponymous (named) lectures are a powerful way of disseminating ideas. Distinguished lecturers can sometimes compress the lessons of their lifetime and foresee some of the future. The NPHT established an annual series of Rock Carling lectures to commemorate one of their Trustees. The Trust published these annually as books and as a young GP in Exeter I read them avidly.

The 1969 lecture was delivered by Sir Denis Hill, a leading psychiatrist. He, via the NPHT, helped general practice greatly by stating at a time when it was not generally respected that: *"The family doctor's role is a difficult one. If it is to be sustained they need to become the most comprehensively educated doctors in the NHS"* (Hill, 1969).

Some of the Rock Carling lectures were internationally important. Professor Archie Cochrane (1972) called his monograph "Effectiveness and efficiency" and set out the case for rational priorities for the NHS. Professor McKeown (1976) in "The role of medicine: Dream, mirage or nemesis?" challenged the over-confidence of the medical profession in the effectiveness of their treatments and suggested that non-medical factors were more important than had been realised. The recent understanding of the importance of social determinants of health (Magnan, 2017) confirms he reached well into the future. Archie Cochrane now has an international legacy with Cochrane centres around the world. However, it was the NPHT Trustees who chose him, paid his fellowship, giving him the platform, he deserved.

The Trust also established a series of fellowships/lecturers in John Fry's honour. Among several valuable contributions, Iona Heath's (1995) "The Mystery of General Practice," became a classic. She identified the importance of GPs "witnessing" key events and sharing important experiences with patients. An example I had is described in Chapter 6, Learning the Craft.

General Practice

On 1 December 1973, the University of Exeter established the first Postgraduate University Department of General Practice in Europe, appointing me as the senior lecturer in-charge. This Department was within the Postgraduate Medical Institute, which the NPHT had funded (Chapter 13, Department/ Institute of General Practice story).

Its funding, direct from the DHSS, occurred because the report of the Royal Commission on Medical Education (1968) had recommended postgraduate training for general practice, similar to the medical specialties. The Chair of that Royal Commission, Lord Todd, was another Nuffield Foundation Trustee in 1950, and he was later Chair of that Trust. As Lord Nuffield invited his trustees personally (McLachlan, 1992), he showed a rare skill in identifying reformers. He personally chose as his Trustees the two Chairs of the two most important reports on medical education in the 20th century: Goodenough (1944) and the Royal Commission on Medical Education (1968). These transformed the place of general practice. The first introduced a compulsory preregistration year; i.e. postgraduate training, and the second postgraduate training for GPs.

By the early 1970s, Ministers approved the recommendations of the Royal Commission, so it was clear that vocational (postgraduate) training for general practice was coming. However, general practice, alone in British medicine, had no experience of teaching its own postgraduate trainees. Ekke Kuenssberg, an outstanding GP leader and Chair of the RCGP Council, identified the need to train a cohort of GP organisers. Supported by Ian Watson, he approached the NPHT, which provided substantial funding for what became known as 'the Nuffield course' (*JRCGP,* 1975e). The RCGP appointed Paul Freeling as the Director of the course, an inspired move. I developed a link with the Trust through attending six residential weeks in the first year of this course in 1974 and attending as a teacher for a week in the second year. It was the most influential course that I ever attended, introducing me to educational theory and personality analysis as well as the experience of being in a group led by Tavistock Institute psychoanalyst Pierre Touquet. I was sensitised for life to the feelings of adult learners.

Michael Ashley-Miller

The next Secretary (Chief Executive) of the Trust was Michael Ashley-Miller (1930–2017). His interest was countering disability. He steered the Trust to raise the profile of disabled people and to fund chairs of disability and rehabilitation. He did much at that time and well deserved his CBE.

I was at a conference with him in 1992 when he made a comment about general practice, which suggested that he was not fully informed. I managed to sit next to him at the conference dinner. It is a standard GP consulting technique to search for shared points of interest, which can form common ground and help working relationships. We got on well, especially after we discovered that he and his wife and Jill and I shared a liking for a hotel in Salcombe. I spoke about the need for facts and figures from general practice, coupling it with the suggestion he might visit our general practice when he next went to Salcombe. He jumped at this opportunity. Subsequently, he and his wife came to stay with Jill and me and his visit to the Practice went well. We showed him how we recorded the diagnosis from every consultation, operated personal lists, and recorded the continuity of care that patients actually achieved with every partner every month.

Later, I realised that Michael had another agenda. John Fry was seriously ill with a respiratory disease from which his father had died so Michael was looking for a possible successor. On 5 March 1993 he invited me as his personal guest to a Trustee dinner on 6 July: "…the food and wine are guaranteed to be of very high standard, as well as the company." These words and four months' notice made it a serious invitation. I saw it as trial by dinner for my suitability as a Trustee. Afterwards, I received a handwritten letter from John Fry (unpublished) telling me that: "I had passed the test with flying colours!" A letter from Sir Maurice Shock then invited me to become a Trustee in 1993. John Fry died on 28 April 1994, so we were trustees together for only a few months. In July 1994 Jill and I had our first dinner with the other Trustees.

I became the only GP Trustee of the Trust for the next nine years. The meetings awarded research grants and it was good to discuss these with sharp minds. There was always a good dinner and rich conversation in-house afterwards.

In my first year, August 1994, I attended as a member of the Trust's UK team, a three-nation conference with Canadian and US leaders for a week at Lincoln College, Oxford. I was asked to prepare and present a paper on primary health care. I greatly enjoyed the setting and discussions (Ashley-Miller *et al.*, 1996).

GP Fundholding in the NHS

GP fundholding was a big initiative of the Thatcher government and Michael Ashley-Miller consulted me about it. Michael spoke with the RCGP President, Alastair Donald, who was not keen. I well understood as in April 1989 when the RCGP Council considered Thatcher's white paper, Donald had castigated GP fundholding, described in Chapter 23, Chair of Council story.

I suggested to Ashley-Miller that he should see the Chair of the RCGP Council, Bill Styles, and we went to the College together. Ashley-Miller offered to fund a national evaluation of GP fundholding, but the meeting went badly. BIll Styles was unhappy about GP fundholding and declined agreement for the RCGP to be involved in a national evaluation. Michael and I were disappointed. Whatever the personal views of its leaders, GP fundholding was an important experiment and the offer of a properly funded, external evaluation, by a national charity, free to the College, was needed and should have been accepted. Whatever the findings, the College needed to know them.

Dinners

The NPHT held regular, high-powered seminars for invited experts and after these and grant-awarding meetings there were dinners. I met many innovators and was fascinated by conversations that were quite different from what I had previously experienced because of the seniority and importance of the Trustees and guests. Two Trustees were former permanent secretaries. Sir Christopher France (1934–2014) told me how he had to spend one weekend dividing up the huge DHSS after Mrs Thatcher split it in two. Sir Maurice Shock in 1994 said that the future of the world would be increasingly influenced by China, not a perspective I had at that time. One fellow Trustee was the Oxford Director of Clinical Studies, Professor John Ledingham, with whom I got on well. I had read an interview with him: "Oxford is traditionally a non-GP producing school. The Oxford view for many years was that there was no academic content in general practice"... (Just GPs). Oxford has changed its mind. Nowadays we get graduates with first-class honours wanting to do general practice. This would have been unheard of five years ago" (Walker, 1978).

Dinners differ from other professional meetings: the timescale is different; it is rare to have an hour or more, one-to-one with a senior colleague in a meeting; most dinners for national leaders are in London; the absence of an agenda widens conversational possibilities; alcohol loosens tongues, and asides are made which would never be said in meetings or conferences; attitudes are much more often revealed; their main value is to leaders. The following stories illustrate how some attitudes emerged at dinners I was at:

> At one Trust dinner, a woman said to me: "How on earth can a GP be knighted?" revealing her attitude to general practice in eight words (Just GPs).
>
> At an NHS dinner, a woman who held a very senior position in the NHS was chatting to me about her daughter who had recently qualified as a doctor. I expressed pleasure whereupon she said that she had persuaded her not to do general practice as: "She is very intelligent, and I don't want her wasting her time seeing coughs and colds" (Just GPs).
>
> As a guest at a London university dinner, in the 21st century, I was seated beside a professor of mathematics who spoke at length about his work. He asked me what I did, and I said I was a professor of general practice. "That's an oxymoron!" (contradiction in terms) he said (Just a GP). This was the shortest and sharpest academic insult to general practice that I encountered. To his surprise, and that of others at the table, I immediately described two examples of world-class original research in general practice. Afterwards, I wrote to the Dean of his medical school, described the incident, and suggested that this professor be barred from teaching medical students as he was so out of date, since half the medical students in that school would have the privilege of becoming GPs. I then received a two-page apology from the professor.
>
> At a Trust dinner when talking with a grade one civil servant as the new GP contract in 2003 was taking GPs away from out-of-hours work. I suggested that the DH would find that an out-of-hours service not run by experienced GP principals would refer more. He was having none of it. He replied in words that rang in my ears for years: "What you have to understand, Denis, is that the out-of-hours service will be better without the GPs!" (Just GPs). I said my family had been doing out-of-hours care for 100 years and that if GPs stopped it, attendances at A&E departments would rise. "Oh no!" he said. "We don't want that, and they won't because A&E consultants will be involved." I realised he had no idea about the service he was managing, why patients seek care out of hours, why they require generalist clinical skills and how their needs relate to care during the week. He did not respect GPs for doing this work, as they had for 200 years. His thinking was not in DH policy documents, which I had dutifully read. It was after that encounter that I formulated the maxim: *Society is exchanging arrogant doctors for arrogant managers.* That evening I went home knowing that attendances at A&E departments and emergency hospital admissions in England would rise relentlessly. They did. This was an insight that the "top of the office," as the DH refers to the Permanent Secretary's office, lacked.

The Name of the Trust

Sir Maurice Shock (1926–2018), Chair in the 1990s, led an initiative to change the name of the Trust. The Nuffield Provincial Hospitals Trust was always a cumbersome title and it had become progressively less appropriate since 1940, as health policy broadened. I thought the emphasis on hospitals was out of date, and so was supportive. The Trustees agreed and proposed the simple name: the Nuffield Trust. Registered charities are not permitted to change their name at will and need permission from the regulator, the Charities Commission, so this was sought and given.

Sir Maurice received a strong protest from the Nuffield Foundation, which claimed the name of the Nuffield Trust was too close to the Nuffield Foundation and a change of name would cause confusion. They pressed hard. We did not know what had happened between them and the Charities Commission. Attempts were made to smooth down this problem, but anger continued. Finally, the Nuffield Trust simply implemented the new name.

Global Health

Global health was a theme of the Trust in the late 1990s. This led me to several conferences in both Canada and the USA. In Washington we had a tour of the Congress. We were welcomed by a senior US Senator who said he had landed on the Omaha beach in 1944 in the Normandy invasion. This was where the Americans had suffered heavy losses. He saw "the Brits" as steadfast allies and he reminded me of my experience with Professor Huygen in the Netherlands who spoke about the RAF rescuing starving Dutch people in the very same year (Chapter 13, Department/Institute of General Practice story). Symbolically, the Grand Duke of Luxembourg when re-entering his country after the war wore the uniform of a junior guards officer in the British Army (*The Times*, 2019). I realised that as long as such senior people and their equivalents in the UK had such shared memories of facing death together, relationships between the allies in the war were secure. I also realised that those bonds were time limited.

Whilst in Washington I visited a socially deprived area nearby. Here I found a district where doctors were unaffordable, where primary care was delivered in emergency departments of public hospitals, and what care there was in the home came from philanthropic organisations and from nuns. The male mortality rate was the same as in a developing country in a place that was in sight of the seat of power of the richest country on earth.

One of the privileges of attending these conferences was meeting several internationally known American doctors. David Blumenthal and Tom Bodenheimer, whom I met at a Robert Wood Johnson conference, are internationally leading thinkers about family practice/primary care. Bodenheimer wrote about the importance of teaching patients how to manage their own illnesses (Bodenheimer *et al.*, 2002). He also identified the need to pay more attention to the well-being of family doctors in what he called the "quadruple aim" (Bodenheimer *et al.*, 2014). I also met Larry Green, one of the outstanding leaders of US family physicians.

The best-known person I met was Don Berwick, whom Obama soon appointed to head an important US institution. I heard him lecture and chatted with him at dinner. He later came to the UK to speak to an RCGP conference and gave much important advice to the NHS. He was appointed an honorary Knight (honorary because he is a US citizen) as KBE. I wondered if I would be isolated in the United States coming from such a different health system. Not so. Many leading doctors expressed admiration of the NHS, especially its universal access.

Once, however, I was completely isolated in a conversation where I felt I was from a different world with a very different perspective. We discussed the then recent deployment of American troops in Afghanistan, and I said the deployment was a strategic mistake and the United States would lose this war. My American colleagues were startled and asked me why. I said the British Empire was the greatest the world had ever seen, controlling about a fifth of the world, with unique experience of fighting around the world. Yet it had fought three wars in Afghanistan and never won. Then, the Russians, who were a world-class military power and geographically very much closer had invaded and they too had had to retreat. The USA had lost its first war in Asia, in Vietnam, and now, I said, it would lose another. This shook my colleagues. One said: "But the US is the biggest military power on earth." I agreed but said that even a great military power would not win a guerilla war in a mountainous country.

The lessons of history were there for all to see but were little known. Nor, sadly, were the Americans alone. The UK defence minister revealingly said as he committed British troops to the war in Afghanistan, that he hoped not a shot would be fired! There were 454 British deaths. In 2021, President Biden after questionable negotiations withdrew allied troops without victory in a humiliating withdrawal leaving some loyal colleagues behind. In August 2021 the Taliban regained control of the country and control of Kabul airport. A Taliban commander caught the essence of the war with a striking simile: *The Americans have watches, but we have time.*

One leading US doctor was Roger Bulger (1933–), an anglophile and head of US teaching hospitals. (Confusingly to British eyes, it was called the Association of Teaching Health Centres.) I caught his attention when giving a lecture in the United States when I said that GPs/family physicians needed to provide as good a quality of care for their patients as specialists and could do so because of their extra knowledge of the patient as a person and the family which could balance the greater knowledge of the disease by specialists, eg GPs, could achieve lower average levels of HbA1c in their diabetic patients than specialists could as specialists had more patients with complications. He said he had never heard a family physician say that before and asked if he could come to my practice and later did so, as described in Chapter 13, Department/Institute of General Practice Story.

One of the successes for the Nuffield Trust was the relationships built with the DH which led to both the Chief Medical Officer, Sir Liam Donaldson, and Richard Grainger, then leading the big DH computer project, to come to Washington with the Trust. The Trust also established good relationships with The Commonwealth Fund of New York. I visited their headquarters and got to know the director, Karen Davis (1942–). Commonwealth Fund finances the Harkness Fellowships. These were established in 1925 to match the Rhodes scholarships (which bring potential leaders to Britain) so enabling potential British leaders to spend up to a year in US centres of excellence.

I knew about these as Kieran Sweeney, one of my partners, was the first GP ever to win one early in the 1990s (Chapter 34, Practice story, 1987–2000) and soon afterwards Martin Marshall from the Exeter University Department of General Practice did the same. The Nuffield Trust facilitated the appointment of the British Harkness fellows by providing rooms and hospitality.

The Chair

By 2002, there was restlessness among the Trustees about the Chair. Sir Maurice was much respected and a former Vice-Chancellor at Leicester and Rector of Lincoln College, Oxford. However, he chaired meetings with more authority than had become usual by the 21st century. He had said he was going to retire when he was 70 but then showed no sign of doing so. I had seen this syndrome in a great man before (Chapter 9, Journal story).

Then Trustees started to talk openly about the need for a new chair. I said nothing as I expected Sir Maurice to produce some Oxford star. Then Don Detmer, the American Trustee, asked me if I would do the job. The background was that the Trust had had a succession of nationally distinguished chairmen: Sir William Goodenough (1867–1945), who had chaired the Goodenough Committee (1944); the Hon Sir Geoffrey Gibbs (1901–1975) who chaired both the Nuffield Foundation and the Trust; and Sir Edgar Williams CBE DSO (1912–1995) who was described as "the best intelligence officer on either side," when aged 29 he anticipated Rommel's moves and gave Montgomery valuable advice in the North African campaign in the World War II. He had become the third Chair of the Trustees and the first when the NPHT was a separate entity. He was followed by Maurice Shock as the fourth Chair in 1988.

I said I would need to consult the other Trustees and did so. Sir Leslie Boriesevicz was influential, and I went to see him as Vice-Principal in Imperial College. I found that there was strong support for me. Some Trustees mentioned my chairing of the Academy of Medical Royal Colleges and having had eight years as a Trustee. Being knighted probably helped since every former chair had been, as well as many former Trustees.

In the autumn of 2002, a formal motion signed by several Trustees, but not by me, came to a Trustee meeting proposing that I should succeed as Chair. I was elected chair-elected *nem con*. Most chairs would have arranged to hand over quite quickly, but Sir Maurice said he would retire the following July. In 2003, I collected donations from all the current, and some previous, Trustees and we were able to buy him a nice piece of silver. After the July meeting we held a dinner to which Jill came and I made a speech of thanks on behalf of the Trust and made the presentation. He had served as Chairman for 15 years and was aged 77 when he stood down (*The Times*, 2003).

My election as Chair was radical. Ever since its separation from the Nuffield Foundation, with Sir Edgar Williams the first Chair, the Nuffield Trust had been chaired by an Oxford don. I was the first medically qualified Chair, let alone the first GP. All the previous chairs had looked for inspiration to the top of Britain's teaching hospitals, whereas I looked for inspiration from personal medical care in the community. Oxford was one of the so called ancient universities and was often ranked first in the world. The University of Exeter was a post–World War II creation. It was quite a change.

In 2003, the Trust was invited to a two-day meeting of the European Foundation (charities) 'Leaders summit,' which I attended as Chair-Elect. This was organised by the European Mercator fund in Brussels. There were 66 foundations present across Europe. Eight were British. I knew almost no one but had a useful discussion with the Director of the Nuffield Foundation. It was ironic that two Nuffield charities, both London based, should meet in Brussels. The keynote address was given by Javier Solana, to whom I was introduced. He was then Secretary General to the Council of the EU, a big figure in the European Union and later its first Foreign Minister. His theme was the desirability of more co-operation between foundations and with the European Union. I thought I detected a hint of the EU seeking influence or control.

Seminars in the Trust

Seminars in the Trust were of very high quality, and I much enjoyed them as a rich source for my continuing education. There was regular attendance from Simon (later Sir, later still Lord) Stevens, then health adviser to the Prime Minister, Tony Blair. He was later appointed Chief Executive of NHS England. Professor Chris Ham also came regularly as he was then leading the DH strategy unit. He was later appointed Chief Executive of the King's Fund and knighted when he retired. Ham had an able GP on the staff of the strategy unit, Tim Wilson, who had done quality assurance work with the College, and they wrote an important article on the contribution of general practice to the NHS (Wilson *et al.*, 2006). Barry McCormick, Chief Economic Adviser to the DH, also came regularly to the seminars. He had been a Harkness fellow and later came to the St Leonard's Practice and gave us research advice.

I was given an important insight in a Trust seminar on privatisation in the NHS. I was chairing and always tried to be strictly balanced when summing up. On this occasion I said that one of the advantages of privatisation, which was then fashionable and common, was that it transferred risk from the state to a private organisation. A lawyer from a leading London law firm said: "not necessarily!" He said that he had written several legal contracts in big privatisations. "Just wait," he said, "until one of these big outsourcing companies goes bust then the risk will fall straight back on to the public sector!" This was new to me, and I realised I had not been thinking hard enough. Later a big company did fail, and Transport for London had to take on risk. Later still, Carillion also failed, leaving central government taking on risk.

Whilst Chair of the Trust, I held two other honorary positions: President of the children's charity, What About the Children? (WATCh?) and Patron of the National Association for Patient Participation (NAPP). I arranged for the Trust to host a seminar and dinner for both these small charities. WATCh? used the opportunity, skilfully arranging for Professor Melhuish, a researcher on the Sure Start programme and Ms Penelope Leach, a national expert, to attend.

One dramatic dinner after a seminar was in 2004 when Tony Blair proposed establishing foundation hospitals in Parliament. He split the Labour Government in doing so. We had several DH guests, and they were on edge, looking at their mobiles during dinner. I quietly spoke to one who told me they thought their jobs were on the line that night! The proposal passed in Parliament, with support from some Conservative opposition votes, but with a majority of only four. They asked me what I thought about foundation hospitals. I said I would answer once they had explained why there were no proposals for foundation general practices or foundation primary care trusts!

A highlight was a seminar with Amartya Sen CH FBA (1933–), the first time I had the privilege of a conversation with a Nobel Laureate. We discussed the Irish potato famine in the 1840s. An Indian expert on the British empire, he said that poor, starving people did not always react with violence. Whilst many able-bodied Irish had emigrated to the United States, taking a hatred of the British with them, the poor mainly starved to death. He asked me if I thought the British Government would have done so little if the famine had been in England!

A moving seminar for me was attended by Professor Ian McWhinney (1926–2012) from Canada, the leading GP academic worldwide. I hugely admired him. I had known him when he was an English GP. I apologised to him, 30 years after the event for my great mistake in dropping him from the Editorial Board of the College *Journal* (Chapter 9, Journal story) in 1972. He was gracious about it. I showed him out of the building knowing we would never meet again.

Publications

John Horder introduced me to John Bunker (1920–2012) and we met several times. He was an American anaesthetist, an intellectual giant, who had pioneered the evaluation of surgery (Bunker *et al.*, 1978) nicknamed "Bunker's Bible," and co-authored a key paper showing that mortality fell when hospitals often did high volumes of an operation (Luft *et al.*, 1979). Bunker became involved with the Trust at the turn of the century when the role of doctors was being debunked. Aged over 80, Bunker wrote *Medicine matters after all: measuring the benefits of medical care, a healthy lifestyle and a just social community,* which the Trust was pleased to publish (Bunker, 2001).

I wrote an article for the *Health Service Journal* and risked some predictions of the future as: "2020 vision." In 2003 I predicted that: "Healthcare in Europe will be more and more about human behaviour and its modification" (DPG, 2003). I foresaw total expenditure on health systems would rise progressively and proposed that the value of a life should be publicised and used by the DH as it is in the Department of Transport. Health expenditure certainly rose but the value of a life is hidden in NICE figures. It remains a key figure for planning and evaluating the value of health care and it is still in the NHS's interest that it be known.

As a UK-wide think-tank I was interested in the results of devolution of health services to Northern Ireland, Scotland and Wales. This four-way variation in policy making was a natural experiment crying out for comparative analyses. It was good the Trust did this (Jervis and Plowden, 2003). I wrote letters to leading newspapers, achieving my first letter in the *Financial Times* (DPG, 2004a), which is harder to achieve than in *The Times*, with a letter "Impact of new pension load set to grow in the future."

In 2004, the Blair family became involved in a political argument about whether their son, Leo, had had the MMR jab (Rogers and O'Reilly, 2004). The press clamoured for the information. I argued that the Blair family should have the usual medical confidentiality. I was also concerned that if Leo had a medical contraindication that false conclusions might be drawn.

Clive Smee CB (1942–2019) had been the Chief Economic Adviser to the DH, initiating economic evaluation there. He had good links with the Trust, and we agreed to encourage h his memoir. He told me how when Tony Blair, skilfully provoked by a Bristol doctor, had made his famous commitment on television that he would bring NHS spending up to the European average there were repercussions. No one knew what that would cost! He was roped in one Sunday morning to provide an estimate. This was huge – about 2% of the GDP. There were stories that Gordon Brown said to Blair: "You have stolen my f........budget!" It was also wittily said that the incident had been the most expensive breakfast in British history! I was lucky to see it live on television. This memoir was published whilst I was chairing as *Speaking Truth to Power: Two Decades of Analysis in the Department of Health* (Smee, 2005).

Royal Visit

The Trust's Patron was the Princess Royal, Princess Anne, and the Trust was offered a royal visit. Royal activities like these are not well understood. At one level they demonstrate recognition by society. At another level they are a highlight, particularly for staff like cleaners, who are often introduced to the Royal Visitor. This may be a lifetime high point for some of them. I always remember the pleasure Prince Charles gave to a group of people with learning disabilities at the RCGP. The British system of deploying about half a dozen members of the Royal Family is more flexible and subtle than the presidential equivalent in countries that are republics. I had met the Queen, Prince Philip, Prince Charles (several times; see Chapter 23, Chair of Council story), and Princess Anne before. I was impressed to read in the subsequent Court circular in the *Times* that she had done three different public engagements that day.

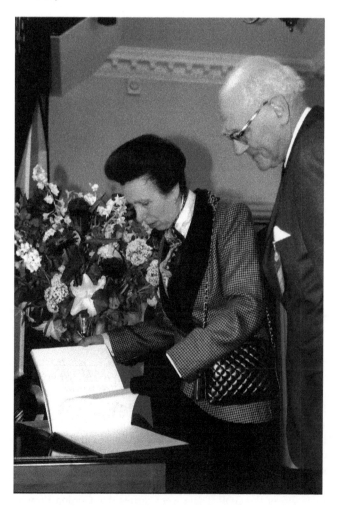

FIGURE 44.1   HRH Princess Anne, with me as Chair Nuffield Trust, 2004.

John Fry Lecture

In 2003, important research emerged in the *Journal of the American Board of Family Medicine* in the United States. I was still a member of the Editorial Board of that *Journal* and so I received a personal copy with this article at home. Shi, Macinko and Starfield *et al.* (2004) examined the relationship between primary care, income inequality and mortality in US states 1980 to 1995. They confirmed that income inequality was significantly associated with mortality across the United States but although important this was not new. What was new was the association between the number of primary care doctors in relation to their population and mortality and the time periods they used – namely 15 consecutive years. Using sophisticated analyses, analysing both contemporary and time-lagged figures, they found that higher numbers of primary care doctors were associated with lower mortality. They dealt with the organisational problem in the United States that there are several different kinds of doctor providing primary care, including specialists, and were able to show that among the primary care subspecialties: "only family medicine was consistently and significantly (P<0.01) associated with lower all-cause mortality for all time periods."

They confirmed what Shi (1992) had first reported that higher numbers of specialist doctors were associated with a higher all-cause mortality in all time periods except 1990. This is difficult to handle medico politically and general practice/primary care has not yet attempted it, but it seems likely that the intensive investigations and the heavy use of hospitals are associated with specialist practice may have more serious adverse effects than is generally realised. One article (McAlister *et al.*, 2007) reported that people with diabetes, even after controlling for morbidity, who saw a specialist as well as a GP, died more often. It is never discussed. Starfield *et al.* (2005) provides powerful evidence underpinning the value of general practice/family medicine in Western societies and gave GPs confidence that, although much is invisible, their work is of great value. Coming out in 2003, it helped me in the Trust to bring Barbara Starfield from the United States to give a big Trust lecture.

As the GP Trustee, I led on the next lecturer for the John Fry lectureship. I wanted the leading person in the world on the evidence on the value of general/family practice, Professor Barbara Starfield (1932–2011) from the Johns Hopkins Medical School, USA. The Trustees approved a lecture fee of £5,000 and business class travel. No other organisation in the UK at that time, including the RCGP could match this for a general practice lecture. I invited her. She knew me as she had cited Sweeney and DPG (1995) in her textbook on *Primary Care* and I had had the privilege as RCGP President of presenting her with the College's honorary fellowship.

To my pleasure, she accepted. My brief to her was to deploy the research on the value of general/family practice on which she was the world's expert. She had shown in the *Lancet* that countries with more primary care orientation had lower overall health system costs (Starfield, 1994) and had later shown that every extra family physician in the United States was associated with 34 lives saved per hundred thousand American citizens (Starfield, 2001). I was optimistic about this lecture and the Trust invited many GP leaders to hear her.

To my disappointment, she gave a different lecture on the importance of health inequalities (she was President of the International Society for Equity in Health). It was well delivered, politely received, and the Trust published it (Starfield, 2003). Two years later, she and colleagues published just what I had sought: "The contribution of primary care to western health systems," an important article which became a classic (Starfield *et al.*, 2005). I do not know what went wrong. As I used to say to our children: "You can't win 'em all!"

2006 DH White Paper

The DH started on a white paper on the community services. The Trust had excellent working relationships with various DH officials, and we offered them a room in the Trust with facilities such as teas/coffees etc. This was more comfortable than the usual Government facilities so much drafting was done in the Trust. Over conversations the civil servants became interested in my experience, as this white paper was on the community, highlighting general practice. I gave them references and a paper called: "A dozen facts about general practice," in which there were statements like: "There are more general practitioners than all consultants combined," and "A British child after birth never sees a paediatrician, most older people never see a geriatrician, most of the mentally ill never see a psychiatrist, and most people with diabetes never see a diabetician, whereas the GP on average sees all these every week."

It transpired that some senior civil servants did not know several of these facts (the first us no longer true) and I was consulted increasingly. They wanted to emphasise how close the average GP surgery is to the average NHS patient (only a kilometre); this is a great strength in a frontline service, especially for poor people without cars. I offered the phrase "within pram-pushing distance." Ministers liked it and incorporated it in the text of the white paper (DH, 2006; DPG, 2006). I reflected on how I had previously spent nearly seven years of my life in democratically elected leadership positions in the RCGP, both as Chair and President, entitling me to speak on behalf of GPs, without ever being consulted like this. Now I had been elected by only nine trustees, none of whom was a doctor let alone a GP and I was being consulted much more.

At a late stage I learned that the white paper was going to refer to the NHS as 'a sickness service' for the NHS. This was and still is a common problem, but it is seriously prejudicial to general practice as it is the hospital service, which is a sickness service. Anyone using this phrase is revealing a hospital orientation and unfairly undervalues the huge contribution general practice makes to personal preventive medicine and anticipatory care. This includes a whole array of immunisations for children, case finding for conditions such as high blood pressure and high cholesterol levels, providing cervical screening and immunisations for children and the elderly, and the most sophisticated anticipatory care: taking into account a ten-year risk in many clinical consultations. I felt strongly about this.

I took Stephen Dunn, a civil servant on the white paper team (now an NHS manager), out to lunch alone. I lobbied him to avoid the 'sickness service,' a phrase meaning Ministers would reveal the hospital orientation and lack of knowledge about general practice. The phrase did not appear in the 2006 white paper. However, attitudes are hard to change and the bias towards hospitals is embedded in Government and DH thinking. Tony Blair, frequently talked of "schools and hospitals," equating hospital care with the whole NHS. I won a battle but did not win the war. Twelve years later, a Secretary of State for Health in a different Government, described the NHS as a 'sickness service.' Surprisingly, Ministers approved my 'dozen facts about general practice' as an appendix. The white paper appeared in 2006 as *Our Health, Our Care, Our Choice* (DH, 2006).

Role of the Chair

I was conscious that I was the first medical Chair of the Nuffield Trust. I knew how non-executive directors may not know all the facts (Chapter 33, non-Executive Directorships story). This can occur in organisations accidentally but sometimes deliberately. I ensured I was fully informed, immersing myself in the Trust's organisation, spending time with all levels of staff, and had detailed discussions one-to-one with the Trust's accountant, the auditor, and solicitors.

I inherited the difficult relationship with the Nuffield Foundation after the change of the Trust's name. The Trustees agreed I should meet the Chair of the Trustees of the Foundation and explore reconciliation. My opposite number was Baroness Onora O'Neill whom I had not met but whom I greatly admired after her BBC Reith lectures (O'Neill, 2002). She had elucidated the importance of trust in the professions and how excessive regulation diminishes it. I took her out to lunch, which was pleasant. However, when I broached the relationship between the two charities, she closed me down saying there was no chance of reconciliation whilst John Wyn Owen was our Secretary. I did not know there were any personal factors involved. My negotiation failed, as I was not informed. As it happened, John

Wyn Owen (1942–2020) left the Trust during my chairmanship but not for any reason connected with the Nuffield Foundation. I became for a time, in the absence of a CEO, executive chair.

Sir Cyril Chantler (1939–), as Chairman of the Trustees of the King's Fund. suggested that the King's Fund and the Nuffield Trust should merge. He said the two organisations were doing similar work, operated geographically close to each other and the merger would save substantially on overheads. I said I would think it over and thought long and hard about the proposal. The case that Chantler was making made me think a 'merger' would be more like a 'takeover' as the King's Fund was older, richer and better known. I saw the advantage to the King's Fund in sidestepping the limitations of its charter and becoming able to operate over the whole of the UK. I saw no counterbalancing advantage for the Nuffield Trust. I politely, but firmly, turned the merger down. The continuing existence of the Nuffield Trust is part of my legacy.

My Retirement

It was agreed when I was elected that I would serve a three-year term and retire in June 2006. The process of identifying my successor was done through a search committee. I was completely relaxed until I heard that a doctor whom I knew well had been identified. There was no doubt about their ability, but this colleague had publicly accepted a high-profile, politically sensitive post for a Government Department for six sessions per week. I doubted if anyone in such a position could be fully independent of Government or be actively involved in publications seriously questioning government policy. This was not a personal objection but a point of principle. I knew Lord Nuffield had wanted rigorous independence. For me, the Trust's independence from Government and the ability to speak honestly and openly about current issues was fundamental. I did not look forward to such a handover. I tried hard to resolve the problem with my fellow Trustees with success. So, I resigned a few weeks before my term was due to end. Dame Fiona Caldecott (1941–2021) was elected interim Chair.

45

Negotiations between the Department of Health and the BMA

After a good negotiation both parties feel satisfied.

Chinese Proverb

Between 1998 and 2006 I was successively Vice-Chair and Chair of the Academy of Medical Royal Colleges, and then Chair of the trustees of the Nuffield Trust. I heard comments from both sides of DH: BMA negotiations. This chapter seeks to piece three stories together.

The British Medical Association (BMA) is the registered medical trade union and undertakes pay and contract negotiations for all doctors. It is a federal body and includes separate groups for GPs, senior hospital doctors, junior doctors and public health physicians. Each has a national conference, a national committee and an executive group which negotiates. The BMA Council, on which I served for four years from 1967–1971 (Chapter 8, LMC/BMA story) co-ordinates policy.

The NHS was nationalised in 1948, which meant that the pay and conditions became a responsibility of a Government minister. Whilst there are other professions working in state-run services, in medicine and nursing it has been generally regarded as unethical to strike. This disadvantages these professions in negotiations, especially as the DH is effectively a monopoly employer.

In the 1950s, after tough negotiations between the GPs and the DHSS, the GPs, led by Solomon Wand, with whom I served on the BMA Council, went to adjudication. Mr Justice Danckwertz (1888–1978) in the High Court, adjudicated in favour of the GPs, awarding them £40 million. My father received a useful sum and the DHSS never agreed to arbitration again.

All this was unsatisfactory. The Government established a Royal Commission to examine how the medical profession should be paid. This Royal Commission on Doctors' and Dentists' Remuneration (1960) was chaired by Sir Harry (later Lord) Pilkington (1905–1983). It proposed a new body, independent of the DHSS and the doctors, the Review Body on Doctors' and Dentists' Remuneration (Review Body) "whose advice would only be exceptionally overruled." This would independently analyse incomes in comparable occupations. This was a logical and civilised suggestion.

The new system started well but an award in the 1960s was rejected by the GPs, triggering 18,000 of them, including me, to send undated letters of resignation from the NHS to the BMA (Chapter 8, LMC/BMA story). A new GP contract was agreed which the same Review Body priced much more highly. Later, the DHSS/DH started 'phasing' the Review Body award, i.e. paying what had been recommended but delayed by six months, reducing the cost to government and the amount received by doctors. Over time the Government/DH progressively downgraded the independence of the Review Body. In the 21st century written instructions were being given to the Review Body stating what percentage increase was Government policy and by implication should not be exceeded. The core principle of comparability was eroded.

DOI: 10.1201/9781032713601-54

(1) DH Negotiations with GPs

In 2001 the Chair of the BMA GP committee and lead negotiator was John Chisholm whom I had known since 1980 (Chapter 13, Department/Institute of General Practice). He adopted a new strategy for the BMA, to enhance quality of care and to seek to ensure that was remunerated. The DH, for the first and only time, uniquely delegated GP negotiations to the NHS Confederation, an NHS employers' body. Its Chief Executive Gill (later Dame) Morgan (1953–) was a doctor and had been to our practice when Chief Executive of our local health authority. I had a dinner alone with her as Chair of the Nuffield Trust. For the first time I knew the leaders of both sides.

The negotiating teams needed experts and were advised by the Manchester GP Department. Their GPs included Martin Marshall, a Professor who had been with me in the Exeter Department for many years (Chapter 13, Department/Institute of General Practice story). The atmosphere of these negotiations was described to me as 'cosy The advisers reported when good GP care was significantly associated with better patient outcomes. The negotiators turned these into measurable targets for GPs, forming the Quality and Outcomes Framework (QOF), which was introduced into the GP contract. This was the RCGP's (1985a) good practice allowance divided into fractions. The targets were not controversial as many of them, such as GPs knowing the smoking status and blood pressures of their patients, were already accepted as good practice.

There were, however, big questions about the terms and conditions of service. Since 1948, NHS general practitioners like my father and me, had 24-hour responsibility for each patient throughout the year. My father's generation delivered that personally, but from the 1970s GPs increasingly shared it, first by inter-practice arrangements and in the 1990s through out-of-hours arrangements. Later these involved GPs in a local area sharing out-of-hours between them. These cooperatives worked well, improving relationships between general practices and, since the service was mainly provided by experienced GP principals, there were few complaints. I believe that the DH should have supported co-operatives rather than abolishing them. Out-of-hours work was always sensitive because working in the evenings, nights, weekends and bank holidays was demanding and affected GPs' personal lives. The BMA was looking to free GPs as much as possible. The core interest of the Confederation, representing the public interest, and the profession were not aligned. Patient representatives were not involved or consulted.

Two key questions were as follows: first, how Saturday morning surgeries were used and valued. In our practice, we saw about 15 patients each Saturday. Amazingly, the NHS Confederation never surveyed this, never modelled how patients used the service, nor estimated where patients would go if the GPs were not available.

Second, the value of a GP accepting responsibility for on-call for a share of out-of-hours work (evenings, nights, Saturdays, Sundays, and bank holidays) was another key issue. My personal, private, judgement was that a fair price was about £15,000 per GP a year. During the negotiations, the price was discussed as there was a figure of what GPs were previously paid under the old contract. This existed because the Review Body had priced it for GPs who, after serious illness, could no longer do night work. What was not understood outside the profession was that the Review Body merely allocated a part of the overall payment that GPs were being paid and it never analysed the value. The sum, moreover, had been pitched low to protect ill GPs and the profession accepted it as a compassionate notional division. The paper price GPs were being paid for out-of-hours work was much too low. It had been ignored because GPs looked at their total payment and the notional figure for out-of-hours work was irrelevant as they mostly did both day and night work. The BMA team understood this: the Confederation team took the current book figure literally.

The DH proposed that GPs should be freed completely from the 24-hour responsibility and out-of-hours work be defined to include both Saturdays and Sundays. The Confederation, remarkably, and with the full backing of the DH, offered GPs a five-day week. No trade union could have declined this offer.

It was necessary to decide what GPs should be paid for accepting responsibility.

The BMA was unusually passive and the DH succeeded, it thought, in winning a bargain price; i.e. any GP taking a share of responsibility of evenings, nights, Saturdays, Sundays and bank holidays would earn only an additional £6,000 a year. This was reported to the DH as a negotiating success. Both sides thought they had won. The Confederation as the sum was so low, and the BMA because it knew that few if any GPs would do out-of-hours care; so there was no danger of splitting the profession. The Confederation and the DH were confident that with the £6,000 from the GPs opting out they could run the out-of-hours services. But they never piloted it.

When GPs saw the proposal they did not consider the £6,000 gross, as most were higher rate (40%) taxpayers, so they considered their after tax, take-home pay which would be only £3,600. Some GPs felt insulted by this offer for the considerable clinical responsibility for evenings, nights and weekend responsibilities. The great majority of GPs stopped out-of-hours at once and most followed later.

A BMA negotiator at a dinner in the Nuffield Trust was cock-a-hoop, saying "Now for the first time the DH will learn what GP out-of-hours work is really worth!" He was right and the DH learned a painful lesson when the NHS CCGs sent urgent messages that they could not run a GP out-of-hours service with the collection of £6,000s. Moreover, fewer GPs were now willing to work out of hours and, moreover, required higher payments as it had was now a commercial matter rather than a shared professional responsibility.

NHS contracting bodies became so short of GPs that they flew them in at weekends from Europe. In the South West some spoke so little English that they consulted with a dictionary in hand and were nicknamed 'the dictionary doctors!' They often did not know NHS arrangements or local phrases used by patients, who received an inferior service. I protested to Finlay Scott, the GMC registrar. There also was a presentation issue. Ministers, when supporting the contract, had boasted that British patients would no longer be seen out of hours by tired British GPs, who were working during the week. Ironically, patients were now being seen by tired European GPs working during the week.

I watched with regret as three years' work in the JCPTGP (Chapter 29, the JCPTGP story) ensuring that British patients were seen only by GPs who had been assessed was bypassed. A disaster was inevitable and occurred in 2008 when a European doctor gave a lethal injection to an NHS patient out of hours. The NHS had approved him working but he was struck off by the GMC in 2010.

The financial consequences for the DH were substantial. The English CCGs had needed rescuing by on average about £1 million each, nationally over £150 million. This was unbudgeted and greatly irritated ministers. I had two conversations with DH staff about this.

At a DH meeting where regret was expressed that GPs would no longer provide Saturday morning surgeries, one upper-class woman said loudly, "I've never been to see my GP on a Saturday morning!" In front of a big group, I replied that I thought Saturday morning surgeries were important and helped to keep patients out of hospital. In Exeter alone, about 200 patients were seen every Saturday morning in GP surgeries and we also provided emergency surgeries at bank holidays. I said, "It's not people like you who come on Saturday mornings, it is mothers worried about children with temperatures, it is carers worried about those they look after, and it's the anxious and depressed who are worried about coping. Closing Saturday morning surgeries will mean more use of A&E departments and higher NHS costs." As I left, a senior civil servant sidled up to me, "I very much hope you are wrong Denis, but I very much fear you will be right!" NHS attendances at A&E departments in England rose 5% in the first year and continued to rise for the next 18 years. A consultation in A&E costs the NHS much more than a GP consultation. With no weekend GP co-operatives left and with general practices closed from 6 pm on Friday until 8am on Mondays, the DH broke the 200-year tradition of patients consulting GPs first. For patients, going to A&E first became much more logical and a new social pattern was set.

The Political Consequences of the 2003 GP Contract

There were big political consequences of the 2003 GP contract. The press presented it as GPs gaining shorter working hours and a big pay increase, with the average full-time GP principal earning over £100,000 a year. Payments to GPs from the Quality and Outcomes Framework were higher than estimated, reaching £1 billion a year. The bailouts for the CCGs cost over £150 million, and A&E attendances as well as hospital attendances rose progressively. The DH never delegated negotiations with the medical profession again.

Clearly the BMA won. However, there is a Chinese proverb that satisfactory negotiations occur only when both parties leave feeling happy. Here the Labour Government, including Prime Minister Gordon Brown, felt very unhappy. The incomes of GPs were progressively reduced and funds clawed back. In real terms GPs in 2014 earned no more than 10 years earlier. The Government's irritation with general practice led to priority being given to the hospital service. Consultant numbers doubled in the decade ending 2016 (Moberly, 2019) crucially overtaking the number of GPs in 2009. Recruitment to general practice withered on the vine. General practice paid a high price for its contractual 'success That Chinese proverb captures a truth.

---

(2) DH Negotiations with Senior Hospital Doctors

DH negotiations with senior hospital doctors took place with a DH-led team. The Secretary of State was Alan Milburn and the lead hospital negotiator was Peter Hawker, a consultant gastroenterologist. The Secretary of State was concerned about consultants' private practice. I was at meetings where Milburn and Peter Hawker were together and noted tension between them. Milburn often patronised Hawker, who to his credit, never responded.

Consultant private practice was a longstanding problem, but only for a small minority of consultants. Ever since 1948, consultants had had the opportunity to choose a so-called 'maximum part-time contract' which meant working nine weekly sessions for the NHS but having two sessions a week for private practice, usually in private consulting rooms or private hospitals. The problem was, particularly in London teaching hospitals, a small number of consultants were taking time out of the NHS to do private practice and Milburn was, reasonably, keen to stop this. My view was that this was a management problem for the chief executive and managers of the hospital concerned who knew when any consultant was out of the hospital and they had authority to deal with it. The hidden problem was that some of these consultants were exceptionally energetic and did much for the hospital as well. Milburn sought maximum control over consultant hours. This skewed the negotiations.

A curious feature was that rather than the DH trying to keep costs down as usual, they seemed to be ready to give consultants a substantial pay increase. Also, whilst I often heard how concerned the DH was about young women doctors working out of hours in general practice, I never once heard concerns about young women doctors working out of hours in hospitals.

The BMA recommended the new contract to its members for a vote. Then a senior DH official gave a lecture to NHS managers. He included a slide claiming that the DH was gaining control over consultants working out of hours. In the audience was a consultant in senior management who circulated the slide, which was copied widely with a strong negative reaction. The BMA was inundated by messages, particularly from younger women consultants, who had sacrificed work-life balance to achieve consultant status and now were determined to retain it. Talking with Peter Hawker he was worried that the contract he had negotiated would be rejected. He was right. English consultants rejected the contract, forcing Hawker's resignation. However, the Scottish consultants accepted it. This gave the BMA a problem, as it likes to work across the UK. The Government quickly implemented the contract in Scotland. The BMA Consultants' Committee elected a new Chair and went back to the DH asking for improvements to the contract, which the Secretary of State refused. There was a stand-off. When Milburn stood down, Tony Blair appointed John Reid in June 2003 as the new Secretary of State for Health. Reid made some more concessions and agreement was finally reached.

However, there were still problems in the hospitals. Hospital chief executives told me that the sums allocated to implement the consultant contract did not cover the real costs. The situation was exacerbated by an understanding amongst consultants that if they worked more than the agreed number of hours they would get paid accordingly. The main problem for the NHS and the chief executives was that many consultants for years had been working well over their contracted hours per week. I knew consultants, like David Mattingly in Exeter, who were regularly working on evenings and weekends seeing patients about whom they were worried. Previous surveys of hours worked by consultants also showed that many were working over their contracted hours.

Emphasising the hours worked partly deprofessionalised consultants. There were awkward discussions about whether some consultants would reduce their hours to the contracted number if there were no additional payments. A grade one civil servant said to me: "Denis, it's extraordinary that we can give one of the highest-paid groups in the Health Service a substantial pay rise and have many of them more discontented than when we started!"

---

(3) DH Negotiations with Junior Doctors

In the BMA, junior doctors are a separate craft with their own national conference and negotiating committee. They negotiate separately from senior hospital doctors. The word 'junior' for hospital doctors means 'in a training post but some hospital doctors can still be 'junior doctors' aged up to 40. Ever since 1948, arrangements for junior hospital doctors were antiquated. In the 1960s, when I was one, I was required to be in the hospital six and a half days out of seven and one colleague was not allowed to leave the hospital! My pay as a pre-registration house officer was about £500 a year. Pay and conditions improved, too slowly: some junior doctors worked 100 hours a week in the 21st century.

Junior doctors were badly treated. Their conditions steadily worsened: doctors' messes were closed so they lost a safe space to relax and talk privately. Accommodation at night was often basic. They were required to apply online for career posts. Having spent years acquiring good CVs, the value of CVs was downgraded. There was a medical training application system, which was an administrative disaster. To add insult to injury the DH asked junior doctors to declare their sexual orientation and then in an extraordinary lapse of data protection published these online! The Secretary of State had to establish an independent inquiry conducted by John Tooke from Exeter, which exposed multiple management failures (Tooke Task Force, 2008).

The Government introduced a new contract for junior doctors in 2016, proposing less favourable working hours. Agreement was not reached despite the conciliation service, ACAS, being involved. This provoked the juniors. Industrial action began, i.e. not working in various ways. The juniors started with three assets: first they had the support of the public, many of whom thought the hours they worked were ridiculous and hoped not to be treated by a tired doctor. Secondly, they had support from the hospital consultants. Thirdly, they had stories of oppressive management, like a young woman telling management that she was to be married in several months' time and requesting time off for her wedding and being told to find her own locum. I knew married couples posted to hospitals miles apart. This was a generation of skilled young people working hard but being undervalued.

The junior doctors stopped work for short periods in the week. They picketed hospital gates with placards, often with the slogan: "Saving the NHS," illustrating how blurred were their objectives for this action. Jeremy Hunt was Secretary of State for Health. When there were no concessions, the juniors escalated their strike with considerable implications in the hospital service. Whilst consultants covered substantially, the British hospital system depends on juniors to run it. The strikes strained the hospitals and anxious messages were sent to the DH by some managers and might well have delivered results. Industrial action was led by the BMA's Junior Doctors' Committee which called for the juniors to strike for around four days a week. However, most junior doctors declined, as many felt it was unethical. The juniors leadership overplayed its hand: the strike collapsed. Two Chairs of the Junior Doctors' Committee had to resign. Jeremy Hunt reduced some hours, improved support, and imposed the contract.

These were some of the most able young people in the country who were NHS employees and their widespread support for industrial action was an indictment of their working conditions, the responsibility of the DH and their employers. The DH won but at high cost. Junior doctors were left angered with their underlying dissatisfaction unresolved.

The first reaction was that they planned their careers differently. The proportion entering higher training halved (Hollis *et al.*, 2020). Applications for GP training, having lagged for years, rose above target. Health Education England saw this as success. General practice management is more flexible than hospital management, for example in our practice one GP principal asked for her room in a new building to be decorated in a different colour from all the others. The managing partners agreed—not a request any consultant could make or be granted. GP management looked more attractive.

Record numbers of graduating GPs chose locum work. Locums provide valuable flexibility, but do not commit to patients or to practices. The Chinese proverb provides understanding. The juniors were left dissatisfied. An interpretation is that a generation of junior doctors sought collectively to improve their conditions. After a political defeat, they were reacting individually and taking more control of their lives. An increased use of locums in general practice will be damaging for patients, for GPs and for the NHS in the future.

ADDENDA

In 2023, junior doctors went on strike again. The unresolved anger from 2016 led to them taking a much harder line this time. They stopped working for much longer periods, five days running, and even refused emergency care. Co-led by a GP trainee, they took a hard-line position.

Also in 2023, consultants voted by 81% with a 71% turnout to take industrial action. The attitudes of hospital doctors have greatly hardened and their relationship with the DHSC is exceptionally bad.

Section X

46

An Unfinished Campaign 2013–2023

Discipline: A branch of learning or scholarly instruction.

Shorter Oxford Dictionary

If a medical school does not teach general practice as a subject, has no GP curriculum and provides no GP reading list, it gives a powerful non-verbal signal that general practice is not important and that there is nothing written from or about general practice which future doctors need to read!.

House of Commons Health Select Committee (2016) ***Primary Care,*** **citing DPG**

In 2013 I made an uncomfortable discovery in the St Leonard's Practice when I was asked to give a tutorial to a couple of GP trainees. In discussion I asked them if they had read anything about general practice as a discipline. Neither had. I then asked them if they had heard of either Professors Ian McWhinney or Barbara Starfield (two of the world's leading thinkers about general practice and prolific writers), but they did not know of either.

I was invited to give a keynote lecture at a conference in Plymouth for all the new GP trainees in Devon and Cornwall. I sat through the day and found that no reading list was given out nor any suggestion made that there were important texts and books on general practice that deserved to be read. Lecturing at another trainee conference in North Devon during questions Michael Balint's name came up. I asked if anyone had read anything about him. In a room with about 100 people present, four hands went up, two were from programme directors or trainers. By 2014, I therefore knew that general practice postgraduate training had lost touch with its own research base. A campaign was needed to get general practice taught as research-based discipline.

In 2015 I had a letter published in the *BMJ* on general practice being a discipline but not being taught as such in medical schools (DPG, 2015b). The *BMJ* made it the lead letter of that week. It drew scathing criticism from the Dean of the new Medical School at Plymouth (Sneyde, 2015). A well-connected colleague told me my letter had caused concern at high levels in the Exeter Medical School too, but it had been decided not to reply. I was told my letter had "not been helpful."

As members of the Tamar Faculty Board, Nick Bradley who was then Provost (President) and I wrote a paper on general practice as a discipline. We were friends as he had been a trainee in the practice in the 1980s. We proposed that local GP teachers should have a reading list for general practice as neither of the two medical schools in the county of Devon issued one to their medical students. We proposed that GP trainers should keep a lever-arch file of key general practice articles and use them to supplement teaching in the practice. The Faculty Board approved the paper.

I wrote a reading list and consulted several medical students. They reported that the eponymous lectures were the most readable and helpful, in particular Iona Heath's (2011) Harveian oration. The Board approved the list.

DOI: 10.1201/9781032713601-56

Lectures

I delivered the keynote lecture in Birmingham at the annual conference of the South of England group of University Departments of General Practice/Primary Care in the spring of 2015 This was later published in the *BJGP* as "Academic general practice: achievements and challenges" (DPG, 2015c). José Valderas, was Professor of Health Services Research in the University of Exeter and did his clinical work in St Leonard's Practice. Hearing this lecture, he invited me to give the inaugural Starfield Memorial Lecture, which he was organising.

This was a great privilege as I had known, and admired Barbara Starfield and it gave me a rare platform to tackle the topic of general practice as a discipline in its own right. In the lecture I set out an outline syllabus for its research-based principles in medical schools. The essence of being a discipline is having a research-based body of knowledge that can be taught. Hence my title was "Towards research-based learning outcomes for teaching general practice in medical schools" (DPG, 2017a, c). I thought would be my last eponymous lecture (wrong) and it was a privilege to give it in Exeter with Jill and family, including Naomi one of my granddaughters, present within days of my 80th birthday.

Alice James, President of the Bristol Student GP Society came. She was the daughter of Sarah Wollaston, the Devon MP and former GP, who chaired the Health Select Committee of Parliament and who also came to the lecture. At the reception afterwards, Sarah Wollaston invited me to give evidence to her Select Committee, which was then reviewing primary care/general practice.

There is a long history of conceptualisation of general practice as a science. Conrad Harris (1970) described general practice as: "The study of the psychological factors that affect the health and treatment of an individual patient in the context of continuing medical care". Amending 'psychological' to 'psychosocial' to embrace the environmental and social context of each patient would update this. He also grasped it was a science, although his suggested descriptor of "innominate" science never resonated. I had described general practice as a behavioural in my Mackenzie Lecture (DPG, 1978) I summarised the 22 principles of general practice in 2017 (Appendix 8).

Select Committee of Parliament on Health and Social Care 2016

I accepted Sarah Wollaston's invitation and wrote formal written evidence to the Health Select Committee at the end of 2015. This was published on the Select Committee's website at the beginning of 2016 (DPG, 2016). It was picked up by the Council of Deans of Medical Schools who wrote to me about it but did not act on it. The Health Select Committee (House of Commons Health Select Committee, 2016) published its report *Primary Care* the same summer citing my evidence twice in paragraphs 143 and 144:

> *143. This view formed part of Sir Denis's wider argument that medical schools actively discriminate against general practice as a discipline. Sir Denis reasoned that evidence of this ranges from medical schools failing to reference general practice in prospectuses to allocating only a small proportion of their teaching budgets to general practice. In addition, he said: If a medical school does not teach general practice as a subject, has no GP curriculum and provides no GP reading list, it gives a powerful non-verbal signal that general practice is not important and that there is nothing written from or about general practice which future doctors need to read! The current generation of medical students are the most able academically ever, usually being selected on very high A level grades. They are thirsty for theory and principles and want to know the hows and whys of medical practice. If in five years they are not taught any theory on the principles of general practice, naturally they will tend to turn away from it or to enter it for other reasons.*

Then in the next paragraph, 144, it at last recommended that general practice should be taught in medical schools "as a subject" (House of Commons Select Committee, 2016). In a university context this means a research-based body of knowledge. I was content.

Resolution of the Council of the RCGP 2016

Meanwhile, in February 2016, the work of the Tamar Faculty Board bore fruit. The long paper Nick Bradley and I had written was considered in successive meetings of the Board and it was agreed that the key message should be condensed into a motion from the Faculty to the Council.

"The Tamar Faculty of the RCGP requests the Council of the RCGP take all reasonable steps to ensure that general practice is taught as a medical specialty within UK medical schools."

This was presented to the Council in writing and by Jonathan White, the Faculty's representative. The Council approved it, so it became the formal policy of the RCGP.

However, after several months, there was no discernible action so I wrote several times to Professor Kamila Hawthorne, hoping the College would write to all the UK medical schools about the College's new policy. Kamila was the educational lead for the College and one of the Vice-Chairs. Finally, Susanna Hill, the Tamar Faculty Chair, arranged a three-way meeting in a café in Bristol. Kamila treated us to a cream tea and agreed that the College would send the letter: the deal was done. A letter went from Helen Stokes-Lampard, Chair of Council, and Kamila Hawthorne to the Deans of British Medical Schools. However, there was no follow up. The RCGP did not have its heart in this.

Bristol research reported what GP academics were actually teaching in UK medical schools (Boon *et al.*, 2017). This was important, revealing there was no consensus around the principles of general practice as a discipline as the teaching varied greatly and reflected mainly the varying interests of local GP academic staff. The biggest branch of the medical profession lacked a syllabus.

Alex Harding, Co-Chair of the Heads of Teaching (HOTs), invited me to their annual meeting and to speak after their dinner. They let me lead a seminar on teaching general practice as a subject. This led to a good discussion and an invitation to visit several medical schools. However, I was anxious as they did not seem equipped to teach general practice as a research-based discipline, as none of them ever spoke about key GP research.

Invitations

During 2016, after this seminar and the Starfield lecture, I received a succession of invitations to meetings and conferences in medical education. These included a conference run by medical students at Bristol where I proposed that medical students needed a syllabus for general practice. This apparently simple idea is highly controversial amongst professional medical educators who look down on 'syllabi' and usually prefer to write about the 'curriculum,' which includes details about how the content should be taught. Universities have curricula and schools have syllabi. Having seen several medical school curricula, I had noted that as far as general practice was concerned the content was skimpy or absent. Hence by concentrating on a syllabus I was trying to direct attention on to *what* should be taught about the principles of general practice rather than *how to* teach. Speaking to about 100 medical students I said that most of them had found syllabi for their 'A' levels useful and had learned them so well that they were medical students! They deserved a GP syllabus. All adult students deserve an outline of the key topics they are expected to learn.

An invitation to lecture at the Leicester Medical School gave me my biggest ever audience. They brought all five years of medical students together. I found myself on a platform in a concert hall with 1,350 medical students. The audience was in three tiers, with hundreds in galleries above me, hundreds more on my eye level, and hundreds more well below me, with the Dean sitting in the front row. Maintaining eye contact was therefore unusually challenging.

A new experience for me was lecturing on general practice as a discipline at the private medical school at the University of Buckingham, my first experience in a private school. Here the students were paying £35,000 a year and I was interested to meet several of them and discuss education with them. I also gave lectures in Bristol Exeter, Plymouth, and Truro to GP trainees and medical students where I presented a 20-point syllabus for general practice summarised on one side of one piece of paper (Appendix 8).

I appreciated invitations to the Cardiff and UCL Medical Schools and discussion with GP teachers at King's College London and Queen's University Belfast. It was disappointing that Queen's, although having a GP who was a professor then, had no GP department with which medical students could identify.

The five key observations from all these contacts were:

- UK medical schools usually did not provide a GP-specific reading list.
- There was usually no protected time in the course for research-based teaching on the principles of general practice.
- GP teaching was mainly outsourced to service general practices, none of whom had a specific GP syllabus to follow.
- The same topic could be taught many times and others not at all.
- There was usually no assessment of general practice as a research-based subject in the medical schools' final examinations.

I realised that none of these medical schools were visualising general practice as a research-based subject needing to be taught in its own right.

GMC 2017

As far as the teaching in medical schools is concerned all roads lead to the GMC as the national regulator of all UK medical schools. I had met its Chair Professor (later Sir) Terence Stephenson (1947–) as he was both a former President of the Royal College of Paediatrics and Child Health and one of my successors as Chair of the Academy of Medical Royal Colleges.

In 2017 I went the GMC to discuss the teaching of general practice. I was encouraged that the GMC Chair chaired it himself with the Director of Standards, Colin Melville, present. I was given an hour. They had my Starfield lecture published that year on "Research-based learning outcomes for general practice in medical schools." We started well as the GMC said it was adopting the term 'learning outcomes' as I had in my Starfield lecture. The GMC was moving towards a national qualifying examination, as in the United States, which I understood as different British medical schools' examinations had different standards.

They gave me plenty of time to present my case that all medical students ought to learn the core principles, such as continuity, family care etc that underpin general practice – the biggest branch of medical practice. However, I made no progress at all. They said they were always being lobbied by groups wanting their special interest included in the curriculum. I argued that general practice was no small interest group but a third of the medical profession.

As the discussion went on my heart sank. The GMC representatives were always courteous but did not accept my case. The Chair said: "You haven't mentioned dementia." I said I had not mentioned any single disease. I wanted medical students to hear about a set of *principles* for general practice so they could choose their branch of practice with an informed mind. These two GMC leaders, both former consultants, could not accept general practice as a discipline in its own right. I failed. They did not offer to pay my expenses.

King's College, London

I had been on the Principal's Advisory Committee for the Doyly Carte Chair of Medicine and the Arts since its inception, and so got to know the Principal, Professor Sir Richard Trainor (1948–). He was succeeded by Professor Ed (Later Sir) Byrne (1952–). I met some educationalists and found King's was similar to the other medical schools I had visited.

I wrote a paper of about 5,000 words suggesting that King's, as the largest training institution in Europe and with the world-famous Institute of Psychiatry and the Florence Nightingale School of Nursing, should teach general practice as a research-based subject. King's had 26 professors of business studies with only one in general practice. This paper went to Professor Sir Robert Lechler (1951–) the Executive Director of King's Health Partners, an academic health sciences centre whom I knew as President of the Academy of Medical Sciences. He sent me a short email dismissing the idea. I got a response from Tim Lancaster, Head of Medical Education, a GP. He listed the strengths of King's but did not suggest teaching the research-based principles of general practice, I had failed again.

Destination General Practice 2017

The Medical Schools Council and the RCGP surveyed over 3,000 British medical students (Medical Schools Council and the RCGP, 2017). It contained disturbing findings, in particular that only 3% of medical students saw general practice having any intellectual challenge! The RCGP had jointly agreed this report and so co-owned it. For some unknown reason, the College dropped the ball and did nothing about it.

Many GPs, including me, did not know it existed. We discovered it in 2019 in the St Leonard's Practice. Molly Dineen, a medical student attached to St Leonard's wrote a protest letter to the *BJGP* saying she was one of the 3% and certainly understood the intellectual challenge. I wrote as well:

> *The finding that only 3% of medical students see general practice as intellectually challenging is the biggest wake-up call for British medical schools since 1948. Medical schools are taking many of the most able students of their generation for five years, but this powerful evidence shows they are failing to introduce their students to some of the most interesting medical research in the world. Students are being denied proper opportunities to analyse this research, although higher education prioritises intellectual analysis.*
>
> *GPs are the biggest branch of the medical profession, and the NHS wants half of all medical students to choose general practice. GPs face the widest range of clinical problems, see the social determinants of health more than other doctors, have the most complex consultations whilst having the longest and deepest working relationships with patients in British medicine. This educational tragedy has occurred through the hidden curriculum and the non-verbal signals from British medical schools, especially by not examining the principles of general practice in their final examinations. This signals to students that the intellectual content of general practice is irrelevant.*
>
> *General practice has its own distinct body of research separate from the medical specialties, which all students need to learn. Even in 2019, the GMC is approving medical schools which neither teach general practice as a research-based discipline, nor examine its principles in their finals. Medical school final examinations and the new planned national, licensing examination GMC should include 15% of questions on these principles.*

The *BJGP* published both letters (Dineen, 2019; DPG, 2019) with mine as the Editor's choice. So the public protest to *Destination General Practice* challenging the 3% finding were in the form of two letters from one general practice.

A National Course on the Research-Based Principles of General Practice

In 2018 a big step in the right direction occurred. Alex Harding, as the new co-Chair of the Heads of Teaching (HOTs) of the Society of Academic Primary Care (SAPC), led on a HOTs document setting out the principles for teaching general practice in UK medical schools. HOTs wisely joined with the RCGP, which published the document (Harding *et al.*, 2018). Alex went on to lead on a further document written by different academic GPs in the medical schools (Harding *et al.*, 2019).

In 2018, I had an editorial in the *British Journal of General Practice* called: "The discipline of general practice." I got into print that I was meeting GP trainees who had never heard of Ian McWhinney or Barbara Starfield – two professors who are amongst the world's deepest thinkers about general practice. Sadly no one in general practice was able to deny this.

> *Confusion exists between the diseases seen in general practice, which are usually well taught, and the principles of general practice, which are often not taught at all. The non-verbal signal to medical students is that general practice principles are of little or perhaps no importance.*

(DPG, 2018a)

In 2017, Stuart Cole, a medical student, did a master's degree in Exeter. He was interested in general practice and how it was taught and so became involved with Alex Harding as Sub-dean and me. He chose GP teaching for his dissertation. Alex facilitated him attending a HOTs meeting at Warwick and they agreed to participate in his survey. He got his MSc in 2018. We strongly supported his article (Cole *et al.*, 2020). It included several anonymous quotations from senior GP teachers in UK medical schools:

- "Above all I would not want to see GPs trying to be separatist as it is viewed/sees itself as being the second cousin/underdog."
- "The prime purpose of our modules has not been to teach general practice, rather to help students with their core skills and gain some insight into general practice en route."
- "Looking backwards to Starfield is not helpful."
- "If we are to have a national curriculum it absolutely must not be a list of things to be covered."
- "Disagree with all statements which include vision as we all see things differently. Leadership in institutions should provide this."

There is no mention of GP research, and the tone is downbeat. There is no pride in general practice or understanding of its distinct qualities. Such leaders may have difficulty showing highly intelligent medical students how to be proud of general practice. Being proud of general practice means understanding how important the work is and why it has some unique features, including knowing when general practice leads the profession as in medical teaching.

For example, personal teaching and professional relationships in the medical profession are now led by GPs. Dame Sally Davies as she left office as Chief Medical Officer, reported that she regularly asked groups of junior hospital doctors how many of them thought their consultants knew their names. She regretted that usually: "few hands went up" (Ross, 2019). Fortunately, this does not happen with GP trainers who now lead on providing student centre teaching.

Many senior GP teachers in medical schools do not value outstanding research in their own field so the logic is a national course provided first for medical school teachers and then cascaded to GP trainers and GP undergraduate teachers. My Starfield lecture "Research based learning outcomes for general practice in medical schools" (DPG, 2017a) sought, but failed, to trigger this discussion.

There is a successful historical precedent. In 1971 general practice faced a new national teaching role with no training or much experience of teaching. Ekke Kuenssberg, Chair of the RCGP, with support from the Nuffield Trust, initiated a national teaching course, directed by Paul Freeling (*JRCGP*, 1975e). This was an outstanding success and was cascaded UK wide.

GPs from a standing start developed, over 30 years, to become the best medical teachers in the medical profession (Goldacre *et al.,* 2008; Paice and Smith, 2009; GMC, 2018; Regional Adviser story). Personal teaching in the medical profession is now led by GPs.

Medical students and GP trainees may never receive a specific reading list for general practice and may remain ignorant about classic GP texts, which still inspire. Most university undergraduates study key texts in their chosen field. Medical schools do not examine the principles of general practice in MB finals, signalling to thousands of medical students that these principles are dispensable. The title of this book, "Just a GP", from my Gale lecture (DPG, 1980a) seeks to generate discussion and hopefully find new counter measures.

Conclusions

Encouraging steps have been the formal recommendation by the Health Select Committee of Parliament (House of Commons Health Select Committee, 2016) that general practice be taught "as a subject," which in a university/medical school context means research based. Similarly, the Harding *et al.* (2018) report was important in leading the profession towards teaching general practice as a distinct subject in UK medical schools. Most of all, new research, like continuity of GP care being associated with lower mortality for patients (Baker *et al.,* 2020) has underlined the importance of general practice in its own right.

However, the great majority of medical students in the UK, whilst undertaking a five-year, mostly full-time, course, never receive even a two-week formal course, taught within their medical school, on the research underpinning the 20 principles of general practice (Appendix 8) Few medical students even receive a reading list specific to general practice explaining the core principles.

Most British medical students choose their branch of medical practice without ever learning enough about what general practice has to offer or why it is so important. General practice will continue to have a recruitment problem until this is rectified. In my McConaghey Lecture in 2022 I offered "the integrating discipline" as a new formulation of the GP's role (DPG, 2023). This campaign to get general practice taught as a research-based discipline is unfinished.

47

Last Hurrah

You win some: you lose some.

After finishing as Chair of the Nuffield Trust in 2006, I was looking forward to researching questions of my own choice in the Practice. I was 70 and assumed my days of meeting cabinet ministers were over. However, I was still to meet a Prime Minister and two cabinet ministers.

Prime Minister at 10 Downing Street

In July 2008, I received a fax from the office of the Prime Minister, Gordon Brown (1951–), inviting me to a meeting at 10 Downing Street. The background was my long-term working relationship with Michael Dixon (1952–) who as a GP trainee who had been at the St Leonard's Practice. We got on well. He was a broad thinker had read philosophy at Oxford before doing medicine and he was an exceptional professional leader.

Over the years, we saw each other intermittently. He had a broad approach to practice and sympathy with alternative approaches, which later led to him being appointed first Medical Adviser to the Prince of Wales and later, the first ever GP to Head of the Royal Medical Household. I gave him advice about researching the effectiveness of a healer in his practice, who was a former patient of mine. In the 1990s he was elected to leader the NHS Alliance. As its Chair for a long time (1998–2015), he was remarkably successful in building links with successive health ministers and senior civil servants.

The invitation, unusually, was to for breakfast followed by a meeting with the PM. I met several leading GPs, including Michael and Sam (later Sir) Everington (1957–). I was a longstanding admirer of him as he had qualified as a barrister before becoming a doctor. He had attacked racial discrimination and opposed excessively long hours for junior doctors, notably by sleeping outside his teaching hospital. As a GP he led the visionary Bromley-by-Bow general practice, which I had visited. There, in deprived East London, he built up a practice with exceptional community involvement and become Chair of his Clinical Commissioning Group (CCG). Jennifer had an attachment there.

Sir John Oldham (1953–) was there too. He had made his name through NHS service development in general practice and had pioneered so called 'advance access.' In 2003, he had become the youngest ever GP knight, aged only 50. There were others there, including the National Association for Primary Care, but a striking absence was the RCGP. I was the only GP with substantial RCGP experience as all the other leaders, Dixon, Everington and Oldham, had risen through the NHS or other organisations. All three had made substantial achievements, had great skill in making the right contacts and speaking up for general practice. The seminar was a culmination of years of skilled lobbying. I had expected to see Ben Bradshaw, not as my Exeter MP, but as a Health Minister, as he had been appointed by Gordon Brown in his first reshuffle the year before. However, he could not come and Ann Keen (1948–), a former district nurse and the Parliamentary Undersecretary of State for Health, the third Minister, represented the DH. The usual civil servants were there.

DOI: 10.1201/9781032713601-57

I had never been to a breakfast at No 10 before and this was a social not a working breakfast, with Gordon Brown mingling amiably. After it, we moved into an adjacent room where the PM took the chair. I was much the oldest person in the room (72) with most of the major players in their early 50s.

I appreciated how special the opportunity was, wondering if it was unique. I did not know of any occasion since the NHS started in 1948 when a Prime Minister in office had held a seminar in No 10 focused exclusively on general practice. It meant he was thinking about it seriously. The preceding breakfast was unusual and a courtesy. Margaret Thatcher's seminar which I had attended in Chequers, twenty years earlier, had been on the NHS as a whole; as had been my meeting with Tony Blair in No 10 six years earlier.

I knew I was likely to get only two to three minutes, so I prepared carefully. Just speaking face to face about general practice with a PM in office is difficult to achieve for a GP leader. Access to the PM is fiercely guarded and there are formal and informal gate keepers. The government system means that senior civil servants and ministers may talk about general practice but what gets passed up the system is filtered by their own views and the perceived importance of general practice. The system assumes that even if important, a topic should normally be handled by the Secretary of State for Health. This was Alan Johnson (1950–) at the time, but he was not present.

Secondary care has long had preferential access. For example, leading NHS hospital managers had access to Tony Blair and lobbied him so successfully that he introduced foundation hospital trusts to give them more clout and resources. As I once said in the Nuffield Trust no one ever even suggested foundation primary care organisations with equivalent privileges.

General practices in financial difficulties are left to go bust, whilst hospitals running up big debts are always rescued by successive governments. One big STP (Sustainable Transformation Partnership) formed to integrate primary and secondary care, used primary care funds to bail out a debt-laden hospital.

General practice has a continuing cultural disadvantage. Whilst ministers repeatedly pay lip service to it as 'the backbone of the NHS,' they give their time and allocate resources preferentially to secondary and tertiary health care. Similarly, NHS management pays hospital managers higher salaries than in primary care/general practice organisations. In Devon and Cornwall, one successful PCT chief executive was appointed to a higher paid and more prestigious post as chief executive of a hospital.

The honours lists are valuable in revealing in public the private, cultural assumptions of the British establishment. Many people miss the subtlety of the messages that honours convey about organisations, as they focus only on the individuals. Many honours, including my own citation: "President of the RCGP," explicitly refer to institutions, which is how the establishment recognises these institutions. When I became Chair of the College, then 35 years old, even GP giants like William Pickles, John Hunt, Ekke Kuenssberg and John Horder were not knighted. Since all four were appointed CBE, with another four RCGP Presidents as well, there is a consensus establishment view about what is appropriate for GP leaders and College presidents. Analysed over time a pattern emerges. Four out of 22 (18%) eligible GP Presidents of the RCGP have been appointed Dame or Knight, whereas in the same years every President of the Royal College of Physicians of London has been awarded that honour.

In addition to the longstanding cultural view of the relativity of primary and secondary care, there is a separate problem of knowledge about the scientific basis of general practice. Politicians and senior civil servants are not usually aware that GPs have the longest and deepest working relationships with patients and so are best placed to help patients care for themselves; i.e. 'enablement' ie empowerment (Howie *et al.*, 1999). GPs are best placed to see first-hand and to understand the social determinants of ill health (Magnan, 2017), to ameliorate social disadvantage (Shi *et al.*, 2003), to minimise hospital admissions for the elderly (the most expensive part of the NHS (Barker *et al.*, 2017), reduce overall costs in the whole health care system (De Maeseneer *et al.*, 2003) and even to reduce mortality (Baker *et al.*, 2020).

Many of the most important NHS objectives can be fulfilled through good general practice but this has not been digested yet at the top of government. Whilst some of this research came out after 2008, this was the background as I understood it in preparing my three precious minutes. My plan was to appeal to Brown's intellect and academic ability (he had a PhD and had written books), as well as his strong socialist interest in reducing social inequality. I wanted a solid research basis such as Starfield *et al.* (2005). I hoped to reach a former socialist Chancellor of the Exchequer with research showing general practice contains overall NHS costs (De Maeseneer *et al.,* 2003) and also partly ameliorate socio-economic disadvantage (Shi *et al.*, 2003).

The format was the same as I had experienced with Margaret Thatcher, with the PM addressing each of us in turn. The seminar proceeded smoothly. I knew I would be the only GP academic summarising key research.

However, a minute after I started speaking the door suddenly opened and one of Gordon Brown's little boys ran into the room (10 Downing Street is the Prime Minister's home as well as his office). Brown turned away and picked him up and cuddled him and started talking to him. He took him out and soon returned, but I was seriously thrown off my stride. I did not know whether to start again (which I should have done) or to continue where I had left off, which I did. My flow had been disrupted and my contribution fragmented. Perhaps at 72, I was not as intellectually flexible as I had previously been. At the end, when I was feeling dissatisfied, Gordon Brown somehow sensed this. "Sir Denis, have you something more to say?" I was therefore given a second bite of the cherry, an example of unusually sensitive chairmanship.

Nevertheless, the seminar was useful in briefing the PM and in July 2008 our hopes were reasonably high that the PM was seriously interested in general practice. Was it at last going to have some important top level attention?

August is a dead month in government, but in September the world changed. On 15 September 2008, only a few weeks afterwards, a big US financial institution, Lehman Brothers, failed. This was a 19th-century institution with revenue of about $20,000 million. A world-wide financial crash occurred because unsatisfactory securities for mortgages had been widely sold around the world. Gordon Brown became a pivotal figure in an international financial crisis as a Prime Minister with ten years' experience in the Treasury and with Britain holding a key role in the G7 international group. He became heavily engaged nationally and internationally. General practice was wiped off his agenda and this rare opportunity was lost. You win some; you lose some!

Rt Hon Ben Bradshaw MP

Following the seminar and with the advantage of having a Minister of Health as our local MP, I suggested a meeting. He came to our home, arriving on his bicycle. I took this rare chance to brief him on the wider aspects of general practice. He stayed a whole hour, which was more than I expected. In 2009, Gordon Brown appointed him to the Cabinet as Secretary of State for Culture. He lost office after only a year when Cameron's coalition government was elected in 2010. When the Labour Party elected Jeremy Corbyn and moved to the political left, Bradshaw became isolated in opposition and was never given a shadow post. He was openly critical of Corbyn. However, even when in later general elections the Southwestern region swung heavily to the Conservatives, he still held Exeter for Labour for 25 years in succession.

Rt Hon Jeremy Hunt MP

My final contact with the Secretary of State for Health in office came a few years later with Jeremy Hunt, now in the Conservative-led coalition government. Michael Dixon, whom I was seeing in Devon, invited me to the annual conference of the NHS Alliance where, as a longstanding Chairman, he was making the annual leader's speech. Jeremy Hunt was the invited speaker.

Subsequently the NHS Alliance teamed up with the National Association of Primary Care and Hunt agreed to come to a meeting. I was invited and had a brief opportunity to speak and I emphasised the growing amount of research on the benefits for patients if GPs can provide continuity of care. His political adviser followed up and I supplied a set of references on the key research.

Jeremy Hunt (1966–) is skilled verbally and makes one feel heard. He understood the importance of continuity of care. He changed the GP NHS contract to ensure that all NHS general practices provided all their patients (including children) with a named GP in the practice who was 'accountable' for their care. He remained as Secretary of State for Health for an unusually long six years adding 'for social care' to his portfolio. He reached the final two in the election for the leadership of the Conservative Party in 2019.

In 2022, when Chair of the Health Select Committee, he was unexpectedly generous in welcoming me as a visitor to his Select Committee.

48

General Practice as a Learning Environment

Education is not the filling of a pail but the lighting of a fire.

WB Yeats (1865–1939)

All organisations exist to fulfil some function but how they do so varies immensely. One big variable is the attitude to people in the organisation, which depends on the management. There are two broad but contrasting approaches. Both seek organisational efficiency.

The first system sees staff as widgets; the aim is maximum control of staff and extracting as much work from them as possible. Management is confident it knows best and the organisation functions through top-down memoranda. This is common in big organisations. In the other main system, the staff are seen as part of the assets of the organisation and nurturing and developing them over time is a management aim. Management is not confident it knows all the answers and so consults regularly. Seniors listen to people on the front line assuming they will generate good ideas, do a better job, and stay in post longer. Such organisations seek to be learning environments. The proof is that people in them grow and develop and are usually happier too. The NHS is a widget system and this book gives evidence of politicians not consulting and not listening to advice (Chapter 38, Chair of the Academy of Medical Royal Colleges).

General practice is privileged in two ways. It works in relatively small units with shorter hierarchies so staff can know and value each other more easily. Senior partners can and do talk easily with junior receptionists. Secondly, GP partners are not salaried employees but are independent contractors (DPG, 1977b) and so managers themselves. They have great privileges in being able to shape the organisation in which they work. The psychology literature (Spector, 1982) reveals that increased "locus of control" improves morale.

GP partners set the management style. This chapter describes one general practice through a learning environment lens for over a century. Many learning activities occur in general practices but it is not always clear how much is learned. One way of knowing if learning has actually occurred is by external validation, i.e. by assessment and an award by an independent, external body.

Degrees Obtained by GPs in the Practice

My grandfather Joseph Pereira set the scene in 1903 in the Practice that he had established in 1895 by passing an examination for the degree of MD Brussels. It is said he was provoked by learning that the title 'doctor' for medical practitioners is only a courtesy. A photo taken of him in 1903 in his MD robes was presented by the City of Exeter police, whose medical officer he was and the inscription refers to his kindness. It hung in my consulting room for years – a non-verbal inspiration to me.

During the next 127 years in the practice two GP partners obtained a taught MSc and another an MMed. Three others obtained the other form of master's degree by research, the MPhil, from the University of Exeter. Another GP partner was awarded a doctorate from the University of London

DOI: 10.1201/9781032713601-58

and another partner honorary doctorates from three different universities. Eight different GP partners were awarded 11 university degrees between them.

Nor was this a medical endeavour only, as the nurse practitioner was awarded an MSc, as was an attached midwife both from the University of Exeter. Also an attached district nurse was awarded a bachelor's degree from the University of Plymouth (Appendix 8).

Awards other than university degrees included a GP partner becoming the ninth GP in the UK to achieve fellowship by assessment of the RCGP (Chapter 24, Fellowship by Assessment story), a practice manager led the Practice to the award of Investors in People, and an attached student won the University of Exeter Quintiles prize for Women in Science. In the Practice, higher university degrees obtained in general practice moved from being a rare event in the first decade of the 20th century to become common in the 1990s, when five successive partners obtained one. In learning environments people mature and grow and influence each other. Five GP partners were appointed professors of the University of Exeter.

Such things cannot be planned or mandated; all depends on the educational atmosphere or culture in the practice. Personal relationships and mutual support are crucial. Helpful steps were constantly valuing learning, fostering colleague aspirations and contributing to university fees from the practice account. Celebrating successes was important. Education is not just about transmitting information but sharing enthusiasm and giving time and encouragement. WB Yeats called this "Lighting a fire".

Philip Evans led a special study unit (SSU) for Exeter medical students on research in general practice. He did this yearly for 14 years, providing nine hours' teaching in each week with individual tuition for every student. The SSU was based on an anonymised database of about 400 patients who had diabetes. It was odd that this was the only SSU of its kind and that the Medical School did not see the need to provide more SSUs for medical students on general practice research. He attracted about six medical students a year, including Ellie White and Molly Dineen. I ran an SSU on advanced communication for several years.

University of Exeter

In 2009, I was appointed an honorary Doctor of Science (DSc) of the University of Exeter, following two other honorary doctorates at De Montfort and Nottingham universities. The Exeter one was most unexpected as it was not usual for former staff to receive honorary degrees. But this was an unusual year as the University was conferring three honorary doctorates for medical work in Exeter. The other two were Professor Robin Ling FRCS (1927–2017), an orthopaedic consultant surgeon who had developed the Exeter hip in conjunction with Clive (later Professor) Lee (1938–2021), a University of Exeter engineer. The Exeter hip proved to be successful because the bone contours were professionally engineered. Clive Lee and his family had been patients of mine for many years and he kept me informed when he consulted about the story of the Exeter hip.

At the lunch before my degree was conferred, I was seated next to Baroness Floella Benjamin (1949–, the Chancellor), and she told me, as she later told the Queen, about how her family had experienced racism when arriving in England by notices: "No dogs, No blacks." Another honorary graduand that day was Professor Sir Lezek Borysievic (1951–), with whom I had been a trustee at the Nuffield Trust and who became Vice-Chancellor of the University of Cambridge. He gave the address whilst his GP wife, Gwen, sat with Jill in the front row. The Dean, of the new Exeter Medical School, Professor Sir John Tooke, gave me a generous citation and the family came in strength including Jonathan, Gay, Elizabeth, Graham and Jennifer. I also received Honorary Fellowship of the Academy of Medical Educators from its President, Professor Sean Hilton, at a very pleasant dinner.

In 2012, an Exeter BSc student, Eleanor White, exercised her option for her academic year's professional placement in general practice. No student had done this before. Her tutor Ginny Russell, a social scientist, knew me and asked about a practice placement. Philip Evans agreed and I met Ellie that year when I took her with me when opening a new general practice building in Somerset. She joined the Practice in September 2013 for an academic year.

A serious student project was required so I offered her the study of patients who had been registered in the practice continuously for 50 or more years. This was original and I had nursed the idea for 15 years since the fiftieth anniversary of the NHS in 1998, when I was a working GP. As this meant asking patients for information, we applied to the NHS Ethics Committee; we went together. The interview was straightforward, but we were given a condition that my name should not appear on the questionnaires even though I was directing the study and supervising her. So much for transparency. The Committee thought that seeing my name would be 'coercive.' Having retired from clinical practice 13 years earlier, this seemed to be OTT. I had enjoyed rich, working relationships with most of my patients and I doubt if some had been surveyed that they would have felt 'coerced'.

Ellie found 190 patients (2.3% of the practice list) who had 50 or more years of continuous registration and identified an age-sex matched control group who had registered in recent years. We found a previously unreported group of patients who had remained registered with a general practice for half a century. The 50-year registered patients were less healthy but were being managed with the same number of GP consultations and prescriptions each year.

She minuted the meetings of the age and deprivation research team and learned much about academic teamwork and environments. I took her with me to the lectures I gave that year including the Forum lecture of the Academy of Medical Sciences and local meetings. She was pleased to meet Professor (later Sir) David Haslam (1949–) at a supper in Exeter. Ellie was awarded the Quintiles Prize for Women in Science in the University of Exeter whilst attached to the Practice. She had her trophy presented by the Chancellor of the Exchequer, George Osborne (1971–), and was introduced to another government minister, Nickie Morgan (1972–; now Baroness). She graduated with first-class honours, including a first-class grade for her dissertation on continuity. At her graduation I was in the university procession and met her parents. The study in *Family Practice* (White *et al.*, 2016) gave her a first-authored publication in a medical journal and 22 citations by 2023.

She extended her contact with the Practice by working when possible in administrative roles in the practice and keeping in touch with us so she was offered several other academic opportunities. Ginny Russell a social scientist and I were jointly her and we discussed medicalisation together involving interesting discussions across the social science/medical science divide. A publication was written by the three of us: "Medicalisation in the UK — Dynamic but ongoing" (DPG *et al.*, 2016a).

Seminar in the Practice for the Vice-Chancellor

The Vice-Chancellor of the University of Exeter and I met on the London train. I invited him and colleagues to come to the Practice for an academic seminar. He came in 2014 for lunch with the Deputy Vice-Chancellor, Professor Janice Kay, and the Dean of the Medical School, Professor Steven Thornton.

The event took place in the Kieran Sweeney seminar room, which was lined with journals and books giving it an academic ambience. The practice staff presented to them in turn for ten minutes each followed by questions. The seminar was planned around the links the practice had with the Medical School. Four GPs spoke: Philip Evans (Managing Partner and Research Fellow), Adrian Freeman (Managing Partner and Professor of Medical Education), Alex Harding (Managing Partner and Community Sub dean) and José Valderas (sessional GP and Professor of Health Services Research). All went well. The VC showed most interest in Alex Harding's talk on integrated longitudinal attachments for medical students, advising him to write it up using quantitative data.

I asked two attached students to speak. Leyla Osman asked poignantly why she only encountered exciting reading material about general practice in the St Leonard's Practice at the very end of her five years, although she had been interested in general practice all through the medical school course? Why hadn't she had a GP reading list? Ellie reported it had taken her time to settle in this placement and suggested that medical students should be given longer to settle in placements and not be moved every week, as was happening on the Exeter course. The Dean heard two big problems of his course neatly articulated in a few minutes each. But nothing changed. I chaired as a former Managing Partner and Emeritus Professor. We included a light lunch. This was probably the only seminar for a University Vice-Chancellor, Deputy Vice-Chancellor and a Medical School Dean run by a practice in a general practice.

Medical Student Education

Alex Harding invited me to join a group writing up a national survey of GP educators. He had been elected Co-chair of the GP Heads of Teaching (HOTs) group of the Society of Academic Primary Care (SAPC) and had skilfully helped to get this survey done. I advised publication in the *BJGP* which all the authors agreed. One author was a local GP trainee, Marwa Al Seaidy, whom I saw several times. I contributed editing skills and the article was published in the *BJGP* (Harding *et al.*, 2015, 49 citations). Two findings were that undergraduate GP teaching had peaked at 13% of the curriculum and the number of GP university departments had fallen seriously.

My article "Down with primary care: up with general practice!" was a *BMJ* blog (DPG, 2017b). Then it was published in an extended form in the printed *BMJ* in September, but the Editors unfortunately reversed the heading to: "Up with general practice: down with primary care" and removed my exclamation mark (DPG, 2017c). This suggested that in medical schools the words 'primary care' were 'weasel words' denying the name of the discipline of general practice, and making it harder for medical students to choose general practice and be proud of it. I got many supportive emails, including one from Marshall Marinker.

GP leaders were writing about being 'exposed to general practice,' meaning teaching in general practice, so Kate and I wrote that 'exposure' has connotations of danger and the need for protection (DPG and Sidaway-Lee, 2018a).

Doctor Continuity and Mortality

This next article (DPG *et al.*, 2018c in *BMJ Open*) was the first systematic review of the relationship between doctor continuity and death rates in patients and is described in Chapter 49, the St Leonard's Research Practice story. We found that 18/22 highly screened articles showed reduced patient mortality. We had two Exeter students, Ellie White and Angus Thorne and they both became so involved that both earned their place as co-authors. Both thus had the unusual student experience of co-authoring an article that went on to have 100,000 downloads and over 500 citations, illustrating the Practice as a learning environment.

Molly Dineen was another Exeter medical student doing an intercalated Exeter master's degree. She had done Phil Evans's SSU and came back to the Practice as her academic base for her master's research project. I suggested choosing family history as a big under-studied theme of family medicine. Phil Evans and I were her supervisors but he led being on the staff of the Medical School now as an Associate Professor. She was the only student of her year to gain ethics approval and only because Philip gave her so much support. Procedures have become overcomplicated and hostile to students. A generation of students with imaginative ideas, at the height of their intellectual powers, are being frozen out of studies, which previous generations of students have been able to do. She worked hard graduating MSc with distinction. At her graduation we were pleased to meet her parents. Three current/former partners from the St Leonard's Practice were in the University's staff procession. She got her study published (Dineen *et al.*, 2021) in *Family Practice*. We empowered four Exeter University students and two junior doctors to become co-authors in eight articles in peer-reviewed medical journals.

Visitors

The many visitors to the Practice (Chapter 49, St. Leonard's Research Practice; Appendix 10) gave us an especially valuable form of continuing education. They included two chief medical officers for England, one from Scotland and one CMO from Wales and two Directors of NHS Research. They came at their own expense in their own time to engage with us in some stimulating discussions. We were continually learning from our visitors in our own work setting. The Practice was an exciting learning environment.

49

The St Leonard's Research Practice: 2002 to 2023

The opportunities for the general practitioner are essential for the investigation of disease and the progress of medicine.

Sir James Mackenzie (1921)

Small is beautiful.

EF Schumacher (1973)

After retiring clinically from the practice on 30 September 2000, I did not see a patient professionally again. This retirement was in two parts: first, six years holding two national chairmanships, the Academy of Medical Royal Colleges (two years), followed by the three years as Chair of the Trustees of the Nuffield Trust, both based in London. These are described in Chapter 38, Chair of the Academy of Medical Royal Colleges, 2000–2002, and Chapter 44, The Nuffield Trust, 1993–2006.

I needed to resolve continuing confusion about my surname. I was christened Denis John Pereira Gray, but in 1962 on returning to Exeter, I found that there were already two GPs called Gray in the city: my father and uncle, Richard Gray. Following my grandfather, I used Pereira Gray as my surname in the Practice and in all professional organisations. However, most of the international databases listed me as Gray DP so in December 2005 I changed my surname by deed poll to Pereira Gray.

St Leonard's Research Practice

Philip Evans invited me to do more in the research wing of the St Leonard's practice. The Practice received funding from the NHS, which Philip had secured in 1997. It employed a series of part-time research fellows: Manjo Luthra, Peter Langley, Christine Wright, and Kate Sidaway-Lee, the last three all had PhDs. We called the research wing of the Practice the 'St Leonard's Research Practice' and it had its own writing paper and bank account. We won four research/teaching grants. This chapter describes my research in the Practice in my clinical retirement.

In 2007 the Practice moved to new purpose-built premises in nearby Athelstan Road. An important gain was that we had a room dedicated to research. The Patient Participation Group (PPG) asked me to write a history of the previous building and the practice, which was printed as *Holmedale–Family Home and Family Practice* (DPG, 2008). I gave copies to the PPG who sold them at £3.00 each for the PPG's funds. It soon sold out. That year I was appointed by the NHS Director of Research to the selection committee for the NHS R&D lead investigators.

We had had success in the Practice before with Kieran Sweeney *et al.*'s (1998) think piece on personal significance in the *Lancet*. In 2008, we had our first original research published.

THE HISTORY . OF
HOLMEDALE

1879 - 2008

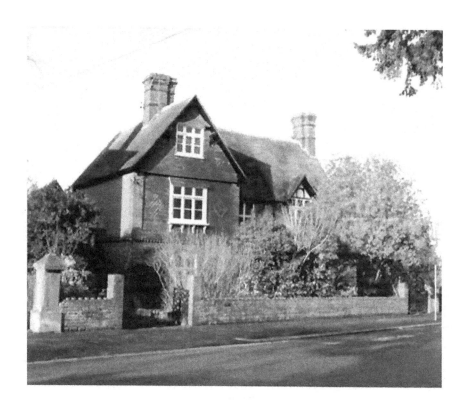

By
Denis Pereira Gray

FIGURE 49.1   Holmedale, 2008 – Family Home and Family Practice.

This showed that GPs could diagnose the majority of their patients with type 2 diabetes before they complained of a single symptom of the disease (Evans *et al.,* 2008). This was achieved by 'clinical opportunistic screening,' meaning the GP used the patient's presence in the consulting room to offer a screening test. Philip led on this with Peter Langley as the Research Fellow. This had some theoretical importance as it revealed that working GPs and their records had valuable data and unrecognised clinical skills. This was the first article to note that GPs make the most diagnoses in the NHS.

Kieran Sweeney was appointed an honorary Professor of General Practice in Exeter in 2008 on the basis of scholarship, an exceptional achievement. Jill and I tried to set up a celebratory dinner with the former staff and spouses at the Institute of General Practice, which had made it possible. However, Kieran dashed abroad for a last precious holiday with his wife Barbara and we could not find a date. Kieran had been both a partner with me in the practice for 14 years and a colleague in the University. He had been medical correspondent for *The Times,* obtained an MD in his 50s and wrote four books. Tragically, he developed mesothelioma soon after being promoted. This terrible disease has a life expectation of less than a year. He wrote a moving article in the *BMJ* (Sweeney *et al.,* 2009) and recorded an even more moving video at a late stage of his disease. I visited him at home several times as he was dying, which was a deeply sad experience. His son wrote an obituary in the *Guardian* (Sweeney, 2010).

Christopher Gardner-Thorpe, Editor of the *Journal of Medical Biography,* invited an editorial. I knew him as an Exeter consultant. I had only one page allocated but squeezed in ideas like the

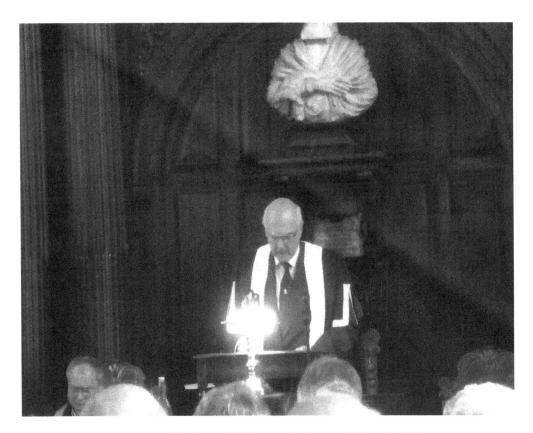

FIGURE 49.2   Winning the Rose Prize for medical history at Apothecaries Hall London, 2013.

first statement of the importance of the duration of registration of patients in general practice. I used my 38 years' service to contrast patterns of clinical experience over different decades (DPG, 2010a).

Ridd *et al.* (2011) from the Bristol Medical School published in the *Annals of Family Medicine*, a leading US GP academic journal, a way of measuring the patient-GP relationship, a major advance. However, the article gave us two problems. First, the Bristol team, including many colleagues we knew, wrote of "a lack of research on continuity improving patient care." Secondly, the questions in their new instrument were strikingly similar to questions in the Reis *et al.* (2008) instrument in the Fetzer study in which I had participated (Chapter 32; Fetzer Institute story). Was this ignorance or plagiarism? This was serious as British academics had been repeatedly undervaluing the research benefits associated with continuity of care and Bristol was a leading research department. So, two West Country academic units in England, only 80 miles apart, did academic battle with each other in an American journal.

Our difficulty was that the *Annals* stated a limit for letters of only 400 words. We drafted an 800-word reply dealing with both problems and I sent a covering letter to Kurt Stange, the Editor, an internationally known family physician. He was generous and published our letter in full, although it was effectively a short article (DPG *et al.*, 2011). Eventually, there was no evidence of plagiarism and as Reis *et al.* had been published in a psychological not a family medicine journal. The duplication of questions was through two separate academic teams reaching similar questions independently. The Bristol team in effect validated the questions in Reis *et al.* (2008).

Having shown that GPs could diagnose type 2 diabetes before symptoms, the next step was obviously to cost this process. I led on this, and we were pleased to have it published in *Diabetic Medicine* (DPG *et al.*, 2012). The finding was that diagnosing diabetes by clinical opportunistic screening (COS) was better value for money than population-based screening through eliminating the costs of arranging appointments. We also found that because GPs keep undertaking clinical opportunistic screening through continuity of care, the numbers of diagnoses they make become comparable with population screening.

The greatest value of COS is by GPs in developing countries, especially in Asia where the prevalence of type 2 diabetes is much higher. Such countries can never afford population-based screening, but often have family physicians with computers. Clinical opportunistic screening on general/family practice is the method of choice in much of the world.

In 2009 I was surprisingly awarded the Honorary Doctor of Science of the University of Exeter (photo). Staff do not usually receive honorary doctorates, but that year Robin Ling and Clive Lee also received ones for the Exeter hip. The family came in strength.

Multidisciplinary Members of the Practice Team

After I finished as Chair of the Trustees of the Nuffield Trust in 2006, I went at my own expense to some of their meetings. At one London meeting, a GP from East Devon, Philip Taylor, a former fellow clinical tutor with me, introduced me to a data manager in the NEW (North East and West) Devon CCG. This was Todd Chenore. I found he was an enthusiast for data analysis and worked close to my home.

I started going to see him in Devon County Hall and discovered he had a master's degree and was a skilled data analyst. He had devised a new 'Devon predictive model' for identifying patients at risk of emergency admission to hospital but was not getting much recognition for this, so I offered collaboration with of the St Leonard's Practice, which he welcomed. We had several meetings and when we needed expert statistical advice, I was able to link with William Henley, a new professor of biostatistics in Exeter. Todd was in touch with a GP registrar, Jim Forrer, doing a specialist GP training post (ST4), so we invited him to join. I mentored him, encouraging him to do a master's degree.

HONORARY GRADUATES

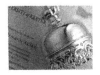

Friday 24 July 2:30pm

PROFESSOR SIR DENIS PEREIRA GRAY (DSC)

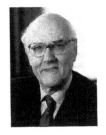

Sir Denis Pereira Gray worked for 38 years in the St Leonard's Medical Practice Exeter, following his father and grandfather. He established the first postgraduate university department of general practice in Europe at the University of Exeter and was later appointed Professor and Director of the Exeter University Postgraduate Medical School. He was twice elected by the registered medical practitioners in England to the General Medical Council.

Sir Denis was elected Chairman of Council and later President of the Royal College of General Practitioners, Chairman of the JCPTPGP a medical regulatory body, and Chairman of the Trustees of the Nuffield Trust. He is the only General Practitioner ever elected Chairman of the Academy of the Medical Royal Colleges of Great Britain and Ireland and is one of 23 British doctors who have been elected to the Institute of Medicine, of the National Academy of Sciences, Washington, USA.

He is currently an Assessor for the Queen's Award for Higher and Further Education, Patron of the National Association for Patient Participation, and President of the charity, What About the Children?

Sir Denis was knighted for services to quality assurance in medicine. He was awarded the Gold Medal of the Hunterian Society, the Gold Medal of the Royal Institute of Public Health, and holds honorary degrees from three British universities.

FIGURE 49.3 University of Exeter Honorary DSc, 2009.

Todd asked me about research in the practice and I spoke about continuity of care. He mused that he had access to the date of first registration of patients with their GP in the database. He then added that fact to the model and found it was a new significant factor: the patients with long-term registration with their GP had a significantly lower rate of emergency admission to hospital. So it was that in a five-minute chat, on another subject, a modest new contribution to the theory of longitudinal continuity of doctor care was made. We were published in the *Journal of Public Health* (Chenore *et al.*, 2013).

This article provided evidence that the Devon predictive model performed better than the leading model: the combined model. We reported for the first time that, in a population of about 750,000, longitudinal continuity of GP care was significantly associated with fewer emergency admissions to hospital. It was not possible to explore the reasons. However, three years later in a publication from the Practice on "Fifty years of longitudinal continuity in general practice" (White *et al.*, 2016), we wrote that longitudinal continuity facilitates relationship building between the patient and the GP but is in itself not enough. It is a necessary – but not sufficient – condition.

After the success of extending the work of the research practice beyond its own population with the publication of the Devon predictive model, one day it dawned on me that there were two big factors that everyone agreed were associated with emergency admissions to hospital: age and social deprivation. But which was the more important and how did they relate? I realised that this relationship could be modelled although I did not have the skills to do it myself.

I invited the team that had done predictive modelling to my home and put the proposition to them. All agreed, and crucially William Henley the statistics professor, was confident he could build a model with the CCG data. We held the subsequent meetings in the Practice. The model was built and proved fascinating. Up to about age 50, social deprivation is the leading factor influencing emergency admissions to hospital, but thereafter age becomes progressively more influential and at older ages heavily outweighs social deprivation. A highlight was publishing five, beautiful, J-shaped curves revealing that the relationship was the same in all groups of social deprivation from the poorest to the most affluent people. We had unravelled a biological fact. Kate Sidaway-Lee was making valuable contributions in the Practice research team, so we invited her to become a co-author.

Knowing the health care system in Ireland proved helpful when we were challenged by an Irish assessor for the journal who had published findings different from ours. We replied that the NHS, unlike the Irish system, gathers details of all hospital admissions across England charging them to the host CCG. So, our rate of hospital admissions was higher than the Irish figures only from Dublin hospitals. The data processing advantages of the NHS are underestimated. We were published in *BMJ Open* (DPG *et al.*, 2017).

Personally, I think this work has high relevance to the NHS, which allocates about £75 billion pounds a year to clinical commissioning groups (CCGs) on a formula that, according to our work, undervalues the contribution of age to hospital admissions. This explains why CCGs with bigger proportions of older people are continually under financial pressure, many with deficits. Moreover, the demographic balance of the population in east Devon models the population of England in 2030. We sent the article to Simon (later Sir; later still Lord) Stevens (1966–), Chief Executive of NHS England, who wrote that he had referred it to the financial allocation group but, as far as we know, the NHS funding allocation formula has not been altered. The article has been ignored academically with only nine citations by 2022 – disappointing.

Peter Orton's MD

Peter Oton had asked me 18 years earlier when I was an active professor, to supervise his MD. His subject "Burnout in GPs" was important and topical. He lived and worked as a GP in Essex. I advised on the method, which he carried out rigorously and he gained ethics approval and several grants in Essex. The local medical committee and local GPs were strongly supportive. He managed the data collection in Essex.

He flew his private plane to Exeter for supervisions. Jill gave him some lunches in our home and he gave me some dinners in Exeter. I sent detailed written reports after each supervision. He worked full-time in general practice and his passion was flying. The MD progressed slowly as it was his third priority. He obtained additional flying skills and then flew the Atlantic alone in his small plane.

I had always taught that a good doctoral thesis should lead to two publications in the peer-reviewed literature and Peter therefore embarked on an article on burnout in GPs. With my love of alliteration, I provided the first words of our title: "Depersonalised doctors…". It was published in *BMJ Open* (Orton *et al.*, 2012). This reported the biggest number of British GPs completing the Maslach burnout inventory. The worrying finding was that about a third were burnt out using the best validated measure of burnout in the world. By 2023 this article had 150 citations. The publication strengthened Peter's work on his thesis in two ways: first, writing to the standards of an international peer-reviewed journal is educational and tightens up a doctoral candidate's work; secondly, being published adds credibility to a thesis. Countries like the Netherlands require doctoral candidates to obtain six peer-reviewed publications and a commentary linking them for a thesis.

When we did that research, there were clues that doctor burnout was associated with worse care for patients and we judged that the sense of depersonalisation would be the most important of the three

Maslach features. Six years later, Panagioti *et al.* (2018) reported that burnt-out doctors did make more mistakes, especially when depersonalised.

After getting the burnout article accepted, Peter moved on another section of the thesis. He had precisely timed 822 GP consultations and had contemporaneous data about the characteristics of the GPs involved. This gave us an opportunity to analyse doctor factors affecting the length of consultations in general practice, an important, under studied topic. Using the Canadian patient-centredness instrument, the key finding was that longer GP consultations were significantly more patient centred. This was circumstantial evidence for continuity, as providing more time through longer consultations is the other way GPs can give patients more time.

Peter got statistical advice in Cambridge. We tussled with the assessors of the journal *Family Practice* as we did not have data on the patients' characteristics and there was some groupthink that patients were the decisive influence on the duration of consultations. This threatened acceptance of the article. Ironically, one of my GP trainees contributed to this thinking as Westcott (1977; 51 citations) found that patients with emotional problems had longer consultations. However, the model built on Peter's data clearly showed that GPs, not patients, are the main influence on the length of consultations. Actually, this is obvious, but was not well understood at the time. Most GPs, most of the time, run their surgery sessions to time regardless of the problems patients bring them. The Orton and DPG paper (2016) was published in *Family Practice*. By 2023 it had 54 citations.

Peter eventually completed his thesis, by which time I had sent him over 900 emails and had six, full, A4 ring-bound folders. His doctoral viva was examined by Professors Brian Hurwitz and Ruth Chambers, and they approved the award of an MD with modest amendments.

He sent a bound copy of the thesis to the RCGP, as its library has the biggest collection of GP theses in the world. There was no academic response. The RCGP did not realise how rare a GP doctoral thesis by a full-time GP from a single practice and done outside a university was. One price of the College's unwise decision to abolish its Research Committee was starkly revealed.

Diabetes Care in General Practice

I was invited in 2013 to the 'summit' conference of the Nuffield Trust where I was assailed by a leading professor of epidemiology, whom I knew, and who was a national authority. He pitched into me about how awful the care of people with diabetes was in general practice (just GPs). I was surprised but read it up and found that the national charity, Diabetes UK, had written about the: "Scandal of GP care for people with diabetes." The criteria assumed that every patient should always receive every recommended intervention. At the time, Peter Langley, the practice Research Fellow, was reporting that the Practice was being accused by auditors of failing to provide some diabetic care when he had written evidence that it had been provided. He had reported this, but it had not been agreed upon. We tackled both problems together, resulting in the publication of "Is the 'scandal' of diabetes care in general practice fact or fiction?" in the *BJGP* (DPG *et al.*, 2014). This pointed out that some diabetic interventions were inappropriate, e.g., if patients were dying, and also that adult patients with mental capacity had a right to decline some care and some did so. We published evidence that the national audit had got our practice figures wrong. Only then was this acknowledged. Across Europe, amputation rates in UK diabetic patients were the fourth best out of 32 countries. I learned that highly regarded national charities can have a perverse incentive to play the blame game, as they gain press publicity and donations from doing so. In addition, even leading epidemiologists can have serious biases.

At a big annual conference in London on diabetes, I was invited to speak in two separate years and went the first year with Ellie White and the second year with Kate Sidaway-Lee, each year giving joint presentations to audiences of about 80–100. Both times *Practical Diabetes* invited editorials afterwards (DPG and Sidaway-Lee, 2018b). That year I was awarded the Rose Prize for medical history and was photographed in the Society of Apothecarie.

In 2017 with Kate, I first lectured about my long-held view that conflicts of interest were a big problem in Britain. I was brought up to believe that the British constitution separated politicians from the judiciary. Only in mid-life did I discover that the Lord Chancellor was a member of the Cabinet at the heart of British politics, whilst being head of the judiciary. It took pressure from the European Union to end this serious conflict of interest leading to the UK establishing an independent Supreme Court. I listed many conflicts of interest in the diabetes world. Ahn *et al.* (2017) found 68% of principal investigators had financial ties to the pharmaceutical industry and that such links were significantly associated with positive findings. Kate presented figures that patients with type 2 diabetes were significantly more socially deprived than other patients and showed comparison of risk factors for patients in the Practice for type 2 diabetes with obesity being comparable to social deprivation (DPG and Sidaway-Lee, 2018b).

Care Quality Commission (CQC) Practice Visits 2013 and 2017

The Practice was visited by the CQC and the provisional report awarded a rating of "good." This undervalued the Practice, so I drafted an appeal using the CQC's own criteria. The award was upgraded to "outstanding" (awarded to 4% of practices). This was the only general practice in England to appeal against the award of "good."

The CQC visited the Practice again in 2017. This time it interviewed the research wing of the practice seriously. Philip, Kate and I were given a good opportunity to display the research, some of which matched our assessors' interests. The award of "outstanding" was repeated.

Philip Evans

In my last year as head of the Institute of General Practice in the University in 2001, I had appointed Phil Evans as the Director of SaNDNet, then the name for the local primary care research network established in the Institute. The NHS repeatedly changed the name, the function, and the geographical area of the network. Philip's leadership style in the network was low key, empowering and effective. The South West emerged under his leadership as the most successful NHS region in England for recruiting patients into trials.

After about 20 years, Philip was appointed to be the lead GP in the NIHR NHS network and cluster lead for primary care, dermatology, public health, social care and mental health with an academic appointment in King's College, London. We were all pleased that in 2022 he was promoted to be Professor of Primary Care Research in the University of Exeter and received a bronze clinical excellence award. These insights increased his input into the research practice. In 2022 he was promoted again to be Deputy Medical Director of the National Institute for Health Services Research (NIHR). Initially, he was funded in the Research Practice with a session a week but over the years the funding was lost and thereafter his contribution was, like mine, voluntary.

Continuity of Doctor Care

In 2016 we had a narrative review of continuity of care published in *InnovAiT*, the journal for GPs in training – an educational journal. Most articles are written for others to read but we suspect this one was not read much by GP trainees. It is behind a paywall for those not inside the RCGP and is not easily accessible. It has only been cited 29 times. However, it was easy for us to write, as we knew the literature. It enabled us to construct a classification of benefits of continuity: for patients, for GPs, and for the health system/NHS and adverse effects of continuity, which helped us later. Ellie and Angus, another Exeter BSc student, were co-authors as students with the core team of Philip, Kate and me on "Improving continuity THE clinical challenge" (DPG *et al.,* 2016b).

After this, it dawned on me that the next big step in the continuity research story would be to undertake in the Practice the first systematic review of the relationship between continuity of doctor care and mortality. We had put down a marker with a letter in the *Lancet* (DPG *et al.* 2016c) noting that general practice could reduce patient mortality. A systematic review would be new but was possible because Kate Sidaway-Lee was a good academic. We had two BSc students from the University of Exeter in the Practice: Ellie White and Angus Thorne. We invited them to join the practice research team. Both were keen and did their share of finding and assessing articles. We registered in the Prospero database. It took us about two years of searches to identify over 700 articles and reduce them to 22 for detailed study, requiring both measured doctor continuity and mortality. We were disappointed that the *New England Journal of Medicine* did not want systematic reviews but were pleased to be accepted by *BMJ Open.* Both students earned their co-authorships and were much encouraged by the outcome.

We were published in June 2018 (DPG *et al.,* 2018c). The balloon went up! On the morning of publication there were reports on our research on the front pages of both *The Times* and *The Guardian.* Press interest was intense and I spent almost a whole day on the telephone for mainly US media, whilst Philip took interviews from 17 local BBC radio stations. We identified research where continuity of specialist care for physicians, psychiatrists and surgeons was also associated with lower mortality. Mortality is a hard outcome and cannot be ignored. I got pleasure from 'beating the system' as I was 82 at the time and this was 17 years after I had been forced to retire on age grounds as a university professor.

This article led the Director of Primary Care in NHS England, Dominic Hardy, and the Chair of the trustees of the Nuffield Trust, Andy McKeon, visiting the Practice. Nikki Kanani, Medical Director of Primary Care in NHS England, and an influential NHS manager Ed Waller, saw us in London. Later Adrian Hayter, the first GP-appointed NHS National Director for the Care of Older People came too. The article continues to attract interest with 617 citations, over 100,000 downloads, and an Altmetric score (measure of general interest) of 2,462, which is high amongst publications from British medical schools.

Our next article measured GP continuity in St Leonard's using the practice system: the **St L**eonard's **I**ndex of **C**ontinuity of **C**are (SLICC, Kate's idea) in the *BJGP.* Of appointments by the over-65s, 65% were with their personal GP (Sidaway-Lee *et al.,* 2019). We followed this with an article on the mechanisms of continuity (Sidaway-Lee *et al.,* 2021).

Health Foundation Improving GP Continuity Programme 2018

In 2018, the Health Foundation tweeted about continuity of care asking: "To whom should we be talking?" Kate thought it was hilarious and teased me when I responded with a formal, typed letter. However, tweet to letter worked as the Practice was selected as one of five centres in England with a grant of £167,000. We ran this grant as a three: Philip Evans, Kate and me.

The aim was to increase continuity of GP care. Our measure of GP continuity, the SLICC, was published in the *BJGP* (Sidaway-Lee *et al.,* 2019). I had invented this system in 1974 (DPG, 1979a). We used it for years with paper records, but it was now computerised. Kate led as she did the monthly returns and developed the template for other practices. Our method in the programme was to emphasise measurement of GP continuity in general practice and showing four collaborating general practices how to do this using the SLICC. We ran 37 workshops for GPs, patients, and the administrative staff, taking over 50 hours, with sophisticated international patient evaluations.

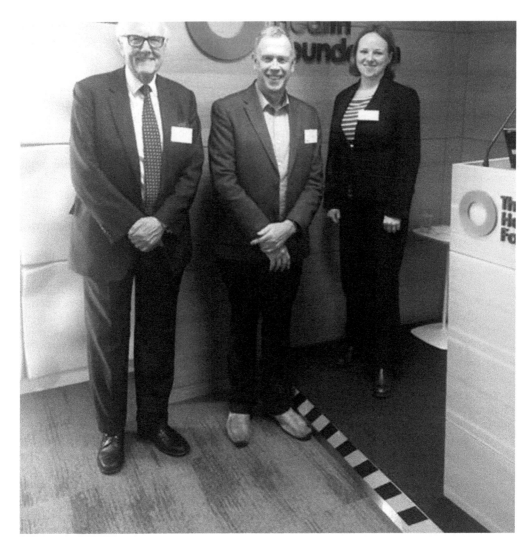

FIGURE 49.4   With Philip Evans and Kate Sidaway-Lee, Health Foundation grant for continuity, 2018.

Our statistical control charts showed that despite falling GP continuity nationally, four of five practices maintained GP continuity and three improved it significantly (Health Foundation, 2022).

Jill died in September 2020. Philip Evans and Joy Choules, who had worked for years in with us both in the College publications office, wrote her obituary in the BJGP (Evans and Choules, 2021).

Other Academic Activities

I went to the farewell lecture of Chris Van Weel (2012) as Professor of General Practice in Nijmegen, the Netherlands and President of the World Association of Family Doctors. I was honoured to be

Life & Times
Lady Pereira Gray:
an appreciation

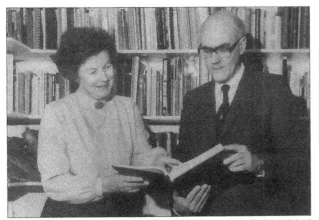

Jill and Denis Pereira Gray, RCGP publications office, Exeter, date unknown. Image obtained by kind permission of Sir Denis.

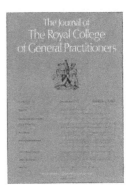

The Journal of the Royal College of General Practitioners, Vol. 32, Issue 235, February 1982 (where Jill's article appeared).

Born 10 May 1937; died 26 September 2020

Lady Jill Pereira Gray, the wife of former Chairman of Council and President of the College Sir Denis Pereira Gray for 58 years, died in September 2020 aged 83 after a long battle with cancer.

Jill used her English degree from the University of London and her academic publishing skills, working alongside Denis as an Assistant Editor in the editorial office of the College, based in their home in Exeter. Jill started working for the RCGP in 1976 and continued for the next 21 years as an Assistant Editor.

Between them they produced the *Journal of the Royal College of General Practitioners* and *Journal* supplements, over 70 Occasional Papers, Reports from General Practice 18–25, the 'white cover' reprinted classic general practice books, and several other books and booklets,

including the annual *RCGP Members' Reference Book* from 1982–1996. Another joint venture was *The Medical Annual* from 1983–1987. As general practice developed rapidly as a discipline, a number of these Occasional Papers and reports were fundamental to the development of our discipline and the development of vocational training for general practice.

Jill wrote an article in the *Journal of the Royal College of General Practitioners* in 1982 about the role of the doctor's family[1] and a chapter in *The Medical Annual 1984* about the medical care of doctors' families.[2]

These were key publications, leading to her giving lectures on the subject. Subsequently, policy and practice changed dramatically, for the better.

Jill supported Denis in his work from starting as a GP through to him being Chair (1987–1990), and then President of the RCGP (1997–2000), and beyond.

The Revd Canon Dr John Searle, a lifetime friend and colleague, in his fitting eulogy identified Jill's overriding passions as being her friends, her family, and her faith.

Jill leaves her husband Denis, their four children Peter, Penny, Liz, and Jen, as well as 14 grandchildren, and four great-grandchildren.

Philip H Evans,
GP and Associate Professor of General Practice and Primary Care, College of Medicine and Health, University of Exeter, Exeter.
Email: p.h.evans@exeter.ac.uk

Joy Choules,
Former Secretary and Editorial Assistant, RCGP Publications 1985–1987; Administrator to NIHR CRN National Specialty Lead for Primary Care, University of Exeter Medical School, Exeter.

DOI: https://doi.org/10.3399/bjgp21X714509

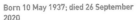

"[Jill wrote] *key publications, leading to her giving lectures on the subject* [on the role and medical care of doctors' families]. *Subsequently, policy and practice changed dramatically, for the better.*"

REFERENCES

1. Pereira Gray J. The doctor's family: some problems and solutions. *J Roy Coll Gen Pract* 1982; **32(235):** 75–79.

2. Pereira Gray J. The health of doctors' families. In: *The Medical Annual 1984.* Bristol: John Wright & Sons, 1984: 213–225.

FIGURE 49.5   Jill's obituary in the *Br. J Gen Practice,* January 2021. (With permission of the Editor.)

called one of his mentors. About 800 attended – more than any British GP professor would get, indicating the strength of Dutch academic general practice.

With Martin Marshall, a former Exeter trainee, now a professor, I wrote a warning editorial in the *BMJ*. We suggested that many strengths of general practice, like continuity, were being eroded, so it should not be assumed that general practice could continue to deliver so much. Was general practice taking a leap in the dark? (Marshall and DPG, 2016).

In January 2020 in the *BJGP* we put measurement of continuity into context, as one of eight key pieces of information which would empower practices to manage themselves more professionally (DPG *et al.*, 2020c). GP computer systems are untapped data gold mines.

We published the third commentary on the use of words. After the first, a critique of the words 'primary care' (DPG, 2017c), followed by a critique of the word 'exposed' for general practice teaching (DPG and Sidaway-Lee, 2018a). The third article challenged the phrase 'the worried well' (DPG *et al.*, 2020d).

I joined two GP professors and Catherine Johns, Chair of the Practice Patient Group, in a *BMJ* editorial on the COVID pandemic. We wrote that patients were being disempowered. We listed benefits associated with continuity and empathy in general practice and hoped general practices would return, after the pandemic, to personal care (DPG *et al.*, 2020e).

In 2022, the RCGP locally through the Tamar Faculty invited me to deliver the McConaghey's Lecture and fortunately in Exeter too. Then the RCGP nationally awarded me its Life-Time Achievement Award. I broke my arm on the journey and was lucky to escape an accident and emergency department. I arrived patched up and with a stitched eyebrow, with 20 minutes to spare, to receive it and make a speech of thanks.

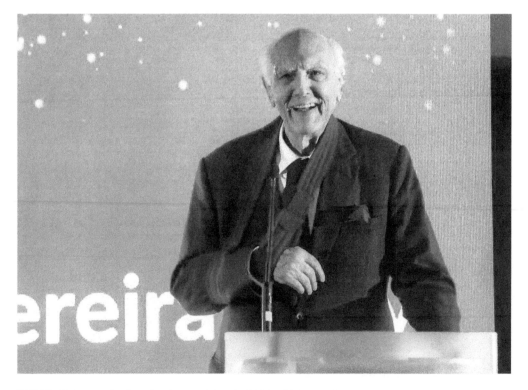

FIGURE 49.6   Speech of thanks after receiving the RCGP Lifetime Achievement Award in 2022, six hours after breaking an arm and having an eyebrow stitched, aged 87.

Letters in Professional Journals

We had 26 letters published in seven professional journals including: the *American Board of Family Medicine, Annals of Family Medicine, British Journal of General Practice, BMJ, Diabetes Medicine*, the *Journal of the Royal Society of Medicine*, and the *Lancet*. Three in the *BMJ* and *BJGP* were the lead letter or 'Editor's Choice.' The most important was a letter with Patricia Wilkie amending the findings of research in the *Lancet*. We re-analysed a table finding that patients, after triage by GPs for requests for new consultations, had a 22% increased use of out of hours compared with patients who were seen by a GP face to face (DPG and Wilkie, 2015; Campbell *et al.,* 2014; Chapter 40, Patient Participation story).

The medical newspaper *Pulse* (2012) reported I was judged the second most influential GP in the last 50 years, behind Julian Tudor Hart and ahead of Donald Irvine. I was also included by Neil Metcalfe (2019), who edited a book with the title *100 Notable Names from General Practice*.

Letters in the Press

I continued to indulge my hobby of seeking to get letters published in *The Times* and or *Financial Times (FT)*. These national newspapers can only accept about 5% of the letters they are offered and provide in their letter pages important daily analyses and commentaries on current affairs. I was fortunate in getting 15 published in *The Times* and in the *FT* between 2017 and 2022.

I had several controversial letters published. One on marriage as a public health issue (DPG, 2010b) was the lead letter of the day and I published more than one critical of vaping (DPG, 2018b; because e-cigarettes contain tobacco and 7% of British children aged 11–17 use them, attracting little concern). I used these platforms to defend general practice and also to publicise several principles of general practice, like continuity (DPG, 2022a) and medical generalisms such as "Breadth and depth" (DPG, 2022c). The *Financial Times* (DPG, 2022d) printed a letter from me on "Why GPs are invaluable to the NHS." These free, influential, international platforms enabled some principles of general practice to be stated for an international readership.

Analysis

The 17 years, 2006–2023, were when I was in clinical retirement. I resumed academic work in a small, happy, research team in the St Leonard's Practice. We had 38 publications in those years, in 16 journals, including eight editorials in four different journals and one chapter in a book, 11 articles presented original empirical data. I authored 29 and my most common co-author was Philip Evans (13). He and I have worked together for 36 years in a variety of roles, including being partners for 13 years and having a doctor–patient relationship for 17 years. The journal accepting the most was the *BJGP,* with 14 publications. That journal published our editorial on GP continuity (DPG *et al.,* 2022b) giving me a 50-year connection and a 50th anniversary of my first editorial in it in January 1972 (*J Roy Coll Gen Pract*, 1972).

Kate Sidaway-Lee arrived at the Practice in October 2014, and her PhD in biological sciences equipped her well to do general practice research. By 2023 she had co-authored 12 articles. She was our third research fellow with a PhD, making the biggest contribution. Early on she said: "You are accepting almost all my suggestions." I agreed and said I wanted her frankest criticism. Academics need four characteristics to succeed: first, adequate intelligence (clear thinking is always needed); second, a work ethic (there are no short cuts in time); third, a love of reading (preferably widely); and fourth, an openness to frank criticism (the least common feature).

I learned in Cambridge that I was not the brightest button on the beach, so I concentrated on the other three features. I believe welcoming criticism is my strongest suit. Kate became a strong critic and a valued colleague. A scientist employed by a general practice and working with enthusiastic GPs is an exciting model and we described her as "researcher in residence" (Marshall *et al.*, 2014). It needs fostering, replicating and researching.

In eight years (July 2006-Sept 2014) the Research Practice had nine publications (1.1 pa). In the 8.75 years with Kate (Oct 2014–June 2023) we had 28, so she was associated with tripling our productivity to an average of 3.2 publications per year. The advantages of working in a small team are huge. Small organisations are undervalued and governments lean towards big ones. Yet 'micro-organisations' (employing 0–9 people) generate one-third of all UK employment and 21% of turnover (House of Commons Library, 2021). For me, Schumacher's (1973, republished 2011) conclusion that "small is beautiful" remains true.

I hope this chapter illustrates the potential for research inside a general practice, supporting Mackenzie's (1921) statement: "The opportunities for the general practitioner are essential for the investigation of disease and the progress of medicine."

The Academic Triad: Service, Teaching, and Active Research

In the Western world, teaching hospitals are based on the academic triad of good service (teaching hospitals achieve better results than other hospitals), research, and teaching. Since 1948 in the UK, medical schools have worked in partnerships with teaching hospitals. The challenge for general practice has always been to match this triad, given the historic disadvantage that the original, 1948, GP NHS contract was research free.

The Practice did undergraduate teaching from 1972 and postgraduate teaching from 1975. It achieved the triad in the 1990s when Russell Steele's fellowship by assessment provided external validation of high-quality care and the practice had several publications with different first authors in the *BJGP*, the *BMJ*, the *Occasional Papers*, and the *Lancet*.

It was in 2016–2022 that the full flowering of the academic triad occurred. Being awarded outstanding by the CQC twice, having a student project undertaken exclusively in the practice and being published in a good journal (White *et al.*, 2016), and a student winning the Quintiles Prize for women in science were important steps. Our systematic review of continuity of doctor care and mortality (DPG *et al.*, 2018c) was the first in the world.

The St Leonard's Practice fulfilled the academic triad on all three professional criteria, and we described this in a letter in the *BJGP* with two former students as co-authors (DPG *et al.*, 2021). What it lacked was recognition or secure funding.

50

Reflections

Life can only be lived forwards but must be understood backwards.

Kierkegaard (1813–1855) Danish philosopher

We die and that may be the meaning of life and we do language and that may be the measure of life.

Toni Morrison (1931–2019; 1993) American writer, acceptance speech for the Nobel Prize for Literature

Of these two quotations, the first is undeniably true and a great insight for biographers. The second is I believe only half true, as one measure of a life in human terms lies in the minds of those we love. But for professional and leadership roles, it is true that what was done and recorded in writing is the measure. Hence, the illustrations of my life with writings and their context.

They come from the generation which experienced a world war with local bombing and food rationing. We learned that a modern European country could organise mass murder in our lifetimes. Cultural revolutions which we have experienced include women gaining control of their own fertility and 75% of mothers with children going to work, both for the first time in thousands of years (DPG *et al.*, 2020b). When Jill and I went to our universities, only 7% of the population did so, and now half of Britain's young people go there.

The ageing society has brought us great benefits. Jill and I never knew our great-grandparents but at the baptism of one of our great-grandchildren, seven of the eight great grandparents were present. The arrival of computers in everyday life and the information age, symbolised by the Internet and the mobile phone, are a revolution comparable to the Industrial Revolution.

Society Changes

The quality and tone of public discourse have deteriorated. Social media have enabled anonymous comments to be publicised, some of which are violent, racist, and sexist and are often aimed at women and racial minorities. Society needs to find a way of stopping, or at least greatly limiting, such personal abuse being 'published' anonymously. Anonymous comments of this kind are not allowed in the publishing world where laws of slander and libel apply. It is currently an important question if Section 230 of the 1996 US *Communications and Decency Act*, which protects social media companies from publishing responsibility, should continue, as I believe they are publishers. Anonymous social media communications have serious adverse effects in society.

One of the world's most influential leaders has been repeatedly making statements which can easily be shown to be untrue – clear evidence of deterioration in public discourse. Society needs to develop new systems, and these are possible. For example, the UK Statistics Commission rebukes government ministers when they misuse statistics. One UK example occurred in 2018 when the Health Secretary wrongly tweeted that the number of GPs had risen when it had in fact fallen. The Statistics Commission required this tweet to be deleted. It has also corrected Boris Johnson when Prime Minister. The tide may be turning. One university professor has successfully sued after a malicious tweet. The British *Malicious Communications Act 1988* is now being used and the French in 2021 have acted against posts on social media, including harassment and discrimination.

The use of foodbanks is high and rising in Britain – an indictment of a modern society. It is extraordinary that so many citizens need them in the sixth richest country in the world. One in six of those using them is in work. As in the 19th century, charities like the Trussell Trust, which fosters foodbanks, have provided an important response.

England in 2020 is in some ways a harsher country in the way it treats the poor than half a century earlier. In 1948, the National Assistance Act provided for those in danger of destitution to receive cash payments from the state. Sadly, government policy is significantly responsible for foodbank use, partly by the withholding of welfare benefits for 5–6 weeks, when GPs since my grandfather's day have known that some poor people have chaotic lifestyles and need to be paid weekly. This policy of delaying benefits was introduced by highly intelligent, well-educated politicians and civil servants who simply had no idea about how some poor people live. Meanwhile, Jill and I receive hundreds of pounds a year for winter fuel, which we give to the Exeter foodbank. The middle classes are subsidised with thousands of pounds, when buying green cars, in a society where some children go hungry. In the USA, the richest country, 9% of citizens are frequently hungry (*Economist*, 2021).

The wider perspective of inequality in society is now fortunately receiving more academic and political attention but is moving too slowly. In the USA, the Congressional Research Service (2021) recently reported that over the *last 40 years* (1979–2019; my italics) incomes for the 10% lowest earners fell in real terms. The group with the biggest fall was white men. The gains from globalisation went to capital rather than labour. In the UK, the payments to leaders of FT100 companies have risen so that chairs are paid about five million pounds pa on average. Poor people need more generous support.

One of my saddest discoveries has been learning how often and how badly men have behaved towards women, especially sexual aggression towards younger women. I saw in my 20s that society was sexist with only three colleges at Cambridge taking women and with women students at Bart's being treated less well than men. But I only slowly understood the size of this problem by my, and previous generations, of men. Much is written about air and water pollution; I suspect that pornography is a comparable problem, damaging attitudes seriously. Domestic violence is mainly a male problem.

Another big change in my life has been the increasing numbers of women in medicine, now a majority in general practice. My editorial "Women general practitioners" in the *JRCGP* (1979) suggested women make better GPs and should be welcomed into general practice. It took years for the underpinning research to emerge when Hojat *et al.* (2002) found women medical students had more empathy than men. Men have to work harder to develop skills, as women have a built-in advantage. When watching couples of opposite sex walking in the road, the women glance at the men two or three times more often than men glance at women.

An Evolutionary Approach to Policymaking

Lessons can be learned from nature. The huge variety of plants and species offer a model. Darwin's (1859) masterpiece *On the Origin of Species,* revealed how success develops over time in the real world by continual change and adaptation. The most successful survive and propagate. Evolution is a fundamental principle with widespread applicability. Similarly, in the world of companies there are always multiple new organisations, but many also fail. Companies that were world-famous in the early FT and Dow indices of 30 years ago, like Kodak, have disappeared. New names are always appearing. Size, reputation and resources are not the key; it is adaptation and development in the real world that matters.

Evolution offers a model of policymaking. Instead of issuing a succession of top-down edicts, governments could instead work from models in the real world. The assumption that politicians have a divine right to rule is outmoded. Government's role would then be fourfold: first, the aims of a service like the NHS would need to be agreed with patients and the professions and be published as high-level aims for the NHS. These might be: patient satisfaction, making early diagnoses, providing good care for long-term illnesses, building high-quality relationships with patients, empowering patients to maximise their own health, optimising the well-being and satisfaction of staff, and providing high-quality teaching and research at reasonable cost.

Second, instead of spending big sums issuing and monitoring instructions, the NHS would develop the best possible systems of evaluation to measure the performance of the different components of the NHS. Third, the NHS would study the characteristics; for example, of general practices, which were associated with significantly above average achievement of these aims. Fourth, the government would reward the most effective organisations, providing an incentive for others to copy them. This nature following approach would respect fieldworkers, value and encourage their innovative abilities and experience, instead of often ignoring hard won experience.

Data are already gathered at great expense, which should be used better than they are at present. Only 4% of NHS general practices are graded 'outstanding' by the Care Quality Commission, but no research has been undertaken to determine if these practices achieve better outcomes for their patients than other practices. Even their characteristics are unpublished, so lessons are not being learned and considerable public expenditure is not being capitalised upon.

Responding to Criticism

I have discovered that responding to criticism is one of the most sensitive indicators of an individual's personality and also of the maturity of an organisation. I have been surprised to find intolerance of criticism among intelligent and successful people. It means insensitivity. Intolerance to criticism is also common in big institutions. The Pentagon Papers (1971) revealed that was practised by the US government and it occurs in big private companies. Disappointingly, it also occurs in the NHS, including in the Great Ormond Street hospital, the best endowed hospital in Britain, where its treatment of a consultant paediatrician in the 'baby P case' was unacceptable.

Criticism needs to be encouraged through systematic education. My first editorial preface in the *Medical Annual* (DPG, 1984e) publicly "invited *criticism*s... (my emphasis), all of which will be acknowledged." In the medical profession, and especially general practice, maintaining multiple audits of performance, which expose day-to-day weaker performance, is helpful in facing deficiencies regularly and dealing with them in a mature way. Whistle blowers have been consistently ill-treated, many of them experiencing managerial vengeance, which should be made a crime. Encouraging tolerance of criticism and protecting whistle blowers are high social priorities.

Four Personal Disappointments

I have been remarkably fortunate in my life and have had interesting and enjoyable experiences in many different settings, several of which allowed me to innovate. However, I have had four, big, professional disappointments, outside the practice. In the chronological order in which they occurred they were:

First, the decision of the Home Office to abandon the Diploma in Prison Medicine, which had been set up voluntarily with such effort by three Medical Royal Colleges and which was an international first and a success (Chapter 26; Prison Medicine).

Second, the abandonment, once I had retired in 2001, by the University of Exeter of Europe's first Institute of General Practice is an enduring disappointment to me (Chapter 13; Department/ Institute of General Practice).

Third, the RCGP, in stopping Fellowship by Assessment, abandoned the measurement of quality in general practice by the profession, removed a big career incentive for hundreds of GPs and weakened the RCGP, which could no longer demonstrate what good general practice looked like (Chapter 24; Fellowship by Assessment).

Fourth, the decision by the RCGP to abandon academic publishing, and especially the production of the *Occasional Papers* reporting new ideas and developments in general practice, has reduced the intellectual stimulation many GPs used to get and still need (Chapter 10; Exeter RCGP Publishing).

The Status of General Practice

When I entered general practice in 1962, it was not an attractive career. Medical schools were run by specialists and provided specialist-dominated teaching, there was no GP vocational training system and no professor of general practice anywhere in the world. Lord Moran's (1958) metaphor of "falling off the ladder" (stated whilst I was a medical student) described general practice as being inferior to specialist medicine and Irvine's brutal (1975) metaphor was that general practice was "the dustbin of medicine."

I nevertheless chose general practice partly because I was disenchanted by how patients were treated in my teaching hospital and in particular because I had the privilege of growing up in the home of a family doctor who obviously valued his job, and I could see first-hand his rich relationships with his patients (Chapter 5; Practice 1962–1975 story). It is no accident that many GP leaders were, like me, the children of GPs, including: Alastair Donald, John Fry, Clare Gerada, Donald Irvine, Irvine Loudon, Ian McWhinney, Lottie Newman, Robin Steel, and Julian Tudor Hart.

My early experience in general practice was uncomfortable as I did not understand the problems the patients were bringing, and they did not seem to have the diseases I had learnt about at Cambridge and Bart's. In time, as relationships built up with my patients, I came to understand patients as people, with more understanding of the context of their lives and I appreciated the private and personal information they were giving me.

The job became progressively more interesting, and I came to believe it is perhaps the most interesting job in Britain. Where else are there such difficult intellectual problems to unravel? Where else in medicine is there such variety, with life and death responsibility, such as possible meningitis in a child? Where else is such emotional satisfaction obtained through partnership relationships, forged with clients/patients – and GP colleagues, some, for me, lasting over 35 years?

I actively supported the RCGP as the one national organisation, which valued general practice and sought to improve it. There have been huge advances, notably in the development of the research wing of general practice with no GP professor in the world when I entered practice, to over 100 professors now. British GP research is amongst the best in the world; much of it underpinning the theory of the job which, in addition, great insights have come from research in the social and behavioural sciences.

Nevertheless, I accept at the end of my professional career that general practice is still not as understood or respected as it ought to be. First of all, specialist medicine simply does not respect the intellectual component of general practice, partly through ignorance, but partly because of an attitudinal block. Generalist doctors learn much about specialty practice and all of them work for at least 18 months in hospital specialist departments. There is an asymmetry in medical education, as specialist doctors never learn the core theory of general practice, many never receive any postgraduate training in general practice, and some still never work as postgraduates in general practice. This has been a long-term failure of the medical postgraduate educational system.

A second obstacle has been the DHSC under its former name of the Department of Health, as in a government-run service it controls the allocation of resources. In the early years, the DH did much to develop general practice and was ahead of the medical schools and universities in understanding its importance and promoting it through vocational training for general practice. It funded the Exeter

University Department of General Practice and other GP initiatives. The DH, now called the DHSC, can be proud of that record. But, after GP postgraduate training was established by law in 1982, it backed off and consistently declined to support many of the developmental innovations that general practice repeatedly requested (RCGP, 1989b; Conference of Academic Organisations, 1996). From 1989 onwards, the College was asking for research training fellowships and support for higher professional training which the DH consistently funded only for specialist medicine. In 2012 the RCGP worked very hard, led by Clare (now Dame) Gerada, and built a cross-specialty consensus on the need for a year's further postgraduate training for GPs Gerada C *et al.*, (2012a and b). The DH and Health Education England rejected this whilst supporting up to eight years' postgraduate training in some medical specialties (just GPs).

The third and an important cause for the lack of respect for general practice lies with GPs themselves; as Shakespeare put it: "The fault dear Brutus lies not in our stars but in ourselves." Some GPs have a professional inferiority complex. This is understandable when they have all been trained in medical schools that are specialist orientated and where even today only 6.5% of the academic staff are generalists (Campbell J *et al.,* 2015b) and 87% of their experience is based on specialists in hospitals (Harding *et al.,* 2015).

The RCGP, the GMC, the medical schools, and GP postgraduate training have not remedied this corporate inferiority complex because they have not tackled the central issue of why general practice is a distinct medical specialty. They do not teach systematically the research explaining this to the most intelligent generation of students ever. Nor do they teach the areas of medical practice where general practice leads the medical profession. Some GPs lack pride in their discipline because many do not know the research on their own core principles and general practice's successes: integrating preventive and curative medicine, integrating mental and physical problems, and integrating physical and social factors to provide sensitive personal care for a precisely defined population (DPG, 2023). GP leaders often acquire their confidence by reading.

Medical students and GP trainees still may never receive a specific reading list for general practice and often do not have the chance to discuss classic GP texts, which still inspire. Meanwhile, other undergraduate university students are supported in studying key texts in their chosen field. Most medical schools do not examine the principles of general practice in MB finals, signalling to all medical students that the principles of general practice are dispensable. General practice recruitment will remain a problem as long as medical students are denied understanding of how exciting and interesting the job is, illuminated by its underpinning research. Many students choose careers in the specialties in ignorance of the full potential of a career in general practice.

Nature of General Practice

GPs refer problem patients to specialists who are better at diagnosing rare diseases, particularly through their access to investigations. So it is an easy, false, shortcut to assume that specialists are generally cleverer and better than GPs. The prioritisation of rare (and so interesting to specialists) diseases over common ones is a prejudice that needs challenging. It is obviously in the interest of most people and the NHS that common conditions are seen as the most important and need to be managed as well as possible and as a high priority in the public interest.

GPs in the front line of the NHS see "undifferentiated" (Balint, 1955, 1957) presentations in all parts of the body and mind. Specialist medicine tends to underestimate and undervalue this function wrongly, assuming that most such presentations are trivial. It is rarely noted in hospitals that diagnoses are more difficult to make in the very early stages of illness.

The generalist function is the most demanding in medicine because the breadth of problems that may be encountered is the widest range in any branch of medicine, being literally from head to toe; i.e. migraine to an ingrowing toe nail. GPs face the greatest uncertainties in medicine. Katerndahl *et al.* (2015) assessed the complexity of family medicine consultations compared with cardiology and psychiatry and found generalist consultations were the more complex.

Any patient can have anything wrong. Diagnostic failures dog GPs, but Professor William Hamilton (Professor of Primary Care Diagnostics) notes that almost every symptom a GP sees might be a first presentation of cancer. Patients with a cough are common but each instance may be cancer or tuberculosis. Some people write that all symptoms must be fully investigated, not understanding the clinical challenge. Even for the limited number of patients with standard, 'red flag' symptoms of cancer risk who are promptly referred by GPs under the 'urgent,' two-week wait system, 93% after detailed testing do not have cancer. The costs of this are already causing concern, whilst policy is that GP referrals should increase referrals to a rate when 97% of patients do not have cancer. Furthermore, one of the main difficulties in cancer diagnosis for GPs is that the early symptoms of a cancer often occur in patients who already have another, different, established disease which causes exactly the same symptom. Medicine is the only science where the study of a part is rated more highly than the study of the whole (person).

Clinical uncertainty is too daunting for some doctors who choose to reduce it by narrowing the clinical field in which they work. In most specialty practice, except accident and emergency medicine and anaesthetics, the vast majority of the patients have been selected into just that one specialty. Some consultants are now one-operation surgeons or like diabetologists, one-disease doctors.

A major reason for the lower respect that many specialists give to general practice is that GPs are seen to be dealing with many psychosocial problems, which specialists do not see as mainline medicine at all. When specialists meet these problems, they often sidestep them or refer patients to social workers. Whereas to GPs seeking to make a three-dimensional diagnosis (integrating physical, psychological, and social factors (Evans and DPG, 1999) they are an integral component of the job. Social determinants matter and social prescribing in general practice has a long history.

Hospital medicine tends to accept a hierarchy with physical diseases being seen as more important than psychological diseases and many staff see social problems as outside their purview. 'Diagnoses' like 'functional condition' indicate a lower priority for some conditions than 'real medicine,' i.e. pathologically based disease. It is disappointing that British medical schools for so many years have produced many doctors who believe that a patient whose symptoms arise from a pathological lesion is more worthy than another patient whose symptoms arise from emotional trauma.

Multimorbidity is an important and growing role for GPs who are best placed to manage it. Learning the patient's priorities is necessary and good working relationships between doctor and patient become essential in learning how best to make management decisions. Long-term diseases need long-term continuity of care. Sometimes the treatment of one condition should be prioritised over treatment of another. The structure of hospitals around single specialty departments is increasingly awkward and inconvenient in helping older people with multiple diseases.

Just a GP

The title of this book, *Just a GP*, is based on my personal experiences described in several chapters which show that successive governments, specialist medicine, and the NHS have often not treated doctors in general practice equally compared with doctors in specialist medicine. I was introduced to this at Cambridge, when as President of the university chess club, a leading specialist said to me: "There is no need for you to be just a GP!" 'Just a GP' is a statement about the relationship between general practice and specialist medicine, in which general practice is perceived as inferior. I used the phrase as the title for my Gale memorial lecture (DPG, 1980a). In choosing it again, 40 years on, for the title of this book, I seek to highlight this little discussed problem, to generate discussion, and hopefully to stimulate counter measures.

In seeking to redress the balance, I am repeating the attempt by Horder (1977) in his lecture "Physicians and family doctors: a new relationship," when he sought to establish general practice as different and equal with specialist medicine. This has been my philosophy too. Horder presented the case for general practice clinically and argued it on the grounds of moral and intellectual equivalence.

I am trying a different approach with research and political evidence interwoven with the story of my life. The fact that I am having to do so 47 years after his attempt indicates that he failed in his aim of achieving equality and that I may do so too. The inferior position of general practice reflects a common view inside and outside the medical profession that specialists are intrinsically superior to generalists. This is understandable as often specialising means acquiring additional skills. The many successes of specialist medicine are striking and well known. My family and I have received some excellent care from specialists. However, the priority is to recognise the unique roles and value of frontline generalist doctors.

In 1948 when the NHS was established, UK medical schools formed a specialist-based partnership with them. General practice was excluded, as it was not then a discipline (established in 1961, DPG, 1989). When specialists received postgraduate training and GPs had none, it was reasonable for specialists to feel superior. In the 1970s, Professor John Ledingham at Oxford, with whom I later got on well as fellow Nuffield trustees, reported that the Oxford University view was that: "General practice had no [original] content" (Walker, 1978). Successive governments thought so little of general practice that for 23 years, from 1948 to 1981, they allowed doctors untrained for general practice to have unlimited clinical responsibility when doing it.

Even 11 years after GP postgraduate training was introduced by law, the NHS (Walford, 1992) funded over 4,500 postgraduate, registrar and training posts in specialist medicine and none for general practice (the sharpest discrimination I had then met (Chapter 14, Regional Adviser story), a statement that general practice was not seen as important or as complex as specialist medicine.

Moreover, medical specialists still undertake longer postgraduate training (up to eight years; ST8s), compared to GPs who have about four to five years; specialists also have a more rigorous training as GP vocational training has currently lost touch with the research base of its own discipline. This perpetuates attitudes.

Asymmetries

There are several asymmetries between general practice and specialist medicine, with most GPs having respect for most specialists. Whilst, as shown in several chapters, as late as the 1990s, leading specialists thought they had a monopoly of academic research and excellence and did not respect general practice as a discipline. GPs rarely dispute research underpinning the various branches of hospital medicine whereas many specialists conceptualise general practice as hospital medicine outside hospital, practised at a more superficial level. Many do not know the underpinning GP research and do not respect general practice as an independent clinical discipline. A Royal College President said as late as 2000 that he could not vote for me for the Chair of the Academy because: "General practice does not have a discipline" (Chapter 36; Vice-Chair, Academy of Medical Royal Colleges). It had then one for 39 years and he was at the top of the medical profession.

Postgraduate education in general practice needs reform so that GP trainees learn the key research in their own discipline. Similarly postgraduate education in the specialties needs to be reformed so that doctors in specialist medicine learn about major research and developments in medicine outside hospitals.

GPs invite specialists thousands of times a year to lecture on advances in their fields, but it is almost unknown for hospital staff to request a GP to lecture on general practice: they don't believe they have anything important to learn. Specialist medicine is good at displaying, sometimes trumpeting, its successes. Whereas general practice successes are less visible and general practice does not have a tradition of broadcasting clinical successes, even though some of them are substantial. The areas listed below where general practice leads the medical profession are rarely discussed.

All doctors make mistakes but there is an asymmetry in the way these are seen and commented on by the two halves of the profession. Both halves see the failures of the other half of the profession. The fact that 100 or more GPs may refer to one hospital means that hospital doctors see the collective mistakes of all those GPs. Such mistakes are inevitably widely discussed by groups of doctors and many nurses, as I have witnessed in both teaching and a non-teaching hospitals. This is not necessarily prejudicial behaviour by hospital doctors but follows from the way hospitals see referrals from many GPs.

However, the mistakes made by hospital doctors are seen by only one general practice and, in personal list general practices, may be understood by only one GP. Furthermore, GPs are much less likely to talk about such mistakes. For many years in practice, I kept a notebook of all serious mistakes made by the practice and those made by the hospital. Hospital mistakes included:

- A child referred to a consultant physician with the diagnosis of scurvy had the diagnosis ridiculed in writing, but it was soon confirmed by a consultant orthopaedic specialist.
- A consultant refusing a brain scan and diagnosing depression for a patient referred with a full history and a strong recommendation for a scan. [Reversed and patient scanned after a vigorous GP protest and a brain lesion found.]
- A consultant advising a child with a shorter leg to have the good leg shortened. The GP refused to endorse this and referred to a London orthopaedic consultant who disagreed with the Exeter specialist's opinion.
- A patient given two cards with two different blood groups (creating the possibility for a potentially lethal blood transfusion) spotted by the GP.
- A patient discharged with asthma on beta-blocker drugs (after a British GP had been prosecuted for manslaughter for doing that).
- A patient with a perforated duodenal ulcer being discharged from an accident and emergency department leading his GP to re-admit urgently.
- A child admitted with probable meningitis, who was observed by junior doctors without calling a consultant, until just before the child died of meningitis.
- A consultant being told by a devout Christian after an operation had gone wrong: "I am trying to forgive you" (a signal of needing to talk) but not understanding or having a private talk with that patient, retaining his retinue of juniors. He was subsequently successfully sued.

The conclusions over more than 25 years, were that big medical mistakes in our practice population were slightly more often made by the hospital than the practice. GPs must accept that as the biggest branch of medicine, if they make mistakes at the same rate as specialists, they will always be responsible in absolute terms for the biggest number of them. Doctors generally are reluctant to discuss the error rate in clinical practice, which is much higher than patients would like. Singh *et al.* (2013) reported a diagnostic error rate of 10.8% for primary care consultations which was the same rate that Vincent *et al.* (2001) found for British patients in hospitals suffering adverse events, a third of which led to "moderate or greater disability or death." [I had previously voted in the Nuffield Trust to fund this research.] Briggs *et al.* (2008) reported a rate of 13% for "major discrepancies" in specialist reports in radiology.

GPs' diagnostic mistakes are often discussed in both medical journals and the lay press, to the advantage of specialist medicine. Failures by specialists are less often discussed. However, more than half of all patients referred by GPs to chest pain clinics are returned without a diagnosis (Dumville *et al.,* 2007) and with a brief note: "No abnormal cardiovascular findings. Discharged." Because specialist medicine defines its mission in terms of pathology only, this escapes comment. Similarly, many patients with medically unexplained symptoms fare the same way: "No abnormal findings in such and such a specialty." GPs have a demanding and continuing role and very rarely discharge patients (put them off the list), even when some patients and some problems are exceptionally difficult. Virtually every criminal and every psychopath is on some GP's list.

Most doctors in all branches of medicine gain professional satisfaction from making a diagnosis. This satisfaction is often enhanced if another doctor has previously missed the diagnosis. Hospital doctors inevitably gain professional satisfaction from making diagnoses GPs have missed or got wrong.

However, the situation is different in general practice. Having sat in a practice common room with GPs for many years seeing test results and hospital letters being read, I noted that a hospital mistake brought little satisfaction. On the contrary, it was often painful for the GP as it usually meant bad news for a well-known patient with whom the GP identified and usually meant extra work. I did see occasional gloating when a GP diagnosis was vindicated, but not as much as I had seen in hospital after GP errors.

Leading the Medical Profession

Prejudice against medical generalists continues, but research evidence has quietly emerged that GPs are leading the medical profession in at least seven important ways. GPs have longer and deeper working relationships with patients than specialists and value them. More patients do not remember the name of their consultant than their GP. The traditional role of the British family doctor being the one known health professional who understands the patient is now under threat, but is still a reality in many general practices.

Dame Sally Davies was interviewed when she retired as Chief Medical Officer for England (Ross, 2019). Disturbingly, she reported she often visited junior doctors in hospitals and asked them if their consultants knew their names. She said that: "It's rare that a hand goes up." This clashes with the attitudes and practices of GP trainers and leaves GPs as the guardians and leaders of human relationships within medical education and the medical profession.

Relationships with patients are often undervalued in hospital medicine since in many specialties care is often episodic and long-term follow up relatively rare. My consultant friends often asked me about what happened to patients they had seen in hospital. The value of general practice was starkly revealed whilst I was a member of the Academy, and the interim Wanless Report (2002) was published. This showed that patients were more satisfied with "Your NHS GP" than with hospital in-patients or outpatients. One specialist Royal College president expostulated to me: "How can this be true when in teaching hospitals (where he worked) we have all the expertise, the investigation equipment and most of the nurses?!" I quietly explained that GPs had the better relationships with patients, were more accessible and better known to patients. In his 60s, and top of his tree, it was this leading consultant's introduction to evidence of the importance of doctor–patient relationships in medicine. Nor was this a new finding as the *British Social Attitudes* survey had reported that patient dissatisfaction with hospital outpatients was more than twice as high as that for general practice, 11 years earlier (Jowell *et al.,* 1991).

General practice has the privilege of being best placed to build partnership relationships with patients over time and the necessary time is available. Patients in Islington, London with multiple long-term conditions, averaged 15 years' duration of relationship with their general practice (Barker *et al.,* 2018).

Another interesting area is postgraduate medical education where general practice, despite a start as late as the 1970s, has quietly overtaken specialist medicine, as shown by three separate sets of evidence. Lamberts and Goldacre (2006) surveyed 5,344 doctors in their first postgraduate year asking eight educational questions and others about management and nursing support. For seven of the eight educational aspects, GP training posts were rated the most highly, all being significantly (P<0.01) better than ratings from junior doctors in hospital training posts. "Being required to perform tasks for which they felt inadequately trained" was the lowest in general practice 6.2% vs. 16.3% in surgical training. Several other ratings were twice as good as those in medical and surgical training posts. Management and nursing support in general practice was also judged better. The next year Paice and Smith (2009) unearthed disturbing evidence of a significant amount of bullying of junior doctors in British postgraduate training in several specialties and minimally in GP training practices.

Thirdly, the GMC (2018) national training surveys, year after year, report that junior doctors in post-graduate training are more satisfied in training general practices than in specialty placements. Despite this the NHS until 2022 paid more to hospitals than to GPs for teaching the same medical students.

General practice leads the medical profession in the integration of physical and mental health whose separation is the great unmentioned, fault-line of specialist medicine. Much specialist mental health is still provided in mental hospitals, well separated from hospitals dealing with physical diseases. Psychiatry still has stigma. Patients go to GPs with physical and emotional problems without stigma and GPs deal with both kinds of problem in the same consultation. This is successful integration and a profession-leading system.

A fundamental realignment of priorities in medicine and health care is now happening as recent research indicates that a huge amount of illness is caused by social factors (so-called social determinants) of ill health. These include the patient's home, family, work and patient's educational and income level. The new importance of these factors when combined may, remarkably, be as important as all medical treatments (Magnan, 2017). This puts general practice in a leadership position in medicine. No other branch of the profession knows these factors better and general practice is best placed to gather more of this information and integrate it best into clinical care.

The costs of modern health care inevitably keep rising but do so at a rate in most countries that is often greater than the annual rate of inflation. This gives those who pay for health care a continuing problem; in the UK this is the Government. Hence, evidence of cost-effectiveness becomes increasingly important. On this factor alone, general practice comes into its own. Several studies have revealed that continuity of GP care is associated with lower costs in the overall health system (De Maeseneer *et al.*, 2003; Bazemore *et al.*, 2023). There are three important research studies from the 1990s in which generalist doctors were compared directly with different kinds of specialists, which I cited in my lecture to the specialist presidents (Chapter 38, Chair of the Academy of Medical Royal Colleges). The Edinburgh depression study (Scott and Freeman, 1992) compared GP care for patients with depression with care from consultant psychiatrists and social workers. There was a marginal gain from consultant care at a big increase in cost. Policies steering depressed patients to psychiatrists ceased. As well, Carey *et al.* (1995) compared family physician care for new backache, randomised against care from specialist orthopaedic surgeons and chiropracters. The outcomes were the same for all three groups. The chiropracters had the best patient satisfaction but through seeing patients far more often than the two kinds of doctor. The orthopaedic specialists had the highest costs through using computerised tomography much more. For policymakers, the conclusion was that family physicians were the most efficient obtaining the same outcomes at far lower costs. Finally, Friedlr *et al.* (1997) compared in a randomised study, GP care to counselling. They concluded: "General-practitioner care is as effective as brief psychotherapy for patients usually referred by doctors to practice-based psychotherapists."

These three studies show that conventional, low-tech, personal and friendly care, with focused consultation skills, encouragement and practical suggestions is more effective than generally recognised and is cost-effective. This efficiency is so great that the cost to the NHS of a patient seeing a GP is lower than the NHS cost of a patient seeing a nurse in a nurse-led walk-in centre (Salisbury *et al.*, 2002). This great cost efficiency is relatively little discussed by policy-makers.

Social inequality is one of the biggest social problems and has been thought to be outside medical practice. Now, however, it has been found that general practice can partially alleviate socio-economic disadvantage. This was first found in the USA but has been confirmed in the UK. The strong association between socioeconomic disadvantage and mortality is reduced by primary care in the USA (Shi, 1992; Shi *et al.*, 2003). Professor Sir Julian Le Grand (1945–), an economist who advised a Prime Minister, concluded that "the distribution of use of [UK] general practitioners (GPs) is broadly equitable, that for specialist treatment is pro-rich" (Dixon, Le Grand *et al.*, 2007). Numerous social and cultural factors impede poor people and more so for hospitals than practices. This important GP achievement is through generalist doctors' practices being local, 'within pram-pushing distances,' being embedded in communities, being more socially aware, seeing patients repeatedly for different conditions over time, and so becoming a more human service. General practice's leading position is confirmed. Hetlevik *et al* (2021) showed that, using educational attainment as a proxy for deprivation, GPs are effective in bridging the inequality divide.

The world is now dominated by machines and is less personal as more activities are undertaken remotely. General practice has long led in rejecting the machine model of medicine (Batten, 1955), which tends to depersonalise patients. Health care is always personal to the patient as illness is a personal threat, so important human behaviour is involved. Patients yearn for care that recognises them as a person rather than being a case of something. Hospital medicine is gradually becoming more technical, and investigation orientated. Many consultants will only see a patient in outpatients after many tests have been completed. The cost-efficiency of this is rarely discussed. Meanwhile GPs manage bigger numbers using fewer investigations. The difference is between generalist doctors who using discretion in requesting investigations and specialists who often request a battery of tests for everyone.

Continuity of Care

GPs have undervalued themselves for years in terms of the importance and effectiveness of continuity of GP care, where the GP's personality, skills and relationship with patients are important (Balint, 1957; "the doctor as drug"). The following findings are statistically significantly associated with continuity of GP care, which is a proxy measure for doctor–patient relationships.

- Better patient satisfaction (Adler *et al.*, 2010)
- Better adherence to medical advice (Youens *et al.*, 2021)
- Better adherence for prescribed medication (Warren *et al.*, 2015)
- Better take-up of personal preventive medicine like immunisations and cervical smear tests (O'Malley *et al.,* 1997; Christakis *et al.*, 2000)
- Better patient GP communication (Katz *et al.*, 2014)
- Lower workload in a practice (Kajira-Montag *et al,* 2024)
- Higher quality of GP care both acute (Granier *et al.*, 1998) and chronic physical illnesses (O'Connor *et al.*, 1998) and chronic mental illnesses (Delgado *et al.,* 2022)
- Lower use of A&E departments (McGovern *et al.*, 2017)
- Lower use of hospital admissions, especially for the elderly with ambulatory care sensitive conditions (where GP care is especially valuable) (Barker *et al.,* 2017).

These nine outcomes include some of the most important in the whole of medical practice, but two more overarching findings have been revealed. General practice/primary care continuity is significantly associated with better outcomes and reduced overall costs in the health system (De Maeseneer *et al.,* 2003; Bazemore *et al.,* 2023) – the Holy Grail for NHS policymakers. Costs are and will remain a challenge for governments in all countries and it is only recently that the relatively high costs of specialist care are becoming visible. One emergency hospital admission lasting more than one night costs the NHS as much as £3,899. Despite a series of experiments to reduce admissions, only continuity of GP care has been repeatedly shown to be linked over time to a lower rate of such admissions. How long will it take for the NHS to realise this?

Two systematic reviews reported that patients have lower mortality with continuity of doctor care (DPG and Sidaway-Lee *et al.*, 2018c) and specifically for primary care staff (Baker *et al.*, 2020). Death is the ultimate outcome and patients, when they learn this, will take it seriously. All this research has not yet been digested by the programme directors running GP vocational training schemes nor by NHS policymakers. How long will it take for the penny to drop?

Generalist Thinking

Generalist thinking is broader than much specialist thinking which, by concentrating on pathology, can become reductionist. It focuses on the individual patient, their priorities. It uses context in its widest sense, the patient's previous experiences including the family and personal environment. Uncertainty in medicine has been queried but, interestingly, quantum physics accepts profound uncertainties in theory and fact, both for the exact position of an element and the power of relationships. Context includes time: a consultation between a GP and patient who have known each other for years can be very different from the same GP seeing a strange patient for the same condition.

GPs working directly with patients in the front line of the NHS have to do their best in real time and often without evidence from randomised trials. They often give advice based "on the balance of probabilities." and use a wide range of social information. The COVID-19 pandemic has provided three interesting examples of the value of generalist v specialist thinking.

First, early in the pandemic, leading public health physicians, speaking at 10 Downing Street, advised against the use of masks because there had not been randomised trials to support their use. It is a common limitation of epidemiological thinking that if there is not a randomised trial in support of a policy it cannot be recommended. Generalist politicians quickly rejected this advice.

Medical specialists often find it more difficult than medical generalists to say they do not know. They are also less willing to use socially based, contextual information to give advice. Facts like COVID-19 is a respiratory virus, and that masks protect others, are much used in countries with the most experience of such diseases, and that are most unlikely to have adverse effects were initially seen as non-scientific but were publicised after adoption of the mask wearing policy.

Second, the biggest policy mistake in the COVID pandemic was discharging patients untested, or with COVID-19, into care homes. If one or two GPs who had patients in care homes had been on Scientific Advisory Group for Emergencies (SAGE) or on the DH staff they might have been able to stop such advice from expert public health doctors/epidemiologists, whose clinical experience was too narrow and whose expectations of care homes were too high.

Third, in 2021, the Joint Committee on Vaccination and Immunisation (JCVI) advised against vaccines for 12–15 year olds. The four UK Chief Medical Officers soon gave the opposite advice; taking school attendance, long COVID, and the risk of children infecting older people into account. The JCVI thus, in effect, stated it was too specialised and too narrowly constituted to advise. Generalist thinking prevailed.

General practice has the longest and deepest relationships with patients in medicine and the best opportunity to provide humane personal care, to integrate physical and psychosocial medicine, and to integrate preventive and therapeutic care. With the best medical teachers and providing the most cost-effective care, the long-term future of general practice is secure, even if the short-term outlook looks bumpy. Far from being seen as inferior, general practice will in time emerge as the branch of the medical profession that is *primus inter pares*.

Our Family

One of the biggest changes in my life has been the growth of our family. Jill was an only child and always wanted a big family. I was one of two boys. Now there are our four children, three sons/daughters-in-law, 14 grandchildren, three of whom have been adopted, and these have given us four grandson/daughters-in-law and six great-grandchildren. Being close to my brother and sister-in-law makes a family group of 35. As in the title of one of the classic books about a GP (Berger and Mohr, 1968), I am a "fortunate man."

Appendices

Appendix 1: Personal Awards

CIVIL HONOURS

1981	OBE	Queen's Birthday Honours List
1999	Knight Bachelor	New Year Honours List

UNIVERSITIES

1997   Honorary Doctor of Science, De Montfort University
2003   Honorary Doctor of Medicine, University of Nottingham
2009   Honorary Doctor of Science, University of Exeter

PROFESSIONAL

1966   Gold Medal of the Hunterian Society
1967   Sir Charles Hastings Prize of the BMA
1969   Gold Medal of the Hunterian Society
1978   George Abercrombie Award for contributions to the literature
1980   Foundation Council Award of the Royal College of General Practitioners
1981   Sir Harry Platt Prize
1989   Silver Medal of the SIMG, Florence, Italy
1997   Honorary Fellow of the Royal Society of Health
1997   Honorary Fellow of the Faculty of Public Health
1999   Gold Medal of the Royal Institute of Public Health and Hygiene
1999   Fellowship of the Royal College of Physicians of London
2000   Honorary Member of the Cuban Association of Family Physicians Cuba
2000   Honorary Member of the Polish Association of Family Physicians, Kracow, Poland
2001   Honorary Fellow of the Royal College of Physicians of Ireland, Dublin
2003   Honorary Fellow of the Faculty of General Dental Practitioners Royal College of Surgeons
2013   Honorary Fellow of the Academy of Medical Educators
2022   RCGP Life-Time Achievement Award

Appendix 2: Eponymous or Equivalent Lectures

Year	Name	Site	Published
1977	James Mackenzie Lecture	RCGP AGM London	DPG (1978) *JRCGP*
1979	Pfizer Lecture	RCGP North-East England Faculty, Newcastle	DPG (1979a) *JRCGP*
1979	Gale Memorial Lecture	RCGP South-West England Faculty, Barnstaple, Devon	DPG (1980a) *JRCGP*
1988	Harvard Davis Lecture	RCGP Welsh Council, Denbigh, Wales	
1988	Haliburton Hume Lecture	Newcastle-Upon-Tyne	
	Eli Lilley Lecture	Ballymoney, Northern Ireland	
1988	McConaghey Memorial Lecture	RCGP Tamar Faculty, Lifton, Devon	DPG (1989) *JRCGP*
1988	Northcott Memorial Lecture	Barnstaple, Devon	
1990	Murray Scott Lecture	North-East Scotland Faculty, of the RCGP, Aberdeen	
1994	Harben Lecture	Royal Institute of Public Health and Hygiene, London	
1995	Sally Irvine Lecture	Association of Managers in General Practice, Ashridge, Herts	
1997	Annual Address	Royal Society of Health	
1998	Albert Wander Lecture	Royal Society of Medicine	
1998	Andrew Smith Lecture	RCGP North of England, Durham	
1999	David Bruce Lecture	Armed Services London	
2000	Reading Oration	Reading	
2002b	Frans Huygen Lecture	Nijmegen, The Netherlands	DPG (2002) *Huisarts en Wetenchap*
2002	Deakin Lecture	Melbourne, Australia	
2002	Long Fox Lecture	Bristol Medical Society, Bristol	
2013	Doreen Goodman Lecture	What About the Children? London	DPG (2013) Published privately
2015	Starfield Memorial Lecture	College of Medicine and Health, University of Exeter	DPG (2017a) *BJGP Open*
2022	McConaghey Memorial Lecture	Tamar Faculty, Royal College of General Practitioners, Exeter	DPG (2023) *Br J Gen Pract*
2023	Gale Memorial Lecture	Severn Faculty, Royal College of General Practitioners, Bristol	

Appendix 3: Publications (in Addition to the Journal) from the RCGP Exeter Publications Office

Reports from General Practice

Reports from General Practice represent RCGP policy. Most were formally adopted by the Council of the College, and a few were judged by the officers of the College to be in accordance with College policy. Twelve separate *Reports from General Practice* were published by the Exeter Publications Office of the RCGP between 1972 and 1997, and four of them, Nos 18–21, were subsequently republished as a combined publication. They were all posted to fellows, members, and associates of the RCGP.

No	Date	Title	Author/Editor	Pages and notes
15	June 1972	*Teaching Practices*	Donald Irvine	43pp
16	March 1973	*Present State and Future Needs of General Practice* *Third edition*	John Fry OBE	63pp
17	June 1976	*The assessment of vocational training for general practice*	PS Byrne CBE	26pp
New format: A4				
18	February 1981	*Health and Prevention in Primary Care*	Chairman of the Main Working Party: John Horder OBE	24pp
19	February 1981	*Prevention of Arterial Disease in General Practice*	Chairman of the Working Party: Julian Tudor Hart	19pp
20	February 1981	*Prevention of Psychiatric Disorders in General Practice*	Chairman of the Working Party: Philip Graham Convenor: Peter Tomson	17pp
21	August 1981	*Family Planning: An Exercise in Preventive Medicine*	Chairman of the Working Party: Allen Hutchinson	7pp
22	1982	*Healthier Children – Thinking Prevention*	Co-Convenors: Christopher Donovan, Denis Pereira Gray	113pp
18–21	September 1984	*Combined Reports on Prevention*		67pp
23	July 1985	*What Sort of Doctor?*	Chairmen of Working Parties: JAR Lawson OBE TPC Schofield	27pp
24	1986	Alcohol – A Balanced View	J Bennison	57pp

(Continued)

No	Date	Title	Author/Editor	Pages and notes
New Format: Two colour cover				
25	March 1987	*The Front Line of the Health Service*	Denis Pereira Gray	24pp
26	April 1995	*The Development and Implementation of Clinical Guidelines*	Allen Hutchinson	31pp
27	January 1996	*The Nature of General Medical Practice*	Nigel Stott	20pp

Supplements to the *Journal of the Royal College of General Practitioners*

Supplements to the *Journal of the Royal College of General Practitioners* were posted to all fellows, members and associates of the College with a copy of the *Journal*. They do not represent the policy of the College; their status is the same as an article in the *Journal* and they were edited to the same standard. The Exeter Publications Office of the RCGP edited and published 11 Supplements between 1972 and 1997.

No	Date	Title	Authors/Editor	Pages and notes
1	August 1972	*General Practitioners and Abortion*	Ann Cartwright, Marjorie Waite	63pp
2	October 1972	*General Practice in the London Borough of Camden*	Victor W Sidel, Margot Jefferys, Peter J Mansfield	26pp
3	September 1972	*General Practitioners and Contraception*	Ann Cartwright, Marjorie Waite	31pp
4	November 1972	*The Renaissance of General Practice*	John H Hunt	20pp
5	February 1973	*Undergraduate Departments of General Practice*	Professor PS Byrne	12pp
6	June 1973 Second edition	*A General Practice Glossary*	The Research Unit of the Royal College of General Practitioners	15pp
7	September 1974	*The Medical Use of Psychotropic Drugs*	Peter Parish, WM Williams, PC Elmes (Eds)	80pp
8	September 1974	*The Hostile Environment of Man*	Yorkshire Faculty	46pp
9	October 1974	*A visit to Australia and the Far East*	George Swift	19pp
10	December 1976	*Prescribing in General Practice*	The Medical Sociology Research Centres, University College of Swansea, Wales	108pp
11	April 1980	*Prescribing for the Elderly in General Practice*	James DE Knox	8pp

Occasional Papers

The *Occasional* Papers were academic manuscripts introduced in 1976. They were submitted to, assessed, accepted, edited and published by the Exeter Publications office in Marlborough Road and then put on sale. There were 75 from the Exeter office and an additional three after the office closed in 1997. All were selected and edited by DPG.

No	Date	Title	Authors/Editors	Pages and notes
1	December 1976	*An International Classification of the Health Problems of Primary Care*	BG Bentzen, WONCA Working Party	41pp
2	December 1976	*An Opportunity to Learn*	EV Kuenssberg CBE	78pp
3	December 1976	*Trends in National Morbidity*	RCGP Birmingham Research Unit	41pp
New format: All green in A4				
4	September1977	*A System of Training for General Practice*	DJ Pereira Gray	Author DPG 29pp
	September 1979	Second edition		
5	July 1978	*Medical Records in General Practice*	LI Zander, Shirley A Beresford, Patricia Thomas	38pp
6	August 1978	*Some Aims for Training for General Practice*	RCGP	17pp
7	December 1979	*Doctors on the Move*	John Bevan, Diane Cunningham, Clifford Floyd	35pp
8	March 1979	*Patients and their Doctors 1977*	Ann Cartwright, Robert Anderson	22pp
9	November 1979	*General Practitioners and Postgraduate Education in the Northern Region*	BLEC Reedy, Barbara Gregson, Margaret Williams	29pp
10	May 1980	*Selected Papers from the Eighth World Conference on Family Medicine*	WONCA	44pp
11	June 1980	*Section 63 Activities*	J Wood, PS Byrne	50pp
12	July 1980	*Hypertension in Primary Care*	John Coope	38pp
13	June 1980	*Computers in Primary Care*	Computer Working Party Chairman: C Kay CBE	19pp
14	September 1980	*Education for Cooperation in Health and Social Work*	Central Council of Education and Training in Social Work, Panel of Assessors for District Nurse Training, Council for the Education and Training of Health Visitors, Royal College of General Practitioners Hugh England (Ed)	31pp
15	March 1981	*The Measurement of the Quality of General Practitioner Care*	CJ Watkins	18pp
16	May 1981	*A Survey of Primary Care in London*	Brian Jarman	138pp
17	June 1981	*Patient Participation in General Practice*	Peter Pritchard (Ed)	40pp
18	October 1981	*Fourth National Trainee Conference, Exeter 1980*	Clare Ronalds, Angela Douglas, Denis Pereira Gray, Peter Selley (Eds)	84pp
19	December 1981	*Inner Cities*	KJ Bolden Dept of General Practice, University of Exeter	13pp

(Continued)

No	Date	Title	Authors/Editors	Pages and notes
20	September 1982	*Medical Audit in General Practice*	Michael G Sheldon	21pp
21	December 1982	*The Influence of Trainers on Trainees in General Practice*	James Freeman, James Roberts, David Metcalfe, Valerie Hillier	17pp
22	May 1983	*Promoting Prevention*	RCGP Colin Waine (Ed)	11pp
23	September 1983	*General Practitioner Hospitals*	RCGP Working Party	12pp
24	January 1984	*Prescribing – A Suitable Case of Treatment*	CM Harris, B Jarman, W Woodman, P White, JS Fry	39pp
25	April 1984	*Social Class and Health Status: Inequality of Difference McConaghey Memorial Lecture 1983*	DL Crombie OBE	15pp
26	May 1984	*Classification of Diseases, Problems and Procedures 1984*	RCGP	68pp
	June 1986	Second edition under title: *The Classification and Analysis of General Practice Data*	RCGP	125pp
27	October 1984	*Clinical Knowledge and Education for General Practice*	HWK Acheson, Margaret Henley	28pp
28	December 1984	*Undergraduate Medical Education in General Practice*	Association of University Teachers in General Practice in the UK and Republic of Ireland	25pp
29	March 1985	*Trainee Projects*	Trainee Syntex Award Winners 1981–1984	52pp
30	1985	*Priorities and Objectives for General Practice Vocational Training*	Oxford Region Course Organisers and Regional Advisers Group	15pp
	1988	Second edition		
31	April 1985	*Booking for Maternity Care: A Comparison of Two Systems*	Michael Klein, Diana Elbourne, Ivor Lloyd	17pp
New format: Two colour				
32	June 1986	*An Atlas of Bedside Microscopy*	JM Longmore	30pp
33	September 1986	*Working Together – Learning Together*	RVH Jones Exeter Department of General Practice	26pp
34	October 1986	Course Organisers in General Practice	AHE Williams	39pp
35	March 1987	*Preventive Care of the Elderly: A Review of Current Developments*	RC Taylor, EG Buckley	53pp
36	September 1987	*The Prevention of Depression: Current Approaches*	P Freeling, LJ Downey, JC Malkin	21pp
37	January 1988	*The Work of Counsellors in General Practice*	June McLeod	13pp

(Continued)

No	Date	Title	Authors/Editors	Pages and notes
38	May 1988	*Continuing Education for General Practitioners*	Alan Branthwaite, Alistair Ross, Ann Henshaw, Charmian Davie	39pp
39	July 1988	*Practice Assessment and Quality of Care*	Richard Baker	30pp
40	1988	*Rating Scales for Vocational Training in General Practice*	Centre for Primary Care Research, Department of General Practice, University of Manchester	40pp
41	December 1988	*Practice Activity Analysis*	DL Crombie, DM Fleming	47pp
42	December 1988	*The Contribution of Academic General Practice to Undergraduate Medical Education*	Robin C Fraser, Elan Preston-Whyte	40pp
43	September 1990	*Community Hospitals – Preparing for the Future*	RCGP, Associations of General Practitioner Community Hospitals	51pp
44	September 1990	*Towards a Curriculum for General Practice Training*	Oliver Samuel	44pp
45	October 1990	*Care of Old People: A Framework for Progress*	RCGP	23pp
46	November 1990	*Examination for Membership of the Royal College of General Practitioners (MRCGP)*	Cameron Lockie	61pp
47	November 1990	*Primary care for People with Mental Handicap*	RCGP Chair Working Party: Martin Barker	50pp
48	November 1990	*The Interface Study COMAC-HSR in Collaboration with European General Practice Research Workshop*	DL Crombie, J van der Zee, P Backer	67pp
49	November 1990	*A College Plan: Priorities for the Future*	RCGP Denis Pereira Gray	54pp
50	November 1990	*Fellowship by Assessment*	RCGP Drafted by DPG	52pp
	1995	Second edition	Michael Pringle	79pp
51	June 1991	*Higher Professional Education Courses in the UK*	JI Koppel, RG Pietroni	21pp
52	1991	*Interprofessional Collaboration in Primary Health Care Organisations*	Barbara Gregson, Ann Cartlidge, John Bond	52pp
53	October 1991	*Annual and Seasonal Variation in the Incidence of Common Diseases*	DM Fleming, CA Norbury, Dl Crombie	24pp
54	November 1991	*Prescribing in General Practice*	JD Gilleghan	36pp
55	March 1992	*Guidelines for the Management of Hyperlipidaemia in General Practice*	RCGP Chairman of Working Party: Colin Waine DPG and P Evans (St Leonard's Practice, Exeter): Members of the Working Party	15pp

(Continued)

No	Date	Title	Authors/Editors	Pages and notes
56	April 1992	*The European Study of Referrals from Primary to Secondary Care: Report to the Concerted Action Committee of Health Services Research for the European Community*	Chair of Project Management Group: DM Fleming *Chef de File:* P Backer	75pp
57	June 1992	*Planning Primary Care*	Denis Pereira Gray	67pp
58	December 1992	*Clinical Guidelines*	Andrew Haines, Brian Hurwitz	91pp
59	April 1993	*Health Checks for People Aged 75 and Over*	W Idris Williams, Paul Wallace	30pp
60	May 1993	*Shared Care of Patients with Mental Health Problems*	Royal College of Psychiatrists, Royal College of General Practitioners	10pp
61	August 1993	*Stress Management in General Practice*	RCGP Chairman of Working Party: Dr Michael King	42pp
62	October 1993	*The Application of a General Practice Database to Pharmaco Epidemiology*	DM Fleming, J Fullerton	21pp
63	December 1993	*Portfolio-Based Learning in General Practice*	RCGP Convenor Working Party: Roger Pietroni	22pp
64	January 1994	*Community Participation in Primary Care*	Zoe Heritage (Ed)	37pp
65	July 1994	*What Is Good General Practice?*	Peter Toon	52pp
66	October 1994	*Report of the Inner City Taskforce*	Maria Lorentzon, Brian Jarman, Madhavi Rajekal, Chair: I Heath	50pp
67	October 1994	*Shared Care for Diabetes: A Systematic Review*	PM Greenhalgh	32pp
68	February 1995	*Influences on Computer Use in General Practice*	Michael Pringle, Paul Dixon, Roy Carr-Hill, Audrey Ashworth	65pp
69	February 1995	*Drug Education*	MM Kochen	46pp
70	March 1995	*Significant Event Auditing*	Michael Pringle, Colin Bradley, Catherine Carmichael, Heather Wallis, Anne Moore	71pp
71	September 1995	*Rural General Practice in the UK*	Jim Cox	49pp
72	November 1995	*The Role of General Practice in Maternity Care*	RCGP Chairman Task Force: John Noakes	14pp
73	October 1996	*Needs Assessment in General Practice*	SJ Gillam, SA Murray	56pp
74	November 1996	*The Role of Counsellors in General Practice*	Bonnie Sibbald, Julia Addington-Hall, Douglas Brenneman, Paul Freeling	19pp
75	February 1997	*Measuring Quality in General Practice*	JGR Howie CBE, DJ Heaney, M Maxwell	32pp

(Continued)

No	Date	Title	Authors/Editors	Pages and notes
Exeter Publishing office closed			**DPG Hon Editor with staff support in London**	
76	April 1998	*The Human Side of Medicine*	M Evans, KG Sweeney KG Sweeney former partner	25pp
77	June 1998	*Genetics in Primary Care*	North West England Faculty	12pp
78	April 1999	*Towards a Philosophy of General Practice: A Study of the Virtuous Practitioner*	P Toon	69pp

The RCGP White Cover Series of Books

Between 1972 and 1997 most of the books published by the RCGP through the Exeter Publications Office were photo reproductions of books judged by the Editor to be general practice 'classics' and after the Editor had negotiated permission from the original publisher to reproduce them. They were then advertised in the College *Journal;* and in all other RCGP publications, and offered for sale from the RCGP headquarters in London.

Date	Title	Author	Notes
1978	*Doctors Talking to Patients*	Patrick S Byrne, Barrie EL Long	Republished with permission from HMSO 1976
1982	*Epidemiology and Research in a General Practice*	GI Watson	Constructed posthumously by Jill Pereira Gray
1982	*To Heal or to Harm: The Prevention of Somatic Fixation in General Practice*	Richard Grol (Ed)	First published in the Netherlands
1984	*Epidemiology in Country Practice*	William Pickles	First published by John Wright & Sons
1984	*Will Pickles of Wensleydale*	John Pemberton	First published by Geoffrey Bles 1970
1985	*Trends in General Practice Computing*	Michael Sheldon, Norman Stoddart	
1986	*Sir James Mackenzie MD: 1853–1925. General Practitioner*	Alex Mair	First published by Dekker and van de Vegt Churchill Livingstone
1986	*In Pursuit of Quality*	David Pendleton, Theo Schofield, Marshall Marinker	
1990	*Family Medicine – The Medical Life History of Families*	FJA Huygen	First published in the Netherlands
1991	*Milestones: Diary of a Trainee GP*	Peter Stott	First published by Pan Books Ltd
1992	*The Longest Art*	Kenneth Lane	First published by HarperCollins
1992	*The Future General Practitioner – Learning and Teaching*	RCGP Working Party Chair: JP Horder	First published by BMJ Publications
1994	*Psychiatry in General Practice*	CAH Watts, BM Watts	Previously published 1953
1996	*The Life of Professor PS Byrne CBE FRCGP*	John Findlater	

Individual Formats

1987	*14 Princes Gate: Home of the Royal College of General Practitioners*	John Horder, Stephen Pasmore	
1992	*The Writings of John Hunt*	J Horder (Ed)	Hardback

Booklets

Several smaller books and booklets were published on clinical, educational and organisational topics.

The RCGP Members' Reference Books

Edited annually by the Exeter RCGP publications office 1982–1997 = 16 editions.

RCGP Books Published Elsewhere

Pullen I, Wilkinson G, Wright A, Pereira Gray D (Eds) (1994) *Psychiatry and General Practice Today.* London: Royal College of Psychiatrists.

Royal College of General Practitioners (1992) *Forty Years On: The Story of the First 40 Years of the RCGP.* Pereira Gray D (Ed). London: Atalink.

Appendix 4: Medical Annuals

	No of pages	No of chapters	No of chapters by DPG and Jill PG
1983	284	28	2
1984	303	26	3 (plus one by Jill)
1985	324	29	2.5
1986	295	25	3.5
1987	241	23	2
Total for the 5 years	1,447	131	13 chapters plus one by Jill (11%)

Appendix 5: Peer-Reviewed Journal Publications by DPG's Students at the St Leonard's Practice

GP Trainees

Surname	First name	Student status	Journal	Year	Title	Vol/Pages
Bradley	Nicholas	GP Trainee	*J Roy Coll Gen Pract.*	1981	Expectations of people who consult in a training practice	31:420–5
Bradley	Nicholas	GP Trainee	*J Roy Coll Gen Pract.*	1983	Sale of cigarettes to children in Exeter	33:559–62
Colmer	Linda, *et al.*	GP Trainee	*Practitioner*	1983	An audit of the care of asthma in general practice	227:196–201
Douglas	Angela	GP Trainee	*BMJ*	1981	From city to coast	282:113–4
Douglas	Angela, *et al.*	GP Trainee	RCGP *Occasional Paper 18* (Ronalds *et al*)	1981	Fourth National Trainee Conference	Exeter: RCGP
Donohoe	Mollie, *et al.*	GP Trainee	*BMJ*	1982	How to get the most out of the trainee year	284:315–6
Kratky	Adrian	GP Trainee	*J Roy Coll Gen Pract.*	1977	An audit of the care of diabetics in one general practice	27:536–43
Mansfield	Brian	GP Trainee	*J Roy Coll Gen Pract.*	1986	How bad are medical records? A review of notes received by a practice	36:405–7
Peppiatt	Roger	GP Trainee	*Resuscitation*	1978	Blood alcohol concentrations in those attending an accident and emergency department	6:37–43
Peppiatt	Roger	GP Trainee	*Practitioner*	1979	Patients' use of general practitioners and consultant accident and emergency departments: general practitioners' expectations	224: 11–14
Selley	Peter, *et al.*	GP Trainee	RCGP *Occasional Paper 18* (Ronalds *et al*)	1981	Fourth National Trainee Conference	Exeter: RCGP
Stubbings	Clive, *et al.*	GP Trainee	*J Roy Coll Gen Pract.*	1979	A comparison of trainer and trainee experience	29:47–52
Westcott	Richard	GP Trainee	*J Roy Coll Gen Pract.*	1977	The length of consultations in general practice	27:552–5

Other Students

Surname	First name	Student status	Journal	Year	Title	Vol/Pages
Illingworth	Charlotte	Pre-registration house officer	*BMJ*	1994	The pre-registration alternative	308:1109
White	Eleanor	BSc Student	*Family Practice*	2016	Fifty years of longitudinal continuity	33:144–53
Dineen	Molly	MSc Student, jointly supervised	*Family Practice*	2021	Family history recording	https://doi.org/10.1093/fampra/cmab117

Analysis 1972–2021. Number of publications = 16 from 13 different students.

Appendix 6: Books/Booklets Written/Edited by the Staff of the Department/Institute of General Practice, University of Exeter

Year	Title	Authors	Publisher
1977	*A System of Training for General Practice* Second edition 1979	DPG	*Occasional Paper 4* RCGP
1978	*Running a Practice* Second edition Third edition	RVH Jones, KJ Bolden DPG, MS Hall	London: Croom Helm Ltd
1981	*Fourth National Trainee Conference*	C Ronalds, A Douglas, P Selley, DPG	*Occasional Paper 18* RCGP
1982	*Training for General Practice*	DPG	Plymouth: Macdonald and Evans
1982	*Healthier Children – Thinking Prevention* *Report from General Practice 22* Second Impression	Ed DPG	RCGP
1983	*A GP Training Handbook* Second and third editions	Ed MS Hall	London: Blackwell
1983	*Medical Annual 1983*	Ed DPG	Bristol: John Wright & Sons
1984	*A Practice Nurse Handbook* Second edition Third edition	KJ Bolden, B Tackle	London: Blackwell
1984	*Medical Annual 1984*	Ed DPG	Bristol: John Wright & Sons
1985	*Medical Annual 1985*	Ed DPG	Bristol: John Wright & Sons
1986	*Working Together: Learning Together*	RVH Jones	*Occasional Paper 36* RCGP
1986	*Medical Annual 1986*	Ed DPG	Bristol: John Wright & Sons
1987	*The Front Line of the Health Service*	DPG	*Report from General Practice 25* RCGP
1987	*Medical Annual 1987*	Ed DPG	Bristol: John Wright & Sons
1988	*Information Handling in General Practice*	R Westcott, RVH Jones	London: Croom Helm Ltd
1989	*Running a Course*	KJ Bolden, R Steele, D Dwyer. R Leete	Abingdon: Radcliffe Later Taylor & Francis
1990	*Fellowship by Assessment*	DPG	*Occasional Paper 50* RCGP
1992	*Planning Primary Care*	DPG	*Occasional Paper 52* RCGP
1992	*Forty Years On: The Story of the first 40 years of the RCGP*	DPG	London: Atalink

(Continued)

Year	Title	Authors	Publisher
1992	*Psychiatry and General Practice Today*	Eds I Pullen, G Wilkinson, A Wright, DPG	London: Royal College of Psychiatrists
1994	*Practice Nursing: Stability and Change*	M Damant, C Martin, S Openshaw	Guildford: Mosby
1996	*Developing Primary Care: the Academic Contribution*	DPG	Conference of Academic Organisations of General Practice RCGP
TOTALS	**22 separate publications**	**Plus 6 later editions**	**28 publications**

The Department/Institute of General Practice existed between 1973 and 2001, i.e. 28 years.

Appendix 7: University Degrees/Awards Obtained from the Practice

1903	Joseph Anthony Pereira	GP partner	MD Brussels by examination	MD(Brux)
1972	Richard Hillier	GP partner	MD University of London	MD
1991	Russell Steele	GP partner	Fellowship by Assessment, Royal College of General Practitioners	FRCGP
1988	Ann Buxton	GP partner	MSc University of Exeter	MSc(Exon)
1992	Keiran Sweeney	GP partner	Harkness Fellowship	
1994	Philip Evans	GP partner	Master's degree by research	MPhil (Exon)
1995	Kieran Sweeney	GP partner	Master's degree by research	MPhil (Exon)
1995	Teony McHale	Attached Midwife	MSc University of Exeter	MSc(Exon)
1998	Tim Smith	Practice Manager	Investors in People	
2000	Russell Steele	GP partner	Masters by research	MPhil (Exon)
2000	Denis Pereira Gray	GP partner	Honorary Doctor of Science, De Montfort University	HonDSc (De Montfort)
2000	Rosemary Stevens	Attached district nurse	Bachelor's degree, University of Plymouth	BSc
2003	Denis Pereira Gray	GP partner	Honorary Doctor of Medicine. University of Nottingham	HonDM (Nott)
2004	Helen Keenan	GP partner	MSc University of Exeter	MSc(Exon)
2007	Dawn Tarr	Nurse Practitioner	MSc University of Exeter	MSc(Exon)
2007	Alex Harding	GP partner	Masters in Medical Education	MMEd
2009	Denis Pereira Gray	GP former partner	Honorary Doctor of Science, University of Exeter	HonDSc (Exon)
2014	Eleanor White	Attached BSc Student	Quintiles Prize for Women in Science (from the practice)	
2015	Philip Evans and Denis Pereira Gray	GP partner and clinically retired partner	ESRC funding via University of Exeter Living Centre	Grant £9,500
2017	Alex Harding	GP partner	Doctor of Education, University of London	Ed D
2018–2021	Denis Pereira Gray Philip Evans Kate Sidaway-Lee	2 clinically retired GPs + Research Fellow	Grant of £167,000 to develop continuity of GP care	
				Total 21

Appendix 8: GP Syllabus – Theory and Principles of General Practice: 20 Features

Handout for medical students used in the Exeter Medical School 2017

Sir Denis Pereira Gray OBE HonDSc FRCP FRCGP FMedSci

*First-contact care	Front door of the NHS.
*Diagnostic process	Integrates the widest range of factors
Behavioural medicine	General practice as a behavioural science
**Patient – GP relationships	Longest and deepest in the medical profession
**Family medicine	DPG had 7% of all patients in four generations
*Generalism	Bridging body and mind, unlike hospital medicine
*Whole-person medicine	Integrating physical, psychological & social factors, especially social determinants of disease
*Responsive attitude	Patients not excluded by "wrong pathology"
**Personal preventive care	Unique integration – "anticipatory care"
*Patient-centred medicine	Tailoring management to the individual Supreme Court Ruling (2015)
*Narrative medicine	Patients' communicate by words & metaphors
*Community care	GPs as lead clinicians in the community
*Geographical proximity to homes	Surgeries often within "pram pushing" distance
*Home visits	Optimum setting to understand a patient
*Cost-effectiveness	Huge value and underpins the NHS
**Independent status/Partnership practice	Unique contract for NHS doctors. A privilege. Locus of control. Partnership practice fosters sharing flexibility. Female GPs have first baby 3 years earlier than doctors in specialist medicine

Plus Four Factors Relatively or Completely Invisible on Student Placements

**Population medicine	Unique in measuring individual uptake rates
*Continuity of care	Like a wonder drug. 6 big advantages for patients. Good for doctors and NHS too
**Reducing socio-economic disadvantage	Hospitals "pro rich": general practice alone "equitable" – reducing health inequalities
*Reducing mortality	Each GP associated with 34 lives saved

* Denotes leading branch of medicine. ** Unique feature in British clinical medicine.

REFERENCE

Pereira Gray D (2017) Towards research-based learning outcomes for general practice in medical schools. Inaugural Barbara Starfield Memorial Lecture *BJGP Open*; **1(1)** [Open Access].

Appendix 9: Chairmanships in the RCGP

Years	Years in office	
1972–1980	9	Editorial Board of the *Journal of the RCGP*
1976–1979	3	South West England Faculty (Last Chair)
1980–1981	1	Publications Committee
1980–1982	2	Co-Convener Healthier Children Working Party
1980–1981	1	Tamar Faculty (First Chair)
1981–1984	3	Communications Division
1987–1990	3.75	The Council
		General Purposes Committee
1993–1996	3	Research Division [2]
1994–1997	3	JCPTGP [2]
1997–2000	3	Annual General Meetings, 1998, 1999, 2000
		Awards Committee [3]
		Fellowship Committee [3]
2006–2012	6	Heritage Committee
	36.75 years	**Number of posts = 14**

[1] The Chair of Council chairs the General Purposes Committee.

[2] The Chairmanships of the Research Division and the JCPTGP overlapped in 1994–1996.

[3] The President chairs the Awards and Fellowship Committees.

Appendix 10: Visitors to the St Leonard's Practice

Dr Michael Abrams CB	Deputy Chief Medical Officer, DHSS
Sir Donald Acheson KBE (1926–2010)	Chief Medical Officer England
Dr Michael Ashley-Miller CBE (1930–2017)	Secretary, Nuffield Provincial Hospitals Trust
Rt Hon Lord Ashley of Stoke	When Labour MP for Stoke-on Trent
Sir Brian Bailey OBE (1924–2018)	Former Chairman South West Regional Health Authority
Rt Hon Sir Ben Bradshaw	MP for Exeter
	Former Secretary of State of Health
Rt Hon Baroness Browning	When a Devon MP
Dr Roger Bulger	Chief Executive Officer of the Association of University Health Centres (US Teaching Hospitals)
Sir Kenneth Calman KCB	Chief Medical Officer England
Sir Geoffrey Finsberg MBE (1926–1996)	Parliamentary Under Secretary, DHSS
Reverend Mrs Miriam Gent	Chair, Devon Family Health Services Authority
Professor Jeannie Haggerty	Research Professor, McGill University Canada
Ms Rebecca Harriot	Chief Officer, NEW Devon CCG
Dr Adrian Haytor	NHS National Clinical Director for Elderly People
Dame Dierdre Hine DBE	Chief Medical Officer, Wales
Dr Richard Horton	Editor, *Lancet*
Sir Donald Irvine CBE (1935–2018)	President, GMC
Lady Irvine	
Professor Janice Kay CBE	Provost, Exeter Medical School
Professor Harry Keen CBE (1925–2013)	Professor of Medicine, Guys Hospital and Chair, British Diabetic Association
Mr Charles Kennedy (1959–2015)	When an MP
	Later leader of the Liberal Party
Professor Rudolf Klein CBE	University of Bath
	Political commentator
Mr Vincent Lawton	Managing Director, MSD
Mrs Judy Leverton	Chair, Strategic Health Authority
Professor Martin Marshall CBE	Chair of Council, RCGP
Professor Barry McCormick CBE	Chief Economic Adviser, DH
Mr Andy McKeon CBE	Principal Private Secretary, Secretary of State DHSS
	Returned 30 years later as Chair of the Trustees of the Nuffield Trust
Dame Gillian Morgan DBE	As Dr Morgan of local Health Authority
	Later Chief Executive, NHS Confederation
Dr David Ower	Lead GP, DHSS
Professor Sir John Pattison (1942–2020)	Director of Research and Analysis, DH
Sir Joe Pilling KCB	When official at DHSS
	Later Permanent Secretary, Northern Ireland office
Sir John Reid KCMG (1926–1994)	Chief Medical Officer, Scotland

(Continued)

Dr Gilbert Smith	Deputy Director, R&D, DH
Sir Steve Smith	Vice Chancellor, University of Exeter
Professor John Swales	Director, NHS R&D
Professor Steven Thornton	Dean, Exeter Medical School
Professor Sir John Tooke	Dean, Peninsula Medical School
Professor Dame Margaret Turner-Warwick DBE (1924–2017)	Past President, Royal College of Physicians and Chair RD&E NHS Trust
Professor William van't Hoff	Chief Executive, National Institute for Healthcare Research (NIHR)
Rt Hon Lord David Willetts	As Principal Private Secretary to Prime Minister (Mrs Thatcher) Later Minister for Universities and member of the House of Lords
World Health Organisation	12 Deans of European Medical Schools with Sir John Reid

Appendix 11: People Met

Heads of State

Person	Role	Place
HM the Queen	UK and Commonwealth	Buckingham Palace
Mary Robinson	President of Ireland	Glasgow
Bromislaw Komorowski	President of Poland	Cracow, Poland

Other Members of the Royal Family

HRH The Duke of Edinburgh	As RCGP President	RCGP, London
HRH Prince Charles	As RCGP President	Princes Gate, London and Kensington Palace London and Highgrove, Gloucs.
HRH Anne the Princess Royal	As Chair of Trustees, Nuffield Trust	London
HRH Prince Edward	At Imperial Society of Knights	London

Prime Ministers before or in Post

Name	Party	Office	Where met
Margaret Thatcher	Conservative	In office	Chequers and 10 Downing Street
Tony Blair	Labour	In office	Cabinet Room 10 Downing Street
Gordon Brown	Labour	In office	10 Downing Street
John Major	Conservative	Cabinet Minister before being PM	Chequers
Julia Gillard	Labour	As Health Minister in Australia before being PM in Australia	Nuffield Trust

Ministers

Paul Boetang		Labour	London	Cabinet Minister
Virginia Bottomley	Later Baroness	Conservative	London	Cabinet Minister
Ben Bradshaw	Later Knight	Labour	Exeter	Cabinet Minister
Kenneth Clarke	Later Lord	Conservative	Exeter	Cabinet Minister
Edwina Currie		Conservative	London	
Paul Dean	Later Knight	Conservative	Exeter	
Frank Dobson		Labour	London	Cabinet Minister
Stephen Dorrell		Conservative Later Liberal Democrat	London	Cabinet Minister

(Continued)

Sir Geoffrey Finsberg		Conservative	Exeter	
Norman Fowler	Later Lord	Conservative	London	Cabinet Minister
Lord Glenarthur		Conservative	Exeter	
Lord Howe		Conservative	London	
Jeremy Hunt		Conservative	London	Cabinet Minister
Philip Hunt	Later Lord	Labour	London	
John Hutton	Later Lord	Labour	London	Cabinet Minister
Andrew Lansley	Later Lord	Conservative	London	Cabinet Minister
Gerry Malone		Conservative	London	
David Mellor		Conservative	Exeter	
Alan Milburn		Labour	London	Cabinet Minister
John Moore	Later Lord	Conservative	London	Cabinet Minister
Tony Newton	Later Lord	Conservative	London	Cabinet Minister
Gisela Stuart	Later Baroness	Labour	London	
Baroness Trumpington		Conservative	Exeter	
Norman Warner	Later Lord	Labour	London	
Anne Widdicombe		Conservative	London	
David Willetts	Later Lord	Conservative	London 10 Downing Street and Exeter	Later Minister and attended Cabinet
Lord Williams		Labour	London	

Appendix 12: Glossary

AcMedSci	Academy of Medical Sciences	
AoMRC	Academy of Medical Royal Colleges	
APC	Academic Policy Committee	University of Exeter
AMGP	Association of Managers in General Practice	Now dissolved
ARM	Annual Representative Meeting	Of the BMA
BJGP	*British Journal of General Practice*	*RCGP Journal*
BMA	British Medical Association	
BMJ	*British Medical Journal*	
BSc	Bachelor of Science	
CBE	Commander of the British Empire	Civil honour, one grade below damehoods/knighthoods
CCG	Clinical Commissioning Group	Local part of the NHS
CMG	Commander of the Order of St Michael and St George	Civil honour equivalent to a CBE
CMO	Chief Medical Officer	One in each of the four home nations
CO	Course organiser	For GP vocational training replaced by TPD
CoAoGP	Conference of Academic Organisations in General Practice	
COGPED	Conference of GP Educational Directors	Formerly Regional Advisers
CoMRC	Conference of Medical Royal Colleges and Faculties	Replaced by the Academy of Medical Royal Colleges
CRAGPIE	Committee of Regional Advisers in England	
DGP	Department of General Practice, University of Exeter	Later became Institute of General Practice
DGPE	Director of General Practice Education	
DH	Department of Health	
DHSC	Department of Health and Social Care	
DHSS	Department of Health and Social Security	Before 1978
DM	Doctorate in Medicine	Used instead of MD in a minority of universities
DPG	Denis Pereira Gray	
DSc	Doctor of Science	
EC	Executive Council	The original NHS body with which GPs were in contract. Abolished & replaced by FHSAs
ECC	Ethics and Confidentiality Committee	Succeeded PIAG
EdD	Doctorate in Education	Higher, third level, university degree obtained by thesis
ECC	Ethics and Confidentiality Committee	Formerly PIAG
FBA	Fellowship by Assessment of the Royal College of General Practitioners	
FDA	Food and Drug Administration	USA
FDS	Faculty of Dental Surgery of the Royal College of Surgeons of England	

(Continued)

FDS RCS	Fellow of Dental Surgery, Royal College of Surgeons	
FGDP	Faculty of General Dental Practitioners of the Royal College of Surgeons of England	
FHSA	Family Health Services Committee	Local part of the NHS before CCGs now abolished
FPH	Faculty of Public Health	
FRS	Fellow of the Royal Society	Most prestigious academic body in the UK
GDC	General Dental Council	UK medical regulator for dentists
GDP	General Dental Practitioner	Dentist
GMC	General Medical Council	UK medical regulator for doctors
GMSC	General Medical Services Committee, BMA	Replaced by the General Practitioners Committee BMA
GP	General Practitioner	
GPC	General Practitioners Committee	Successor to the GMSC
	General Purposes Committee	Executive committee of the Council of the RCGP
HF	Health Foundation	London-based health charity
HoTs	Heads of Teaching for general practice	In UK medical schools
HRT	Hormone replacement therapy	
HSR	Health Services Research	Compared with biomedical research
IGP	Institute of General Practice, University of Exeter	Successor to DGP
IoM	Institute of Medicine	Washington USA, now the National Academy of Medicine
JCC	Joint Consultants Committee	
JCPTGP	Joint Committee for Postgraduate Training for General practice	Competent Authority for GP Training
JRCGP	*Journal of the Royal College of General Practitioners*	After 1991 called the *British Journal of General Practice*
KBE	Knight in the Order of the British Empire	High Civil honour
KCB	Knight in the Order of the Bath	Usually awarded to senior civil servants
KCMG	Knight in the Order of St Michael and St George	High Civil honour
KF	King's Fund	Charity in London
MASC	Medical Academic Staff Committee	Of the BMA
MBE	Member of the Order of the British Empire	Civil honour
MBTI	Myers Briggs Type Inventory	Classification of personality
MD	Doctor of Medicine	Higher, third level university degree obtained by thesis
MoH	Medical Officer of Health	Now abolished
MPhil	Master's degree	Usually by research
MRB	Members' Reference Book of the RCGP	Included the RCGP annual report
MRC	Medical Research Council	Agency for research, mainly biomedical
MRCP	Member of the Royal College Physicians	Obtained by examination
MRCS LRCP	Member of the Royal College of Surgeons and Licentiate of the Royal College of Physicians	A basic medical qualification
MSC	Medical Schools Council	Attended by the Heads of Medical Schools
MSc	Master of Science	
NAM	National Academy of Medicine	Washington, DC, USA Formerly Institute of Medicine
NAPP	National Association for Patient Participation	
NHS	National Health Service	UK system of health care

(Continued)

NICE	National Institute of Health and Social Care Excellence	
NIGB	National Information Governance Board	Since abolished
NMC	Nursing and Midwifery Council	UK regulator
NPHT	Nuffield Provincial Hospitals Trust	Later renamed the Nuffield Trust
NT	Nuffield Trust	Replaced the Nuffield Provincial Hospitals Trust
OBE	Office in the Order of the British Empire	Civil honour, middle grade
OP	Occasional Papers	Series of academic papers published by the RCGP
Oxbridge	Oxford and Cambridge universities	
PAcMedSci	President, Academy of Medical Sciences	
PCMD	Peninsula College of Medicine and Dentistry of the Universities of Exeter and Plymouth	Dissolved
PCT	Primary care trusts	Local part of the NHS now abolished
PGMI	Postgraduate Medical Institute of the University of Exeter	Became the Postgraduate Medical School
PGMS	Postgraduate Medical School of the University of Exeter	Later absorbed within the Exeter Medical School
PhD	Doctor of Philosophy	Highet, third level, university degree obtained by thesis
PIAG	Patient Information and Advisory Group	Changed to ECC
PMETB	Postgraduate Medical Education and Training Board	Since abolished
PPG	Patient Participation Group	Usually in relation to a general practice
PPS	Principal private secretary	High flying junior civil servant
PRCGP	President of the Royal College of General Practitioners	Highest elected post
PRCOG	President of the Royal College of Obstetricians and Gynaecologists	
PRCP	President of the Royal College of Physicians	
PRCPI	President of the Royal College of Physicians of Ireland	
PRCSEd	President of the Royal College of Surgeons of Edinburgh	
PRCSEng	President of the Royal College of Surgeons of England	
PRCSI	President of the Royal College of Surgeons in Ireland	
Princes Gate	Former Headquarters of the RCGP	London
RA	Regional Adviser in General Practice	After mid-1990s Director of GP Education
RAE	Research Assessment Exercise	For British universities quality assurance exercise
RCA	Royal College of Anaesthetists	
RCGP	Royal College of General Practitioners	
RCP	Royal College of Physicians	
RCPI	Royal College of Physicians in Ireland	
RCP	Royal College of Physicians of London	
RCPsych	Royal College of Psychiatrists	
RCS Ed	Royal College of Surgeons of Edinburgh	
RCSEng	Royal College of Surgeons of England	
RCSI	Royal College of Surgeons in Ireland	
RGPEC	Regional General Practice Education Committee of the University of Bristol	Now abolished
RHA	Regional Health Authority	Now abolished
RoSL	Royal Overseas League	London club

(*Continued*)

RSH	Royal Society of Health	Charity promoting public health
RSM	Royal Society of Medicine	London club
RSPHH	Royal Society of Public Health and Hygiene	Later merged to become the RSH
SAGE	Scientific Advisory Group in England	Advised Government during the Covid-19 epidemic
SAS	Special Air Service	Elite counter terrorism group
SHHD	Scottish Home and Health Department	Former HQ for the Scottish Office Abolished
SHO	Senior House Officer	Junior hospital doctor
SIMG	Society Internationale Medicine Generale	European academic society for GPs; Later merged with WONCA Europe
SLMP	St Leonard's Medical Practice, Exeter	Medical Practice in Exeter
SLRP	St Leonard's Research Practice, Exeter	The research wing of the St Leonard's Practice
SPM	Serious professional misconduct	The most serious charge brought by the GMC against doctors
STA	Specialist Training Authority	Abolished
STP	Sustainable and Transformation Plans	Local NHS policy groups later abolished
STV	Single transferable vote	Voting system in which a vote for a losing candidate moves on to another candidate
SWGPT	South West General Practice Trust	Charity to promote academic general practice in the South West of England
SWRHA	South Western Regional Health Authority	Abolished
TPD	Training Programme Director --for general practice training	Replaced course organisers
UKCC	UK Regulator for Nursing and Midwifery	Now the Nursing and Midwifery Council
UoB	University of Bristol	
UoC	University of Cambridge	
UEMO	Medico-political group for European GPs	
UoE	University of Exeter	
UoNott	University of Nottingham	
VC	Vice Chancellor	Head of a university
VTS	Vocational Training Scheme	Usually refers to general practice
WATCh?	What About the Children?	Children's charity fostering the emotional health of the under threes
Westminster		Collective term for UK parliamentarians
Whitehall		Term for the British civil service
WHO	World Health Organisation	Has HQ in Geneva and Regional Office in Copenhagen
WO	Welsh Office	Former Department of State Replaced by the Welsh Assembly
WONCA	World Organisation of National Colleges/Academies for General Practice/Family Medicine	World Organisation of Family Doctors

References

Academy of Medical Royal Colleges (2000) *Annual Report 1999/2000*. London: AoMRC.

Academy of Medical Royal Colleges (2001) *Evidence to the GMC on Revalidation*. London: AoMRC.

Academy of Medical Sciences (AMS) (2011) *A New Pathway for the Regulation and Governance of Health Research*. Chair, Prof Sir Michael Rawlins. London: AcMedSci.

Adler, R., Vasiliadis, A. and Bickell, N (2010) The relationship between continuity and patient satisfaction: a systematic review. *Family Practice*; **27(2)**:171–8.

Ahn R, Woodbridge AR, Abraham A *et al.* (2017) Financial ties of principal investigators and randomised controlled trial outcomes. *BMJ*; **356**:i6770.

Allen J, Evans A, Foulkes J *et al.* (1998) Simulated surgery in the summative assessment of general practice training: Results of a trial in the Trent and Yorkshire regions. *Br J Gen Pract*; **48(430)**:1219–23.

Almond B (2006) *The Fragmenting Family*. Oxford: Oxford University Press.

Ames J (2019) Brain-damaged boy wins £30m for hospital negligence. *The Times*, 31 Oct.

Anderson, S.R., Gianola, M., Medina, N.A., Perry, J.M., Wager, T.D. and Losin, EAR (2023) Doctor trustworthiness influences pain and its neural correlates in virtual medical interactions. *Cerebral Cortex*; **33(7)**:3421–36.

Argyle M (1975) *Bodily Communication*. New York: International Universities Press.

Ashley-Miller M (1993) Personal letter re-invitation to first Trustee dinner. March.

Ashley-Miller M, Barkun H, Bulger R (Eds) (1995) *Changes in Health Needs and Health Services Provision by 2005. The Role and Training of Doctors. A Report of a Trilateral Seminar Held 27 August–3 September 1996*. London: Nuffield Provincial Hospitals Trust.

Austurbaejar G (1957) *Fourth World Student Team Championship*. Iceland: Reykjavik.

Ayanian JZ, Weissman JS (2002) Teaching hospitals and quality of care: A review of the literature. *Millbank Q*; **80(3)**:569–93.

Baker R, Freeman GK, Haggerty JL *et al.* (2020) Primary medical care continuity and patient mortality: A systematic review. *Br J Gen Pract*; **70(698)**:e600–e611.

Balint M (1955) The doctor, his patient, and the illness. *Lancet*; **268(6866)**:683–8.

Balint M (1957) *The Doctor, His Patient, and the Illness*. London: Tavistock Publications.

Barber H (1985) Higher degrees in general practice. In *The Medical Annual*. Bristol: John Wright & Sons.

Barker I, Steventon A, Deeny SR (2017) Association between continuity of care in general practice and hospital admissions for ambulatory care sensitive conditions: Cross sectional study of routinely collected, person level data. *BMJ*; **356**:j84.

Barker I, Steventon A, Williamson R *et al.* (2018) Self-management capability in patients with long-term conditions is associated with reduced healthcare utilisation across a whole health economy: Cross-sectional analysis of electronic health records. *BMJ Qual Saf*; **27(12)**:989–99.

Barley SL (1981) The nurturing of a medical journal. Editorial. *J R Coll Gen Pract*; **31(222)**:5.

Barlow J, Parsons J, Stewart-Brown S (2005) Preventing emotional and behavioural problems: The effectiveness of parenting programmes with children less than 3 years of age. *Child Care Health Dev*; **31(1)**:33–42.

Batten L (1955) *Lecture to medical students at St Bartholomew's Hospital*. London: Privately published.

Bazemore, A, Merenstein, Z, Handler, L and Saultz, JW (2023) The Impact of Interpersonal Continuity of Primary Care on Health Care Costs and Use: A Critical Review. The Annals of Family Medicine; 21(3):274–79.

Beale N, Nethercott S (1988a) The nature of unemployment morbidity. 1. Recognition. *J R Coll Gen Pract*; **38(310)**:197–9.

Beale N, Nethercott S (1988b) The nature of unemployment morbidity. 2. Description. *J R Coll Gen Pract*; **38(310)**:200–2.

Bellis M, Hughes K, Hardcastle K *et al.* (2017) The impact of adverse childhood experiences on health service use across the life course using a retrospective cohort study. *J Health Serv Res & Policy*; **22(3)**:168–77.

Belsky J, Rovine MJ (1988) Nonmaternal care in the first year of life and the security of infant-parent attachment. *Child Dev*; **59(1)**:157–67.

Belsky J, Vandell DL, Burchinall M *et al.* (2007) Are there long-term effects of early child care? *Child Development*; **78(2)**:681–701.

Beral V, Peto R, Pirie K *et al.* (2019) Menopausal therapy and 20-year breast cancer mortality. *Lancet*; **394(10204)**:1139.

Berger J, Mohr J (1968) *A Fortunate Man*. London: Penguin Press.

Black Report (1985) *Review of the Arrangements for Health Care in Guernsey*. States of Guernsey.

BMA Planning Unit (1970) *Planning Primary Medical Care*. Chair, Prof Margot Jefferys. London: BMA.

BMJ (1990) Report of the meeting of the GMSC 27 January.

Bodenheimer T, Lorig K, Holman H, Grumbach K (2002) Patient self-management of chronic disease in primary care. *JAMA*; **288(19)**:2469–75.

Bodenheimer T, Sinsky C (2014) From triple to quadruple aim: Care of the patient requires care of the provider. *Ann Fam Med*; **12(5)**:573–6.

Bolden KJ, Dwyer D, Leete R *et al.* (1988) *Running a Course*. [Foreword DPG]. Oxford: Radcliffe Medical Press.

Bolden KJ, Lewis AP (1990) A joint course for general practitioner and practice nurse trainers. *Br J Gen Pract*; **40(338)**:386–7.

Bolden KJ, Takle B (1984) *Practice Nurse Handbook*. London: Blackwell.

Boon V, Ridd M, Blythe A (2017) Medical undergraduate primary care teaching across the UK: What is being taught? *Educ Prim Care*; **28(1)**:23–28.

Bradley NCA (1981) Expectations and experience of people who consult in a training practice. *J R Coll Gen Pract*; **31(228)**:420–5.

Bradley NCA (1983a) Sale of cigarettes to children in Exeter. *J R Coll Gen Pract*; **3(254)**:559–62.

Bradley NCA (1983b) Time and the general practice consultation. In *The Medical Annual*. Bristol: John Wright & Sons.

Brain R (1951) Letter to Dr John Hunt on behalf of the Royal Colleges of Physicians, Surgeons and Obstetricians. In the RCGP archives and reprinted in Pereira Gray D (Ed). *Forty Years On: The Story of the First 40 Years of the RCGP*. London: Atalink, 1992.

Briggs GM, Flynn PA, Worthington M *et al.* (2008) The role of specialist neuroradiology second opinion reporting: Is there added value? *Clinical Radiology*; **63(7)**:791.

Briggs Myers I (1993) *Gift Differing: Understanding Personality Type*. Palo Alto, CA: Consulting Psychologists Press.

Brimblecombe FS (1965) A progress report on the Postgraduate Medical Institute of the University of Exeter. *Postgrad Med J*; **41(474)**:169–71.

Bristol Evening Post (1964) Gray v Clapp. 10 October.

British Medical Journal (BMJ) (1990) From the GMSC: Committee blocks debate on sanctions ballot. Anger at RCGP's inroad into contractual matters. *BMJ Affairs*; **300**:265.

British Medical Journal (BMJ, Clinical Research Edition) (1983) From the CCCM: Community physicians and merit awards. Sir Stanley Clayton addresses committee. **286**:412.

British Medical Journal (BMJ, Clinical Research Edition) (1986) From the LMC Conference: GPs reject good practice allowance. **293**:1384.

Bunker JP (2001) *Medicine Matters After All: Measuring the Benefits of Medical Care, a Healthy Lifestyle, and a Just Social Environment*. London: Nuffield Trust.

Bunker JP, Hinkley D, McDermott WV (1978) Surgical innovation and its evaluation. *Science*; **200(4344)**:937–41.

Byrne PS, Long BEL (1984) *Doctors Talking to Patients*. [First published London: HMSO, 1976.] Republished Exeter: RCGP.

Calman K (1997) *On the State of the Public Health 1996*. London: Department of Health.

Calman K (1998a) *On the State of the Public Health 1997.* London: Department of Health.

Calman K (1998b) *A Review of Continuing Professional Development in General Practice: A Report by the Chief Medical Officer.* London: Department of Health.

Cambridge Correspondent (1955) Cambridge letter, p20. *The Exonian:* Exeter School.

Campbell JL, Fletcher E, Britten N *et al.* (2014) Telephone triage for the management of same-day consultation requests in general practice (the ESTEEM trial): A cluster-randomised controlled trial and cost-consequence analysis. *Lancet;* **384(9957)**:1859–68.

Campbell J, Hobbs FDR, Irish B *et al.* (2015b) UK academic general practice and primary care. Editorial. *BMJ;* **351**:h4164.

Campbell J, Warren F, Taylor R, *et al.* (2015a) Patient perspectives on telephone triage in general practice. Authors' reply. *Lancet;* **385(9969)**:688.

Campbell LM (1996) The development of a summative assessment system for vocational trainees in general practice. MD thesis. Glasgow: University of Glasgow.

Campbell LM, Howie JG, Murray TS (1993) Summative assessment: A pilot project in the west of Scotland. *Br J Gen Pract;* **43(375)**:430–4.

Campbell LM, Howie JGR, Murray TS (1995) Use of videotaped consultations in summative assessment in general practice. *B J Gen Pract;* **45(392)**:137–41.

Campbell LM, Lough JRM, Murray TS (1996) Summative assessment in general practice. Letter. *BMJ;* **313**:1556–7.

Campbell LM, Murray TS (1996) Summative assessment of vocational trainees: Results of a three-year study *Br J Gen Pract;* **46(408)**:411–14.

Care Quality Commission (2022) Report on maternity services. London: CQC.

Carey TS, Garrett J, Jackman A *et al.* (1995) North Carolina Back Pain Project. The outcomes and costs of care for acute low back pain among patients seen by primary care practitioners, chiropractors, and orthopedic surgeons. *N Eng J Med;* **333(14)**:913–17.

Carne S (1984) Serious illness in children. In *The Medical Annual.* Bristol: John Wright & Sons.

Carnell D (1996) Summative assessment in general practice. Editorial. *BMJ;* **313**:638.

Cartwright A, Waite M (1972a) *General Practitioners and Abortion.* Evidence to the committee on the working of the Abortion Act. *J Roy Coll Gen Pract;* **22(Suppl)**:1–24.

Cartwright A, Waite M (1972b) *General Practitioners and Contraception in 1970–71. J R Coll Gen Pract;* **22(Suppl2)**:1–31.

Centre for Social Justice (2008) *Breakthrough Britain: The Next Generation.* Chair, Dr Samantha Callan. London: CSJ.

Chalker L (1980) Maternity grants. Quoted in Medical News. *J R Coll Gen Pract;* **30(216)**:438–9.

Charon R (2001) The patient-physician relationship. Narrative medicine: A model for empathy, reflection, profession, and trust. *JAMA;* **286(15)**:1897–1902.

Chenore T, Pereira Gray DJ, Forrer J *et al.* (2013) Emergency hospital admissions for the elderly: Insights from the Devon Predictive Model. *J Pub Health (Oxf);* **35(4)**:616–23.

Christakis DA, Mell L, Wright JA *et al.* (2000) The association between greater continuity of care and timely measles-mumps-rubella vaccination. *Am J Public Health;* **90(6)**:962–5.

Clarke PH (1959) World Student Team Championship 1959. *British Chess Magazine.*

Clark MS, Reis HT (1988) Interpersonal processes in close relationships. *Ann Rev Psychol;* **39**:609–72.

Clayton S (1982) Advisory Committee on Distinction Awards. *BMJ;* **284**:157–8.

Clyne MB (1961) *Night Calls: A Study in General Practice.* Mind and Medicine Monograph. London: Tavistock Publications.

Cochrane A (1972) *Effectiveness and Efficiency: Random Reflections on Health Services.* Rock Carling Lecture 1972. London: NPHT.

Cogwheel Report (1967) *First Report of the Joint Working Party on the Organization of Medical Work in Hospitals.* London: HMSO.

Cohen Committee (1950) *General Practice and the Training of the General Practitioner. The Report of the Committee of the Association.* Chair, Sir Henry Cohen. London: BMA.

Colditz GA, Hankinson SE, Hunter DJ *et al.* (1995) The use of estrogens and progestins and the risk of breast cancer in postmenopausal women. *N Engl J Med;* **332(24)**:1589–93.

Cole SR, Harding A, Pereira Gray D (2020) What factors influence the introduction of a national undergraduate general practice curriculum in the UK? *Educ Prim Care*; **31(5)**:270–80.

College of General Practitioners (CGP) (1965) *Special Vocational Training for General Practice. Report from General Practice 1*. Chair, Dr WH Hylton. London: CGP.

College of General Practitioners (CGP) (1966) *Evidence of the College of General Practitioners to the Royal Commission on Medical Education. Report from General Practice 5*. London: CGP.

Collings JS (1950) General practice in England today: A reconnaissance. *Lancet*; **1**:555–85.

Colmer LJ, Pereira Gray D (1983) An audit of the care of asthma in a general practice. *Practitioner*; **227(1376)**:271–9.

Committee of Vice Chancellors and Principals (CVCP) (1994) *Annual Report*. London: CVCP.

CONCHA Report (1996) *The Reality of Continuity of Care Workshop 1996–1997*. Chairs: Prof B Livesley, Dr B Jones. West Sussex: Continuity of Care Home Association.

Conference of Academic Organisations in General Practice (1994) *Research and General Practice*. Chair, Dr W McN Styles. Exeter: RCGP.

Conference of Academic Organisations in General Practice (1996) *Developing Primary Care: The Academic Contribution*. Chair, Prof D Pereira Gray. Exeter: RCGP.

Conference of Postgraduate Advisers in General Practice Universities of the United Kingdom (1995) *Summative assessment for GP registrars completing vocational training after 1 September 1996*. Winchester: South and West Regional Health Authority.

Congressional Research Service (2021) *The US Income Distribution: Trends and Issues*. Washington: CRS, 13 January.

Coulter AN, Bradlow JE, Martin-Bates CH *et al.* (1991) Outcome of general practitioner referrals to specialist outpatient clinics for back pain. *Br J Gen Pract*; **41(352)**:450–3.

Council of the Royal College of General Practitioners (1975) Evidence of the RCGP to the Select Committee of Parliament on the Abortion (Amendment) Bill. *J R Coll Gen Pract*; **25(159)**:774–6.

Court Committee (1976) *Fit for the Future* Chair, Professor Donald Court. London: DHSS, DES and the Welsh Office.

Cronin AJ (1937) *The Citadel*. London: Golancz.

Culyer Task Force (1994) *Supporting Research and Development in the NHS, a Report to the Minister of Health by a Research and Development Task Force*. Chair, AJ Culyer. London: HMSO.

Dahrendorf R (1982) *On Britain*. London: BBC.

Damant M, Martin C, Openshaw S (1994) *Practice Nursing. Stability and Change*. London: Mosby.

Darwin C (1859) *On the Origin of Species by Means of Natural Selection*. London: John Murray.

De Maeseneer JM, De Prins L, Gosset C, Heyerick J (2003) Provider continuity in family medicine: Does it make a difference for total health care costs? *Ann Fam Med* **1(3)**:144–8.

Delgado J, Evans PH, Pereira Gray D *et al.* (2022) Continuity of GP care for patients with dementia: Impact on prescribing and the health of patients. *Br J Gen Pract*; **72(715)**:e91–e98.

Department of Health (1989) *Working for Patients. Cm 555*. Foreword by Mrs Thatcher. London: HMSO.

Department of Health (2000) *The General and Specialist Medical Practice (Education, Training and Qualifications) Order. "Postgraduate Medical Education and Training Board"*. London: DH.

Department of Health (2006) *Our Health, Our Care, Our Say: A New Direction for Community Services*. London: DH.

Department of Health and Social Security (DHSS) (1986) *Primary Health Care: An Agenda for Discussion*. Cmnd 9771. London: HMSO.

Department of Health and Social Security (DHSS) and the Welsh Office (1972) Appointment of regional advisers in general practice. *Circular HM(72)75*. London: DHSS.

Department of Health and Social Security (DHSS), Department of Education and Science, and Welsh Office (1976) *Fit for the Future. Report of the Committee on Child Health Services*. Vols 1 & 2. Chair, Prof SDM Court. Cmnd 6684. London: HMSO.

Department of Health and Social Security (DHSS), the Joint Computer Group and Exeter University Department of General Practice (1986) *Micros in Practice*. London: HMSO.

Department of Health and Welsh Office (1989) *General Practice in the National Health Service. A New Contract.* London: DH.

Di Blasi Z, Harkness E, Ernst E *et al.* (2001) Influence of context effects on health outcomes: A systematic review. *Lancet*; **357(9528)**:757–62.

Diabetes UK (2012) *Care. Connect. Campaign. State of the Nation 2012 England.* London: DUK.

Digby A (1999) *The Evolution of British General Practice 1850–1948.* Oxford: OUP.

Dineen M (2019) *Raising the profile of academic general practice to our medical students.* Letter. *Br J Gen Pract*; **69(685)**:381.

Dineen M, Sidaway-Lee K, Pereira Gray D *et al.* (2021) Family history recording in UK general practice: The lIFeLONG study. Fam Pract; **39(4)**:610–15. https://doi.org/10.1093/fampra/cmab117

Dixon A, Le Grand J, Henderson J *et al.* (2007) Is the British National Health Service equitable? The evidence on socioeconomic differences in utilization. *J Health Serv Res & Policy*; **12(2)**:104–9.

Donabedian A (1966) Evaluating the quality of medical care. *Milbank Mem Fund Q*; **44(3)**:166–206.

Donohoe M, Courtney P (1982) How to get the most out of the trainee year. *BMJ (Clin Res Ed*; **284(6312)**: 315–6.

Douglas A (1981) Profiles of practices: From city to coast. *BMJ (Clin Res Ed); **282(6258)**:113–14.

Dressler WW, Evans P, Pereira Gray D (1992) Status incongruence and serum cholesterol in an English general practice. *Soc Sci Med*; **34(7)**:757–62.

Dumville JC, MacPerson H, Griffith K *et al.* (2007) Non-cardiac chest pain: A retrospective cohort study of patients who attended a Rapid Access Chest Pain Clinic. *Fam Pract*; **24(2)**:152–7.

Economist (2021) The hunger wanes. 18 September.

Edwards JR, Graham-Bonnalie FE, Pereira Gray DJ (1966) Practice premises. Letter. *BMJ*; **1**:236.

Electoral Reform Ballot Services (1992) *Your choices for the future.* 99–104. London: GMSC.

Engel GL (1977) The need for a new medical model: A challenge for biomedicine. *Science*; **196(4286)**:129–36.

Enthoven AC (1985) *Reflections on the Management of the National Health Service. An American looks at incentives to efficiency in health services management in the UK.* London: Nuffield Provincial Hospitals Trust.

Ernst E (1995a) St. John's Wort, an anti-depressant? A systematic, criteria-based review. *Phytomedicine*; **2(1)**:67–71.

Ernst E (1995b) A leading medical school seriously damaged: Vienna 1938. *Ann Intern Med*; **122(10)**: 789–92.

Ernst E (2015) *A Scientist in Wonderland: A Memoir of Searching for Truth and Finding Trouble.* Exeter, UK: Imprint academic.

European Council [Medical Directive] (1995) Title 1V, 93/16/EEC April 1993. *Official Journal of the European Committee.*

Evans PH (1995) *Hyperlipidaemia in General Practice.* MPhil Dissertation. Exeter: University of Exeter.

Evans PH, Choules J (2021) Lady Pereira Gray. *Br J Gen Pract*; **71**:30.

Evans P, Langley P, Pereira Gray D (2008) Diagnosing type 2 diabetes before patients complain of diabetic symptoms—clinical opportunistic screening in a single general practice. *Fam Pract*; **25(5)**:376–81.

Evans P, Pereira Gray D (1994) Value of screening for secondary causes of hyperlipidaemia in general practice. *BMJ*; **309(6953)**:509–10.

Evans PH, Pereira Gray D (1999) Three dimensional care? Editorial. *Eur J Gen Pract*; **5**:135–6.

Fehr B, Sprecher S, Underwood LG (Eds.) (2009) *The Science of Compassionate Love: Theory, Research and Applications.* London: Wiley-Blackwell.

Feinmann J (1989) Profile: Professor Denis Pereira Gray. *Pulse*, 7 April.

Findlater J (1996) *The Life of Professor PS Byrne CBE FRCGP: A Career "with Bells on".* Exeter: RCGP.

Firth J (1986) Levels and source of stress among medical students. *BMJ*; **292**:1177–80.

Fisher M and Croft p (2022) *Making it Happen: The Influence of One General Practice on Academic Primary Care in North Staffordshire and Keele University* p16. Newcastle-under-lyme: Published privately.

Fitter MJ (1986) *A Prescription for Change: A Report on the Long-Term Use and Development of Computers in General Practice.* London: TSO.

Florence A (1960) Is thalidomide to blame? *BMJ letter ii*; 30 December.

Ford S, Barnes S (2013) Midwifery regulation needs overhaul, says ombudsman. *Nursing Times*; **109(51)**:5.

Forman JAS (1971) Personal and continuing care in group practice. *Update Plus.*

Forman JAS, Fairbairn E (1968) *Social Casework in General Practice.* London: Nuffield Provincial Hospitals Trust.

Forrest Report (1986) *Breast Cancer Screening: Report to the Ministers in England, Wales, Scotland and Northern Ireland.* Chair, Prof Sir Patrick Forrest. London: HMSO.

Fountain S (1986) Management in practice. In *The Medical Annual.* Bristol: John Wright & Sons.

Francis R (2013) *Report of the Mid Staffordshire NHS Foundation Trust Public Inquiry.* Vol 1. Analysis of evidence and lessons learned (Part 1). Chair, Robert Francis QC. London: TSO.

Freeman G, Hughes J (2010) *Continuity of Care and the Patient Experience.* London: King's Fund.

Friedlr K, King MB, Lloyd M, Horder J (1997) Randomised controlled assessment of non-directive psycho-therapy versus routine general-practitioner care. *Lancet*; **350(9092)**:1662–5.

Fry J (1961) *The Catarrhal Child.* London: Butterworth.

Fuller CJ (1963) A postgraduate medical institute at Exeter. *Postgrad Med J*; **39(449)**:119–20.

Furedi A (1999) The public health implications of the 1995 'pill scare'. *Hum Reprod Update;* **5(6)**:621–6.

Gaffney D, Pollock AM (1999) Pump-priming the PFI: Why are privately financed hospital schemes being subsidized? *Pub Money Manag*; **19(1)**:55–62.

General Medical Council (GMC) (1967) *Recommendations as to Basic Medical Education.* London: GMC.

General Medical Council (GMC) (1995) *Good Medical Practice.* London: GMC.

General Medical Council (GMC) (2018) *National Training Survey.* London: GMC.

Gerada C, Riley B (2012a) The 2022 GP: Our profession, our patients, our future. Editorial. *Br J Gen Pract*; **62(604)**:566–7.

Gerada C Riley B and Simon C (2012b) Preparing the future GP: The case for enhanced GP training: RCGP report. www.rcgp.org.uk/Opolicy/rcgp-policy-areas/-media/Files/Policy/Z%20policy/Case_for_enhanced_GP_training.ashx

Gillie A (1969) *Do Something about That Middle Age.* London: Howard Baker.

Gillie Report (1963) *The Field of Work of the Family Doctor.* Chair, Dr Annis Gillie. London: HMSO.

Giving USA (2019) *The Annual Report on Philanthropy for the Year 2018* available for download at www.givingusa.org.

Glanville, J, Kendrick, T, McNally, R, Campbell, J and Hobbs, FR (2011) Research output on primary care in Australia, Canada, Germany, the Netherlands, the United Kingdom, and the United States: biblio-metric analysis. *BMJ*; **342**:d1028

Godber G (1968) *General practice, past and present.* Second Monckton Copeman Lecture. *J R Coll Gen Pract*; **16(3)**:175–90.

Godber G (1983) General practice in the NHS. In *The Medical Annual.* Bristol: John Wright & Sons.

Goldacre MJ, Davidson JM, Lambert TW (2008) The first house officer year: Views of graduate and non-graduate entrants to medical school. *Med Educ*; **42(3)**:286–93.

Goldberg D, Bridges K, Duncan-Jones P *et al.* (1985) Detecting anxiety and depression in general medical settings. *BMJ*; **297**:897–9.

Goodenough Committee (1944) *The Training of Doctors. Report of the Interdepartmental Committee on medical schools.* Chairman, Sir William Goodenough. London: HMSO.

Goodman D (1992) Letter. *Guardian.*

Gore J (2020) *The Terror Raids of 1942: The Baedeker Blitz.* Barnsley: Pen and Sword.

Granier S, Owen P, Pill R *et al.* (1998) Recognising meningococcal disease in primary care: Qualitative study of how general practitioners process clinical and contextual information. *BMJ*; **3**:276–9.

Gray DJP (1959) The British Student Team at Budapest. *Chess* **24**:342–5.

Gray K (1990) Pride of place. Letter. *The Times*, 16 February.

Gray S, Smith L (2000) All primary care beacons for clinical governance in South West have research funding and fellowship by assessment. Letter. *BMJ*; **320(7227)**:121.

Greengross S (1987) The role of the general practitioner in the care of the elderly. In *The Medical Annual.* Bristol: John Wright & Sons.

Greenhalgh T, Hurwitz B (1999) Narrative based medicine: Why study narrative? *BMJ*; **318(7175)**:48–50.

Grol R (Ed) (1988) *To Heal or to Harm? The Prevention of Somatic Fixation in General Practice.* Republished Exeter: RCGP. First published in Dutch, 1981.

Hall MS, Dwyer D, Lewis T (Eds) (1983) *The GP Training Handbook.* London: Blackwell.

Hall MS, Pereira Gray D (2005) Obituary for Robert Vernon Holmes Jones. *BMJ*; **326**:40.

Harding A, Hawthorne K, Rosenthal J (2018) *Teaching General Practice: Guiding Principles for the Undergraduate General Practice Curricula in UK Medical Schools.* London: RCGP and SAPC.

Harding A, Rosenthal J, Al-Seaidy M, Pereira Gray D *et al.* (2015) Provision of medical student teaching in UK general practices: A cross-sectional questionnaire study. *Br J Gen Pract*; **65(635)**:e409–17.

Harding AM, Rosenthal J, Hawthorne K (2019) *Learning General Practice.* London: RCGP.

Harris CM (1970) Innominate science, the specialty of general practice. *J R Coll Gen Pract*; **20(99)**:194–201.

Hart G (1995) Public health advocacy. Letter. *Lancet*; **345(8956)**:1050

Haslam D (1987) Behavioural problems in children. In *The Medical Annual.* Bristol: John Wright & Sons Ltd.

Hawgood D (2012) Herbert Nicholas Chilcote MRCS (1840–86). Obelisk in St Marychurch, Devon. *J Med Biog*; **20(2)**:85–86.

Hayden B (1965) West of England Congress. Coast v Gray. *British Chess Magazine* **85(6)**:166.

Health Foundation (2022) *Report on the Improving GP Continuity Programme. Includes Continuity Counts, the Report from the St Leonard's Research General Practice.* Exeter. London; HF.

Heath I (1995) *The Mystery of General Practice.* London: Nuffield Provincial Hospitals Trust.

Heath I (2011) Divided we fail. Harveian Oration of the RCP 2011. *Clin Med (Lond)*; **11(6)**:576–86.

Helman CG (1981) Disease versus illness in general practice. *J R Coll Gen Pract*; **31(230)**:548–52.

Hetlevik Ø, Holmas TH, Monståd K (2021) Continuity of care, measurement and association with hospital admission and mortality: A registry-based longitudinal cohort study. *BMJ Open*; **11**:e051958.

Hewitt H, Gafaranga J, McKinstry B (2010) Comparison of face-to-face and telephone consultations in primary care: Qualitative analysis. *Br J Gen Pract*; **60(574)**:e201–e12.

Hill D (1969) *Psychiatry in Medicine. Rock Carling Monograph.* London: Nuffield Provincial Hospitals Trust.

Hobfoll SE, Johnson RJ, Ennis N, Jackson AP (2003) Resource loss, resource gain, and emotional outcomes among inner city women. *J Pers Soc Psychol*; **84(3)**:632–43.

Hodges A (2014) *Alan Turing: The Enigma.* London: Vintage, Random House.

Hoffenberg Report (1989) *Prison Medical Service in England and Wales: Recruitment and of Doctors.* Chair, Prof Sir Raymond Hoffenberg PRCP. London: Royal College of Physicians.

Hoffenberg R, Todd IP, Pinker G (1987) Joint statement from the Presidents of the Royal College of Physicians, the Royal College of Surgeons, and the Royal College of Obstetricians and Gynaecologists. Letter. *Lancet*; 12 December; **330(8572)**:1411.

Hoggart R (1957) *The Uses of Literacy.* London: Chatto and Windus.

Hojat M, Gonnella JS, Mangione S *et al.* (2002) Empathy in medical students as related to academic performance, clinical competence and gender. *Med Educ*; **36(6)**:522–7.

Holden J (2013) Fellowship by Assessment six years on: A personal view. *RCGP News,* April, p8.

Holden J, Kay A (2005) Fellowship by Assessment: 15 years of peer assessment of high-quality general practice. *Qual Prim Care*; **13**:3–7.

Hollis AC, Streeter J, van Hamel C *et al.* (2020) The new cultural norm: Reasons why UK foundation doctors are choosing not to go straight into specialty training. *BMC Med Educ*; **20(1)**:282.

Honigsbaum F (1972) Quality in general practice. A commentary on the quality of care provided by general practitioners. *J R Coll Gen Pract*; **22(120)**:429–51.

Hope-Simpson RE (1965) The nature of herpes zoster: A long-term study and a new hypothesis. *Proc R Soc Med*; **58(1)**:9–20.

Hopkins RJ (1990) The Exeter Care Card: A CP8-based global health care record for the United Kingdom's National Health Service. Editorial. *J Med Syst*; **14(3)**:150–4.

Horder J (Ed) (1992) *The Writings of John Hunt.* Exeter: RCGP.

Horder JP (1977) Physicians and family doctors: A new relationship. *J R Coll Gen Pract*; **27(180)**:391–7.

Horder JP (1980) From the Dart to the Tagus. First McConaghey Memorial Lecture. *J R Coll Gen Pract*; **30(219)**:585–92.

Horder JP (1983) General practice in 2000: Alma Ata declaration. *BMJ (Clin Res Ed)*; **286(6360)**:191–4.

Horder JP, Pasmore S (1987) *14 Princes Gate. Home of the Royal College of General Practitioners*. Preface by DPG. Exeter: RCGP.

Hospital Doctor (1997) Quoting J Johnson speaking at the Hospital Doctors Conference May

Hospital Doctor (2000) Donald on the defensive. 11 February.

House of Commons Health Select Committee (2016) *Primary Care*. Chair, Dr Sarah Wollaston MP. London: House of Commons.

House of Commons Library (2021) *Business statistics. Research Briefing*. London: House of Commons.

Howie JG, Heaney DJ, Maxwell M (1997) *Measuring quality in general practice. Pilot study of a needs, process and outcome measure. Occasional Paper 75*. London: RCGP.

Howie JGR, Heaney DJ, Maxwell M *et al.* (1999) Quality at general practice consultations: Cross sectional survey. *BMJ*; **319(7212)**:738–43.

Howie JG, Porter AM, Heaney DJ, Hopton JL (1991) Long to short consultation ratio: A proxy measure of quality of care for general practice. *Br J Gen Pract*; **41(343)**:48–54.

Humphreys LR (2010) *Hoffenberg: Physician and Humanitarian*. London: Royal College of Physicians.

Hunt JH (1973) The foundation of a College. The conception, birth and early days of the College of General Practitioners. James Mackenzie Lecture 1972. *J R Coll Gen Pract*; **23(126)**:5–20.

Huygen FJA (1990) *Family Medicine: The Medical Life History of Families*. Republished Exeter: RCGP. First published: Nijmegen, The Netherlands: Dekker & Van de Vegt: 1978.

Illingworth C (1994) The pre-registration alternative *BMJ*; **308**:1109.

Illman J (1989) Thatcher's secret nine. *Medical Monitor*, 28 April.

Ipsos Mori (2019) *Trust in the professions*. London: IM.

Irvine D (1972) *Teaching Practices. Report from General Practice 15*. Exeter: RCGP.

Irvine D (1975) 1984: The quiet revolution. William Pickles Lecture 1975. *J R Coll Gen Pract*; **25(155)**:399–407.

Irvine D (1983) Quality of care in general practice: Our outstanding problem. *J R Coll Gen Pract*; **33**:521–3.

Irvine D (2003) *The Doctor's Tale: Professionalism and Public Trust*. Abingdon: Radcliffe Medical Press [President GMC, 1995–2002].

Irvine D (2006) A short history of the General Medical Council. *Med Ed*; **40**:202–11.

Irvine D (2017) *Medical Professionalism and Public Trust: Reflections on a Life in Medicine*. London: RCGP.

Irvine S (1992) *Balancing Dreams and Discipline: Managing in Practice*. Exeter: RCGP.

Irvine D, Pereira Gray D, Bogle I (1990) Vocational training: The meaning of 'satisfactory completion'. Letter. *Br J Gen Pract*; **40**:434.

Jarman B (1983) Identification of underprivileged areas. *BMJ (Clin Res Ed)*; **286(6379)**:1705–9.

Jarman B (1985) Social security benefits and general practice. In *The Medical Annual*. Bristol: John Wright & Sons.

Jarman B (2000) The quality of care in hospitals. Harveian Oration 1999. *J Roy College of Physicians of London*; **34(1)**:75–91.

Jarman B, Pereira Gray D (1986) Undergraduate teaching and examination of general practice. In *The Medical Annual*. Bristol: John Wright & Sons.

Jenkins RM (1996) Why not the FBA way? In *RCGP Members' Reference Book 1996*. London: Sterling Publications.

Jervis P, Plowden W (2013) *The impact of political devolution on the UK's Health Services*. London: Nuffield Trust.

Johnson N, Hasler J (1997) Content validity of a trainer's report: Summative assessment in general practice. *Med Educ*; **31**:287–92.

Johnson N, Hasler J, Toby J, Grant J (1996a) Consensus minimum standards for use in a trainer's report for summative assessment in general practice. *Br J Gen Pract*; **46(404)**:140–4.

Johnson N, Hasler J, Toby J, Grant J (1996b) Content of a trainer's report for summative assessment in general practice: Views of trainers. *Br J Gen Pract*; **46(404)**:135–9.

Johnson J (1997) *Health Services Journal*; May.

Johnson Samuel (1755) Preface. *Dictionary of the English Language*. London: Consortium.

Joint Committee on Postgraduate Training for General Practice (JCPTGP) (1976) *Criteria for the Selection of Trainers*. London: JCPTGP.

Joint Committee on Postgraduate Training for General Practice (JCPTGP) (1995) *Minute of Meeting in November 1995*. London: JCPTGP.

Joint Committee on Postgraduate Training for General Practice (JCPTGP) (1996a) Annual Report. In *RCGP Members' Reference Book*. London: Sterling Publications.

Joint Committee on Postgraduate Training for General Practice (JCPTGP) (1996b) Summative assessment of vocational training for general practice—a second position paper. In *RCGP Members' Reference Book*. London: Sterling Publications.

Joint Prison Service and NHS Executive (1999) *The Future Organisation of Prison Health Care*. London: Department of Health.

Jones RV (1986) *Working Together: Learning Together. Occasional Paper 33*. Exeter: RCGP.

Jones RVH, Bolden KJ, Pereira Gray D, Hall MS (1978) *Running a Practice*. First edition. Second edition 1981, third edition 1985. London: Croom Helm Ltd.

Jones RV, Greenwood B (1994) Breast cancer: Causes of patients' distress identified by qualitative analysis. *Br J Gen Pract*; **44(385)**:370–1.

Jones RV, Hansford J, Fiske J (1993) Death from cancer at home: The carers' perspective. *BMJ*; **306(6872)**:249–51.

Journal of the Royal College of General Practitioners (JRCGP) (1972a) Out of debt. Editorial. [Anonymous, DPG]; **22(114)**:4–5.

Journal of the Royal College of General Practitioners (JRCGP) (1972b) Si monumentum require, circumspice. Editorial. [Anonymous, DPG]; **22(114)**:3–4.

Journal of the Royal College of General Practitioners (JRCGP) (1972c) First English chair. Editorial. [Anonymous, DPG]; **22(115)**:68–69.

Journal of the Royal College of General Practitioners. (JRCGP) (1972d) Michael Balint. Editorial. [Anonymous, DPG]; **22(116)**:133–5.

Journal of the Royal College of General Practitioners (JRCGP,1972e) Quality in question. Editorial. [Anonymous by DPG]; **22(120)**:425–6.

Journal of the Royal College of General Practitioners (JRCGP) (1973a) Continuity of care. Editorial. [Anonymous, DPG]; **23(136)**:749–50.

Journal of the Royal College of General Practitioners (JRCGP) (1973b) Confidentiality in general practice. Editorial. [Anonymous, DPG]; **23(137)**:833–9.

Journal of the Royal College of General Practitioners (JRCGP) (1974a) Patient power. Editorial. [Anonymous, DPG]; **24(138)**:1–3.

Journal of the Royal College of General Practitioners (JRCGP) (1974b) What is a patient? Editorial [Anonymous DPG]; **24(145)**:513.

Journal of the Royal College of General Practitioners (JRCGP) (1975a) Obituary Sydney Joseph Pereira Gray. [Anonymous DPG]; **25(155)**:439.

Journal of the Royal College of General Practitioners (JRCGP) (1975b) The maternity grant—room for reform. Editorial. [Anonymous DPG]; **25(151)**:81.

Journal of the Royal College of General Practitioners (JRCGP) (1975c) Is there discrimination in the BMA? Editorial. [Anonymous DPG]; **25(159)**:706–7.

Journal of the Royal College of General Practitioners (JRCGP) (1975d) Mac. Editorial. [Anonymous DPG]; **25(158)**:627–9.

Journal of the Royal College of General Practitioners (JRCGP) (1975e) The Nuffield experiment. Editorial [Anonymous DPG]; **25(157)**:547–8.

Journal of the Royal College of General Practitioners (JRCGP) (1977) Is sickness a sin? Editorial. [Anonymous DPG]; **27(178)**:259.

Journal of the Royal College of General Practitioners (JRCGP) (1979) Women general practitioners. Editorial. [Anonymous, DPG]; **29(201)**:195–8.

Journal of the Royal College of General Practitioners (JRCGP) (1980a) What kind of journal? Editorial. [Anonymous DPG]; **30(221)**:707–9.

Journal of the Royal College of General Practitioners (JRCGP) (1980b) Family doctors for doctors' families. Editorial. [Anonymous DPG]; **30(221)**:709–11.

Journal of the Royal College of General Practitioners (JRCGP) (1988) News: College action in the North East Thames Region. **38(310)**:239.

Jowell R, Brook L, Taylor B (1991) *British Social Attitudes*. 8th Report. London: Dartmouth Publishing Co.

Judicial Committee of the Privy Council (1999) Dr John Roylance versus the GMC Appeal, No 49 of 1998. Delivered 24 March.

Kahana E, Stange KC, Meehan R *et al.* (1997) Forced disruption in continuity of primary care: The patients' perspective. *Sociological Focu*s; **30(2)**:177–87.

Kajira-Montag H Freeman M and Scholtes S (2024) Continuity of care increases physician productivity in primary care. *Management Science*. https://doi.org./10.1287/mnsc.2021.02018

Kaplan SH, Greenfield S, Ware JE Jr (1989) Assessing the effects of physician-patient interactions on the outcomes of chronic disease. *Med Care*; **27(3 Suppl)**:S110–27.

Katerndahl D, Wood R, Jaén CR (2015) Complexity of ambulatory care across disciplines. *Healthcare*; **3(2)**:89–96.

Katz DA, McCoy K, Sarrazin MV (2014) Does improved continuity of primary care affect clinician–patient communication in VA? *J Gen Intern Med*; **29(Suppl2)**:682–8.

Kelsey Frances. In photo in John F Kennedy Presidential Library and Museum (1962) Kennedy signing the 1962 Drug Act on October 1962 with Dr Frances Kelsey of the FDA present.

Kendall-Gallagher D, Aiken LH, Sloane DM *et al.* (2011) Nurse specialty certification, inpatient mortality, and failure to rescue. *J Nurs Scholarsh*; **43(2)**:188–94.

Kennedy I (2001) *Report of the public inquiry into children's heart surgery at the Bristol Royal Infirmary 1984–1995. Learning from Bristol.* Cm 5207(II). Chair, Sir Ian Kennedy. London: HMSO.

Kent A (1986) How democratic is democracy? *BMA News Review;* August, p15.

Kessler D, Lloyd K, Lewis G, Pereira Gray D (1999) Cross-sectional study of symptom attribution and recognition of depression and anxiety in primary care. *BMJ*; **318(7181)**:436–40.

Kotsopoulos J (2019) Menopausal hormones: Definitive evidence for breast cancer. Editorial. *Lancet*; **394(10204)**:1116–8.

Kratky AP (1977) An audit of the care of diabetics in one general practice. *J R Coll Gen Pract*; **27(182)**:536–43.

Kuenssberg EV (1976) *Opportunity to Learn. Occasional Paper 2*. Exeter: RCGP.

Kuenssberg EV, Simpson JA, Stanton JB (1961) Is thalidomide to blame? Letter. *BMJ*; **1**:291.

Lamberts TW, Goldacre MJ (2006) Doctors' views about the first postgraduate year in UK medical practice: House officers in 2003. Table 2. *Med Educ*; **40**:115–22.

Lancet (1962) A new postgraduate medical institute. Editorial. i, 367.

Lancet (1978) General-practice training, Exeter style. Editorial. **311(8056)**:134–5.

Lancet (1980) Personal doctoring. Editorial. **315(8162)**:239.

Lane Committee (1974) *Report of the Committee on the Working of the Abortion Act*. Chairman, The Hon Mrs Justice Lane. Vols 1, 2 and 3. London: HMSO.

Lane E (1985) *Hear the Other Side: The Autobiography of England's first Woman Judge*. London: Butterworths.

Lane K (1992) *The Longest Art*. Republished Exeter: RCGP. First published Sydney, Australia: Allen & Unwin, 1969.

Lassagna L (1960) Thalidomide – a new non barbiturate sleep-inducing drug *J Chronic Diseases*; **11**:627–31.

Lawson JAR (1983) The development of general practice/family medicine throughout the world. In *The Medical Annual*. Bristol: John Wright & Sons.

Lee M, Saunders K (2004) Oak trees from acorns? An evaluation of local bursaries in primary care. *Primary Health Care Research and Development*; **5(2)**:93–95.

Lefroy J, Bruce F, Glen J *et al.* (2014) *Holding the Centre: Social Stability and Social Capital*. London: House of Commons.

Levitt HN (1964) Diagnostic facilities for general practitioners in England and Wales. Table 1. *J Coll Gen Pract*; **8**:312–321.

Lewis AP, Bolden KJ (1989) General practitioners and their learning styles. *J R Coll Gen Pract*; **39(322)**:187–9.

Lings P, Evans P, Seamark D *et al.* (2003) The doctor-patient relationship in US primary care. *J Roy Soc Med*; **96(4)**:180–4.

Lings P, Pereira Gray D (2002) Professional development for general practitioners through fellowship by assessment. *Med Educ*; **36(4)**:360–5.

Lord Moran C (1958) Evidence to the Royal Commission on Doctors' and Dentists' Remuneration. *BMJ*; **1**(Suppl):27–30.

Loudon I, Horder JP, Webster C (Eds) (1998) *General Practice under the NHS 1948–1997: The First 50 years*. Table D6 p310. Oxford: Clarendon Press.

Loudon K, Loudon I (1986) *Medical Care and the General Practitioner, 1750–1850*. Table D Oxford: Oxford University Press.

Lough JR, McKay J, Murray TS (1995a) Audit and summative assessment: Two years' pilot experience. *Med Educ*; **29(2)**:101–3.

Lough JRM, McKay J, Murray TS (1995b) Audit and summative assessment: A criterion-referenced marking schedule. *Br J Gen Pract*; **45(400)**:607–9.

Lough JRM, McKay J, Murray TS (1995c) Audit: Trainers' and trainees' attitudes and experiences. *Med Educ*; **29(1)**:85–90.

Lough JRM, Murray TS (1997) Training for audit: Lessons still to be learned. *Br J Gen Pract*; **47(418)**: 290–2.

Luft HS, Bunker JP, Enthoven AC (1979) Should operations be regionalized? The empirical relation between surgical volume and mortality. *N Engl J Med*; **301(25)**:1364–9.

Lydall R (2005) Family friendly pledge for the Thames Gateway: Schools and GPs within 'pram-pushing distance *Evening Standard* p16 23 November

Mackenzie J (1921) A defence of the thesis that "the opportunities of general practitioner are essential for the investigation of disease and the progress of medicine". *BMJ*; **I**:797–804.

Magnan S (2017) Social determinants of health 101 for health care: Five plus five. Discussion paper. Washington: NAM Perspectives.

Mainous AG 3rd, Baker R, Love MM *et al.* (2001) Continuity of care and trust in one's physician: Evidence from primary care in the United States and the United Kingdom. *Fam Med*; **33(1)**:22–27.

Mair A (1986) *Sir James Mackenzie MD: 1853–1925. General Practitioner*. Republished Exeter: RCGP. First published Edinburgh and London: Churchill Livingston, 1973.

Mallick Report (1993) *Report of the Review of the London Renal Services*. Chair: NP Mallick. London: HMSO.

Malone G (1996) [As Minister of State] Letter to Chairman of JCPTGP [DPG] September 1995. In *RCGP Members' Reference Book*. London: Sterling Publications.

Mansfield B (1986) How bad are medical records? A review of notes received by a practice *J R Coll Gen Pract*; **36**:405–7.

Mant Committee (1997) *Research and Development in Primary Care: National Working Party Report*. Chair, Prof David Mant London: NHS Executive.

Marinker M (1984) Through a glass darkly – learning with video. In *The Medical Annual*. Bristol: John Wright & Sons.

Marinker M, Pereira Gray D, Maynard A (1986) The doctor, the patient, and their contract. II. A good practice allowance: Is it feasible? *BMJ (Clin Res Ed)*; **292(6532)**:1374–6.

Marinker ML (1973) On the boundary. Gale Lecture 1972. *J R Coll Gen Pract*; **23(127)**:83–94.

Marshall M, Pagel C, French C *et al.* (2014) Moving improvement research closer to practice: The Researcher-in-Residence model. *BMJ Qual Saf*; **23(10)**:801–5.

Marshall M, Pereira Gray D (2016) General practice is making a leap in the dark. Editorial. *BMJ*; **355**:i5698.

Marsh GN, Kaim-Caudle PR (1976) *Team Care in General Practice*. London: Croom Helm Ltd.

Martin E (1984) Comparison of medical care in prisons and in general practice. *BMJ (Clin Res Ed)*; **289(6450)**:967–9.

Martin E (1985) Medical care in prisons. *Lancet*; **326(8461)**:942.

Martin E (1986) The medical care of prisoners. In *The Medical Annual*. Bristol: John Wright & Sons.

Martin E (1987) News: Council. *J R Coll Gen Pract*; **37(296)**:137.

Maynard A, Marinker M, Pereira Gray D (1986) The doctor, the patient, and their contract. III. Alternative contracts: Are they viable? *BMJ (Clin Res Ed)*; **292(6533)**:1438–40.

McAlister FA, Majumadar SR, Eurich DT *et al.* (2007) The effect of specialist care within the first year on subsequent outcomes in 24,232 adults with new onset diabetes mellitus: Population-based cohort study. *Qual Saf Health Care*; **16**:6–11.

McCartney M (2020) Medicine before Covid-19 and after. *Lancet*; **395**:1248–9.

McEwan J (1983) The role of the general practitioner in preventive medicine. In *The Medical Annual*. Bristol: John Wrights & Sons.

McGovern CM, Redmond M, Arcoleo K *et al.* (2017) A missed primary care appointment correlates with subsequent emergency department visit among children with asthma. *J Asthma*; **54(9)**:977–82.

McKee M, Dunnell K, Anderson M *et al.* (2021) The changing health needs of the UK population. *Lancet*; **397(10288)**:1979–91.

McKeown T (1976) *The Role of Medicine: Dream, Mirage or Nemesis? Rock Carling Lecture*. London: Nuffield Provincial Hospitals Trust.

McLachlan G (1992) *A History of the Nuffield Provincial Hospital Hospitals Trust 1940–1990*. London: NPHT. Foreword by Williams E on Lord Nuffield.

Medical (Professional Performance) Act (1995) *Amendment to Medical Act 1983*. London: HMSO.

Medical Research Council (MRC) (1997) *Primary Health Care: MRC Topic Review*. Chair, Prof Nigel Stott. London: MRC.

Medical Research Council (MRC) Working Party (1985) MRC trial of treatment of mild hypertension: Principal results. *Br Med J (Clin Res Ed)*; **291(6488)**:97–104.

Medical Schools Council and Royal College of General Practitioners (RCGP) (2017) *Destination GP. Medical students' experiences and perceptions of general practice*. London: MSC and RCGP.

Merrifield N (2015) Barts placed in special measures following damning CQC report. *Nurs Times*; **111(13)**:5.

Merrison Committee (1975) *Report of the Merrison Committee into the Regulation of the Medical Profession*. Cmnd 6018. Chair, Dr AW Merrison. London: HMSO.

Metcalfe N (Ed) (2019) *100 Notable Names from General Practice*. Florida: CRC Press.

Mitchell D (1992) *25 Years. An Interim History of the Royal College of Physicians of Ireland 1963–88*. Dublin: RCPI. P.35.

Moberly T (2019) More doctors are taking a break from training after foundation programme. *BMJ*; **364**:1842.

Moore R (1994) *The MRCGP Examination: A Guide for Candidates and Teachers*. Exeter: RCGP.

Moore R (1998) *The First Hundred Fellows by Assessment*. Exeter: RCGP.

Moran C [Lord] (1958) Evidence to the Royal Commission on Doctors' and Dentists' *Remuneration BMJ*; **1**(suppl):27–30.

Morrell DC, Evans ME, Morris RW, Roland MO (1986) The "five minute" consultation: Effect of time constraint on clinical content and patient satisfaction. *Br Med J (Clin Res Ed)*; **292(6524)**:870–3.

National Association of Health Authorities and Trusts (1992) Prison medical service. Data briefing. *Health Serv J*; **102(5323)**:41.

National Audit Office (2018) *PFI and PF2*. London: NAO.

National Information Governance Board for Health and Social Care (NIGB) (2009) *The NHS Constitution for England*. London: DHSC.

Newbould J, Abel G, Ball S *et al.* (2017) Evaluation of telephone first approach to demand management in English general practice: Observational study. *BMJ*; **358**:j4197.

Newman L (1992) Second among equals. James Mackenzie Lecture 1991. *Br J Gen Pract*; **42(355)**:71–74.

NHS Confederation and BMA (2003) *Investing in General Practice: New GMS Contract*. London: BMA/ NHS Confederation.

NHS Executive (1994) *Developing NHS Purchasing: Towards a Primary Care Led NHS*. Leeds: NHSE.

NHS Management Executive (1990) *The Care Card: Evaluation of the Exmouth Project* London: HMSO

Nimnuan C, Hotopf M, Wessely S (2001) Medically unexplained symptoms: An epidemiological study in seven specialties. *J Psychosom Res*; **51(1)**:361–7.

Nimzowitsch A (1950) *My System. A Chess Treatise.* London: G Bell & Sons.

Nissen, SE (2005) Halting the progression of atherosclerosis with intensive lipid lowering: results from the Reversal of Atherosclerosis with Aggressive Lipid Lowering (REVERSAL) trial. *Am J Med*; **118(12)**:22–7.

O'Connor PJ, Desai J, Rish WA *et al.* (1998) Is having a regular provider of diabetes care related to intensity of control? *J Fam Pract*; **47**:290–7.

O'Malley AS, Mandelblatt J, Gold K *et al.* (1997) Continuity of care and the use of breast and cervical cancer screening services in a multi-ethnic community. *Arch Int Med*; **157(13)**:1462–70.

O'Neill O (2002) *A question of trust. Reith Lecture 2002.* London: BBC.

Office of Health Economics (OHE, 1987) *Compendium of Health Statistics*; London: OHE.

Orton P, Orton C, Pereira Gray D (2012) Depersonalised doctors: A cross-sectional study of 564 doctors, 760 consultations and 1876 patient reports in UK general practice. *BMJ Open*; **2(1)**:e000274.

Orton PK, Pereira Gray D (2016) Factors influencing consultation length in general/family practice. *Family Practice* **33(5)**:529–34.

Paice E, Smith D (2009) Bullying of trainee doctors is a patient safety issue. *Clinical Teacher*; **6(1)**:13–17.

Panagioti M, Geraghty K, Johnson J *et al.* (2018) Association between physician burnout and patient safety, professionalism, and patient satisfaction: A systematic review and meta-analysis. *JAMA Intern Med*; **178(10)**:1317–31.

Pater JE (1981) *The Making of the NHS.* London: King's Fund.

Pemberton J (1984) *Will Pickles of Wensleydale. The life of a country doctor.* Republished Exeter: RCGP. First published London: Geoffrey Bles, 1970.

Pendleton D, Schofield T, Marinker M (Eds) (1986) *In Pursuit of Quality. Approaches to Performance Review in General Practice.* Exeter: RCGP.

Penrose LS (1939) Mental disease and crime: Outline of a comparative study of European Statistics *Br J Med Psychol*; **18(1)**:1–15.

Pentagon Papers (1971) Report of the Office of the Secretary of Defence Vietnam Task Force. Revealed by Daniel Ellsberg. *New York Times.*

Peppiatt R (1980) Patients' use of GPs or accident and emergency departments. *The Practitioner*; **224(1339)**:11–14.

Peppiatt R, Evans R, Jordan P (1978) Blood alcohol concentrations of patient attending an accident and emergency department. *Resuscitation*; **6(1)**:37–43.

Pereira JAW (1903) Tapeworm as a cause of chorea. *Lancet*; **162(4177)**:824.

Pereira JAW (1915) The treatment of acute lobar pneumonia. Letter. *Lancet*; **184(4793)**:94.

Pereira Gray D (DPG) (1966/67) The role of the general practitioner in the early detection of malignant disease. Gold Medal Essay. *Trans Hunter Soc*; **25**:135–79.

Pereira Gray D (DPG) (1969/70) The care of the handicapped child in general practice. Gold Medal Essay 1969. *Trans Hunter Soc*; **28**:121–75.

Pereira Gray D (DPG) (1977a) *A System of Training for General Practice. Occasional Paper 4.* First edition. Second edition 1979. Exeter: RCGP.

Pereira Gray D (DPG) (1977b) General practitioners and the independent contractor status. *J R Coll Gen Pract*; **27(185)**:746–52.

Pereira Gray D (DPG) (1978) Feeling at home. James Mackenzie Lecture 1977. *J R Coll Gen Pract*; **28(186)**:6–17.

Pereira Gray D (DPG) (1979a) The key to personal care. Pfizer Lecture. *J R Coll Gen Pract*; **29(208)**:666–78.

Pereira Gray D (DPG) (1979b) General practice. In *The Medical Annual 1979/80*. Bodley Scott R, Fraser J (Eds). Bristol: John Wright & Sons.

Pereira Gray D (DPG) (1980a) Just a GP. Gale Memorial Lecture 1979. *J R Coll Gen Pract* **30(213)**:231–9.

Pereira Gray D (DPG) (1980b) Patients in the RCGP. *Pulse.*

Pereira Gray D (DPG) (1982) *Training for General Practice.* Plymouth: Macdonald and Evans.

Pereira Gray D (DPG) (1984a) Selecting general practitioner trainers. *BMJ*; **288**:195–8.

Pereira Gray D (DPG) (1984b) The year in general practice. In *The Medical Annual.* Bristol: John Wright & Sons.

Pereira Gray D (DPG) (1984c) A study of preventive care in one general practice. In *The Medical Annual*. Bristol: John Wright & Sons.

Pereira Gray D (DPG) (1984d) The World Health Organization and general practice. In *The Medical Annual*. Bristol: John Wright & Sons.

Pereira Gray D (DPG) (1984e) Editor's preface. In *The Medical Annual*. Bristol: John Wright & Sons.

Pereira Gray D (DPG) (1985) Practice annual reports. In *The Medical Annual*. Bristol: John Wright & Sons.

Pereira Gray D (DPG) (1986a) AIDS. In *The Medical Annual*. Bristol: John Wright & Sons.

Pereira Gray D (DPG) (1986b) Nakedness in medicine. In *The Medical Annual*. Bristol: John Wright & Sons.

Pereira Gray D (DPG) (1987) RCGP Spring Meeting Edinburgh: Chairman of Council's report. *J R Coll Gen Pract*; **37(298)**:230–2.

Pereira Gray D (1987b) Screening for Breast Cancer. In *The Medical Annual*. Bristol: John Wright & Sons.

Pereira Gray D (DPG) (1988) Spring General Meeting 1988: Chairman's report. *J R Coll Gen Pract*; **38(311)**:285–92. ["avalanche of change"]

Pereira Gray D (DPG) (1989) The emergence of the discipline of general practice, its literature and the contribution of the College *Journal*. McConaghey Memorial Lecture 1988. *J R Coll Gen Pract*; **39(323)**:228–33.

Pereira Gray D (DPG) (1991a) Good general practice: Fellowship of the RCGP by assessment. Editorial. *Br J Gen Pract*; **41(346)**:182–3.

Pereira Gray D (DPG) (1991b) Research in general practice: Law of inverse opportunity. *BMJ*; **302(6789)**:1380–2.

Pereira Gray D (Ed) (DPG) (1992a) *Forty Years On: The Story of the First 40 Years of the RCGP*. London: Atalink.

Pereira Gray D (DPG) (1992b) Celebrating a general practitioner thesis the Nijmegen way. Christmas Miscellany. *Br J Gen Pract*; **42(365)**:534–5.

Pereira Gray D (DPG) (1992c) *Planning Primary Care. Occasional Paper 57*. Exeter: RCGP.

Pereira Gray D (DPG) (1995a) The Conference of Academic Organizations in General Practice. In *RCGP Members' Reference Book 1995*. London: Sterling Publications.

Pereira Gray D (DPG) (1995b) Research general practices. Editorial. *Br J Gen Pract*; **45(399)**:516–17.

Pereira Gray D (DPG) (1995c) Primary care and the public health. 1994 Harben Lecture. *Health and Hygiene*; **16**:49–62.

Pereira Gray D (DPG) (1996a) Research general practices. *RCGP Members' Reference Book 1996*. London, *Sterling Publications*.

Pereira Gray D (DPG) (1997a) The challenge of change. Keynote address to 1996 Trainers' Conference in Devon and Cornwall. *Educ Gen Prac*; **8**:72–81.

Pereira Gray D (DPG) (1997b) Summative assessment of vocational training to be required by law. *Br J Gen Pract*; **47(423)**:608–10.

Pereira Gray D (DPG) (1997c) Health promotion and primary care. Annual Address. *J Roy Soc Health*; **117(1)**:250–9.

Pereira Gray D (DPG) (2001) Proposed new law on manslaughter: Implications for the NHS and doctors. *Br J Gen Pract*; **51(463):**156–7.

Pereira Gray D (DPG) (2002) Deprofessionalising doctors? Editorial. *BMJ*; **324(7338):**627–8.

Pereira Gray D (2002) Fourth Franz Huygen Lecture Onderzoek in de huisartsgeneeskunde, de rol van academische netwerken *Huisarts en Wetenschap*; **45(9)**:459–62.

Pereira Gray D (DPG) (2003) 2020 vision. *Health Serv J*; **113(5875)**:18–19.

Pereira Gray D (DPG) (2004a) Impact of new pension load set to grow in the future. *Financial Times* 13 February.

Pereira Gray D (DPG) (2006) Appendix: A dozen facts about general practice/primary care. In Department of Health (2006) *Our Health, Our Care, Our Say: A New Direction for Community Services*. London: DH.

Pereira Gray D (DPG) (2008) *Holmedale: Family Practice and Family Home*. Exeter: published privately.

Pereira Gray D (DPG) (2010a) Biographies in theory and in practice. Editorial. *J Med Biogr*; **18(2)**:63.

Pereira Gray D (DPG) (2010b) Support for marriage is a public health issue. *The Times* 12 April. [Lead letter].

Pereira Gray D (DPG) (2013) *It's the relationships stupid! 2013 Goodman Lecture.* Exeter: WATCh?

Pereira Gray D (DPG) (2015a) Postgraduate medical school of the University of Exeter. Letter. *J Roy Soc Med*; **108(12)**:472.

Pereira Gray D (DPG) (2015b) Research and teaching in general practice/primary care. Letter. *BMJ*; **351**:h4737.

Pereira Gray D (DPG) (2015c) Academic general practice: Viewpoint on achievements and challenges. *Br J Gen Pract*; **65(640)**:e786–8.

Pereira Gray D (DPG) (2016) *Evidence to the Health Select Committee of Parliament.* London: House of Commons.

Pereira Gray D (DPG) (2017a) Towards research-based learning outcomes for general practice in medical schools: Inaugural Barbara Starfield Memorial Lecture. *BJGP Open*; **1(1)**.

Pereira Gray D (DPG) (2017b) Down with "primary care," up with "general practice". BMA Opinion. *BMJ*; 13 March.

Pereira Gray D (DPG) (2017c) Up with "general practice": Down with "primary care". *BMJ;* 30 Sept.

Pereira Gray D (DPG) (2018a) The discipline of general practice: Recognition and teaching. Editorial. *Br J Gen Pract*; **68(670)**:212–13.

Pereira Gray D (DPG) (2018b) Switching to vaping. Letter. *The Times,* 31 October.

Pereira Gray D (DPG) (2019) Absence of intellectual challenge in medical schools. Letter. *Br J Gen Pract*; **69(685)**:378.

Pereira Gray D (DPG) (2022a) Sajid Javid's plan to nationalise GPs. Letter. *The Times,* 31 January.

Pereira Gray D (DPG) (2022b) Medicine must harness mind-body interactions. Letter. *Financial Times,* 7 March.

Pereira Gray D (DPG) (2022c) Breadth and Depth. Letter. *The Times,* 27 April.

Pereira Gray D (DPG) (2022d) Invaluable GPs. *Financial Times.*

Pereira Gray D (2023) General Practice: the Integrating Discipline. Editorial *Br J Gen Pract*; **73(734)**:388–90.

Pereira Gray D, Bolden KJ (1985) Learning in small groups. In *The Medical Annual.* Bristol: John Wright & Sons.

Pereira Gray D, Dean D, Dean PM (2020a) Childcare outside the family for the under-threes: Cause for concern. *J R Soc Med*; **113(4)**:140–2.

Pereira Gray D, Dean D, Dineen M *et al.* (2020b) Science versus society: Is childcare for the under threes a taboo subject? Editorial. *Epigenomics*; **12(14)**:1153–5.

Pereira Gray D, Dineen M, Sidaway-Lee K (2020d) The worried well. *Br J Gen Pract*; **70(691)**:84–85.

Pereira Gray D, Evans P, Sweeney K, Steele R (1996) HRT prescribing—a paradigm for the complexity of prescribing in general practice. *RCGP Members' Reference Book 1996.* London: Sterling Publications.

Pereira Gray D, Evans P, Sweeney K, Lings P, Seamark D, Dixon M, and Bradley, N (2003) Towards a theory of continuity of care. *J R Soc Med*; **96(4)**:160–6.

Pereira Gray D, Evans P, Wright C, Langley P (2011) Patient-doctor depth-of-relationship scale: Development and validation. Letter. *Ann Fam Med*; **9(6)**:538–45.

Pereira Gray DJ, Evans PH, Wright C, Langley P (2012) The cost of diagnosing type 2 diabetes mellitus by clinical opportunistic screening in general practice. *Diabet Med*; **29(7)**:863–8.

Pereira Gray D, Freeman G, Johns C *et al.* (2020e) Covid-19: A fork in the road for general practice. Editorial. *BMJ*; **370**:m3709.

Pereira Gray D, Goble R, Openshaw S *et al.* (1993) Multiprofessional education at the Postgraduate Medical School, University of Exeter, United Kingdom. *Ann Comm Oriented Educ*; **6**:181–90.

Pereira Gray D, Henley W, Chenore T *et al.* (2017) What is the relationship between age and deprivation in influencing emergency hospital admissions? A model using data from a defined, comprehensive, all-age cohort in East Devon, UK. *BMJ Open*; **7(2)**:e014045.

Pereira Gray D, Langley P, White E, Evans P (2014) Is the 'scandal' of diabetes care in general practice fact or fiction? *Br J Gen Pract*; **64(623)**:300.

Pereira Gray D, Marinker M, Maynard A (1986c) The doctor, the patient, and their contract. I. The general practitioner's contract: Why change it? *BMJ (Clin Res Ed)*; **292(6531)**:1313–5.

Pereira Gray Report (1992) Report of the Royal College of Physicians, the Royal College of General Practitioners and the Royal College of Psychiatrists, Education and Training of doctors on the Healthcare Service for Prisoners on the Prison Medical Service. Chairman, Professor Denis Pereira Gray. London: The Home Office.

Pereira Gray D, Sidaway-Lee K (2018a) When I say exposure. *Med Ed*; **52(9)**:894–5.

Pereira Gray D, Sidaway-Lee K (2018b) National standard setting and local developments in the care of type 2 diabetes. Editorial. *Practical Diabetes*; **35(1)**:7–9.

Pereira Gray D, Sidaway-Lee K, Evans P (2016c) The role of general practice in reducing mortality. Letter. *Lancet*; **388(10058)**:2354.

Pereira Gray D, Sidaway-Lee K, White E *et al.* (2018c) Continuity of care with doctors - a matter of life and death? A systematic review of continuity of care and mortality. *BMJ Open*; **8(6)**:e021161.

Pereira Gray D, Sidaway-Lee K, Evans P (2022a) *How to Implement and Manage Personal Lists in General Practice: A Guide for GPs and Practice Managers*. Exeter: St Leonard's Research Practice.

Pereira Gray D, Sidaway-Lee K, Evans P (2022b) Continuity of GP care using personal lists Editorial. *Br J Gen Pract*; **72**:208–09.

Pereira Gray D, Sidaway-Lee K, Kingdon H *et al.* (2020c) Core management data in general practice. *Br J Gen Pract*; **70(690)**:36–37.

Pereira Gray D, Sidaway-Lee K, White E *et al.* (2016b) Improving continuity: The clinical challenge. *InnovAiT*; **9(10)**:635–45.

Pereira Gray D, Sidaway-Lee K, White E, Dineen M, Harding A, and Evans P (2021) The academic triad in general practice. Letter. *Br J Gen Pract*; **71(708)**:301.

Pereira Gray D, Steele R, Sweeney K, Evans P (1994) Generalists in medicine. Editorial. *BMJ*; **308(6927)**:486–7.

Pereira Gray D, Steele R Sweeney K, Evans P (1996c) HRT Prescribing: A paradox for the complexity of prescribing in general practice *RCGP Members' Reference Book 1996* London: Atalink

Pereira Gray D, Steele R, Sweeney K *et al.* (1996c) HRT prescribing—a paradigm for complexity of pre-scribing in general practice In *RCGP Members' Reference Book 1996* London: Sterling Publications.

Pereira Gray D, White E, Russell G (2016a) Medicalisation in the UK: Changing dynamics, but still ongoing. *J Roy Soc Med*; **109(1)**:7–11.

Pereira Gray D, Wilkie P (2017) Patient perspectives on telephone first system. Letter. *BMJ*; **359**:j4925.

Pereira Gray D, Wilkie P (2015) Patient perspectives on telephone triage in general practice. Letter. *Lancet*; **385(9969)**:687–8.

Pereira Gray D, Wright A, O'Dowd T Dunn, G, Hannay, D, King, M, Kinmonth, AL, Taylor, R, Waine, C and Wilmot, J (1997d) The discipline and literature of general practice. Editorial. *Br J Gen Pract*; **47(416)**:139–43.

Pereira Gray J (1982) The doctor's family: Some problems and solutions. *J R Coll Gen Pract*; **32(235)**:75–79.

Pereira Gray J (1984) The health of doctors' families. In *The Medical Annual*. Bristol: John Wright & Sons.

Pereira Gray Report (1992) *Three Medical Royal Colleges Report on Prison Medicine* Chairman, Professor Denis Pereira Gray London: Home Office.

Pew-Fetzer Task Force (1994) *Relationship Centered Health Care*. San Francisco, CA: Pew Health Professions Commission.

Pickering G (1962) Postgraduate medical education: The present opportunity and the immediate need. *BMJ*; **1(5276)**:421–5.

Pickles WN (1984) *Epidemiology in Country Practice*. Republished Exeter: RCGP, 1984. First published Bristol: John Wright & Sons, 1939.

Pollak M (1984) Family practice and child development. In *The Medical Annual*. Bristol: John Wright & Sons.

Pond D (1985) Counselling in primary care. In *The Medical Annual*. Bristol: John Wright & Sons.

Postgraduate Medical School (1994) Academic Plan for 1995/6 to 1997/8. Drafted by DPG. Exeter: PGMS.

Postgraduate Medical School of the University of Exeter (1989) *Annual Report 1990/91*. Exeter: PGMS.

Postgraduate Medical School of the University of Exeter (1990) *Annual Report 1989/90*. Exeter: PGMS.

Preece JF, Gillings DB, Lippman ED *et al.* (1970) An on-line record maintenance and retrieval system in general practice. *Int J Biomed Comput*; **1(4)**:329–37.

Pringle M (1987) Assessing consultations. In *The Medical Annual*. Bristol: John Wright & Sons.

Pritchard P (1983) Patient participation in general practice. In *The Medical Annual*. Bristol: John Wright & Sons.

Pritchard PMM (1981) *Patient Participation. Occasional Paper 17*. Exeter: RCGP.

Pullen I, Wilkinson G, Wright A, Pereira Gray D (Eds) (1994) *Psychiatry and General Practice Today*. London: Royal College of Psychiatrists.

Pulse (2012) Survey on influential GPs.

Reis HT, Clark MS, Pereira Gray DJ *et al.* (2008) Measuring responsiveness in the therapeutic relationship: A patient perspective. *Basic and Applied Social Psychology*; **30(4)**:339–48.

Review Advisory Committee of Department of Health (1993) *Special Health Authorities: Research Review*. London: HMSO.

Richards Independent Task Force (1997) *Clinical Academic Careers*. Chairman, Sir Rex Richards. London: CVCP.

Ridd MJ, Lewis G, Peters TJ, Salisbury C (2011) Patient-doctor depth-of-relationship scale: Development and validation. *Ann Fam Med*; **9(6)**:538–45.

Rix S, Paykel ES, Lelliott P *et al.* (1999) Impact of a national campaign on GP education: An evaluation of the Defeat Depression Campaign. *Br J Gen Pract*; **49(439)**:99–102.

Rodgers R, Hammerstein O (1949) *South Pacific*. USA: Broadway.

Rogers L, O'Reilly J (2004) Baby Blair had MMR jab after outcry. *Sunday Times* 29 February.

Roland MO, Bartholomew J, Courtenay MJ *et al.* (1986) The "five minute" consultation: Effect of time constraint on verbal communication. *Br Med J (Clin Res Ed)*; **292(6524)**:874–6.

Ronalds C, Douglas A, Pereira Gray D *et al.* (1981) *Fourth National Trainee Conference. Occasional Paper 18*. Exeter: RCGP.

Rose FM, Hunt JH (1951) A College of General Practice. Letter. *BMJ*; **2**:908.

Ross N (2019) The role of the chief medical officer in conversation with Dame Sally Davies. *Commentary*; October, pp10–11.

Royal College of General Practitioners (1967) Royal Charter. London: RCGP.

Royal College of General Practitioners (RCGP) (1972a) Quality in General Practice. Press statement. *J R Coll Gen Pract*; **22(123)**:705.

Royal College of General Practitioners (RCGP) (1972b) Evidence of the College submitted to the Lane Committee on the Working of the Abortion Act [drafted by DPG]. *J R Coll Gen Pract*; **22(121)**:543–6.

Royal College of General Practitioners (1972c) *The Future General Practitioner: Learning and Teaching*; London: BMJ.

Royal College of General Practitioners (RCGP) (1974) *Oral Contraception and Health*. London: RCGP.

Royal College of General Practitioners (RCGP) (1975) evidence of the RCGP to the Select Committee of Parliament on the Abortion (Amendment) Bill. *J Roy Coll Gen Pract*; **25(159)**:774–6.

Royal College of General Practitioners (RCGP) (1978) College Policy: The care of children. *J R Coll Gen Pract*; **28(194)**:553–6.

Royal College of General Practitioners (RCGP) (1980a) *Selected Papers from the Eighth World Conference on Family Medicine. Occasional Paper 10*. Exeter: RCGP.

Royal College of General Practitioners (RCGP) (1980b) *Health and Prevention in Primary Care. Report from General Practice 18*. Chair, Dr J Horder. Exeter: RCGP.

Royal College of General Practitioners (RCGP) (1982) *Healthier Children-Thinking Prevention. Report from General Practice 22. Co-Convenors*, Donovan C, Pereira Gray D. Exeter: RCGP.

Royal College of General Practitioners (RCGP) (1985a) *Quality in General Practice. Policy Statement 2*, para 35. Exeter: RCGP.

Royal College of General Practitioners (RCGP) (1985b) *What Sort of Doctor? Assessing Quality of Care in General Practice. Report from General Practice 23.* Exeter: RCGP.

Royal College of General Practitioners (RCGP) (1986) *Prevention and the Primary Care Team.* Chair: Dr C Waine. Exeter: RCGP.

Royal College of General Practitioners (RCGP) (1987a) *The Front Line of the Health Service. Report from General Practice 25.* Exeter: RCGP.

Royal College of General Practitioners (RCGP) (1987b) *The Future General Practitioner–Learning and Teaching.* Republished Exeter: RCGP. First published London: BMJ. 1972.

Royal College of General Practitioners (RCGP) (1987c) Report of the AGM. In *RCGP Annual Members' Reference Book.* London: Sterling Publications.

Royal College of General Practitioners (RCGP) (1989a) College statement on White Paper. In *RCGP Members' Reference Book.* London: Sterling Publications.

Royal College of General Practitioners (RCGP) (1989b) *A College Plan. Occasional Paper 49.* Exeter: RCGP.

Royal College of General Practitioners (RCGP) (1990) *Fellowship by Assessment. Occasional Paper 50.* First edition [Written by DPG]. Second edition 1995. Exeter: RCGP.

Royal College of General Practitioners (1994) *Members' Reference Book* Ed Pereira Gray D; London: Sterling Publications.

Royal College of General Practitioners (1996) *Members' Reference Book Ed* Pereira Gray D. *Report of the JCPTGP Report on the Research Network* London: Sterling Publications.

Royal College of General Practitioners (RCGP) (1996) *RCGP Members' Reference Book. Research Network* pp 48–54 *JCPTGP Report* 195–213 London: Sterling Publications.

Royal College of General Practitioners (RCGP) (1997) *Removal of Patients from GPs' lists.* London: RCGP.

Royal College of General Practitioners (RCGP) (2021) Paper on continuity London: RCGP.

Royal College of General Practitioners (RCGP) (2021) *The power of relationships: what is relationship-based care and why is it important.* General practice COVID-19 recovery. London: RCGP.

Royal College of General Practitioners and the General Practitioners Committee (2001) *Consultation on Criteria for Revalidation.* London: RCGP and GPC.

Royal College of Physicians, Royal College of General Practitioners, Royal College of Psychiatrists (1994) *Three Medical Royal College Report on Prison Medicine.* Education and Training of Doctors in the Health Care Service for Prisoners. Chair, Prof Denis Pereira Gray. London: Home Office.

Royal Commission on Doctors' and Dentists' Remuneration (1960) Chair, Sir Harry Pilkington. London: HMSO.

Royal Commission on Medical Education (1968) Report. Chair, Lord Todd. London: HMSO.

Sajtar J (1959) *The VIIth World Student Chess Championship, Budapest, Hungary 30 June to 14 July 1959.* Prague, Czechoslovakia: International Union of Students.

Salisbury C, Chalder M, Manku-Scott T *et al.* (2002) *The National Evaluation of NHS Walk-in Centres. Final report.* Bristol: University of Bristol.

Salmon Report (1966) *Committee on Senior Nursing Staff Structure.* London: HMSO.

Sandeman DD, Shore AC, Tooke JE (1992) Relation of skin capillary pressure in patients with insulin-dependent diabetes mellitus to complications and metabolic control. *N Engl J Med*; **327(11)**:760–4.

Sapper H (2008) *The Presidents Portraits.* London: RCGP.

Schumacher EF (2011) *Small is Beautiful: A Study of Economics as if People Mattered.* London: Random House.

Scott P (1965) Letter to DPG, 17 August.

Scott AI, Freeman CP (1992) Edinburgh primary care depression study: Treatment outcome, patient satisfaction, and cost after 16 weeks. *BMJ*; **304(6831)**:883–7.

Seale J (1964) Medical emigration from Great Britain and Ireland. *BMJ*; **1 (5391)**:1173–8.

Secretary of State for Health (2000) *The NHS Plan: A Plan for Investment. A Plan for Reform.* The government's response to the Royal College on long-term care. Cm 488–11. London: HMSO.

Secretary of State for Health [Patricia Hewitt] (2006) *Our Health Our Care Our Say: a new direction for community services* London: HM Government and Department of Health

Select Committee of Parliament on Public Administration (2004) *Reformed Honours System*. London: House of Commons.

Select Committee on Science and Technology (1995) *Subcommittee 1 Minutes of Evidence heard in public 24 January 1995*. London: House of Lords.

Selley WG, Roche MT, Pearce VR *et al.* (1995) Dysphagia following strokes: Clinical observations of swallowing rehabilitation employing palatal training appliances. *Dysphagia*; **10(1)**:32–35.

Seward C (1947) *Bedside Diagnosis*. First edition. Edinburgh: E&S Livingstone.

Sheldon MG, Stoddart N (Eds) (1985) *Trends in General Practice Computing*. Exeter: RCGP.

Shepherd M (1983) Social psychiatry and the primary care of psychosocial disorder. In *The Medical Annual*. Bristol: John Wright & Sons.

Shi L (1992) The relationship between primary care and life chances. *J Health Care Poor & Underserved* **3(2)**:321–35.

Shi L, Macinko J, Starfield B *et al.* (2003) The relationship between primary care, income inequality, and mortality in US States, 1980–1995. *J Am Board Fam Pract*; **16(5)**:412–22.

Shipman Inquiry (2004) *Safeguarding Patients: Lessons from the Past. Proposals for the Future*. Chair, Dame Janet Smith. pp. 1023–176. London: Stationery Office.

Sidaway-Lee K, Pereira Gray D, Evans P (2019) A method for measuring continuity of care in day-to-day general practice: A quantitative analysis of appointment data. *Br J Gen Pract*; **69(682)**:e356–e362.

Sidaway-Lee K, Pereira Gray D, Harding A, Evans P (2021) What mechanisms could link GP relational continuity to patient outcomes? *Br J Gen Pract*; **71(707)**:278–81.

Silen W, Cope Z (2010) *Cope's Early Diagnosis of the Acute Abdomen*. 22nd ed. Oxford: OUP.

Singh H, Giardina TD, Meyer AN *et al.* (2013) Types and origins of diagnostic errors in primary care settings. *JAMA Intern Med*; **173**:418.

Smee C (2005) *Speaking Truth to Power: Two Decades of Policy Analysis in the Department of Health*. London: Nuffield Trust.

Smith CF, Drew S, Ziebland S *et al.* (2020) Understanding the role of GPs' gut feelings in diagnosing cancer in primary care: A systematic review and meta-analysis of existing evidence. *Br J Gen Pract*; **70(698)**:e612–21.

Smith D, Pearce L, Pringle M, and Caplan R (1995) Adults with a history of sexual abuse: Evaluation of a pilot therapy service. *BMJ*; **310**:1175–78.

Sneyde JR (2015) Plymouth medical school is committed to producing GPs of the future. Letter. *BMJ*; **351**:h5130.

Snow CP (1963) *The Two Cultures: And a Second Look: An Expanded Version of the Two Cultures and the Scientific Revolution*. From The Rede Lecture 1959. Cambridge, Cup.

Soumerai SB, Avorn J (1990) Principles of educational outreach ('academic detailing') to improve clinical decision making. *JAMA*; **263(4)**:549–56.

Spector, P.E. (1982) Behavior in organizations as a function of employee's locus of control. *Psychological Bulletin*; **91(3) 2**:482.

St Leonard's Research Practice (2022) *Report of the Improving GP Continuity Programme*. London: The Health Foundation.

Stallworthy JA, Moolgaoker AS, Walsh JJ (1971) Legal abortion: A critical assessment of its risks. *Lancet*; **298(7736)**:1245–9.

Starfield B (1994) Is primary care essential? *Lancet*; **344(8930)**:1129–33.

Starfield B (1998) *Primary Care: Balancing Health Needs, Services, and Technology*. New York: OUP.

Starfield B (2001) New paradigms for quality in primary care. *Br J Gen Pract*; **51(465)**:303–9.

Starfield B (2004) Contributions of evidence to the struggle towards equity. Research report. Nuffield Trust.

Starfield B, Shi L, Macinko J (2005) Contribution of primary care to health systems and health. *Milbank Q*; **83(3)**:457–502.

Steele RJFS (2000) Can educational methods developed for general practitioners in the UK be transferred to doctor and nurses in primary care in Hungary? MPhil Dissertation. Exeter: University of Exeter.

Stevens R. (1966) *Medical Practice in Modern England*. London: Yale University Press.

Stevens S (2004) Reform strategies for the English NHS. *Health Aff (Millwood)*; **23(3)**:37–44.

Stewart M (2005) Reflections on the doctor-patient relationship: From evidence and experience. Mackenzie Lecture 2004. *Br J Gen Pract*; **55(519)**:793–801.

Stolper E, van Royen P, Dinant GJ (2010) The 'sense of alarm' ('gut feeling') in clinical practice. A survey among European general practitioners on recognition and expression. *Eur J Gen Pract*; **16(2)**:72–74.

Stott P (1991) *Milestones: The Diary of a GP Trainee.* Exeter: RCGP.

Stott NCH, Davis RH (1979) The exceptional potential in each primary care consultation. *J R Coll Gen Pract*; **29(201)**:201–5.

Stroke Prevention in Atrial Fibrillation (SPAF) (1991) Stroke prevention in atrial fibrillation study. Final results. *Circulation*; **84(2)**:527–39.

Stubbings CA, Gowers JI (1979) A comparison of trainee and trainer clinical experience. *JR Coll Gen Pract*; **29(198)**:47–52.

Styles W (1995) Letter as Chair COAGP to Sir Dai Rees of the Medical Research Council 21 Sept

Summers H (2021) Prison guards get counselling after baby dies in cell but not mother. *The Observer,* 26 September.

Sung, YF, Tsai, CT, Kuo, CY, *et al.* (2022) Use of hormone replacement therapy and risk of dementia: a nationwide cohort study. *Neurology*; **99(17)**:1835–42.

Supreme Court of the UK (2015) Montgomery v Lanarkshire Health Board. Law Reports. *Times.*

Supreme Court of the US (1973) Roe v Wade.

Sweeney K (son) (2010) Dr Kieran Sweeney. Obituary. *Guardian,* 22 January.

Sweeney K, Pereira Gray D, Steele R, Evans P (1995) Use of warfarin in non-rheumatic atrial fibrillation: A commentary from general practice. *Br J Gen Pract*; **45(392)**:153–8.

Sweeney KG (1996) *The Use of Focus Groups for Assessing Consumers' Views on Miscarriage and Minor Surgery.* MPhil Dissertation. Exeter: University of Exeter.

Sweeney KG, MacAuley D, Pereira Gray D (1998) Personal significance: The third dimension. *Lancet*; **351(9096)**:134–6.

Sweeney KG, Pereira Gray D (1995) Patients who do not receive continuity of care from their general practitioner – are they a vulnerable group? *Br J Gen Pract*; **45(392)**:133–5.

Sweeney K, Toy L, Cromwell J (2009) A patient's journey. *BMJ*; **339**:b2862.

Swift G (1968) A course in vocational training for general practice in Wessex. *Brit J Med Educ*; **2**:63–70.

Talbot M (1985) Practice managers. In *The Medical Annual.* Bristol: John Wright & Sons.

Tanner JM (1983) Monitoring growth and development – An essential part of primary care. In *The Medical Annual.* Bristol: John Wright & Sons.

Tartakover S (1950) In Nimzovitsch A *My System: a Chess Treatise*; London: G Bell & Sons.

Taylor M (2022) Crumbling NHS. Letter. *The Times,* 6 May.

Taylor S (1954) *Good General Practice.* London: OUP.

Thatcher M (1993) *The Downing Street Years.* London: HarperCollins. p611.

Thompson A (1963) *Is general practice outmoded? Annual Address to the Royal Society of Health 1962.* London: Royal Society of Health.

Times (1994) John Fry. Obituary. [Anonymous DPG] 21 May.

Times (2003) Dinner for Sir Maurice Shock. 26 July, p4.

Times (2019) Jean, Grand Duke of Luxembourg. Obituary. 24 April.

Times (2020) Mr Tom McDonald. Obituary. 3 January.

Times (2021) Dame Margaret Booth. Obituary. 26 January

Tooke J (2008) *Aspiring to Excellence: Findings and Recommendations of the Independent Inquiry into Modernising Medical Careers.* Chair: Prof Sir John Tooke. London: MMC Inquiry. www.mmcinquiry.org.uk

Tudor Hart J (1971) The inverse care law. *Lancet*; **297(7696)**:405–12.

Tudor Hart J (1975) The management of high blood pressure in general practice. Gold medal essay. *J R Coll Gen Pract*; **25(152)**:160–92.

UK Nursing and Midwifery Council (2022) Nationality of new nurse registrations London: UKCC.

Universities Funding Council Joint Medical Advisory Committee (1995) *NHS University Interactions.* London: UFC.

University of Exeter 1995/96 *Calendar.* Exeter: UoE.

University of Exeter Department of General Practice Prospectus (1979) Exeter: UoE.

Van den Bruel A, Thompson M, Buntinx F *et al.* (2012) Clinicians' gut feeling about serious infections in children: Observational study. *BMJ*; **345**:e6144.

Van Weel C (1985) Hypertension and the general practitioner: Task or challenge. In *The Medical Annual*. Bristol: John Wright & Sons.

Van Weel C (2012) *Atlas, Keeper of Knowledge: An Analysis of the Effectiveness of Primary Care.* Farewell Lecture, 30 November 2012. Nijmegen, the Netherlands: University of Nijmegen.

Vincent C, Neale G, Woloshynowych M (2001) Adverse events in British hospitals: Preliminary retrospective record review. *BMJ*; **322(7285)**:517–19.

Wade R (1957) The Oxford Cambridge chess match. *British Chess Magazine.*

Waine Report (1992) *Guidelines for the Management of Hyperlipidaemia in General Practice. Towards the primary prevention of coronary heart disease. Occasional Paper 55.* Chair of Working Party, Dr Colin Waine. Exeter: RCGP.

Waine C, Hammond M (1983) The literature of general practice. In *Medical Annual*. Bristol: John Wright & Sons.

Waine C, Pereira Gray D, Smith T (1981a) Asthma I: Managing the acute attack. *BMJ (Clin Res Ed)*; **283(6284)**:110–12.

Waine C, Pereira Gray D, Smith T (1981b) Asthma II: Long-term management. *BMJ (Clin Res Ed)*; **283(6285)**:199–201.

Wakeford R, Foulkes J, McManus C, Southgate L (1993) MRCGP pass rate by medical school and region of postgraduate training. Royal College of General Practitioners. *BMJ*; **307(6903)**:542–3.

Walford D (1992) [As Medical Director NHS Management Executive] NHS and academic and research quotas for career registrars. Letter. EL(92)32. 18 May.

Walker A (1990) *Physiotherapy in Primary Care*. MPhil Dissertation. Exeter: University of Exeter.

Walker I (1978) Oxford University. *GP,* 13 January.

Walker JH (1983) The MRCGP examination. In *The Medical Annual*. Bristol: John Wright & Sons.

Walton R, Sawyer B (1987) Paying partners by personal lists. In *The Medical Annual*. Bristol: John Wright & Sons.

Wanless Report (2002) *Securing our Future Health: Taking a Long-Term View.* London: HM Treasury.

Warren HV (1972) Variations in the trace element contents of some vegetables. *J R Coll Gen Pract*; **22(114)**:56–60.

Warren JR, Felster MO, Tran B *et al.* (2015) Association of continuity of primary care and statin adherence. *PLOS One*; **10(10)**:e01.40008

Watson GI (1982) *Epidemiology and Research in a General Practice.* Exeter: RCGP. [Published posthumously]

Watts CAH, Watts BM (1994) *Psychiatry in General Practice.* Republished Exeter: RCGP.

Wellcome Trust (2009) *Towards Consensus for Best Practice.* London: Wellcome Trust.

Wells JE, Browne MO, Aguilar-Gaxiola S *et al.* (2013) Dropout from out-patient mental healthcare in the World Health Organization's World Mental Health Survey Initiative. *Br J Psych*; **202(1)**:42–49.

Westcott R (1977) The length of consultations in general practice. *J R Coll Gen Pract*; **27(182)**:552–5.

White ES, Pereira Gray D, Langley P, Evans PH (2016) Fifty years of longitudinal continuity in general practice: A retrospective observational study. *Fam Pract*; **33(2)**:148–53.

White KL, Williams TF, Greenberg BG (1961) The ecology of medical care. *N Engl J Med*; **265**:885–92.

Wild G Alder R Weich S et al (2022) The Penrose hypothesis in the second half of the 20th century: Investigating the relationship between psychiatric bed numbers and prison population in England between 1960 and 2018–2019 *Br J Psych*; **220** 295–301

Wilkinson MJB, Rapley DM, Gadsby R, Cohen MA (1997) Does the BJGP need more fizz and pop? A Midland Faculty readership survey. *Br J Gen Pract*; **47(416)**:145–9.

Williams D (1990) *As Chairman of the Conference of Medical Royal Colleges and Faculties.* Letter to the Secretary of State for Health. London: CoMRC.

Williams E (1992) Foreword. In McLachlan G (ed). *A History of the Nuffield Provincial Hospitals Trust 1940–1990.* London; NT

Wilson A (1977) Patient participation in a primary care unit. *BMJ*; **1**:398.

Wilson A, Childs S (2002) The relationship between consultation length, process and outcomes in general practice: A systematic review. *Br J Gen Pract*; **52(485)**:101–20.

Wilson T, Roland M, Ham C (2006) The contribution of general practice and the general practitioner to NHS patients. *J R Soc Med*; **99(1)**:24–28.

Winyard Report (1995) *SIFT into the Future. Future arrangements for allocating funds and contracting for NHS service support and facilities for teaching undergraduate medical students.* London: Department of Health.

Wivel A (1998) Abortion policy and politics on the Lane Committee of Enquiry 1971–1974. *Soc Hist Med*; **11(1)**:109–35.

World Health Organisation (WHO) (1984) *Primary Health Care in Undergraduate Medical Education: Report on a WHO Meeting Exeter 1983.* Copenhagen: WHO.

World Health Organisation (WHO) and UNICEF (1978) *Alma Ata Declaration.* Geneva: WHO.

Yodfat Y (1985) Theoretical models in family medicine. In *The Medical Annual.* Bristol: John Wright & Sons.

Youens D, Doust J, Robinson S *et al.* (2021) Regularity and continuity of GP contacts and use of statins amongst people at risk of cardiovascular events. *J Gen Intern Med*; **36(6)**:1656–65.

Young M [Lord] (1985) The expectations of patients. In *The Medical Annual.* Bristol: John Wright & Sons.

Index

Note: Page numbers in *italics* refer to illustrations in the text.

abortion 73–4, 252
Abortion Act (1967) 72
    50th anniversary 75
Abrams, Michael 135
academic general practice 209
    professors 210–11
Academic Medicine Group 159–60
academic plan for general practice 305
Academic Primary Care: The Academic Contribution
    309
academic triad 384
Academy of Medical Royal Colleges 178, 261, 282–3
    Belfast dinner 295
    Chair 226, 279–80, 282, 286–302
    confidential letter 300
    constitution 289–90
    dinners 302
    GMC constitution 289
    and Joint Consultants' Committee 279
    liaison committee with Deans 298
    meeting Tony Blair 299–300
    NHS University 293
    officers (1998) 277–8
    offices 295
    patient group 301–2, 318
    policy papers 278
    policy on revalidation 288–9
    proposed ousting 295–8
    team building 290–1
    Vice-Chair 263–5, 277–80, 307
    VIPs for seminars 290
    visiting other leaders/organisations 291
    writing 292
Academy of Medical Sciences 324
Acheson, Sir Donald 117, 135, 151, 168, 184, 268
acute abdomen, diagnosis 20–1
Addison, Joseph 51
Addition for Clinical Teaching (ACT) 209
Afghanistan 338–9
AIDS 135–6
Aiken, Professor Linda 294
Aitken, JM 13
Al Seaidy, Marwa 369
Albert Wander lectures 271
Alberti, Sir George *187*, 261, *267*, 279, 282, 289, 290–1,
    296
Alderhey scandal 294–5
Alexander, CHO'D (Hugh) 13
Allen, Justin 213, 217, *222*
allied professions 82

Almond, Professor Brenda 330
Annals of Family Medicine 374
Annals of Internal Medicine 198
annual reports 123–4
Aristotle 277, 296
Armstrong, Peter 289
Ashley-Miller, Michael 249, 336
Ashton, Jill 82
atrial fibrillation 245–6
audiography, in general practice 28, 34
Australia, exchange visits 220–1

Baedeker raids 6–7
Bailey, Sir Brian 117
Baker, Maureen 319
Baker, Professor Richard 172
Balancing Dreams and Discipline (Irvine) 63
Balint, Michael 99, 120, 328, 355
Ball, John 130, 146, 159, 165
Barber, Professor Hamish 121
Barley, Simon 58, 59
Barnes, Dame Josephine 75
Barry, Suzie 81
Bart's
    attitudinal weaknesses 17
    as junior doctor 19–20
    as medical student 15–16
Batchelor, Professor Sir Ivor 72, 74
Battye, Roger 318
Baum, Professor 203
Baylis, Sir Richard 131, 305
Bedside Diagnosis 198
Behenna, Barry 79, 192–3
Belfast 295
Belloc, Hilaire 22, 44
Belsky, Professor J 330
Belton, Andrew 144–5
Benjamin, Baroness Floella 367
Benko, Pal 11
Berwick, Don 338
Bevan, Aneurin 68, 143, 240, 303–4
Bible, Luke 7 303
Biden, President Joe 339
Black, Sir Douglas 131
Blair, Leo 341
Blair, Sir Tony 292–3, 299–300, 323–4, 340–1, 344, 349
Bletchley Park 13
Blumenthal, David 338
Blythe, Andrew 101
BMA, *see* British Medical Association

BMJ Open 379
Bodenheimer, Tom 338
Boetang, Rt Hon Paul 188
Bogle, Ian 281–2, 284, 302
Bolden, Keith 80, 81, 83, 84, 86, 88, *92*, 94, 97–9, 109,
        247, *265*
Boorman, Edwin 233
Booth, Dame Margaret 136
Borland, RE 9
Borman, Ed 281
Boryesievic, Professor Sir Lezek 339, 367
Bourne, Dr Alec 20, 21, 22
Box, Graham 318
Boyd, Sir Robert 298
Brackenbury, Sir Henry 308
Bradley, Nick 116, 120, 355, 357, 410
Bradshaw, Sir Ben 362, 364
Brain, Sir Russell 68
breast cancer, and HRT 252, 254
Brimblecombe, Professor Freddie 70, 79, 80, 129, 191,
        192, 195
Bristol cardiac surgery case 231
Bristol Medical School 357
Bristol University 108, 196
British Chess Federation 10, 11–12
British Diabetic Association 94
British Journal of General Practice (BJGP) 57, 167, 360,
        379, *381*, 382
British Medical Association (BMA) 27, 44, 46–8
    Annual Representative Meeting 283–4
    'BMA Guild' 45
    Council 47, 261, 346
    distinction awards for GPs 311–12
    Exeter Division Chair 46–7
    farewell 48
    General Medical Services Committee (GMSC) 44,
        132, 140, 141–2, 160, 164
    General Practitioners Committee 96, 288, 311, 347
    Junior Doctors' Committee 291, 350
    negotiations with DH 346–51
    Planning Unit 47
    and RCGP 163–5
    stance on revalidation 288
British Medical Journal (BMJ) 22–3, 83
    articles on GPA 140–1
    letter on general practice as a discipline 355
    letter to Michael Wilson (1990) 165
British Paediatric Association 165
British Universities' Chess Association (BUCA) 11–12
Broadhurst, Dawn 248
Brown, Rt Hon Gordon 288, 341–2, 349, 362–4
Browne, Professor Judith Bell 237, 238
Browse, Sir Norman 279, 311–12
Bruce, Dick 108, 109, 111
Bruce, Fiona MP 331
Buckingham Palace 262, *263*
Buckley, Graham 57, 166
Bulger, Roger 339
Bunker, John 341

Burdon, John 52, 123, 125
burnout in GPs 376–7
Burtt, Margaret 184
Butterfield, Lord John 157–8, 333
Butterworth Gold Medal Essay 29, 51
Buxton, Ann 30, 31, 244, 246, 414
Byrne, Professor Patrick 40, 55, 63, 68, 81, 131, 305

Cairncross, Robin 222
Caldicott, Dame Fiona 323, 345
Calman, Sir Kenneth 186–7, *198*, 199
Cambridge
    professor of general practice 210–11
    St John's College 14–15
    University chess club 10
Cambridge half blue blazer *262*
Cameron, Sir James 44, 45, 213, 308
Campbell, Professor John 319
Canavan, Desmond 272, 297
cancer registries, patient data 320, 321
Capener, Norman 191
capitation fees 303–4
Care Quality Commission (CQC) 299, 387
    visits to the Practice 378
Carne, Stuart 58, 59, 70, 121, 122, 160–1,
        165–6, *260*
Carter, Professor Yvonne 211, 266, *267*
Cartwright, Ann 60, 74
cataract surgery 290–1
Cates, Joe 97
Catto, Sir Graeme 234
ceremonial dinners 264–5
Cervantes, Miguel de 225
Chair of Complementary Medicine 196–7
Chair of Council 151–65
    election 137, 147–8
    retirement 168
    working dinners 180
Chair of Research Network 207–11
Chalker, Lynda 55
Chambers, Professor Ruth 377
Chantler, Sir Cyril 157–8, 232, *268*, 320, 345
Chapman, Helen 29
Charities Commission 338
Charles III, King 63, *64*, 167, 211, 269, *270*
Charlton, Professor Rodger 61
chess 8, 9
    Cambridge 10
    Exeter 12–13
    international 11–12
    junior championships 9
    tournaments 10
    University of London 12
    value of 13
Chief Medical Officer (CMO) 41, 166, 168, 177, 184,
        201, 279
    confidential paper to Academy 300
    Consultant Adviser to 135–7
    GMC report 234

postgraduate medical school *198*, 199
prison medicine 184
task force on litigation 299
Chilcote, Sir John Nicholas 327
child care
in general practice 129–30
parental 329, 330
children (of DPG) 28, 47, 57, 123, 146
China, College proposed visit 164–5
Chisholm, John 213, 218, 232, 284, 288, 302, 311, 347
Choules, Joy 57, 65, 66, 111
civil honours 398
civil servants 103–4, 344
Clapp, Brian 12
Clark, Chris 176
Clark, Margaret 237, 238
Clarke, Peter 12
Clarke, Lord Kenneth 142, 143, 153–4, 160, 163–4, 273, 305
Council dinner with 161
Clayton, Harry 322–3
Clayton, Sir Stanley 73, 74, 304
Clement, Rosemary 293
clinical commissioning groups (CCGs) 376
Clinical Excellence Scheme 312–13
clinical opportunistic screening (COS) 374
Clinical Standards Board 168
clinics in general practice 242–3
Clubb, John 111
Cochrane, Professor Archie 335
Cogwheel Report 163
Cohen, Sir Henry 96
Cole, Jack (uncle) 295
Cole, John (grandfather) 3
Cole, Nelson 7
Cole, Stuart 360
College of General Dental Practitioners 225
College of General Practitioners 17, 28
Chairman of the Faculty Board 42–3
Council 41
Deputy Chairman of the Board 42
formation 68–9, 96
Gale Memorial Lecture 40–1, 43
South West England Faculty Board 40–1
tutor 41
see also Royal College of General Practitioners
College of Ophthalmologists 290–1, *291*
College of Pathologists 287–8
Collings, Joseph 333–4
Collins, MF 9, 10
Colmer, Linda 116, 410
Colville, Bob 171
Commission for Social Capital 330–1
Committee on the Safety of Medicines 252
Commonwealth Fund of New York 339
communication
GP consultation 33, 35
non-verbal 35
Communications Division, Chair 126–8, 317

complementary medicine 167, 193, 196–9, 306
computing in general practice 88–9, 248
Conference of Academic Organisations of General Practice 180–3
inaugural meeting 181, *181*
publications 182–3
Conference of General Practice Educational Directors (COGPED) 105–6
Conference of Medical Royal Colleges and Faculties 160–1, 180, 226, 305–6, 313
conference of senior hospital doctors 281–2
confidential information 320
confidentiality, breaches 253
conflicts of interest 278, 378
consultant referrals 35, 389–90
consultants
medical student days 16–17
negotiations with DH 349–50
private practice 349
remuneration systems 303
consultations (GP)
communication 33, 35
generational 36–7
length of 222–3, 224, 377
contextual healing effect 237–8
Continuing Care at Home (CONCHA) 89
Continuity Counts 239
continuity of GP care 20–1, 30, 238–9, 246, 369, 374, 378–9
and emergency hospital admissions 375–6, 395
findings associated with 395
Health Foundation Improving GP Continuity Programme 379–80, *380*
measurement 382
and mortality 379
systematic reviews 379, 395
contraceptive advice 29, 74, 140
Cooper, Nick 93
cortisol levels 331
cost-effectiveness of care 394–5
course organisers 165
Court Committee 70
COVID-19 pandemic 382, 396
Cox, Ivan 207
Cox, Jim 208
Cox, John 289
CRAGPIE 102, 104
criticism, response to 387
Cronin, AJ 328
Cuba, 2000 visit 271–2
Culyer Committee 209
Culyer, Tony 209
Cumberlege, Baroness Julia 140
Curry, Edwina 156

D&Cs, infection rate audit 16–17
Dahrendorf, Lord 40
Dain, Sir Guy 308
Dalal, Hayes 176
Danckwertz, Mr Justice 346

Dartington, Lord Young 121
Darwin, Charles 386
data collection, patient consent 320–2
Davies, Dame Sally 360, 393
Davis, Karen 339
Dawson, Sir Anthony 153
De Montfort University, Honorary DSc 261, 268
deafness, diagnosis in general practice 28, 34
Dean, Alan 211
Dean, Diana 329, 330, 331
Dean, Philip 331
Deans of the Medical Schools 298
debates, future of pathology services (Exeter) 137
Denham, Rt Hon John 286
Dennis, Nancy 127, 317
dentistry 225–6
    College established 225, 228
    Faculty of RCSEng 225–6
    General Dental Council 226–7, 231
    Nuffield Trust seminars 227–8
Department of General Practice, Exeter University 79,
        108–9, 334
    academic staff team 86–8
    becomes Institute of General Practice 92–4, *92*, 95
    closure 95
    computers in general practice 88–9
    establishment 79–80
    funding 335
    MSc in Healthcare 88
    multi-professional staff team 82
    personal chair 89, 143–5
    publications 83–4, 412–13
    research 89–92
    retirement 94, *94*, 95
    Spring 1978 RCGP meeting 82
    vocational training scheme 80–2
    WHO seminar 85–6, *86*, 117
Department of Health (DH)
    brush over 2000 White paper 286–7
    distinction awards for GPs 312–13
    meetings organised by 264
    negotiations with GPs 347–9
    negotiations with junior doctors 349–50
    negotiations with senior hospital doctors 349–50
    NHS University 293
    review of research in general practice 209
    and status of general practice 388–9
    White papers, *see* White papers
Department of Health and Social Security (DHSS) 79, 96
    Department of General Practice Exeter 79, 80, 84
    Primary Health Care: An Agenda for Discussion
        140, 145, 151–2, 155
depression
    diagnosis 37, 133
    GP vs. hospital care 394
    research 195, 307
deputising services 130
Destination GP 134
Detmer, Professor Don 339

*Developing NHS Purchasing: Towards a Primary Care-
        Led NHS* 182
Developing Primary Care – The Academic Contribution
        182
Devon Area Health Authority, non-executive
        directorship 240–1
Devon Family Health Services Authority 177–8, 241–2
Dexter, Sir Michael 300
Dezateux, Professor Carol 324
diabetes, diagnosis and care 116, 249, 339, 373, 374,
        377–8
Diabetes UK 318, 377
Diabetic Medicine 374
diagnostic mistakes 390, 391–3
Dickenson, John 180
Difford, Frederick 109, 111
Digby, Anne 266
Dineen, Molly 331, 359, 367, 369, 411
Director of GP education 102–6
disappointments, personal 387–8
discipline, definition 355
Disraeli, Benjamin 191, 194, 286, 297
distinction awards, consultants 304
distinction awards for GPs 168, 278, 298, 304
    Academy of Medical Royal Colleges 309–10
    attempt to introduce 304
    external support 309
    and Institute of General Practice 307
    obstacles 308
    proposal 310–11
    RCGP policy (1989) 305
    and trends 1980s-2000 307–9
Dixon, Michael 93–4, 238, 362
Doar, John 14
Dobson, Rt Hon Frank 251, 264, 300–1
"doctor first" system 319
doctor–patient relationship 35, 120, 393
    context effect 237–8
    Fetzer Institute 237–8, 239
    hospital medicine 393
    prison medicine 185
doctorates
    general practice 207–8
    honorary (DPG) 261, 268, 367, *375*, 399
doctors, trust in 302
Doctors Talking to Patients 62
Donabedian, Professor Avedis 63, 100
Donald, Alastair 70, 71, 125, 126, 161, *260*, 262, 325
Donaldson, Sir Liam 177, 234, 290, 339
Donohoe, Mollie 116, 410
Donovan, Chris 129
Dorothy Mackenzie Trust 82
Douglas, Angela 82, 84, 93, 115–16, 230, 410
Downing Street, invitations 167, 292–3, 299–300,
        362–4
drinking, in medical students 17
drugs, limited prescribing list 136
Drury, Professor Sir Michael 144–5, 146, 154, *260*, 277,
        308

Duke of Edinburgh 68, 69
Duncan Smith, Ian 330
Dunn, Stephen 344
Duthie, Sir Herbert 230–1
Dwyer, Declan 83

early experiences 27–9, 388
East Quay Practice, Somerset 175, *176*
Eastman, Jane 286, 290
Edinburgh depression study 394
Education for Primary Care 83
educational paradigm 81
educational theory 98–9
Egypt, conference on family medicine (2000) *93*, 94
Eliot, TS 325
Elizabeth (daughter) 47, 53, *260*, 261, 262, 329, 367
epidemiologists, use of patient data 322
Epidemiology in Country Practice (Pickles) 62
Epidemiology and Research in a General Practice
          (Watson) 62
epigenetics 331–2
Epigenomics 331
eponymous or equivalent lectures 84, 139, 261, 400
          Nuffield Trust 335
Ernst, Professor Edzard 197–8, *198*, 203, 237–8, 306
ESTEEM study 319
Ethics and Confidentiality Committee (ECC) 323, 324
European Council Medical Directive (1995) 220–1
European Foundation (charities) 'Leaders summit' 340
European Union (EU) 220–1
Euwe, Max 9
Evans, Professor Philip
      the Practice 90, 111, 239, 242, 244, 246–7, *248*,
          254–5, 313, 327, 331, 367
      St Leonard's Research Practice 378, 379–80, *380*
Evans, Sir John Grimley 14
Everington, Sir Sam 362
evolution 386–7
Evolution of British General Practice, The 266
Exeter
      chess club 12–13
      wartime bombing 6–7
Exeter GP trainers' course 15
Exeter hip 367, 374
Exeter and Plymouth postgraduate medical schools 203
Exeter RCGP Publications office 60–6, 401–8
      books 61–4, 407
      Members' Reference Book 64–5, 65–6
      Occasional Papers 56–7, 61, 66, 83, 84, 402–7
      publications catalogue *65*
      workload 64–5
Exeter University
      Department of General Practice, *see* Department of
          General Practice
      honorary doctorate 367, *375*
      Postgraduate Medical School 89, 191–9
      Vice-Chancellor 368–9
Expert Advisory Group on AIDS 135–6
external examiner 90

Eyles, Marion 28
Eynon-Lewis, Andrew 326

Faculty of Dental Surgery 225–6
      honorary fellow 227–8
family (of DPG) 28, 47, 57, 123, 146, 367, 396
Family Health Service Authorities (FHSAs) 241, 243
Family Medicine: The Medical Life History of Families
          (Huygen) 62
Family Practice 368, 369, 377
Family Practitioner Committees (FPCs) 165
Farmer, Professor Andrew 210
Farrar-Brown, Lesley 333
Fellowship by Assessment (FBA) 168, 171–9, 242, 264
      abolished 178–9
      development 172–6
      empowerment of College members 175–6
      impact outside College 177–8
      patient representatives 175, 178–9
      pilots 171–2
      proposal 171
      publications on 176–7
      three-person assessment team 174
Ferguson, John 310
Fetzer Institute (USA) 236–9
Field Work of the Family Doctor, The 308
Financial Times 341, 383
Findlater, John 63
Fit for the Future 70
Folkestone Royal Victoria Hospital 22–3
Food and Drug Administration (FDA US) 23
foodbanks 386
Ford, John 325
Forman, Sholto 41
Forrer, Jim 374
Foundation Council Award 59
foundation hospitals 340–1
Fowler, Norman 141
Fowler, Professor Godfrey 210
Fox, Molly 64
France, Sir Christopher *267*, 337
Francis Report (2013) 294
Freeland, Chrystia 67
Freeling, Paul 81, 122, 133, 166, 335, 361
Freeth, Malcolm 213, *222*
French, Murray 85, 194
Fritchie, Baroness *92*, *198*
Froggatt, Clive 42, 157–8
Fry, John 57, 133, 145, 166–7, 333, 335, 336
Fulford, Mrs Betty 6
Fuller, Clifford 191, 334
Future General Practitioner—Learning and Teaching 62

Gale Memorial Lecture 40–1, 43, 212, 222
Gardner, Gladys (aunt) 272–3
Gardner-Thorpe, Christopher 373–4
Garrett, Diana 286, 295, 296
Garvie, Douglas 124, 139, 144
Gayle, Forman 362

gender discrimination 17
General Dental Council (GDC) 226–7, 231
General Medical Council (GMC) 96, 115–16, 229,
    229–30
  Bristol cardiac surgery case 231
  Conduct Committee 231
  constitution 289
  developments 233–5
  disciplinary function 214, 229, 230, 233, 348
  election for Presidency 230–1
  establishment 229
  first GP as President 306
  Medical Data 2000 232–3
  national training surveys 394
  revalidation 231–2, 281–5
  Standards Committee 218, 230, 232, 320
  teaching of general practice 358
  vote of no-confidence 281–2, 284, 288
General Medical Services Committee (GMSC) 44, 132,
    140, 141–2, 160, 164
general practice
  asymmetry with specialist medicine 391–3
  cost-effectiveness 394
  as a discipline 355–6
  leading medical profession 393–5
  management styles 366
  nature of 389–90
  pride in 360, 389
  status of 388–9
General Practice Finance Corporation (GPFC) 29
general practice (GP) fundholding 163, 250–1, 336
General Practice under the NHS 1948–1997 266
general practitioner (GP) contract
  1965–1966 changes 29
  1990 163–4
  first NHS 27, 44
  out-of-hours work 337
General Purpose Committee (GPC) 67, 138, 144, 145,
    151
generalist thinking 396
genes and environment interaction 238, 331
Gent, Reverend Miriam 241
George Abercrombie Award 53, 70, 271, *271*
Gerada, Dame Clare 389
Gibbs, Sir Geoffrey 334, 339
Gibbs, Sir Roger 334
Gibson, Sir Ronald 47, 308
Gillie, Dame Annis 41, 53–4, 67, 167, 308, 326–7
Gillie report 41
Gillings, Dennis 87
Gipslis, Aivars 11
Gittins, Hilla 213, 221, *222*, 266
Giving USA 236
Glasgow Royal College of Physicians and Surgeons 269,
    269
glaucoma, diagnosis 22
GlaxoSmithKline 324
Gligoric, Svetozar 13

global health, Nuffield Trust 338–9
Goble, Rita 82, *86*, *198*
Godber, Sir George 28, 41, 70, 72
Goldsmith, James (Jimmy) 167
Golombek, Harry 9
Good Medical Practice 218
good practice allowance (GPA) 131–2, 139–43,
    154, 155
Goodenough, Sir William 333, 339
Goodman, Doreen 330
Goodman lecture 330
Goodwin, Shirley 294
Goss, Brian 161
government
  relationship with medical profession 143, 153–6
  role of 386–7
GP trainers 15, 96, 97, 99, 101
  national survey 369
  selection 169, 170
GP 'trainer's grant' 165, 304
A GP Training Handbook (Hall ed.) 83
Grabham, Sir Anthony 230, 312
Graham, Professor Philip 129–30
Grainger, Richard 339
Gray, Jonathan (brother) 6, 7, 30
Gray, Todd 6
Greengross, Baroness 122
Greenhalgh, Professor Trish 32, 268, *268*
Greenspan, Alan 229
Gretsky, Wayne 126
Grol, Professor Richard 62
The Guardian 379
Guernsey medical services 131
Gundry, Bob 171
Gunn, Professor 186
"gut feelings" 37–8

Haines, Professor Sir Andrew 321
Hall, Michael 42, 81, 82, 83, 88, 93–4, 97, 102, 109, *198*,
    265, 317
Ham, Professor Chris 286–7, 340
Hamilton, Professor William 390
Hammond, Margaret 120, 133, 325
Hannaford, Professor Philip 211
Hannam, Sir John 79
Harben lecture 249, 268
Harding, Professor Alex 218, 248, 313, 357, 360, 368,
    369, 414
Hardy, Dominic 379
Hargreaves, Tom 137
Harkness Fellowships 93, 236, 245, 294, 339, 340
Harris, Andrew 323, 324
Harris, Professor Conrad 122
Harrison, Sir David 89, 197
Hart, Graham 104
Hart, Mary 192
Hart, Robert 89, 192
Harveian lecture 266

Haslam, Sir David 121–2, 261, 266, 326
Hasler, John 127, 132, 166, 216, 317
    elected Chair of Council 138–9
    resignation from Chair 146–8
Hastings, Sir Charles 29
Hattersley, Professor Andrew 199, 203
Hawker, Peter 282, 349
Hawker, Professor Ruth 81, 241
Hawthorne, Professor Kamila 357
Hayden, Jacky 105, 171, 217
Hayter, Adrian 379
heads of state met 419
Heads of Teaching (HOTs) 357, 360
Health Education England 351, 389
health expenditure 341
Health Foundation 379–80
Health Select Committee, House of Commons 355,
    356–7, 361
Health Service Journal 341
Health and Social Care Act (2001) 321
health visitors 29
    complaints against 253
Health Visitors Association 294
Healthier Children – Thinking Prevention 70, 129–30,
    165
Healthier Children Working Party 120
heart transplant, Britain's first 29
Heath, Iona 36, 266, 327, 335, 355
Hedley, Robert 186
Henley, Professor William 374, 376
Herbert, Eddie 241
Heritage Committee (RCGP) 325–8
    downgrading 328
    heritage plaques 326–7, 328
    last meeting 327
    oral history of general practice 327
Higgins, Dame Joan 321, 322, 323
Higgins, Peter 122
higher training for highflyers 217
Hill, Peter 171, 302
Hill, Sir Denis 335
Hillier, Richard 30, 414
Hilton, Professor Sean 367
hip fracture 35
Hippocrates 27, 32, 34, 81
history of general practice (1948-1997) 266
Hoffenberg, Professor Sir Raymond 152–3
Holden, John 172, 177
Holland, Sir Geoffrey *200*
Holmedale 4, 5
    history of 371, *372*
    redesign of 30
Home Office 185, 186, 189
home visits 254, 291
    insights 38–9
Honigsbaum, F 55–6
Honiton general practice 208
honorary awards 266–9, *267–9*, 367, *375*

honours
    civil 399
    professional 399
honours system 67–8, 82
Hope-Simpson, Edgar 270–1, *271*
Hopkins, Robin 88, 89
Horder, John 60, 63, *64*, 82, 129, *260*, 277, 363, 390
hormone replacement therapy (HRT) 252, 253–4
hospital admissions, and continuity of GP care 375–6,
    395
Hospital Doctor 289
House of Lords 301
House of Lords Select Committee on Science and
    Technology 210
Hove General Hospital 20–1
Howie, Professor John 84, 209
Hoyte, Sheila 29
Huckle, Mavis 81
Hughes, Roddy 99, 108, 109
Hull University 199
Hume, John 273
Humphreys, Idris 213, 214
"hunches" 37–8
Hunt, Lord John 17, 40, 51, 53, 56, 65, 123, 124, 207, 334
    honours 67–8, 363
Hunt, Rt Hon Jeremy 350, 364–5
Hunter, Paul 291, 295–6, 298
Hunterian Gold Medal 28, 29, 52
Hunterian Museum 325
Hurwitz, Professor Brian 377
Hutton, Lord John 290
Hutton, Professor Peter 300, 302
Huygen, Professor Frans 62, 90, 338
Hylton, WH (Bill) 41
hyperlipidaemia 246–7

Ibrahimovic, Zalatan 207
Ibsen, Henrik 281
Illingworth, Charlotte 411
In Pursuit of Quality (Pendleton *et al.*) 63, 100
Index Medicus 51, 159, 326
industrial action 351
InnovAiT 378–9
Institute of Clinical Sciences 199
Institute of General Practice (Exeter) 92–4, *92*, 202
    and Fetzer Institute 239
Institute of Health Service Managers (IHSM), honorary
    fellowship 268
Institute of Medicine of Washington, Overseas Associate
    274
Investor in People 254
Iranian Embassy siege (1980) 71
Ireland 272–3, 295
    potato famine 341
Irish College of General Practitioners 181
Irvine, Edward 29
Irvine, Sally (née Fountain) 63, *92*, 121, 131, 144, 145,
    147, 207

Irvine, Sir Donald 47, 53, 67, 99, 117, 268, *268*
   Chair of Council 130–2, 138, 169
   General Medical Council Presidency 230–1, 234, 235
   Good Medical Practice 218
   knighthood 308–9
   President of GMC *170*, 306
   retirement 302
Irwin, Professor George 208

Jackson, Claire 325, 327
Jackson, Laurence 207
Jackson, Sir Barry 226, 279–80, 286, 289, 295–7
Jacobs, Adrian 80–1
Jakeaway, Sir Derek 240
James, Alice 356
James Mackenzie lecture 239, 259
   DPG 33, 36, 56, 69–70, 84, 139
Jarman, Sir Brian 121, 122, 126, 266, 308–9
JCPTGP, *see* Joint Committee on Postgraduate Training
   for General Practice
Jeffreys, Professor Margot 47
Jenkins, Professor Rachel 195, 250
Jennifer (daughter) 262, *265*, 298, 362, 367
John Fry lecture 343
John Wright & Sons (publishers) 119
Johns, Catherine 382
Johnson, Rt Hon Alan 363
Johnson, Rt Hon Boris 386
Johnson, Jim 164, 279, 283, 312, 313
Johnson, Samuel 60
Joint Committee on Postgraduate Training for General
   Practice (JCPTGP) 64, 98, 102, 104, 129, 212,
   292
   1995 developments 218–19
   chairmanship 102, 213–14
   distinction awards for GPs 307
   and EC Medical Directive 220–1
   establishment 212
   final meeting as Chair 221–3
   higher training for high flyers 217
   multi-Chairmen letter to Ministers 219
   North-East Thames region 158, 159
   RCGP in 212
   recording of policies 221
   staffing 213
   structure 212
   summative assessment of vocational training 214–17,
      219–20
   teamwork 217–18
Joint Committee on Vaccination and Immunisation
   (JCVI) 396
Joint Consultants' Committee (JCC) 212, 279, 283, 298,
   312
Jones, Bob 81, 83, 88–9, 94, 213
Jones, Ivor 44
Jones, Professor Roger 111, 210, 247
Joseph, Sir Keith 72, 79
Josse, Eddie 158, *222*

Journal of the American Board of Family Medicine 131,
   343
Journal of Basic and Applied Psychology 238–9
Journal of Medical Biography 373–4
Journal of Public Health 375
Journal of the Royal College of General Practitioners
   (JRCGP) 51–9
   articles 55–6
   British Journal of General Practice (1978) 57
   editorial board 53–4, 59
   editorial work 54
   editorials 54–5
   editor's pay 306
   editorship 30, 42, 52–3, 64–5, 66
   Jill appointed to staff 57–8
   members' attitudes survey 59
   news section 56
   occasional papers 56–7, 61, 66, 83, 84, 402–7
   Reports from General Practice 60–1, 401–2
   resignation as editor 58–9
   role of RMS McConaghey 326
   Supplements 60, 402
Journal of the Royal Society of Medicine 331
Jowett, Dymoke *276*
JRCGP, *see Journal of the Royal College of General*
   Practitioners
junior doctor (DPG as)
   Barts 19–20
   formal reprimand 21–2
   Hove General Hospital 20–1
   Royal Victoria Hospital, Folkestone 22–3
junior doctors
   negotiations with DH 350–1
   rating of postgraduate education 393–4
"Just a GP/just GPs" 102, 107, 209, 211, 222, 226, 337,
   390–1

Kay, Alison 177
Kay, Harry 80
Kay, Professor Janice 368
Keele University, academic general practice 84–5
Keen, Ann 362
Keenan, Helen 248, 414
Keene, Professor Harry 249
Keighley, Brian 218–19, 232, 283
Kelsey, Frances 23
Kennedy, President John F 23
Kessler, Professor David 90, 307
Kierkegaard 385
Kilpatrick, Lord Robert 230
King, David 192, 194
Kingman, Sir John 107, 110
King's College London 359
King's Fund 82, 239, 333, 345
Kinmonth, Professor Ann-Louise 181, 211, 309
Kirby, Professor Brian 186, 192, *198*, 202
Kitto, FEA 9, 12
Kleijnen, Professor Jos 237–8

knighthood 202, 255, *255*, 262, *263*
knighthoods, appointment of GPs 308–9
Kratky, Adrian 115, 116, 410
Kuenssberg, Ekke 52, 53, 61, 69–70, 82, 229, 335, 361, 363

Labour government 251, 288, 292–3, 299–301, 362–4
Laing Foundation 196–8, 306
Laing, Sir James 196
Lancaster, Professor Tim 359
Lancet 34, 83, 237, 253–4, 379, 383
    ESTEEM study 319
    influential letters 152–3
    three Presidents's letter 180
Lane Committee 60, 67, 72–5
    membership 72–3, 75
    report 75
    role of DPG 74–5
Lane, Dame Elizabeth 72–5
Lane, Kenneth 62
Langley, Peter 371, 373, 377
Lawrence, Tony 293
Laws, Sir John 211
Lawson, John 52, 120, 122, 127, *222*
Le Grand, Professor Sir Julian 394
learning the craft
    from father 35–6
    from grandfather 34
    from own experience 36–8
    home visits 38–9
Lechler, Professor Sir 359
Ledingham, Professor John 337, 391
Ledward, Rodney 232
Lee, Professor Clive 367, 374
Leech, Penelope 330
Lefroy, Jeremy 331
Leicester Medical School 357
Lennard, Michael 96–7, 99
leukaemia 16, 36
Lewis, Tony 87–8, *87*, 171, 250–1
life-course theory 33, 250
Lifetime Achievement Award 382, *382*
Lilleyman, Professor John 281–3, 287–8, 295, 296–7, 302
limited list of drugs 136
Lincoln, Abraham 259, 261
Ling, Professor Robin 367, 374
Lings, Pamela 239
Lippmann, W 151
listening 33
literacy, prisons 188
litigation, costs 166
litigation in NHS, task force 299
Lloyd George Act 4
Lloyd, Keith 195, 203, 251
Lloyd, KW 10
local government, in NHS administration 240–1

Local Medical Committees (LMC)
    Conference 45–6, 141–3, 154, 162
    Devon 44–5
locum work 351
Longest Art, The (Lane) 62
Longfield, Mike 184, 186
Loudon, Irvine 266

Macara, Sir Sandy 232, 259, 278, 284, 288, 311, 313
MacAuley, Domhnall 93
McAleese, Mary 269
McCartney, Margaret 317
McConaghey memorial lecture 42, 43, 59, 159, 168, 361, 382
McConaghey, RMS (Mac) 41, 207, 326
    College journal 51, 52, 53–4, 326
    death 56
    heritage plaque 326
McConaghey, Gussie 53, 54, 159
McConaghey, Dr Paddy 54, 59, 168, 326
McCormick, Barry 340
MacDonald, Tom 71
McEwen, Professor James *269*, 279
McHale, Teony 248, 414
MacKay, Norman 216, *269*
Mackenzie, Sir James 63, 371
Mackenzie-Ross, Keith 14
McKeon, Andy 249, 379
McKinley, David 128, 325, 326
McLachlan, Gordon 334
McNeish, Sandy 266
MacSween, Professor Sir Roddy 263, *267*, 277–8, 282–3
McWhinney, Professor Ian 53, 341, 355, 360
Mainous, Professor Arch 239
Major, Sir John 158, 165, 301
Malleson, Joan 72
Mallick, Professor Sir Netar 307
Mallison, HV 12
Malone, Beverly 294
management styles 366
Mann, Professor Anthony 195
Mansfield, Brian 410
Mant, Professor David 111, 208–9, 209
Mardle, DV 13
Marinker, Marshall 40–1, 53, 121, 131, 140–1, 144, *268*, 305, 328
Marks, John 229
Marsh, Geoffrey 53
Marshall, Martin 93, 245, 347, 382
Martin, Edwin 121, 184–5
Martin, Sheila 53
Mason, Alastair 101–2, 107
Mason, Pamela 107, *198*
maternity care, failures 299
maternity grant 55
Mattingly, Professor David 41, 79, 97, 109, 191–2, 240, 350
Maynard, Professor Alan 140, 141

Maynard School, Exeter 7
MDs, in general practice 207–8
Medical Academic Staff Committee (MASC) 310
Medical Act (1858) 229
Medical Act (1978) 68
Medical Annual 119–22
Medical Data 2000 232–3
medical mistakes 299, 391–2
    made by GPs 391–2
    made by hospitals 392
medical politics 41
Medical (Professional Performance) Act (1995) 218
medical records
    management standards 101, 158, 159, 249
    prisons 185
Medical Register 229
    striking off of doctors 214, 230, 233, 348
Medical Research Council (MRC) 208, 209, 236
    General Practice Research Framework 208
medical student (DPG)
    Bart's 15–16
    consultants 16–17
    final examinations 17–18
    St John's College 14–15
medical students
    reading lists for general practice 355, 356, 361, 389
    survey on general practice 359
medically unexplained symptoms 33–4
medico-political crisis 44–5
Melhuish, Professor Edward 329–30
Mellor, Dame Julie 299
Melville, Colin 358
membership of the Royal College of General
    Practitioners (MRCGP)
    as endpoint assessment for training 215–16
    for GP trainers 96, 97, 99, 101, 159, 177
    prison doctors 188
'men in grey suits' 146–7, 296
Merck Sharpe and Dohme (MSD) 131, 249, 304–5
Merrison Committee 229
Merrison, Sir Alec 229
Messenger, Sharon 327, 328
Messent, Catherine 213
metaphors in medicine 37
Metcalfe, David 305
Metcalfe, Neil 383
Micros in Practice 88
Mid-Staffordshire NHS Foundation Trust 15, 243
Milburn, Alan 273, 288, 290–1, 292, 294–5, 349
Miles, John 53
Milestones 63
Miller, Adrian 109
Miller, Sir Jonathan 14
ministers met 419–20
Mitchell, Margaret 117
Moore, John 153, 157
Moore, Richard 177
Moran, Lord 17, 40, 68, 142–3, 235, 303–4, 388
Morgan, Baroness Nicky 368

Morgan, Dame Gillian 254, 347
Morpurgo, Sir Michael 330
Morris, William (Viscount Nuffield) 333
Morrison, Toni 385
mortality
    and continuity of care 379
    and professional activity 294
Moss, Sir Sterling 295
Mostyn, Lord Williams 188
mothers, working 329
Mould, Alastair 175
MRCGP, *see* membership of the Royal College of
    General Practitioners
MSD Foundation 268, *268*, 304–5
multimorbidity 390
Murray, Professor Stuart 215, 216, 217, *265*
Mutkin, HG 10
Myers Brigg Type Inventory (MBTI) 98, 99

nappy rash, hospital admission 39
narrative medicine 32–4, 37
National Association for Patient Participation (NAPP)
    317, 318–19, 340
National Audit Office, PFI 301
National Children's Committee 195
National Health Service (NHS) Act (1977) 69
National Information Governance Board (NIGB)
    322–3
National Institute for Health and Care Excellence
    (NICE) 264
Netherlands Conference on Dietary Advice *262*
Neuberger, Baroness *268*
Neville, Julia 177–8, 242
New England Journal of Medicine 195, 253, 379
New Zealand 220–1, 299
    lecture tour (1981) 84
Newman, Lotte 158, 230, 259, *260*, 325
NHS Act (1990) 103
NHS Act (2000) 156
NHS Alliance 362, 365
NHS funding 152
NHS Litigation Authority 322
NHS Plan (2000) 286–7, 312
NHS University 293
night calls 115, 116
Nijmegen University
    PhD external examiner 90, *91*, 247
    Professor Van Weel farewell lecture 380, 382
non-executive directorships
    clinics in general practice 242–3
    Devon Area Health Authority 240–1
    Devon Family Health Services Authority 241–2
    role of 243
non-verbal communication 35
North-East Thames region (1988) 158–9
Nottingham University
    Diploma in Prison Medicine 186–7
    Honorary Doctorate 268
Nuffield Health and Social Service Fund 333

Nuffield Provincial Hospitals Trust (NPHT) 79, 191, 333
    capital and income 334
    change of name 337–8
    dinners 336–7
    general practice 335–6
    GP Trustee 336
    lectures 335
    medical education in Britain 334–5
    Oxford conference (1961) 96
    postgraduate medical school 191, 334
    review of general practice 333–4
    Trustees 333, 338
Nuffield Trust 264
    2006 DH White paper 343–4
    Chair 330–40
    and Department of Health (DH) 343–4
    global health 338–9
    John Fry lecture 343
    patient consent 320
    publications 341–2
    retirement 345
    role of the Chair 344–5
    royal visit 342, *342*
    seminars 340–1
    seminars for dentists 227–8
nurses, practice 27, 29, 367
nursing 293–5

obstetrics, junior doctor experience 22–3
occasional papers 56–7, 61, 66, 83, 84, 402–7
Office for Students 234
Oldham, Sir John 362
on-cost charges 103–4
on-line publishing 125
O'Neill, Baroness Onora 344
oral contraceptive pill 140, 252
oral history of general practice 327
organisations, attitudes to staff 366
Orr, Julie 42
Orton, Peter 376–7
Osborne, Rt Hon George 368
Osborne, Rt Hon George 368
Osler, Sir William 101, 244
Osman, Leyla 368
out-of-hours work 337, 347
Owen, John Wyn 344–5
Owens, George 240
Ower, David 117, 135
Oxford University, professor of general practice
    210–11

paediatrics, in general practice 70
Paine, Tim 317
parental care of children 329, 330
Parliament Act (1911) 4
Parrott, Richard 171
Pasmore, Stephen 63
Patel, Sir Naren 261, 263, 277
pathology 32–3
    effectiveness in general practice 34

Exeter debate 137
GP access to 28
patient complaints
    Devon Family Health Services Authority 241, 242
    the practice 252–3
    violent 251
patient death, first experience 16
Patient Information Advisory Group (PIAG) 232–3,
    321–3
Patient Liaison Group (RCGP) 127–8, 317, 318
patient participation 317–19
    GMC 234
    theory 317–18
patient representatives, FBA 175, 178–9
patients
    aggressive 19–20, 318
    families 36–7
    psychosocial factors 33
    removal from GP's lists 318
patients' feelings 15–16
pay, *see* remuneration
Peckham, Sir Michael 200, *200*
Peguy, Charles 79
Pendleton, David 127
Penelope (Penny) (daughter) 59, 70, 123, 131, 146, 147,
    260, 261, 262, *265*
Peninsula Medical School 95
Penrose, Jonathan 12, 13
Penrose, LS 185
people met 419–20
Peppiatt, Roger 84, 116, 410
Percy, David 105, 216, 293
Pereira Gray, Alice Evelyn (Kit) (mother) 4, 5–6
Pereira Gray, Grace Blanche (née Frances,
    grandmother) 3
Pereira Gray, JAW (grandfather) 3–4, *5*, 34, 366
Pereira Gray, Jill (née Hoyte, wife of DPG) *4*, 13, 14, 18
    BMA 47
    death and obituary 66, 380, *381*
    Exeter general practice 28, 30
    Exeter Publications Office 64, *64*, 66
    as Exeter-based PA 151–2
    family of 396
    Institute of General Practice dinner *92*
    Knighthood of DPG 262, *263*
    Medical Annual 119, 121
    meets HRH Prince of Wales (King Charles III) 63, *64*
    a premonition 23
    in Presidential portrait 275–6
    RCGP *Journal* role 53, 57–8, 59, 63, *64*, 66
    at RCGP President inauguration *260*
    WONCA conference, Switzerland 70–1
    writing 70
Pereira Gray, Professor Sir Denis
    birth 3
    parents 3, 4–6
    Chair, Academy of Medical Royal Colleges 286–302
    Chair of Council RCGP 151–65
    Chair, Nuffield Trust 339–40

childhood 5, 6–7
appointed OBE 82
chess 8
formal reprimand 21–2
junior doctor 19–23
knighthood 202, 255, *255*, 262, *263*
marriage *4*
medical student days 14–18
President of RCGP 260–1, *260*
school education 7–8
Pereira Gray, Richard 7
Pereira Gray, Dr Sydney (father) 4–5, *4*, 7, 8
    BMA AGM (1970) 48
    death 31
    learning from 35–6
    retirement plans 29–30
personal lists 30, 37, 117, 267
Peter (son) *260*, 262, 266
Peters, Sir Keith 210–11
Pew–Fetzer Task Force 236
pharmaceutical industry 323–4, 378
physiotherapy 251
Pickersgill, Trevor 291
Pickles, William 62, 63, 68, 217, 363
Pidgeon, Clive 225
Pietroni, Patrick 271–2
Pilkington, Lord Harry 346
Pilling, Sir Joseph (Joe) 136, 248–9, 273
Pinker, Sir George 152
Pinsent, Robin 51, 53
Pisicano, Nicholas 131
placebo effect 237
Plato 129
Platt, Sir Harry 14, 17
Plymouth Postgraduate Medical School 202, 203
Pocklington, Susan 250–1
policymaking, evolutionary approach 386–7
Pollak, Margaret 121
Pollock, Professor Allyson 301
Pond, Professor Sir Desmond 121, 122
Ponsford, Christine 329
portrait, Presidential 179, 275–6, *276–7*
postgraduate medical deans 102–3
Postgraduate Medical Education Training Board
        (PMETB) 292
Postgraduate Medical School, Exeter 191–9, 334
    academic consultant physician 194–5
    Chair of Complementary Medicine 196–7
    closure 203
    departments within 193–4
    Directorship 89, 192–3, 196
    as model for clinical scientist 199
    national reviews 201
    staff honours 203
    teaching and research 194, 203
Postgraduate University Medical Departments,
        Conference 199
poverty 386
Practical Diabetes 377

the Practice 7, 27–31, 115–18
    complaints by patients 252–3
    continuing education 250
    fundholding 250–1
    Holmedale 4, 5, 30, 371, *372*
    home visits 38–9, 254
    innovations to improve care 251
    internal audits 249–50
    Investor in People award 254
    Kieran Sweeney 90, 93, 117–18, 210, 239, 247, *248*,
        256
    management 244–6
    master's degrees by research 246–8
    medical student education 369
    move to new premises 371
    partnership difficulty 116
    personal lists 117
    Philip Evans 90, 111, 239, 244, 246–7, *248*, 254–5,
        313, 327, 331, 367, 414
    retirement from 255–6, 371
    Russell Steele 115, 116, 118, 245, 247–8, *248*
    seminar for Exeter University Vice-Chancellor 368–9
    service, teaching, research triad 254–5
    staff 27, 29
    staff clinical excellence awards 313
    team development 248
    University degrees/awards obtained from 366–7, 414
    visitors 116–17, 248–9, 370
    vocational training 115–16
    see also St Leonard's Research Practice
practice nurses 27, 29, 367
Preece, John 87
President of the RCGP
    ceremonial dinners 264–5
    Cuba 2000 271–2
    faculty visits 261
    honours 261–2
    inauguration 260–1, *260*
    portrait 179, 275–6, *276–7*
    Spring General Meeting of College 265–6
    successor 274–5
Price, Pat 28, 46, 47
'primary care' 369
Primary Care (Health Select Committee) 356–7
primary care networks 209
Primary Dental Care 228
Primary Health Care: An Agenda for Discussion
        (DHSS) 140, 151–2, 155
    College response 145
Prime Ministers met 419
    see also named Prime Ministers
Prince Philip, Duke of Edinburgh 68, 69
Prince of Wales (King Charles III) 63, *64*, 167, 211, 269,
        270
*14 Princes Gate: Home of the Royal College of General
        Practitioners* 63
Princes Gate
    final lecture at 327
    occupation of No 15 165–6

Princess Royal, Princess Anne 342, *342*
principles of general practice 415
    national teaching course 360–1
Pringle, General Sir Steuart 200
Pringle, Professor Michael 121–2, 160, 171, 172, 177, 268, *268*, 287, 288, 296, 300, 302
Prison Medical Service, role 185
prison medicine 184–90
    Diploma 186–7, *187*
    failure of 190
    three Royal Colleges Working Party 185–6, 188–9
    training 188–9
Pritchard, Peter 317
private finance initiatives 300–1
private medical school (University of Buckingham) 358
private practice 134, 303–4
privatisation, in NHS 340
professionalism in medicine 292
Professor of General Practice (Exeter University) 89, 143–5
professors of general practice 210–11
Project 2000 157
psychiatric consulting 251
Psychiatry in General Practice 62
Psychiatry and General Practice Today 133
psychosocial factors 33, 390
public discourse, quality 385–6
public health 308, 311
public orator 200–1, *200*
Publications Committee 123–5
Pulse 161, 163, 383
Purdy, Professor Sarah 93, 245
Pyke, David 153

Quality in General Practice (RCGP Policy Statement) 132, 139
quality initiatives 130–2, 169–71
    practice awards 177
Quality and Outcomes Framework (QOF) 155, 347, 349
Queen Mary College honorary fellowship 266, *267*
Quintiles Prize for Women in Science 368

Rafferty, Dame Anne Marie 294
Ramsbottom, Sir David 189, 273
Rashid, Ali 261
Rawlins, Sir Michael 264, 324
Read, Professor Alan 107
reading lists, for general practice 355, 356, 361, 389
Reagan, Nancy 72
"Red Book" 163
Reed, John 293
Reed, Professor Lesley 79
referrals, to specialists 35, 389–90
Regional Adviser in General Practice 96–100, 170, 242
regional advisers in general practice, as a group 106
Regional General Practice Educational Committee (RGPEC) 98, 100–1, 102, 105, 107, 108, 170
regional health authorities 103–4

Regional Medical Officer 101–2
regional plan for general practice 100–2, 107–8, 165
registrar quotas 102
Reid, Sir John 85–6, 135
Reis, Professor Harry 237, 238–9
Reith, Bill 328
remuneration 303–4, 346
    DH and BMA negotiations 347–9
    DH negotiations with junior doctors 350–1
    DH negotiations with senior hospital doctors 349–50
    JCPTGP chair 222
    JRCGP editor 306
    merit/distinction awards 304
    nurses 294
    salaried systems 303
Reports from General Practice 60–1, 401–2
Research Assessment Exercise (RAE) 211
Research Ethics Committee 324
Research and General Practice 182
Research Network (RCGP) 207–11
Research Paper of the Year (RCGP) 211
responsiveness 238
revalidation 231–2, 281–5
    Academy of Medical Royal Colleges policy 288–9
Review Body on Doctors' and Dentists' Remuneration 304, 346
Reynolds, Martin 100, 107
Richards, Clive 42
Richards Independent Task Force 181, 182, 309, 313
Richards, Jane 46, 47
Richards, Sir Rex *200*, 309
Richardson, Lord John 109, 110, 111
Ricketts, Frederick Joseph 29
Rivett, Geoffrey 140
Roberts, Michael 99, 100, 107–8, 109
Robinson, Kenneth 45
Rock Carling lectures 335
Rodgers, E and Hammerstein, O 19
Roe versus Wade ruling 73
Ronalds, Clare 84, 128, 213
Rose, Fraser 326, 334
Rose, General Sir Michael 71
Rose Prize 325, *373*, 377
Ross, Donald 29
Rotunda Hospital, Dublin 16–17
Rowland, Tiny 243
Royal College of General Practitioners (RCGP)
    AGM 1980 71
    annual reports 123–4
    archives 327
    Awards Committee 271
    and BMA 163–5
    book publishing 61–4, 66
    Butterworth essay competition 29
    Chair of Council 137, 147–8, 151–65, 180
    Chairmanships held by DPG 416
    changes over time 134
    Chief Examiner 144–5
    College cabinet 67–71

Communications Division 126–8, 317
constitutional issues 166–7
Council Executive 129, 132, 261
Council special meeting (1989) 161–3
distinction awards for GPs 305
electoral system 138–9
evidence to Lane Committee 73
Exeter publishing, *see* Exeter RCGP Publications
    Office
formation 68–9
General Medical Council 229–30
General Purpose Committee (GPC) 67, 138, 144,
    145, 151
Heritage Committee 325–8
international group 127, 128
last lecture in Princes Gate 327
library 134
Lifetime Achievement Award 382, *382*
Members' Reference Book 64, 65–6, 124, 221
membership, *see* membership of the Royal College of
    General Practitioners (MRCGP)
new members' and trainees' group 127–8
Nuffield course for course organisers 81
occupying No 15 Princes Gate 165–6
Patient Liaison Group 126–7, 128, 317, 318
Presidency 259–76
Presidents' honours 363
quality initiatives 130–2, 169–71
representation of faculties 167
research general practices 208–9
Research Network 207–11
Royal Charter 68, 169, 172–3
royal Presidents 68–9, 167
royal visit 269, *270*
South West England Faculty 40–3, 79
Spring General Meeting 82, 156–7
Tamar Faculty 43, 59, 159, 171–2, 275, 326, 357, 382
triennial dinner (2000) 273
White Cover Series Books 61–4, 407
Royal College of Nursing (RCN) 294
Royal College of Obstetricians and Gynaecologists
    (RCOG) 68, 74, 75, 277, 290
Royal College of Physicians of Ireland 272–3, 295, 297
Royal College of Physicians (RCP) 153, 159–60, 184,
    289, 291, 321–2
    fellowship 266, *267*
Royal College of Psychiatrists 133, 152, 166, 289, 307
Royal College of Surgeons of Edinburgh 226
Royal College of Surgeons of England (RCSEng) 68,
    277, 279, 289, 290, 296, 301–2
    Faculty of Dental Surgery 225–6, 227
Royal College of Surgeons in Ireland 295, 298
Royal Colleges, medical 152, 226
    charitable status 169
    relationship with government 189–90
    specialist Presidents 155–6
Royal Commission on Doctors' and Dentists'
    Remuneration (1960) 346

Royal Commission on Medical Education (1968) 80, 96,
    304, 335
Royal family, members met 63, *64*, 68, 69, 167, 211, 269,
    270, 342, *342*, 419
Royal Institute for Public Health and Hygiene 249,
    266–7
Royal Society of Health
    annual address 261
    Honorary Fellow 261
Royal Society of Medicine 261, 331
Ruscoe, Michael 106
Russell, Ginny 367, 368
Russell, Professor Ian 84

Sabbagh, Karl 131
St John-Stevas, Norman 72
St Leonard's Index of Continuity of Care (SLICC) 379
St Leonard's Research Practice 371–4
    academic triad 384
    analysis of academic work 383–4
    Care Quality Commission visits 378
    continuity of doctor care 378–9
    diabetes care in general practice 377–8
    Health Foundation grant for continuity 379–80, *380*
    letters in press 383
    letters in professional journals 383
    multidisciplinary team members 374–6
    part-time research fellows 371
    peer-reviewed publications by students 383, 384,
        410–11
    Peter Orton's MD 376–7
    Philip Evans 378
    visitors 417–18
salaried systems 303
Sales, KD 10
Salmon Report (1966) 15
Sancha, Carlos Luis 275–6
Savage, Wendy 233
Sawyer, Brenda 88, *92*
Scawn, Irene 42, 52, 54, 159, 326
Schumacher, EF 371
Scotland Act (1998) 273
Scotland, Alastair 290
Scott, Finlay 233
Scott, Julian 225, 226
Scott, Noy *46*
Scott, Sir Ronald Bodley 16, 119
Scown, Professor Sir Eric 16
screening tests 34
Seamark, Clare 242
Seamark, David 208
Seccombe, Sir Vernon 107, 110
secretarial support, general practice 28
Seel, Derek 225–6
self-regulation, medical profession 284–5
Selley, Peter 84, 410
Selley, Wilfred 87, 225
Sen, Amartya 341

Seward, Charles 198
sexism 386
sexual abuse, diagnosis 250
Shakespeare, William 389
Shepherd, Professor Michael 120
shingles research 271
Shipman, Harold 232
Shipman Inquiry 234
Shock, Sir Maurice 336, 337–8, 339–40
Shore, Angela 195, 203
Sibbald, Robert 171
Sidaway-Lee, Kate 371, 376, 377–8, 379, *380*, 383–4
single transferable vote (STV) 278
Sir Charles Hastings Prize (BMA) 48
Smee, Clive 341–2
Smerdon, Geoffrey 99, 171
Smith, Colin 310
Smith, Dame Janet 234
Smith, Lindsay 176
Smith, Pam 81
Smith, Sir Adrian *267*
Smith, Tim 254, 414
smokers 267–8
Snow, CP 17
social inequality 38–9, 378, 386
social media 385–6
Society of Academic Primary Care (SAPC) 210, 360, 369
    Heads of Teaching (HOTs) 357, 360
Society of Apothecaries 325, *373*, 377
society changes 385–6
Solana, Javier 340
South West General Practice Trust (SWGPT) 107–11
    continuing role 110–11
    a registered charity 109–10
    University GP departments 108–9
South West NHS/Universities Liaison Committee 99–100
South West regional plan for general practice 100–2, 107–8
South Western NHS Management Executive 105–6
South Western Regional Health Authority (SWRHA) 107, 108
Southgate, Dame Lesley 186, *187*, 274–5, *274*, 296
Spassky, Boris 11
Special Increment for Teaching (SIFT) 209
specialist medicine 34, 389–90, 391
Specialist Training Authority 292
Stallworthy, Professor Sir John 73–4
Stange, Professor Kurt 374
Starfield Memorial Lecture 356, 360–1
Starfield, Professor Barbara 118, 246, 343, 355, 356, 360
statistics, use of 385–6
Stead, Jonathan 89
Steel, Robin 146, 147, 388
Steele, Russell 115, 116, 118, 245, 247–8, *248*, 384, 414

Stephenson, Sir Terence 235, 358
Sterling Publications 63–4, 123–4
Stevens, Deborah 248, 293
Stevens, Rosemary 274, 414
Stevens, Sir Simon 235, 290, 300, 340, 376
Stewart, Professor Moira 236–7, 239
Stewart-Brown, Professor Sarah 330
Stokes-Lampard, Professor Dame Helen 357
Stokoe, Ian 52
storytelling 32
Stott, Professor Nigel 98, 182, 209
Straw, Rt Hon Jack 189
Strunin, Leo 263, 277, 279
Stuart, Baroness Gisele 273
Stubbings, Clive 116, 410
Styles, Bill 131, 133, 138, *162*, 182, 207, 210, 211, 213, 217, 336
substance abuse, prisons 185
suicides 116
summative assessment, vocational training 214–17
Summers, Michael 124
Swansea University 199
Sweeney, Professor Kieran 90, 93, 117–18, 210, 239, 247, *248*, 339, 414
    Harkness Fellowship 93, 245, 339
    illness and death 256, 373
Swift, George 52, 68, 80
Sykes, Sir Richard 324
syllabus for general practice 357, 415
symptoms, medically unexplained 33–4
System of Training for General Practice 15, 83, 291

Tackle, Barbara 83
Tal, Mikhail 11, 13
Talbot, Mary 121
Taliban quotation 27, 244, 250, 339
Tamar Faculty 43, 59, 159, 171–2, 275, 326, 357, 382
Tanner, Professor Norman 120
Tarr, Dawn 414
Taylor, Lord Stephen 333, 334
Taylor, Philip 374
telephone triage 319
television appearances 54, 74–5, 161
ten-minute appointments 222–4
Terence 107
terms and conditions of service 347
thalidomide 22–3
Thatcher government 135, 142–3, 336
    White paper (*Working for Patients*) 154, 160, 161–3, *162*, 181
Thatcher, Margaret 135, 153, 160
    10 Downing Street meeting 167
    Chequers meeting 157–8
Thewlis, Sarah 259–60
Thomas, ARB 12
Thompson, Sir Arthur 40, 261

Thorne, Angus 369, 379
Thornton, Professor Steven 368
time, appreciation in general practice 30–1
The Times 6, 9, 379, 383
To Heal or To Harm? (Grol) 62
Toby, John 133, 217, 261, 277
Todd, Chenore 374–5
Todd, Sir Ian 152, 154, 160–1
Tooke, Professor Sir John 92, 194–5, 196, *198*, 199, 203, 350, 367
Touquet, Pierre 335
Townsend, Sheila 232
Training for General Practice (Pereira Gray) 83, 99
Trainor, Professor Sir Richard 359
Trends in General Practice Computing 63
triage 319, 383
Tripp, John 192, 196, *198*
Trollope, Anthony 119
Tudor Hart, Julian 62, 115, 140, 383, 388
Turnberg, Sir Leslie 308–9
Turner-Warwick, Dame Margaret 164, 184, 185–6, 197, *198*, 200–1, 278, 305

Ulster University 199
Underwood, Lynn 236, 239
United States (USA)
    foundations (charitable) 236
    non-licensing of thalidomide 23
University Funding Council, Medical Advisory Committee 309
University of Leeds 89
University of London, chess club 12
Upjohn Travelling Fellowship 53

Valderas, Professor José 313, 356
value of a life 341
VAMP GP recording system 211
van Weel, Evelyn *91*
van Weel, Professor Chris 98, 121, 122, *262*, *265*, 380, 382
vaping 383
'vexatious litigant' 242
vocational training, endpoint assessment 214–17
voting methods 278
Vuori, Professor 131

Wade, Bob 11–12
Waine, Colin 70, 120, 124, 128, 129, 130, 145, 147, 168
    Chair of Council 133, 182
Walford, Diana 84, 209
Walker, Anne 82, 251
Walker, Philip 320
Walker, Professor John 120, 145
Waller, Ed 379
Walton, Robert 122
Wand, Solomon 346
Wanless Report (2002) 143, 393
Ward, Dorothy 158, *222*

ward rounds, as medical student 15–17
ward sisters, Bart's 15
Washington conference 338
Watkins, Steve 326
Watson, GI (Ian) 52, 53, 62, 335
Watt, Admiral Sir James 196
Watts, CAH and BM 62
Weatherall, Sir David 268
Webster, Charles 266
wellbeing 238
Wellcome Trust 195, 300, 325, 333, 334
Wells, HG 86
Welsh Office 70, 164
Westcott, Richard 84, 116, 410
What About the Children? (WATCh?) 329–32, 340
What Sort of Doctor 169
whistleblowers 387
White Cover series books (RCGP) 61–4, 407
White, Eleanor (Ellie) 367–8, 369, 377, 379, 411, 414
White, Jonathan 357
White papers
    NHS Plan: Plan for Investment; Plan for Reform (2000) 286–7, 312
    Our Health, Our Care, Our Choice (2006) 343–4
    Working for Patients (1989) 154, 160, 161–3, *162*, 181
Whitfield, Michael 108, 109, 110
Wilkie, Patricia 318–19, 383
Willetts, Lord David 156, 249
Williams, Professor Sir Dillwyn 154, 277, 305, 313
Williams, Sir Edgar 339, 340
Wilson, Lord Harold 138, 147
Wilson, Michael 142, 163–4
Wilson, Professor Nairn 227
Wilson, Tim 340
Windmill theatre 17
Winyard, Graham 104
Winyard Report 209
witness role of GPs 36
wives of GPs 28, 46–7
Wollaston, Sarah 356
women in medicine 17, 386
Wood, BH 11
Wood, James 57
Wool, Rosemary 184
words, use of 264, 369, 382
Working for Patients (1989) 154, 160, 161–3, *162*, 181
World Conference of Family Doctors (WONCA) 70–1, 121, 127
World Health Organization (WHO) 85–6, *86*, 117
World Student Chess Championships 11–12
World War II 6–7
Wright, Alastair 306
Wright, John 53
Writings of John Hunt, The (Horder) 63

Yeats, WB 366
Yes Minister television programme 240
Yodfat, Professor Yair 121, 122

For Product Safety Concerns and Information please contact our EU
representative GPSR@taylorandfrancis.com
Taylor & Francis Verlag GmbH, Kaufingerstraße 24, 80331 München, Germany

www.ingramcontent.com/pod-product-compliance
Ingram Content Group UK Ltd.
Pitfield, Milton Keynes, MK11 3LW, UK
UKHW050930180425
457613UK00015B/353